CELLULAR
RECEPTORS
for
ANIMAL VIRUSES

COLD SPRING HARBOR
MONOGRAPH SERIES

The Lactose Operon
The Bacteriophage Lambda
The Molecular Biology of Tumour Viruses
Ribosomes
RNA Phages
RNA Polymerase
The Operon
The Single-Stranded DNA Phages
Transfer RNA:
    Structure, Properties, and Recognition
    Biological Aspects
Molecular Biology of Tumor Viruses, Second Edition:
    DNA Tumor Viruses
    RNA Tumor Viruses
The Molecular Biology of the Yeast *Saccharomyces:*
    Life Cycle and Inheritance
    Metabolism and Gene Expression
Mitochondrial Genes
Lambda II
Nucleases
Gene Function in Prokaryotes
Microbial Development
The Nematode *Caenorhabditis elegans*
Oncogenes and the Molecular Origins of Cancer
Stress Proteins in Biology and Medicine
DNA Topology and Its Biological Implications
The Molecular and Cellular Biology of the Yeast *Saccharomyces:*
    Genome Dynamics, Protein Synthesis, and Energetics
    Gene Expression
Transcriptional Regulation
Reverse Transcriptase
The RNA World
Nucleases, Second Edition
The Biology of Heat Shock Proteins and Molecular Chaperones
Arabidopsis
Cellular Receptors for Animal Viruses

CELLULAR
RECEPTORS
for
ANIMAL VIRUSES

$C - 5828$

Edited by

Eckard Wimmer
School of Medicine
State University of New York at Stony Brook

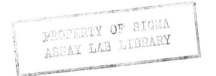

COLD SPRING HARBOR LABORATORY PRESS
1994

CELLULAR RECEPTORS for ANIMAL VIRUSES

Monograph 28
© 1994 by Cold Spring Harbor Laboratory Press
All rights reserved
Printed in the United States of America
Book design by Emily Harste

ISBN 0-87969-429-7
ISSN 0270-1847
LC 94-79112

All Cold Spring Harbor Laboratory Press publications may be ordered directly from Cold Spring Harbor Laboratory Press, 10 Skyline Drive, Plainview, New York 11803. Phone: 1-800-843-4388 in Continental U.S. and Canada. All other locations: (516) 349-1930. FAX: (516) 349-1946.

Contents

Preface, ix

INTRODUCTION AND OVERVIEW

1   **Introduction, 1**
     E. Wimmer

VIRAL RECEPTORS

2   **Human Receptors for Retroviruses, 15**
     R.A. Weiss

3   **CD4: The Receptor for HIV, 33**
     S.C. Harrison

4   **Cellular Receptors for Type C Retroviruses, 49**
     J.M. Cunningham and J.W. Kim

5   **A Protein Related to the LDL Receptor Is a Cellular
     Receptor Specific for Subgroup A Avian Leukosis
     and Sarcoma Viruses, 61**
     J.A.T. Young, H.E. Varmus, and P.F. Bates

6   **Receptors for Picornaviruses, 75**
     R.L. Crowell and R.P. Tomko

7   **Poliovirus Receptors, 101**
     *E. Wimmer, J.J. Harber, J.A. Bibb, M. Gromeier, H.-H. Lu,
     and G. Bernhardt*

8   **Entry of Minor Group Human Rhinoviruses
     into the Cell, 129**
     *D. Blaas, F. Hofer, M. Gruenberger, H. Kowalski, H. Machat,
     E. Kuechler, and M. Huettinger*

9   Cellular Receptors for Alphaviruses, 141
     *J.H. Strauss, T. Rümenapf, R.C. Weir, R.J. Kuhn, K.-S. Wang,
     and E.G. Strauss*

10   Membrane Cofactor Protein (CD46) Is a Receptor for
     Measles Virus That Determines Viral Host Specificity, 165
     R.E. Dörig, A. Marcil, and C.D. Richardson

VIRUS/RECEPTOR INTERACTION

11   Receptor Binding and Membrane Fusion by Influenza
     Hemagglutinin, 187
     *J.J. Skehel, D. Steinhauer, S.A. Wharton, P.A. Bullough,
     F.M. Hughson, S.J. Watowich, and D.C. Wiley*

12   Interaction of Rhinovirus with Its Receptor, ICAM-1, 195
     J.M. Greve and M.G. Rossmann

EARLY STEPS IN VIRAL UPTAKE

13   The Endocytic Pathway and Virus Entry, 215
     M. Marsh and A. Pelchen-Matthews

14   Activation Cleavage of Viral Spike Proteins
     by Host Proteases, 241
     H.-D. Klenk and W. Garten

15   Fusion of Influenza Virus in Endosomes: Role
     of the Hemagglutinin, 281
     J.M. White

16   The Influenza A Virus M2 Ion Channel Protein and Its Role
     in the Influenza Virus Life Cycle, 303
     R.A. Lamb, L.J. Holsinger, and L.H. Pinto

17   Expression of Viral Receptors and the Vectorial
     Release of Viruses in Polarized Epithelial Cells, 323
     S.P. Tucker, E. Wimmer, and R.W. Compans

18   Early Steps in Reovirus Infection of Cells, 341
     M.L. Nibert and B.N. Fields

19   Early Events in Human Herpesvirus Infection of Cells, 365
      N.R. Cooper

VIRUS RECEPTORS AND PATHOGENESIS

20   Interaction of Reovirus with Eukaryotic Host: Pathogenesis
      and Host Immune Response, 389
      A.B. Georgi and B.N. Fields

21   Specificity of Coronavirus/Receptor Interactions, 403
      K.V. Holmes and G.S. Dveksler

22   Distribution of the Poliovirus Receptor in Human Tissue, 445
      M. Freistadt

23   Transgenic Mouse for the Study of Poliovirus
      Pathogenicity, 463
      S. Koike, J. Aoki, and A. Nomoto

24   Lymphocyte Homing Receptor CD44 and Poliovirus
      Attachment, 481
      M.P. Shepley

25   Antibody-dependent Enhancement of Infection: A
      Mechanism for Indirect Virus Entry into Cells, 493
      S.B. Halstead

Index, 517

Preface

In November 1991, a Banbury Conference entitled "Receptor-mediated Virus Entry into Cells" brought together specialists of different disciplines of biological and medical sciences: virology, structural biology, cell biology, pathology, immunology, pharmacology, and others. The program, organized by R.A. Weiss and myself, was as complex as it was exciting. Subsequent to the Banbury Conference, it was decided to gather the most relevant information about viral receptors and viral cell invasion and publish it in the form of a book. In two ways, however, these proceedings are not a chronicle of the Banbury Conference. First, not all participants were able to contribute a summary of their work. Second, several important chapters were written by colleagues who could not attend the meeting, or who had barely started to decipher the complexities of interactions between virion and host cell surface in the viral system of their choice. During the last two years, a deluge of discoveries of viral invasion has swept the literature. We are very fortunate that important discoveries, published as recently as September 1994, have found their way into this volume.

The chapters were broadly grouped under three topics: description of viral receptors, viral attachment and uptake, and receptor-related virus-host interactions. There are some overlaps, of course, but they should serve to expand the treatise of a specific subject.

As the success of a Banbury Conference at the Cold Spring Harbor Laboratory in 1991 is the basis for the present book, we are grateful to Jan A. Witkowski and his colleagues at the Banbury Center for their valuable suggestions and impeccable efficiency in putting together the meeting. I am deeply indebted to John R. Inglis, Nancy E. Ford, Patricia Barker, and Inez Sialiano and their colleagues at the Cold Spring Harbor

Laboratory Press for their suggestions and unbounded patience during the long and sometimes tedious process of collecting the manuscripts. Most importantly, my thanks go to all contributors who have put aside the time, however painfully, to summarize their research results or to give an account of an entire field. I hope that these authors will feel rewarded when presented with the *Gesamtwerk*, as I trust that the volume will be favorably received by students in the biological and medical sciences. Finally, I hope that this book will stimulate research aimed at developing novel chemotherapeutica able to prevent or cure deadly viral diseases such as AIDS or influenza, and mild but ever so frequent recurrent syndromes like the common cold.

E. Wimmer

1

Introduction

Eckard Wimmer
Department of Molecular Genetics and Microbiology
School of Medicine
State University of New York at Stony Brook
Stony Brook, New York 11794

> *I know death has ten thousand several doors...*
> John Webster
> ca. 1610

To escape their existence as mere chemicals, viruses must find cellular receptors to invade a host cell and, thus, enter the life cycle of reproduction. Invasion of the host cell by viruses leads, in most cases, to destruction of the cell, even to the death of the host organism. The receptor, the first cellular molecule encountered by the virus, is an all-essential component of the cellular gate that, unbeknown to the cell, will allow entry of a deadly agent.

Whereas finding the host cell is a chance encounter, the steps of docking onto the cellular receptor, penetration, and uncoating follow elaborate viral strategies. A most surprising discovery in studies of these early events of infection has been the diversity of cellular receptors that viruses have selected for entry. It seems as if any cell-surface molecule, regardless of its structure and cellular function, can facilitate attachment for a specific viral species. To be sure, attachment per se does not necessarily lead to uptake and productive infection, but most viruses are clever enough to have chosen only receptors that are expressed on cells suitable for uptake and replication.

Several years ago, it seemed plausible that certain classes of abundant cell-surface molecules, such as proteins belonging to the immunoglobulin superfamily, might provide the preferred menu from which a virus is likely to choose its receptor (White and Littman 1989). However, a deluge of new data has shown that this is not the case. As the number of known viral receptors is rapidly growing, the most unlikely cell-surface molecules, such as aminopeptidase N, cationic amino acid transporter, α_2-macroglobulin receptor/LDL-receptor-related protein, decay-accelerating factor (CD55), to name a few, have emerged as viral receptors that may be added to the long list of Ig-related proteins, of integrins, and of the carbohydrate moieties of glycoproteins and glycolipids (Table 1) (Bergelson and Finberg 1993; White 1993; Haywood 1994; see also tables in Chapters 1 and 13, and several chapters describing details of viral receptors in this volume).

Not only do viruses of different virus families choose different receptors, even members of the same genus of a virus family may select entirely different chemical entities for cell attachment (Fig. 1). This is most strikingly illustrated by two genera of Picornaviridae. The genus Rhinovirus consists of two groups of human viruses, the major receptor group and the minor receptor group. Both major and minor group virions are closely related in structure and physical properties, and all rhinoviruses cause a similar disease syndrome, the common cold. Yet the major receptor group rhinoviruses have selected as receptor ICAM-1, an Ig-like polypeptide, whereas the minor receptor group rhinoviruses chose an LDL receptor-related protein (Fig. 1) (see Greve and Rossmann; Blaas et al., both this volume). Similarly, polioviruses, ECHO virus type 1, and ECHO virus type 7, which belong to the genus Enterovirus of Picornaviridae, use as receptors an Ig-like protein (PVR), the integrin VLA-2 (a collagen-laminin receptor; Bergelson et al. 1992), and decay-accelerating factor (CD55; Bergelson et al. 1994), respectively. Other examples of receptor diversity are illustrated in Figure 1.

In contrast to receptor diversity of closely related viruses, some agents that belong to entirely different virus families have adopted the same receptor. Examples are coxsackie B3 virus, an RNA enterovirus that shares an unknown cell receptor with adenovirus type 2, a DNA virus (Lonberg-Holm et al. 1976; most recently, it has been suggested that the receptor for coxsackie B viruses is related to nucleolin; R. Kandolf, pers. comm.), and human immunodeficiency virus (HIV), a retrovirus that shares the CD4 receptor with human herpesvirus 7, a DNA virus (Lusso et al. 1994).

The identification of a cell-surface protein as virus receptor has frequently led to a swift recognition of the cellular function of the molecule, based simply on available data provided previously by cell biologists. However, since viruses hardly resemble the natural ligands or substrates of plasma membrane proteins, knowledge of cellular function of a virus receptor has been of little help in identifying the molecular parameters of virus/receptor interaction. Only tedious analyses of receptor and virus variants combined with the elucidation of macromolecular structures at the atomic level have, for instance, led to an understanding of the interaction between influenza virus and the carbohydrate moiety (sialic acid) of the glycoprotein receptor. So far, no studies in other virus/receptor systems have reached this level of sophistication. The interaction of ICAM-1 with the canyon of human rhinovirus 14, or of CD4 with gp120 of HIV, however, are likely to soon be solved at the atomic level (Harrison; Greve and Rossmann, both this volume).

Details of the docking process between virion and receptor reveal little of the events that will occur downstream from viral attachment to the cell surface. Indeed, the steps of "entry" (into endocytotic vesicles), "penetration" (through the plasma membrane), and "uncoating" (activation of the genetic machinery of the virus) are still obscure for most viral systems. Even the question of whether a virus/receptor complex is endocytosed remains unsolved in many cases (see Marsh and Pelchen-Matthews, this volume). Again, research with influenza virus has advanced the understanding of the mechanisms of these earliest steps in viral infection to a knowledge unmatched by that of any other viral system. Here, the uptake into cytotic vesicles, the structural changes of the HA molecule under the influence of low pH, the exposure of a hydrophobic moiety suitable for membrane insertion, the influx of hydrogen ions into the viral core particle through the M2 channel to facilitate uncoating, and, finally, the process of membrane fusion, have been studied in great detail for many years (see various chapters in this volume). Particularly striking are the structural rearrangements that are likely to occur in the HA trimer at low pH, findings very recently published by Bullogh et al. (1994).

Despite its apparent complexity, the invasion of the host cell by influenza virus may be viewed as relatively straightforward in comparison to, e.g., entry of human herpes simplex virus. This virus makes use of at least three different viral glycoproteins for the invasion of the host cell, and more than one cellular macromolecule appears to be required for uptake. After receptor docking, a cascade of interactions between different viral and cellular components appears obligatory for downstream entry into the host cell (Spear 1993; Cooper, this volume).

A prerequisite for the uptake of most enveloped viruses is a prior activation of the viral spike proteins by proteolytic cleavage. Processing of the viral glycoprotein into fragments (that remain associated) is catalyzed by cellular proteases during viral maturation, an event that, depending on the specificity of proteases or the emergence of viral variants, may influence the progression of uptake or spread in the host (see Klenk and Garten, this volume).

For most viruses, the interaction between virion and cellular receptor (as studied, e.g., by using soluble receptor molecules) is of little consequence for the integrity of structure of the viral particle. Here, the

Table 1 A listing of viral receptors

Receptor (binding subunit)	Virus (family)	References
Immunoglobulin-like molecules		
VCAM-1	EMC-D (Picornaviridae)	Huber (1994)
ICAM-1 (first domain)	major group HRVs, CAV 13, 18, 21 (picornaviridae)	Colonno et al. (1986); Greve et al. (1989); Staunton et al. (1989); Tomassini et al. (1989)
PVR (first domain)	polioviruses (Picornaviridae)	Koike et al. (1990); Mendelsohn et al. (1989)
CD4 (first domain)	HIV-1, 2; SIV (Lentiviridae)	Dalgleish et al. (1984); Klatzmann et al. (1984)
	human herpesvirus 7	Lusso et al. (1994)
CEA, several members, (first domain)	mouse hepatitis virus (Coronaviridae)	Williams et al. (1991)
MHC I	Semliki Forest virus? (Togaviridae)	Helenius et al. (1978); Oldstone et al. (1980)
	lactate dehydrogenase virus	Inada and Mims (1984)
	mouse cytomegalovirus (Herpesviridae)	Wykes et al. (1993)
	SV40	Breau et al. (1992)
MHC II	Visna virus (Lentiviridae)	Dalziel et al. (1991)
Integrins		
VLA-2 (α-chain)	ECHO virus 1,8 (Picornaviridae)	Bergelson et al. (1992, 1993)
? (RGD-binding protein)	FMDV (Picornaviridae)	Fox et al. (1989); Mason et al. (1994)
$\alpha_v\beta_3$ (vibronectin)	CAV 9, ECHO virus 22 [?] (Picornaviridae)	Roivainen et al. (1994)
Transport proteins		
phosphate transporter analogon	gibbon ape leukemia virus (Retroviridae)	Johann et al. (1992)
	amphotropic murine leukemia virus (Retroviridae)	Miller et al. (1994)
cationic amino acid transporter	ecotropic murine leukemia virus (Retroviridae)	Albritton et al. (1989)
Signaling receptors		
LDL receptor protein family	minor group HRVs (Picornaviridae)	Hofer et al. (1994)
	subgroup A avian leukosis and sarcoma virus (family ?)	Bates et al. (1993); Conolly et al. (1994)
acetylcholine receptor (α-1)	rabies virus (Rhabdoviridae)	Lentz (1990)
EGF receptor	vaccinia virus (Poxviridae)	Marsh and Eppstein (1987)
leukocyte differentiation antigen [CD9]	feline immunodeficiency virus (Lentiviridae)	Willett et al. (1994)

Table 1 (Continued)

Receptor (binding subunit)	Virus (family)	References
Others		
aminopeptidase N	human corona virus 229E (Coronaviridae)	Yeager et al. (1992)
	TGEV (Coronaviridae)	Delmas et al. (1992)
complement receptor CR2	EBV (Herpesviridae)	McClure (1992)
high-affinity laminin receptor	sindbis virus (Togaviridae)	Wang et al. (1992)
decay-accelerating factor [CD55]	ECHO viruses 7 (6,11,12, 20, 21 ?)	Bergelson et al. (1994)
membrane cofactor protein	measles virus (Morbilliviridae)	Dörig et al. (1993)
moesin	measles virus (Morbilliviridae)	Dunster et al. (1994)
glycophorin A	EMCV (Picornaviridae)	Allaway and Burness (1986)
	reovirus (Reoviridae)	Paul and Lee (1987)
galactosylceramide	HIV-1 (Lentiviridae)	Bhat et al. (1991)
erythrocyte P antigen	Parvovirus B19 (Parvoviridae)	Brown et al. (1993)
BLVRcp 1	bovine leukemia virus (Retroviridae)	Ban et al. (1993)
sialoglycoprotein GP-2	sendai virus (Paramyxoviridae)	Suzuki et al. (1985)
sialic acid	influenza virus (Orthomyxoviridae)	Herrler et al. (1985)
	Reoviridae (Reoviridae)	Fernandes et al. (1994)
	group A porcine rotavirus (Rotaviridae)	Rolsma et al. (1994)
	human coronavirus OC43, bovine coronavirus (Coronaviridae)	Vlasak et al. (1988)
heparan sulfate	human cytomegalovirus (Herpesviridae)	Compton et al. (1993)
	HSV	WuDunn and Spear (1989)

A question mark indicates that the exact identity of the receptor is not known or that there is only circumstantial evidence for a virus binding the receptor listed. Abbreviations used: (VCAM) vascular cell adhesion molecule; (PVR) poliovirus receptor; (CEA) carcinoembryonic antigen; (EMCV) encephalomyocarditis virus; (HRV) human rhinovirus; (CAV) Coxsackievirus A; (FMDV) foot-and-mouth disease virus; (HSV) herpes simplex virus; (TGEV) transmissible gastroenteritis virus; (EBV) Epstein-Barr virus.

receptor may simply serve as attachment device and for the transport of the viral particle for downstream processing. For other viruses, however, the receptor performs more than the function of attachment. In the case of poliovirus, a stable particle able to survive very harsh conditions (pH 2, proteases, EDTA combined with 1% SDS), the poliovirus receptor

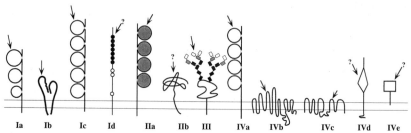

Figure 1 Schematic representation of some plasma membrane molecules that serve as receptors for viruses. Roman numerals indicate that the receptors are used by some members of the following virus families: (I) Picornaviridae; (II) Coronaviridae; (III) Orthomyxo- and Paramyxoviridae; (IV) Retroviridae. (Ia) poliovirus receptor (PVR; an Ig-like protein of unknown function; polioviruses); (Ib) integrin VLA-2 (ECHO virus 1,8); (Ic) ICAM-1 (major group rhinoviruses); (Id) LDL receptor (minor group rhinoviruses); (IIa) murine biliary glycoprotein (related to the human carcinoembryonic antigen family; murine hepatitis coronavirus); (IIb) aminopeptidase N (a metalloprotease; porcine and human coronaviruses); (III) glycoproteins of which sialic acid residues interact with the virion (orthomyxo- and paramyxoviruses); (IVa) CD4 (T-cell surface glyco-protein; HIV); (IVb) mouse cationic amino acid transporter (MCAT-1; ecotropic murine leukemia virus); (IVc) sodium-dependent phosphate transporter (gibbon ape leukemia virus); (IVd) protein of unknown function (bovine leukemia virus); (IVe) an LDL-related protein with an extracellular domain of only 83 amino acids (subgroup A avian leukosis and sarcoma viruses). The arrows mark proposed virus-binding sites. See Table 1 for references; also Weiss (this volume).

(PVR) has the dual function of docking and destabilizing the virion. By a mechanism not yet understood, PVR converts the poliovirion at 37°C and pH 7.5 to a subviral particle (A particle) that lacks the capsid protein VP4, is sensitive to proteases, and is more hydrophobic than the virion. The formation of A particles can thus be considered the first step of un-coating (Wimmer et al., this volume). In view of the virus-modifying function of PVR, it is not surprising that attempts to bypass PVR, that is, to achieve infection of PVR-negative cells with opsonized virions via Fc receptors, have failed (Mason et al. 1993).

Can viruses use more than one distinct receptor? The answer is clear-ly yes, but currently, there are only very few convincing examples that can be cited. In principle, every virus species could have evolved to select attachment sites for different cell-surface proteins. This may be clever to avoid host-range restriction, but is it necessary? Available evi-dence suggests that poliovirus uses only one receptor entity, and that this receptor is expressed in primates only. Yet poliovirus spreads so efficiently from human to human that until this century (which brought us general hygiene), a very high proportion of the human population was infected with poliovirus at an early age. Other viruses, such as influenza virus or sindbis virus, have adapted receptor entities that are ubiquitously expressed. These viruses do not suffer from lack of opportunity to infect cells. Thus, the search for alternative receptors would be of little advantage. In addition, it should be noted that viruses have adapted not only to certain receptors, but also to a cell-internal environment that should provide favorable conditions for replication. Therefore, an alternative receptor is only advantageous if expressed on cells that meet the requirements for proliferation.

The short list of viruses engaging more than one receptor, discussed below, is likely to grow as more information is gathered. Convincing evidence has been published suggesting HIV can utilize more than one receptor entity. Whereas CD4 is likely to be the main HIV receptor, the glycolipid galactosyl ceramide, a molecule expressed on neuronal cells and intestinal epithelium, provides an alternative cellular attachment site. Although the affinity of the GalCer glycolipid to HIV is much lower than that between CD4 and HIV, its interaction with the virus may play a role in the neuropathogenesis of HIV-1 infection (see Weiss, this volume).

Coxsackievirus A9 (CAV 9), a human enterovirus, uses vitronectin $\alpha_v\beta_3$ (an integrin) as viral receptor (Roivainen et al. 1994). The vitronectin attachment site of CAV 9, which includes an RGD motif common in the recognition by integrins, was found to be destroyed by cleavage with trypsin (Roivainen et al. 1991). Treatment of CAV 9 with trypsin, however, did not abolish infectivity, an observation suggesting that a second (yet unknown) receptor entity can function in CAV 9 uptake. It makes sense that CAV 9 uses the alternative receptor while passing through the protease-rich gastrointestinal tract, whereas when spreading to other tissues that lack the ability to proteolytically process the virion, it will recognize vitronectin.

Many viruses have the ability to hemagglutinate erythrocytes. The receptors on these cells remain unknown for the most part; in any case, they may not be the same molecular entities that a virus uses in productive infection of host cells. This has been demonstrated for encephalomyocarditis virus, a cardiovirus of Picornaviridae, which attaches to glycophorine A on erythrocytes and to VCAM-1 on cells allowing replication (see Crowell and Tomko, this volume).

Cell-surface proteins have recently been described that play an essential role in viral entry without serving as attachment proteins (receptors) for the virus. For example, adenovirus binds to the host cell to an as yet unidentified receptor (possibly a nucleolin-related polypeptide; see

8 E. Wimmer

above) via the viral fiber protein. However, downstream from the event of attachment, the penton base of the virus must interact with vitronectin for the infection to proceed (Wickham et al. 1993). Unfortunately, there are publications in which vitronectin has been declared to be a receptor for adenovirus. This is misleading. Vitronectin is more appropriately called an essential *entry accessory factor* functioning in the cascade of adenoviral invasion. A similar dependence on a cellular factor exists for HIV infections mediated by CD4: Whereas CD4 functions as receptor for the virus, another as yet unidentified cellular component (an entry accessory factor?), specific for primate cells, plays an essential role for viral uptake. This serves to explain why rodent cells expressing human CD4 can bind HIV but cannot internalize the virus (see Weiss, this volume). Finally, available evidence suggests that herpes simplex virus uses glycosaminoglycans (principally heparan sulfate) as receptors of host cells. Other cellular proteins, such as the mannose-6-phosphate receptor (Brunetti et al. 1994), may play a role downstream from attachment in the progression of HSV infection, and they, too, are likely to function as entry accessory factors.

Antibodies to the lymphocyte homing receptor CD44 have been found to block infection of HeLa cells with type 2 poliovirus; blockage is less pronounced for type 1, and virtually absent for type 3 polioviruses. Currently, the role of CD44 in poliovirus infection is obscure (Shepley, this volume). On the basis of work with hybrid poliovirus receptors (Bernhardt et al. 1994), it is unlikely that CD44 is an essential entry accessory factor in poliovirus infection, but it may play a role in modulating infection of specific tissue cells, thereby influencing pathogenicity of the virus.

New viruses with an expanded host range may emerge naturally by adaptation to second receptors. Such may be the case with a variant of coxsackievirus A 24 (CAV 24v), an enterovirus causing acute hemorrhagic conjunctivitis. CAV 24v appeared first in 1971 in Singapore (Ishii et al. 1989). At the same time, another enterovirus (enterovirus 70; EV70) emerged, most likely out of Africa, that caused a pandemic of acute hemorrhagic conjunctivitis affecting tens of millions of people (Ishii et al. 1989). The receptors for these viruses have not been identified. CAV 24 causes only mild upper respiratory illness; CAV 24v may have adopted an additional receptor such that its tissue tropism was extended. However, CAV 24 does not seem to share a receptor with EV 70 (N. Takeda, pers. comm.). Similarly, swine vesicular disease virus (SVDV), first isolated in 1966 in Italy, and currently the cause of frequent epidemics among pigs in Europe and in Asia, is a genetic variant of human coxsackievirus B5 (CBV 5) (Zhang et al. 1993). Whether CBV

5 and SVDV compete for the same receptor on human and pig cells has not yet been determined.

A special case of virus/host cell invasion is the antibody-dependent enhancement of viral infection that bypasses viral entry normally mediated through the cognate virus receptor. Instead of attachment to the viral receptor, ligand-coated virions find entry into host cells via receptors specific not for the virus, but for the ligand. Generally, the ligands are IgG or IgM immunoglobulins, and the receptors are Fc and complement receptors. The phenomenon of infection of cells of mononuclear phagocyte lineage by antibody/virion complexes mediated by Fc or complement receptors has profound consequences for the progression of many viral diseases. These include hemorrhagic fever caused by dengue virus and possibly also AIDS caused by HIV (see Halstead, this volume).

An interesting question is the distribution of viral receptors on the surface of the plasma membrane of the host cell. Studies using polarized epithelial cells have shown that viral receptors may be specifically localized at the apical or basolateral surface. Even in the case where the receptor may be distributed evenly between both surfaces, release of progeny virus might be vectorial, a phenomenon of interest for studies of viral pathogenesis (see Tucker et al., this volume).

The events leading to viral infection of a host cell do not reveal the astounding complexity of mechanisms that determine viral pathogenicity in a host organism. Numerous questions still lack answers. Which cells are affected during primary infection, and how does the virus spread to other target tissues? Is tissue tropism governed mainly by the distribution of the cognate receptor or by other factors such as virus stability or cell-internal restriction? What are the viral determinants that contribute to pathogenicity? As far as possible, studies addressing these questions have been carried out in experimental animals (see Georgi and Fields, this volume). With human viruses whose host range is restricted to primates, investigations of pathogenicity are limited to experiments with monkeys. Until recently, this was also the case for studies with poliovirus. Now, however, the generation of transgenic mice expressing the poliovirus receptor has dramatically simplified studies of poliovirus pathogenicity (see Koike et al., this volume).

Apart from a basic interest in molecular mechanisms underlying virus infection, there is an urgent need to identify new targets for the development of novel antiviral drugs. Complete blockage either of viral attachment, penetration, or uncoating would seem the most effective means of preventing viral disease. Surprisingly, only a single drug is currently on the market whose inhibitory action affects early stages of a viral infection (inhibition of uncoating of influenza A virus by amantadine; for effects other than virus uncoating of amantadine and its derivative, see Lamb et al., this volume). It is apparent that the understanding of the viral and cellular components involved in viral invasion into the host cell, combined with a comprehension of the mechanisms that govern this process, will greatly expand the possibilities of chemotherapeutic intervention of viral disease (Kim et al. 1993; see also Weiss; White, both this volume). It is hoped that the summary of the early events of viral infection provided in this volume, however incomplete, will stimulate basic research as well as the search for antiviral chemotherapy.

ACKNOWLEDGMENTS

I thank G. Bernhardt and T. Pfister for help in assembling Table 1, J. A. Bibb for drawing Figure 1, and A. Wimmer for editing the manuscript.

REFERENCES

Albritton, L.M., L. Tseng, D. Scadden, and J.M. Cunningham. 1989. A putative murine ecotropic receptor gene encodes a multiple membrane-spanning protein and confers susceptibility to virus infection. *Cell* **57**: 659.

Allaway, G.P. and A.T.H. Burness. 1986. Site of attachment of encephalomyocarditis virus on human erythrocytes. *J. Virol.* **59**: 768.

Ban, J., D. Portetelle, C. Altaner, B. Horion, D. Milan, V. Krchnak, A. Burny, and R. Kettmann. 1993. Isolation and characterization of a 2.3-kilobase-pair cDNA fragment encoding the binding domain of the bovine leukemia virus cell receptor. *J. Virol.* **67**: 1050.

Bates, P., J.A. Young, and H.E. Varmus. 1993. A receptor for subgroup A Rous sarcoma virus is related to the low density lipoprotein receptor. *Cell* **74**: 1043.

Bergelson, J.M. and R.W. Finberg. 1993. Integrins as receptors for virus attachment and cell entry. *Trends Microbiol.* **1**: 287.

Bergelson, J.M., M.P. Shepley, B.M. Chan, M.E. Hemler, and R.W. Finberg. 1992. Identification of the integrin VLA-2 as a receptor for echovirus 1. *Science* **255**: 1718.

Bergelson, J.M., M. Chan, K.R. Solomon, N.F. St. John, H. Lin, and R.W. Finberg. 1994. Decay-accelerating factor (CD55), a glycosylphosphatidylinositol-anchored complement regulatory protein, is a receptor for several echoviruses. *Proc. Natl. Acad. Sci.* **91**: 6245.

Bergelson, J.M., N. St. John, S. Kawaguchi, M. Chan, H. Stubdal, J. Modlin, and R.W. Finberg. 1993. Infection by echoviruses 1 and 8 depends on the α2 subunit of human VLA-2. *J. Virol.* **67**: 6847.

Bernhardt, G., J.J. Harber, A. Zibert, M. deCrombrugghe, and E. Wimmer. 1994. The poliovirus receptor: Identification of domains and amino acid residues critical for virus binding. *Virology* **203**: 344.

Bhat, S., S.L. Spitalnik, F. Gonzalez-Scarano, and D.H. Silberberg. 1991. Galactosyl ceramide or a derivative is an essential component of the neural receptor for human immunodeficiency virus type 1 envelope glycoprotein gp120. *Proc. Natl. Acad. Sci.* **88**: 7131.

Breau, W.C., W.J. Atwood, and L.C. Norkin. 1992. Class I major histocompatibility proteins are an essential component of the simian virus 40 receptor. *J. Virol.* **66:** 2037.

Brown, K.E., S.M. Anderson, and N.S. Young. 1993. Erythocyte P antigen: Cellular receptor for B19 parvovirus. *Science* **262:** 114.

Brunetti, C.R., R.L. Burke, S. Kornfeld, W. Gregory, F.R. Masiarz, K.S. Dingwell, and D.C. Johnson. 1994. Herpes simplex virus glycoprotein D acquires mannose 6-phosphate residues and binds to mannose 6-phosphate receptors. *J. Biol. Chem.* **269:** 17067.

Bullough, P.A., F.M. Hughson, J.J. Skehel, and D.C. Wiley. 1994. Structure of influenza haemagglutinin at the pH of membrane fusion. *Nature* **371:** 37.

Colonno, R.J., P.L. Callahan, and W.J. Long. 1986. Isolation of a monoclonal antibody that blocks attachment of the major group of human rhinoviruses. *J. Virol.* **57:** 7.

Compton, T., D.M. Nowlin, and N.R. Cooper. 1993. Initiation of human cytomegalovirus infection requires initial interaction with cell surface heparan sulfate. *Virology* **193:** 834.

Conolly, L., K. Zingler, and J.A. Young. 1994. A soluble form of a receptor for subgroup A avian leukosis and sarcoma viruses (ALSV-A) blocks infection and binds directly to ALSV-A. *J. Virol.* **68:** 2760.

Dalgleish, A.G., P.C.L. Beveriev, P.R. Clapham, D.H. Crawford, M.F. Greaves, and R.A. Weiss. 1984. The CD4 (T4) antigen is an essential component of the receptor for the AIDS retrovirus. *Nature* **312:** 763.

Dalziel, R.G., J. Hopkins, N.J. Watt, B.M. Dutia, H.A. Clarke, and I. McConnel. 1991. Identification of a putative cellular receptor for the lentivirus visna virus. *J. Gen. Virol.* **72:** 1905.

Delmas, B., J. Gelfi, R. L'Haridon, L.K. Vogel, H. Sjöström, O. Noren, and H. Laude. 1992. Aminopeptidase N is a major receptor for the enteropathogenic coronavirus TGEV. *Nature* **357:** 417.

Dörig, R.E., A. Marcil, A. Chopra, and C.D. Richardson. 1993. The human CD46 molecule is a receptor for measles virus (Edmonton strain). *Cell* **75:** 295.

Dunster, L.M., J. Schneider-Schaulies, S. Löffler, W. Lankes, R. Schwartz-Albiez, F. Lottspeich, and V. ter Meulen. 1994. Moesin: A cell membrane protein linked with susceptibility to measles virus infection. *Virology* **198:** 265.

Fernandes, J., D. Tang, G. Leone, and P.W. Lee. 1994. Binding of reovirus to receptor leads to conformational changes in viral capsid proteins that are reversible upon detachment. *J. Biol. Chem.* **269:** 17043.

Fox, G., N.R. Parry, P.V. Barnett, B. McGinn, D.J. Rowlands, and F. Brown. 1989. The cell attachment site on foot-and-mouth disease virus includes the amino acid sequence RGD (arginine-glycine-aspartic acid). *J. Gen. Virol.* **70:** 625.

Greve, J.M., G. Davis, A.M. Meyer, C.P. Forte, S.C. Yost, C.W. Marlow. M.E. Kamarck, and A. McClelland. 1989. The major human rhinovirus receptor is ICAM-1. *Cell* **56:** 839.

Haywood, A.M. 1994. Virus receptors: Binding, adhesion strengthening, and changes in viral structure. *J. Virol.* **68:** 1.

Helenius, A., B. Morein, E. Fries, K. Simons, P. Robinson, V. Schirrmacher, C. Terhorst, and J.L. Strominger. 1978. Human (HLA-A and HLA-B) and murine (H-2K and H-2D) histocompatibility antigens are cell surface receptors for Semliki forest virus. *Proc. Natl. Acad. Sci.* **74:** 3846.

Herrler, G., R. Rott, H.-D. Klenk, H.-P. Müller, A.K. Shukla, and R. Schauer. 1985. The receptor-destroying enzyme of influenza C virus is neuraminate-O-acetylesterase. *EMBO J.* **4:** 1503.

Hofer, F., M. Grünberger, H. Kowalski, M. Hüttinger, E. Küchler, and D. Blaas. 1994. Members of the low density lipoprotein receptor family mediate cell entry of a minor-group common cold virus. *Proc. Natl. Acad. Sci.* **91:** 1839.

Huber, S.A. 1994. VCAM-1 is a receptor for encephalomyocarditis virus on murine endothelial cells. *J. Virol.* **68:** 3453.

Inada, T. and C.A. Mims. 1984. Mouse Ia antigen are the receptors for lactate dehydrogenase virus. *Nature* **309:** 59.

Ishii, K., Y. Uchida, K. Miyamura, and S. Yamazaki, eds. 1989. *Acute hemorrhagic conjunctivitis. Etiology, epidemiology and clinical manifestations.* University of Tokyo Press, Japan.

Johann, S.V., J.J. Gibbons, and B. O'Hara, B. 1992. GLVR1, a receptor for gibbon ape leukemia virus, is homologous to a phosphate permease of *Neurospora crassa* and is expressed at high levels in the brain and thymus. *J. Virol.* **66:** 1635.

Kim, K.H., P. Willingmann, Z.-X. Gong, M.J. Kremer, M.S. Chapman, I. Minor, M.A. Oliveira, M.G. Rossmann, K. Andries, G.D. Diana, F.J. Dutko, M.A. McKinley, and D.C. Pevier. 1993. A comparison of the anti-rhinoviral drug binding pocket in HRV14 and HRV1A. *J. Mol. Biol.* **230:** 206.

Klatzmann, D., E. Champagne, S. Chamaret, J. Gruest, D. Guetard, T. Hercend, J.-C. Gluckman, and L. Montagnier. 1984. T lymphocyte T4 molecule behaves as the receptor for human retrovirus LAV. *Nature* **312:** 767.

Koike, S., H. Horie, I. Ise, A. Okitsu, M. Yoshida, N. Iizuka, K. Takeuchi, T. Takegami, and A. Nomoto. 1990. The poliovirus receptor protein is produced both as membrane-bound and secreted forms. *EMBO J.* **9:** 3217.

Lentz, T.L. 1990. Rabies virus binding to an acetylcholine receptor alpha-subunit peptide. *J. Mol. Recognit.* **3:** 82.

Lonberg-Holm, K., R.L. Crowell, and L. Philipson. 1976. Unrelated animal viruses share receptors. *Nature* **259:** 679.

Lusso, P., P. Secchiero, R.W. Crowley, A. Garzino-Demo, Z.N. Berneman, and R.C. Gallo. 1994. CD4 is a critical component of the receptor for human herpesvirus 7: Interference with human immunodeficiency virus. *Proc. Natl. Acad. Sci.* **91:** 3872.

Marsh, Y.V. and D.A. Eppstein. 1987. Vaccinia virus and the EGF receptor: A portal for infectivity? *J. Cell. Biochem.* **34:** 239.

Mason, P.W., E. Rieder, and B. Baxt. 1994. RGD sequence of foot-and-mouth disease virus is essential for infecting cells via the natural receptor but can be bypassed by an antibody dependent enhancement pathway. *Proc. Natl. Acad. Sci.* (in press).

Mason, P.W., B. Baxt, F. Brown, J. Harber, A. Murdin, and E. Wimmer. 1993. Antibody-complexed foot-and-mouth disease virus, but not poliovirus, can infect cells via the Fc receptor. *Virology* **192:** 568.

McClure, J.E. 1992. Cellular receptor for Epstein-Barr virus. *Prog. Med. Virol.* **39:** 116.

Mendelsohn, C.L., E. Wimmer, and V.R. Racaniello. 1989. Cellular receptor for poliovirus: Molecular cloning, nucleotide sequence, and expression of a new member of the immunoglobulin superfamily. *Cell* **56:** 855.

Miller, D.G., R.H. Edwards, and A.D. Miller. 1994. Cloning of the cellular receptor for amphotropic murine retroviruses reveals homology to that for gibbon ape leukemia virus. *Proc. Natl. Acad. Sci.* **91:** 78.

Oldstone, M.B., A. Tishon, F.J. Dutko, S.I. Kennedy, J.J. Holland, and P.W. Lampert. 1980. Does the major histocompatibility complex serve as a specific receptor for Semliki Forest virus? *J. Virol.* **34:** 256.

Paul, R.W. and P.W.K. Lee. 1987. Glycophorin is the reovirus receptor on human erythrocytes. *Virology* **159:** 94.

Roivainen, M., T. Hyypia, L. Piirainen, N. Kalkkinen, G. Stanway, and T. Hovi. 1991. RGD-dependent entry of coxsackievirus A9 into host cells and its bypass after cleavage of VP1 protein by intestinal proteases. *J. Virol.* **65:** 4735.

Roivainen, M., L. Piirainen, T. Hovi, I. Virtanen, T. Riikonen, J. Heino, and T. Hyypiä. 1994. Entry of coxsackievirus A9 into host cells: Specific interactions with $\alpha_v\beta_3$ integrin, the vitronectin receptor. *Virology* **203:** 357.

Rolsma, M.D., H.B. Gelberg, and M.S. Kuhlenschmidt. 1994. Assay for evaluation of rotavirus-cell interactions: Identification of an enterocyte ganglioside fraction that mediates group A porcine rotavirus recognition. *J. Virol.* **68:** 258.

Spear, P.G. 1993. Entry of alphaherpesviruses into cells. *Semin. Virol.* **4:** 167.

Staunton, D.E., V.J. Merluzzi, R. Rothlein, R. Barton, S.D. Marlin, and T.A. Springer. 1989. A cell adhesion molecule, ICAM-1, is the major surface receptor for rhinoviruses. *Cell* **56:** 849.

Suzuki, Y., Y. Hirabayashi, T. Suzuki, and M. Matsumoto. 1985. Occurence of O-glycosidically peptide-linked oligosaccharides of poly-N-acetyllactosamine type (erythroglycan II) in the I-antigenically active Sendai virus receptor sialoglycoprotein GP-2. *J. Biochem.* **98:** 1653.

Tomassini, J.E., T.R. Maxson, and R.J. Colonno. 1989. Biochemical characterization of a glycoprotein required for rhinovirus attachment. *J. Biol. Chem.* **264:** 1656.

Vlasak, R., W. Luytjes, W. Spaan, and P. Palese. 1988. Human and bovine coronaviruses recognize sialic acid-containing receptors similar to those of influenza C virus. *Proc. Natl. Acad. Sci.* **85:** 4526.

Wang, K.-S., R.J. Kuhn, E.G. Strauss, S. Ou, and J.H. Strauss. 1992. High-affinity laminin receptor is a receptor for Sindbis virus in mammalian cells. *J. Virol.* **66:** 4992.

White, J.M. 1993. Integrins as virus receptors. *Curr. Biol.* **3:** 596.

White, J.M. and D.R. Littman. 1989. Viral receptors of the immunoglobulin superfamily. *Cell.* **56:** 725.

Wickham, T.J., P. Mathias, D.A. Cheresh, and G.R. Nemerow. 1993. Integrins $\alpha_v\beta_3$ and $\alpha_v\beta_5$ promote adenovirus internalization but not virus attachment. *Cell* **73:** 309.

Willett, B.J., M.J. Hosie, O. Jarrett, and J.C. Neil. 1994. Identification of a putative cellular receptor for feline immunodeficiency virus as the feline homologue of CD9. *Immunology* **81:** 228.

Williams, R.K., G.-S. Jiang, and K.V. Holmes. 1991. Receptor for mouse hepatitis virus is a member of the carcinoembryonic antigen family of glycoproteins. *Proc. Natl. Acad. Sci.* **88:** 5533.

WuDunn, D. and P.G. Spear. 1989. Initial interaction of herpes simplex virus with cells is binding to heparansulfate. *J. Virol.* **63:** 52.

Wykes, M.N., G.R. Shellam, J. McCluskey, W.M. Kast, R.B. Dallas, and P. Price. 1993. Murine cytomegalovirus interacts with major histocompatibility complex class I molecules to establish cellular infection. *J. Virol.* **67:** 4182.

Yeager, C.L., R.A. Ashmun, C.B. Cardellichio, L.H. Shapiro, A.T. Look, and K.V. Holmes. 1992. Human aminopeptidase N is a receptor for human coronavirus 229E. *Nature* **357:** 420.

Zhang, G., G. Wilsden, N.J. Knowles, and J.W. McCauley. 1993. Complete nucleotide sequence of a coxsackie B5 virus and its relationship to swine vesicular disease virus. *J. Gen. Virol.* **74:** 845.

2

Human Receptors for Retroviruses

Robin A. Weiss
Chester Beatty Laboratories
Institute of Cancer Research
London SW3 6JB, United Kingdom

Interest in human retrovirus receptors has recently been given new impetus for two main reasons. First, the emergence of human immunodeficiency virus type 1 (HIV-1) as a major pathogen has fueled the
search for inhibitors of retroviral replication, including the early steps in
infection. Second, the utility of retroviruses as vectors for gene transfer
and gene therapy is stimulating interest both in natural receptors and in
artificially targeted retroviral vectors. Thus, a greater understanding of
retrovirus attachment and entry will enhance two important areas of
medical research.

Different types of retrovirus recognize an extraordinary variety of receptors. In recent years, some of these receptors have been molecularly
defined, but the selectivity of retrovirus/receptor interactions has been
known since the 1960s, on account of the specificity of host range and
receptor interference properties of retroviral pseudotypes bearing different envelope glycoproteins (Weiss 1993). In initiating infection, the
outer, surface (SU) envelope glycoproteins of retroviruses carry the binding sites for receptor recognition, whereas the transmembrane (TM) envelope protein is thought to effect membrane fusion. The envelope spikes
visualized by electron microscopy are trimers or tetramers of SU/TM
units.

A number of conformational changes occur following the initial binding to receptors before membrane fusion and internalization is achieved.
These events have been studied in most detail with HIV-1, which appears
to require secondary receptors accessory to the principal binding receptor, CD4, to achieve viral entry. With the C-type retroviruses that are
used as gene vectors, however, there is no evidence to date for the involvement of more than one kind of cellular receptor. The route of entry
by retroviruses may be both by direct cell fusion at the plasma membrane
and by receptor-mediated endocytosis (Grewe et al. 1990; Marsh and
Pelchen-Matthews, this volume). The majority of retroviruses do not re-

quire the low pH of endosomes to effect fusion (Fig. 1), although endo-somal proteinases may play a role in the entry of ecotropic murine leukemia virus (MLV-E) in some cell types (Andersen 1987; McClure et al. 1990).

DIVERSITY OF RETROVIRUS RECEPTORS

Several cell-surface receptors for retroviruses are now known. Ten years ago, the CD4 differentiation antigen was identified as an important cell-surface molecule for HIV-1 entry by screening antibodies to T-lymphocyte surface antigens for their ability to block infection (Dal-gleish et al. 1984; Klatzmann et al. 1984). The importance of this recep-tor was confirmed by CD4 gene transfer, whereby human cells such as HeLa are rendered susceptible to HIV-1 infection (Maddon et al. 1986). An alternative binding receptor for HIV-1 SU protein gp120, however, is the glycolipid galactosyl ceramide, expressed on neuronal cells and in-testinal epithelium (Bhat et al. 1991; Fantini et al. 1993), but whether it functions as an efficient receptor for HIV-1 entry remains uncertain. Using a selective expression cloning strategy, Albritton et al. (1989) identified the murine receptor for MLV-E, which is a multispan mem-brane protein serving as a basic amino acid transporter (Cunningham and Kim, this volume). Similar methods were used to identify the receptors for gibbon-ape leukemia virus (GALV) (O'Hara et al. 1990), bovine leukosis virus (BLV) (Ban et al. 1993), and avian leukosis virus sub-group A (ALV-A) (Bates et al. 1993; Young et al., this volume). Recent-ly, the receptor for amphotropic murine leukemia virus (MLV-A) has also been identified as a molecule related to the GALV receptor (Miller et al. 1994).

It is remarkable that several of these receptors represent quite dif-ferent families of membrane proteins (Fig. 2). CD4 belongs to the im-munoglobulin superfamily. The MLV-E receptor serves as a permease for basic amino acids (Cunningham and Kim, this volume). The ALV-A receptor is related to the low density lipoprotein receptor. The BLV receptor is a novel type of protein. The GALV and MLV-A receptors, like that for MLV-E, resemble transporter molecules, with distant homol-ogy to a phosphate transporter of *Neurospora crassa* (Johann et al. 1992).

Using receptor-blocking experiments based on syncytial and pseudo-type assays, Sommerfelt and Weiss (1990) classified some twenty strains of oncovirus into seven human receptor groups (Table 1). The CD4 receptor for immunodeficiency lentiviruses represents an eighth receptor, and the human foamy virus receptor may comprise a ninth group. As al-

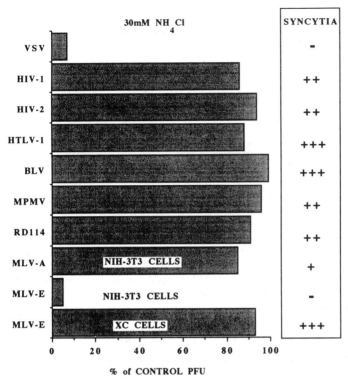

Figure 1 Sensitivity of vesicular stomatitis virus pseudotypes with retroviral envelopes to raised endosomal pH. Cells were treated with 30 mM NH_4Cl for 1 hr before and 3 hr after challenge with virus. The efficiency of plating was calculated from the VSV plaque titer compared to that on cells incubated in control medium. The cells were human sarcoma cells (HT1080) except where stated to be murine NIH-3T3 cells. The sensitivity to cell fusion on cocultivation with cells producing the retrovirus is also indicated. Whereas VSV in its own envelope was dependent on low endosomal pH, only MLV-E among the retroviral envelope pseudotypes was pH-dependent, for NIH-3T3 cells but not for XC cells. Data from McClure et al. (1990). (Reprinted, with permission, from Weiss 1993.)

ready mentioned, the molecular nature of some of these receptors (MLV-A, GALV, and HIV) is known. Others remain to be unequivocally identified. Since murine cells are resistant to infection by human T-cell leukemia virus type I (HTLV-I), we used human/mouse cell hybrids to show that a gene carried on the long arm of human chromosome 17 determines receptor susceptibility to HTLV-I (Sommerfelt et al. 1988). A putative HTLV-I receptor has been identified with a monoclonal antibody to an antigen that maps to human chromosome 17q (Gavalchin et al. 1993). The receptor gene for D-type simian viruses was allocated to

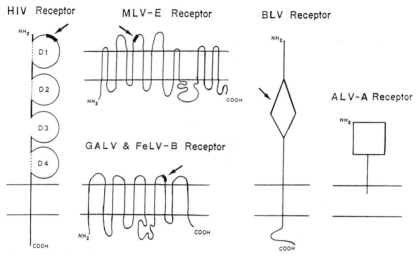

Figure 2 Molecular representation of retrovirus receptors. The arrows mark the virus-binding sites or sites of crucial specificity; the HIV receptor is the CD4 molecule; the MLV-E receptor is an amino acid transporter; the GALV/FeLV-B receptor may be a PO_4 transporter; the MLV-A receptor (not shown) has a similar configuration to the GALV/FeLV-B receptor; the BLV receptor is a novel protein; the ALV-A receptor resembles an LDL receptor motif.

the long arm of human chromosome 19 (Sommerfelt et al. 1990), but the receptor itself remains to be identified.

One unexpected result of our comparative study of human receptors (Sommerfelt and Weiss 1990) was that GALV and the feline leukemia virus type B (FeLV-B) cross-interfered, although their SU glycoproteins are not more closely related to each other than to other C-type retroviruses utilizing different receptors. A common receptor for FeLV-B and GALV was confirmed (Takeuchi et al. 1992) after the GALV receptor was cloned. Thus, two distinct C-type retroviruses may have independently adopted the same receptor. Indeed, quite unrelated microorganisms may share common receptors, e.g., ICAM-1 is shared by rhinoviruses and malaria parasites, and CD4 by HIV and human herpesvirus 7 (Lusso et al. 1994).

Mutational analysis of the GALV/FeLV-B receptor revealed that mutations in the virus recognition site (Johann et al. 1993) yield differential susceptibilities to GALV, FeLV-B, and simian sarcoma-associated virus (SSAV) (Tailor et al. 1993). We have even generated a mutant receptor that functions for FeLV-B entry but not for GALV, a phenotype not found in wild-type receptors of different mammalian species. Single amino acid changes affect the susceptibility of transfected cells to the different retroviruses.

Table 1 Receptor interference groups of retroviruses infecting human cells

Receptor group	Virus	Type	Host species	Origin[a]
1	SRV-1	type D	rhesus macaque	exo
	SRV-2	type D	black macaque	exo
	MPMV	type D	rhesus macaque	exo
	SRV-4	type D	cynomolgus monkey	exo
	SRV-5	type D	rhesus monkey	exo
	PO-1-Lu	type D	spectacled langur	endo
	SMRV	type D	squirrel monkey	endo
	RD114	type C	domestic cat	endo
	BaEV	type C	baboon	endo
2	MLV-A	type C	mouse	exo
3	MLV-X	type C	mouse	endo
4	FeLV-C	type C	domestic cat	exo
5	FeLV-B	type C	domestic cat	exo
	SSAV	type C	woolly monkey	exo
	GALV	type C	gibbon ape	exo
6	BLV	tax-rex	cattle	exo
7	HTLV-1	tax-rex	human	exo
	HTLV-2	tax-rex	human	exo
	ChTLV	tax-rex	chimpanzee	exo
	STLV	tax-rex	bonnet macaque	exo
8	HIV-1	lenti	human	exo
	HIV-2	lenti	human	exo
	SIV_{mac}	lenti	rhesus macaque	exo
	SIV_{smm}	lenti	sooty mangabey	exo
	SIV_{agm}	lenti	green monkey	exo

Data from Sommerfelt and Weiss (1990).
[a](exo) Exogenous; (endo) endogenous.

HIV ENTRY

CD4 is the principal binding receptor not only for HIV-1 (Dalgleish et al. 1984; Klatzmann et al. 1984), but also for HIV-2 and for simian immunodeficiency viruses (SIV) isolated from three host species (Table 1) (Sattentau et al. 1988). The binding site on CD4 for HIVs and SIVs is well conserved among primate CD4 antigens (McClure et al. 1987), but these viruses do not bind to murine and rat CD4 (Maddon et al. 1986). The HIV-binding site has been mapped by site-specific mutagenesis to amino acids 40–52 in the amino-terminal globular domain (D1) of CD4. The epitope resembles the complementarity-determining region 2 (CDR2) of immunoglobulin light chains and is discussed by Harrison (this volume).

The CDR3 region of D1 was also thought to be involved in HIV recognition (Camerini and Seed 1990; Eiden and Lifson 1992). However, the data of Camerini and Seed were inconsistent with those of McClure et al. (1987) and with recent studies by Broder and Berger (1993). Moreover, substitution of the human CDR2 sequence alone into rat CD4 is sufficient to convert it into a functional receptor for HIV binding and entry into cells (Simon et al. 1993).

Following the binding of HIV to its receptor, a complex series of conformational changes takes place in the gp120/gp41 tetrameric spikes of HIV, and also of CD4. These events are not yet well understood and have been reviewed elsewhere (Klasse et al. 1993; Moore et al. 1993; Signoret et al. 1993). Although the CDR2 region of D1 on CD4 is sufficient for binding gp120 of HIV, antibodies specific to epitopes on D2 and D3 can inhibit HIV entry and syncytium formation without affecting virion binding (Moore et al. 1992). The inhibitory effect is thought to occur through interference with a flexible hinge region at the D2-D3 junction, which may be required for the HIV envelope glycoproteins to interact with the cell membrane (Healey et al. 1990). Chimeric receptor molecules in which CD8 regions are substituted for D3 and D4 also slow down HIV entry (Poulin et al. 1991). The cytoplasmic region of CD4 is not essential for entry. Truncations or mutations to CD4 that remove the serine residue on which phosphorylation by phosphokinase C triggers endocytosis still function as HIV receptors for binding, membrane fusion, and entry in HeLa cells (Bedinger et al. 1988; Maddon et al. 1988). Indeed, the tethering of the external domains of CD4 to the outer lipid bilayer of the cell membrane through a glycolipid anchor still allows efficient HIV infection (Diamond et al. 1990; Kost et al. 1991).

The CD4-binding site on gp120 is complex (Klasse et al. 1993). gp120 is divided into relatively conserved regions (C1–C4) and regions (V1–V5) that are highly variable between different strains and isolates of HIV-1 (Leonard et al. 1990). The C4 region is an important part of the CD4-binding site, but other regions also affect gp120/CD4 interaction as deduced by mutational analysis and antibody inhibitor studies. Pollard et al. (1992) constructed a "minimal" CD4-binding protein from gp120 by making truncations of V1, V2, and V3 regions. However, these variable regions are important in determining HIV tropisms (Shioda et al. 1991; Takeuchi et al. 1991; Hwang et al. 1992; Boyd et al. 1993) and as binding sites of neutralizing antibodies (Weiss 1993; Moore et al. 1994). Since neutralization and cellular tropism appear to be determined through events occurring after primary binding to CD4 but before virion/cell-membrane fusion, the variable regions are important in HIV entry.

The binding of CD4 or recombinant soluble CD4 (sCD4) to gp120 at physiological temperature triggers a number of conformational changes eventually leading to the exposure of the hydrophobic domain at the amino terminus of the transmembrane protein, gp41, which is believed to effect membrane fusion (Moore et al. 1993). Allan et al. (1990) first observed that sCD4 treatment of SIV virions activates infection rather than inhibiting it, although we now believe that this enhancement follows the capacity of activated SIV and HIV-2 to infect cells via an alternative receptor to CD4 (Clapham et al. 1992), as discussed below. It was then observed that with syncytium-inducing (SI) strains of HIV-1, sCD4 uncouples gp120 from gp41, leading to irreversible inactivation or neutralization of infection (Moore et al. 1990). However, non-syncytium-inducing (NSI) strains of HIV-1, which represent the majority of primary isolates, do not shed gp120 on sCD4 treatment (Moore et al. 1992), and that may explain why they require much higher sCD4 doses to achieve virus neutralization (Daar et al. 1990). The affinity of sCD4 binding to monomeric gp120 derived from SI and NSI HIV-1 strains does not differ remarkably, whereas the effect of the soluble receptor molecule on virions does, reflecting a difference between binding and conformational shifts in oligomeric gp120/gp41 spikes. There may be cooperativity in sCD4 binding to gp120 on the same spike (Earl et al. 1992). It is clear that HIV-1 virions that do not shed gp120 altogether on binding CD4 or sCD4 remain fusigenic (Thali et al. 1992; Moore et al. 1993), and presumably the CD4 still effects a series of changes that permit exposure of the gp41 fusigen. However, it is also clear that for virion fusion and entry, interaction with cell membrane components accessory to CD4 must also occur.

SECONDARY RECEPTORS FOR HIV

In most cell types, CD4 expression appears to be necessary but not sufficient for HIV-1 entry. This first came to light when Maddon et al. (1986) showed that human cells expressing a CD4 construct were rendered sensitive to HIV-1 infection, whereas murine cells were not. Virions bound to both cell types but fusion, entry, and infection by VSV(HIV-1) pseudotypes only occurred in the CD4+ human cells. It appears that the mouse cells lack an essential component rather than inhibit fusion, because human/mouse heterokaryons expressing CD4 are permissive to HIV-1 entry (Dragic et al. 1992; Broder et al. 1993). Examination of a number of nonhuman cells expressing human CD4 showed that nearly all are refractory to HIV-1 fusion and infection (Ashorn et al. 1990; Clapham et al. 1991). In fact, some human cells also remain resistant to

HIV-1 infection after CD4 transfection, e.g. the astroglial cell lines, U87 and U373 (Chesebro et al. 1990; Clapham et al. 1991; Harrington and Geballe 1993). Again, fusion of nonpermissive CD4$^+$ human cells with CD4$^-$ HeLa or B cells provides HIV-1-permissive hybrids (Hoxie et al. 1988; Harrington and Geballe 1993).

Our studies also showed that different CD4$^+$ cells exhibit remarkably different susceptibility to fusion and infection by HIV-1, HIV-2, and SIV, respectively (Clapham et al. 1991; McKnight et al. 1994). Thus, the secondary components necessary to effect HIV and SIV entry can distinguish between the different major types of immunodeficiency viruses.

These secondary receptors remain to be identified. A putative gp41 receptor has been reported (Henderson and Qureshi 1993). However, because the sequence of the V3 loop of gp120 determines a selective tropism operating at a post-CD4-binding, pre-entry stage for different human cell types such as T-lymphocytic cell lines and macrophages, it is thought that V3 may recognize the secondary receptor. One idea that we espoused is that the accessory receptor might be a cell-surface proteinase which cleaves the V3 loop (Fig. 3) (Clements et al. 1991; Weiss 1993). Hattori et al. (1989) had suggested that a cell-surface tryptase may be involved in HIV-1 entry, and V3 amino acid sequences near the top of the loop resemble peptide inhibitors that occupy the active site of tryptic enzymes (Kido et al. 1991).

Our mutational analysis of the V3 loop of the HXB2 infectious molecular clone of HIV-1 LA1 strain (IIIB) showed that mutation of the arginine at the GPGR β turn to a noncleavable residue rendered the virus noninfectious (Schulz et al. 1993). Neutralizing antibodies to the V3 loop also block thrombin and cathepsin E cleavage (Schulz et al. 1993). The chymotryptic, cathepsin-cleavage site is two amino acids carboxy-terminal to the tryptic site. However, if a proteinase is crucial for viral entry, its substrate requirements on V3 appear to be complex, as many HIV-1 strains lack the thrombin site (Schulz et al. 1993). Given the selective tropism of HIV-1 strains for different human CD4$^+$ cell lineages such as T-lymphocytes and macrophages, and the differential behavior of HIV-1, HIV-2, and SIV for CD4-transfected cell lines alluded to above, one would have to postulate the involvement of several cellular proteinases, or proteinases with multiple specificities, to explain V3-determined viral tropism.

Recently, one cell-surface proteinase, the aminopeptidase known as CD26, has been reported to act as the secondary receptor for HIV-1 entry (Callebaut et al. 1993). Using a short-term assay for p24 *gag* expression, these authors claimed that doubly transfected CD4$^+$, CD26$^+$ mouse cells were permissive for HIV-1 replication. Several laboratories have been

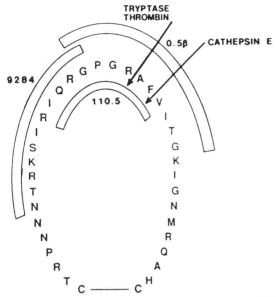

Figure 3 Sequence of the V3 loop of HIV-I IIIB (LAI) showing the binding epitopes of three monoclonal antibodies (0.5β, 9284, 110.5) and proteolytic cleavage sites (*arrows*). The site for tryptase and thrombin is tryptic and that for cathepsin E is chymotryptic. (Reprinted, with permission, from Clements et al. 1991.)

unable to confirm these studies. Our own transfection analysis of mink cells, which are much more permissive to HIV-1 replication once entry is achieved, were also negative, as shown in Table 2 (Patience et al. 1994).

ALTERNATIVE RECEPTORS FOR HIV

A number of cell-surface molecules other than CD4 have been reported to act as HIV receptors. Antibodies to the cell adhesion molecule LFA-1 block cell fusion (Hildreth and Orentas 1989), although if cells are inhibited from adhering to one another, a block to subsequent cell fusion is not surprising. Anti-LFA-1 is probably a nonspecific effect, and the evidence that it blocks cell-free infection by HIV-1 is weak. A number of "CD4⁻" cell lines can be infected by HIV-1 (Clapham 1991; Weiss 1993). Some of these cells do express CD4 at levels below those detected by immunofluorimetric assays, but nonetheless, infection can be inhibited by pretreating the cells with anti-CD4 antibodies. Other cell lines, however, genuinely show CD4-independent susceptibility to HIV infection, although much higher doses of virus are usually required for infection than for $CD4^+$ cells.

Table 2 CD26 does not confer susceptibility to HIV-1 infection

Virus	Mink	Mink-CD4	Mink-CD4-CD26	HeLa-CD4
HIV-1	0	0	0	$10^{4.3}$
HIV-2	0	$10^{2.8}$	$10^{2.6}$	$10^{4.2}$

Mink cells readily replicate HIV-1 provided the viruses penetrate, as previously shown by Canivet et al. (1990) utilizing pseudotypes and by Clapham et al. (1991) utilizing polyethylene-glycol-induced fusion. Expression of human CD4 renders mink cells permissive for HIV-2 infection (McKnight et al. 1994) but is not permissive for HIV-1. Expression of human CD4 with human CD26 is still not sufficient for HIV-1 infection. The virus titers were measured as HIV antigen focal units, as described by Clapham et al. (1991). 100% of mink-CD4 and CD4-CD26 cells expressed human CD4 at the cell surface, and ~ 70% of CD4-CD26 cells also expressed human CD26 at the cell surface. Data from Patience et al. (1994).

We have found that some CD4$^-$ human cell lines are highly sensitive to cell fusion and infection by HIV-2 (Clapham et al. 1992); namely, the RD/TE671 rhabdomyosarcoma cell line, and the B-lymphoblastoid Daudi and Raji cells. Several T-cell lines also appear to express this alternative receptor for HIV-2 (and for SIV), as anti-CD4 does not block infection. These are the cells for which sCD4 enhances infection (Allan et al. 1990). Most strains of HIV-2 require sCD4 to activate the envelope to fuse via the non-CD4 receptor, but we have selected a substrain of HIV-2 RoD which spontaneously fuses these cells (Clapham et al. 1992). This receptor has not yet been identified; it does appear to be the galactosyl ceramide receptor, as antibodies to GalCer do not block HIV-2 infection of these cells or bind to them.

The GalCer glycolipid is a high-affinity receptor for HIV-1 gp120 (Bhat et al. 1991). Anti-GalCer antibodies inhibit infection of CD4$^-$, GalCer$^+$ neuronal cells (Harouse et al. 1991) and colonic mucosal cells (Fantini et al. 1993). Although gp120 binds to GalCer with almost equal affinity (10^{-10} M) as to CD4, this glycolipid seems to be approximately 1000-fold less effective as a route of HIV entry. Even if GalCer is not a major receptor for HIV infection, the interaction of gp120 with the glycolipid may play a role in the neuropathogenesis of HIV-1 infection. Recently, transgenic mice expressing HIV-1 gp120 in astroglial cells through the promoter for glial fibrillar acid protein (GFAP) have been found to undergo brain degeneration resembling that seen in AIDS dementia (Toggas et al. 1994).

HIV RECEPTORS AND THERAPY

The early hope that soluble CD4 acting as a receptor decoy might be a therapeutic agent in HIV infection has not been borne out in preliminary therapeutic trials (Moore and Sweet 1993). Various soluble CD4 constructs have been devised, including chimeric molecules bearing the Fc portion of immunoglobulin molecules (Capon and Ward 1991), which confer a relatively long plasma half-life to the protein. However, the observations that primary isolates of HIV-1 are much more resistant to the inactivating properties of sCD4 than the laboratory isolates adapted to growth in T-cell lines placed the therapeutic dose of such a recombinant protein beyond practical pharmacology (Daar et al. 1990). However, the alacrity with which pharmaceutical companies dropped sCD4 trials in 1991 may have been as premature as the announcement 3 years earlier that heralded soluble receptors as the new cure for AIDS. Tersmette et al. (1989) have shown that SI variants of HIV arise in approximately 50% of HIV-infected patients late in infection, but shortly before AIDS is diagnosed. It is these SI variants that are particularly sensitive to sCD4 inactivation due to irreversible shedding of gp120 from virions (Moore et al. 1990; Bugelski et al. 1991). If the evolution of SI variants in vivo indeed plays a causal role in the development of "full-blown" AIDS (Schuitemaker et al. 1992), then sCD4 therapy may be useful in delaying AIDS in these individuals.

Other reagents also block early, pre-entry steps in HIV infection. CD4 antibodies competitively block the receptor, and there has been some exploration (with disappointing results) of anti-idiotypes to anti-CD4 as antiviral agents. Peptides that antagonize gp120/CD4 interactions might also be developed as antiviral agents, although results have been disappointing to date (Jameson et al. 1988; Moore and Sweet 1993). Sulfated sugars such as dextran sulfate inhibit HIV infection (Baba et al. 1988) and may bind to positively changed epitopes on the virion, such as the V3 loop. However, there is little evidence that these compounds act specifically against HIV (Baba et al. 1988; McClure et al. 1992). Certain 2-indolinone derivatives inhibit HIV infection (Smallheer et al. 1993), possibly by inhibiting gp120/CD4 interaction. As the structural aspects of this interaction become better understood, we may expect a more rational design of receptor inhibitors. However, elucidating the crystallographic structure of gp120 at high resolution is still awaited.

EXPLOITING OTHER RECEPTORS FOR RETROVIRUSES

With the increasing use of retroviral vectors for gene delivery, specific targeting of retroviruses is of growing interest. Most of the retroviral vectors for gene therapy utilize the amphotropic envelope of murine leukemia virus. It is by no means clear, however, that the receptor for MLV-A is the most appropriate for efficient delivery to human hematopoietic stem cells, lymphocytes, epithelia, and other targets for gene therapy. Therefore, packaging cells employing alternative envelopes recognizing other receptors may well come to supersede the amphotropic envelope. For example, we have found that the envelope of the feline endogenous C-type retrovirus is much more resistant to inactivation by human complement and may therefore be more useful for in vivo delivery (Takeuchi et al. 1994). This envelope utilizes the Group 1 receptor (Table 1), which is well expressed on diverse human cell types.

Modification of retroviral envelopes to recognize novel receptor types will also be exploited for gene therapy. Neda et al. (1991) showed that simple chemical modification to place lactose adducts on MLV-E gp70 allowed virions to bind to and infect liver parenchyma expressing the asialoprotein receptor. Battini et al. (1992) have delineated sites on gp70 that tolerate the insertion of peptide epitopes without loss of infectivity or virion uncoating. Thus, the insertion of ligands for receptors to which retroviruses do not normally bind may allow specific targeting to selective cell types.

REFERENCES

Albritton, L.M., L. Tseng, D. Scadden, and J.M. Cunningham. 1989. A putative murine ecotropic retrovirus receptor gene encodes a multiple membrane-spanning protein and confers susceptibility to virus infection. *Cell* **57:** 659.

Allan, J.S., J. Strauss, and D.W. Buck. 1990. Enhancement of SIV infection with soluble receptor molecules. *Science* **247:** 1084.

Andersen, K.B. 1987. Cleavage fragments of the retrovirus surface protein gp70 during virus entry. *J. Gen. Virol.* **68:** 2193.

Ashorn, P., G. England, M.A. Martin, B. Moss, and E.A. Berger. 1990. Anti-HIV activity of CD4-pseudomonas exotoxin on infected primary human lymphocytes and monocyte/macrophages. *J. Infect. Dis.* **163:** 703.

Baba, M., R. Snoeck, R. Pauwels, and E. De Clercq. 1988. Sulfated polysaccharides are potent and selective inhibitors of various enveloped viruses, including herpes simplex virus, cytomegalovirus, vesicular-stomatitis virus, and human immunodeficiency virus. *Antimicrob. Agents Chemother.* **32:** 1442.

Ban, J., D. Portetelle, C. Altaner, B. Horion, D. Milan, V. Krchnak, A. Burny, and R. Kettman. 1993. Isolation and characterisation of a 2.3-kilobase-pair cDNA fragment encoding the binding domain of the bovine leukosis virus cell receptor. *J. Virol.* **67:** 1050.

Bates, P., J.A.T. Young, and H.E. Varmus. 1993. A receptor for subgroup A Rous sarcoma virus is related to the low density lipoprotein receptor. *Cell* **74:** 1043.

Battini, J.-L., J.M. Heard, and O. Danos. 1992. Receptor choice determinants in the envelope glycoproteins of amphotropic, xenotropic, and polytropic murine leukemia viruses. *J. Virol.* **66:** 1468.

Bedinger, P., A. Moriarty, R. von Borstel II, N.J. Donovan, K.S. Steimer, and D.R. Littman. 1988. Internalization of the human immunodeficiency virus does not require the cytoplasmic domain of CD4. *Nature* **334:** 162.

Bhat, S., S.L. Spitalnik, F. Gonzalez-Scarano, and D.H. Silberberg. 1991. Galactosyl ceramide or a molecule derived from it is an essential component of the neural receptor for HIV-1 envelope glycoprotein gp120. *Proc. Natl. Acad. Sci.* **88:** 7131.

Boyd, M.T., G.R. Simpson, A.J. Cann, M.A. Johnson, and R.A. Weiss. 1993. A single amino acid substitution in the V1-loop of human immunodeficiency virus type 1 gp120 alters cellular tropism. *J. Virol.* **67:** 3649.

Broder, C.C. and E.A. Berger. 1993. CD4 molecules with a diversity of mutations encompassing the CDR3 region efficiently support HIV-1 envelope glycoprotein-mediated cell fusion. *J. Virol.* **67:** 913.

Broder, C.C., D.S. Dimitrov, R. Blumenthal, and E.A. Berger. 1993. The block to HIV-1 envelope glycoprotein-mediated membrane fusion in animal cells expressing human CD4 can be overcome by a human cell component(s). *Virology* **193:** 483.

Bugelski, P.J., H. Ellens, T.K. Hart, and R.L. Kirsh. 1991. Soluble CD4 and dextran sulphate mediate release of gp120 from HIV-1: Implications for clinical trials. *J. Acquired Immunne Defic. Syndr.* **4:** 923.

Burkly, L.C., D. Olson, R. Shapiro, G. Winkler, J.J. Rosa, D.W. Thomas, C. Williams, and P. Chisholm. 1992. Inhibition of HIV entry by a CD4 domain 2 specific monoclonal antibody: Dissecting the basis for its inhibitory effect on HIV-induced cell fusion. *J. Immunol.* **149:** 1779.

Callebaut, C., B. Krust, E. Jacotot, and A.G. Hovanessian. 1993. T cell activation antigen, CD26, as a cofactor for entry of HIV in CD4+ cells. *Science* **262:** 2045.

Camerini, D. and B. Seed. 1990. A CD4 domain important for HIV-mediated syncytium formation lies outside the virus binding site. *Cell* **60:** 747.

Canivet, M., A.D. Hoffman, D. Hardy, J. Sernatinger, and J.A. Levy. 1990. Replication of HIV-1 in a wide variety of animal cells following phenotypic mixing with murine retroviruses. *Virology* **178:** 543.

Capon, D.J. and R.H.R. Ward. 1991. The CD4-gp120 interaction and AIDS pathogenesis. *Annu. Rev. Immunol.* **9:** 649.

Chesebro, B., R. Buller, J. Portis, and K. Wehrly. 1990. Failure of human immunodeficiency virus entry and infection in CD4-positive human brain and skin cells. *J. Virol.* **64:** 215.

Clapham, P.R. 1991. Human immunodeficiency virus infection of non-haematopoietic cells. The role of CD4-independent entry. *Rev. Med. Virol.* **1:** 51.

Clapham, P.R., D. Blanc, and R.A. Weiss. 1991. Specific cell surface requirements for infection of CD4-positive cells by human immunodeficiency virus type 1, type 2 and simian immunodeficiency virus. *Virology* **181:** 703.

Clapham, P.R., A. McKnight, and R.A. Weiss. 1992. Human immunodeficiency virus type 2 infection and fusion of CD4-negative human cell lines: Induction and enhancement by soluble CD4. *J. Virol.* **66:** 3531.

Clapham, P., A. McKnight, G. Simmons, and R. Weiss. 1993. Is CD4 sufficient for HIV entry? Cell surface molecules involved in HIV infection. *Philos. Trans. R. Soc. Lond. B Biol. Sci.* **342:** 67.

Clements, G.J., M. Price-Jones, P.E. Stephens, C. Sutton, T.F. Schulz, P.R. Clapham, J.A. McKeating, M.O. McClure, S. Thomson, M. Marsh, J. Kay, R.A. Weiss, and J.P. Moore. 1991. The V3 loops of the HIV-1 and HIV-2 surface glycoproteins contain proteolytic cleavage sites: A possible function in viral fusion? *AIDS Res. Hum. Retroviruses* **7:** 3.

Daar, E.S., X.L. Li, T. Moudgil, and D.D. Ho. 1990. High concentrations of recombinant soluble CD4 are required to neutralize primary human immunodeficiency virus type 1 isolates. *Proc. Natl. Acad. Sci.* **87:** 6574.

Dalgleish, A.G., P.C.L. Beverley, P.R. Clapham, D.H. Crawford, M.F. Greaves, and R.A. Weiss. 1984. The CD4 (T4) antigen is an essential component of the receptor for the AIDS retrovirus. *Nature* **312:** 763.

Diamond, D.C., R. Finberg, S. Chaudhuri, B.P. Sleckman, and S.J. Burakoff. 1990. Human immunodeficiency virus infection is efficiently mediated by a glycolipid-anchored form of CD4. *Proc. Natl. Acad. Sci.* **87:** 5001.

Dragic, T., P. Charneau, F. Clavel, and M. Alizon. 1992. Complementation of murine cells for human immunodeficiency virus envelope/CD4-mediated fusion in human/murine heterokaryons. *J. Virol.* **66:** 4794.

Earl, P.L., R.W. Doms, and B. Moss. 1992. Multimeric CD4 binding exhibited by human and simian immunodeficiency virus envelope protein dimers. *J. Virol.* **66:** 5610.

Eiden, L.E. and J.D. Lifson. 1992. HIV interactions with CD4: A continuum of conformations and consequences. *Immunol. Today* **13:** 201.

Fantini, J., D.G. Cook, N. Nathanson, S.L. Spitalnik, and F. Gonzalez-Scarano. 1993. Infection of colonic epithelial cell lines by type 1 human immunodeficiency virus is associated with cell surface expression of galactosylceramide, a potential alternative gp120 receptor. *Proc. Natl. Acad. Sci.* **90:** 2700.

Gavalchin, J., N. Fan, M.J. Lane, L. Papsidero, and B.J. Poiesz. 1993. Identification of a putative cellular receptor for HTLV-1 by a monoclonal antibody, Mab 34-23. *Virology* **194:** 1.

Grewe, C., A. Beck, and H.R. Gelderblom. 1990. HIV: Early virus-cell interactions. *J. Acquired Immune Defic. Syndr.* **3:** 965.

Harouse, J.M., S. Bhat, S.L. Spitalnik, M. Laughlin, K. Stefano, D.H. Silberberg, and F. Gonzalez-Scarano. 1991. Inhibition of entry of HIV-1 into neural cell lines by antibodies against galactosyl ceramide. *Science* **253:** 320.

Harrington, R.D. and A.P. Geballe. 1993. Cofactor requirement for human immunodeficiency virus type 1 entry into a CD4-expressing human cell line. *J. Virol.* **67:** 5939.

Hattori, T., A. Koito, K. Takatsuki, H. Kido, and N. Katunuma. 1989. Involvement of tryptase-related cellular protease(s) in human immunodeficiency virus type 1 infection. *FEBS Lett.* **248:** 48.

Healey, D., L. Dianda, J.P. Moore, J.S. McDougal, M.J. Moore, P. Estess, D. Buck, P.D. Kwong, P.C.L. Beverley, and Q.J. Sattentau. 1990. Novel anti-CD4 monoclonal antibodies separate HIV infection and fusion of CD4+ cells from virus binding. *J. Exp. Med.* **172:** 1273.

Henderson, L.A. and M.N. Qureshi. 1993. A peptide inhibitor of human immunodeficiency virus infection binds to novel human cell surface polypeptides. *J.Biol. Chem.* **268:** 15291.

Hildreth, J.E.K. and R.J. Orentas. 1989. Involvement of a leukocyte adhesion receptor (LFA-1) in HIV-induced syncytium formation. *Science* **244:** 1075.

Hoxie, J., B. Haggarty, S. Bonser, J. Rackowski, H. Shan, and P. Kanki. 1988. Biological characterization of a simian immunodeficiency virus-like retrovirus (HTLV-IV): Evidence for CD4-associated molecules required for infection. *J. Virol.* **62:** 2557.

Hwang, S.S., T.J. Boyle, H.K. Lyerly, and B.R. Cullen. 1992. Identification of envelope V3 loop as the major determinant of CD4 neutralization sensitivity of HIV-1. *Science* **257:** 535.

Jameson, B.A., P.E. Rao, L.I. Kong, B.H. Hahn, G.M. Shaw, L.E. Hood, and S.B.H. Kent. 1988. Location and chemical synthesis of a binding site for HIV-1 on the CD4 protein. *Science* **240:** 1335.

Johann, S.V., J.J. Gibbons, and B. O'Hara. 1992. GLVR1, a receptor for gibbon ape leukemia virus, is homologous to a phosphate permease of *Neurospora crassa* and is expressed at high levels in the brain and thymus. *J. Virol.* **66:** 1635.

Johann, S.V., M. van Zeijl, J. Cekleniak, and B. O'Hara. 1993. Definition of a domain of GLVR1 which is necessary for infection by gibbon ape leukemia virus and which is highly polymorphic between species. *J. Virol.* **67:** 6733.

Kido, H., A. Fukutomi, and N. Katunuma. 1991. Tryptase TL-2 in the membrane of human T4$^+$ lymphocytes is a novel binding protein of the V3 domain of HIV-1 envelope glycoprotein gp120. *FEBS Lett.* **286:** 233.

Klasse, P.J., J.P. Moore, and B.A. Jameson. 1993. The interplay of the HIV-1 envelope complex, gp120 and gp41, with CD4. In *HIV molecular organization, pathogenicity and treatment* (ed. W.J.W. Morrow and N.L. Haigwood), p. 241. Elsevier, Amsterdam.

Klatzmann, D., E. Champagne, S. Chamaret, J. Gruest, D. Guetard, T. Hercend, J.-C. Gluckman, and L. Montagnier. 1984. T-lymphocyte T4 molecule behaves as the receptor for human retrovirus LAV. *Nature* **312:** 767.

Kost, T.A., J.A. Kessler, I.R. Patel, J.G. Gray, L.K. Overton, and S.G. Carter. 1991. Human immunodeficiency virus infection and syncytium formation in HeLa cells expressing glycophospholipid-anchored CD4. *J. Virol.* **65:** 3276.

Leonard, C.K., M.W. Spellman, L. Riddle, R.J. Harris, J.N. Thomas, and T.J. Gregory. 1990. Assignment of intrachain disulfide bonds and characterization of potential glycosylation sites of the type 1 recombinant human immunodeficiency virus envelope glycoprotein (gp120) expressed in Chinese hamster ovary cells. *J.Biol. Chem.* **265:** 10373.

Lusso, P., P. Secchiero, R.W. Crowley, A. Garzino-Demo, Z.N. Berneman, and R.C. Gallo. 1994. CD4 is a critical component of the receptor for human herpesvirus 7: Interference with human immunodeficiency virus. *Proc. Natl. Acad. Sci.* **91:** 3872.

Maddon, P.J., A.G. Dalgleish, J.S. McDougal, P.R. Clapham, R.A. Weiss, and R. Axel. 1986. The T4 gene encodes the AIDS virus receptor and is expressed in the immune system and brain. *Cell* **47:** 333.

Maddon, P.J., J.S. McDougal, P.R. Clapham, A.G. Dalgleish, S. Jamal, R.A. Weiss, and R. Axel. 1988. HIV infection does not require endocytosis of its receptor, CD4. *Cell* **54:** 865.

McClure, M.O., M.A. Sommerfelt, M. Marsh, and R.A. Weiss. 1990. The pH independence of mammalian retrovirus infection. *J. Gen. Virol.* **71:** 767.

McClure, M.O., Q.J. Sattentau, P.C.L. Beverley, J.P. Hearn, A.K. Fitzgerald, A.J. Zuckerman, and R.A. Weiss. 1987. HIV infection of primate lymphocytes and conservation of the CD4 receptor. *Nature* **330:** 487.

McClure, M.O., J.P. Moore, J.P. Blanc, P. Scotting, G.M.W. Cook, R.J. Keynes, J.N. Weber, D. Davies, and R.A. Weiss. 1992. Investigations into the mechanism by which sulphated polysaccharides inhibit HIV infection *in vivo*. *AIDS Res. Hum. Retroviruses* **8:** 19.

McKnight, A., P.R. Clapham, and R.A. Weiss. 1994. HIV-2 and SIV infection of non-primate cell lines expressing human CD4: Restrictions to replication at distinct stages. *Virology* **201:** 8.

Miller, D.G., R.H. Edwards, and A.D. Miller. 1994. Cloning of the cellular receptor for amphotropic murine retroviruses reveals homology to that for gibbon ape leukemia virus. *Proc. Natl. Acad. Sci.* **91:** 78.

Moore, J.P. and R.W. Sweet. 1993. The HIV gp120-CD4 interaction: A target for pharmacological or immunological intervention? *Perspect. Drug Disc. Des.* **1:** 235.

Moore, J.P., B.A. Jameson, R.A. Weiss, and Q.J. Sattentau. 1993. The HIV-cell fusion reaction. In *Viral fusion mechanisms* (ed. J. Bentz), p. 234. CRC Press, Boca Raton,

Florida. (In press.)

Moore, J.P., J.A. McKeating, R.A. Weiss, and Q.J. Sattentau. 1990. Dissociation of gp120 from HIV-1 virions induced by soluble CD4. *Science* **250:** 1139.

Moore, J.P., Q.J. Sattentau, R. Wyatt, and J. Sodroski. 1994. Probing the structure of the human immunodeficiency virus surface glycoprotein gp120 with a panel of monoclonal antibodies. *J. Virol.* **68:** 469.

Moore, J.P., J.A. McKeating, Y. Huang, A. Ashkenazi, and D.D. Ho. 1992. Virions of primary human immunodeficiency virus type 1 isolates resistant to soluble CD4 (sCD4) neutralization differ in sCD4 binding and glycoprotein gp120 retention from sCD4-sensitive isolates. *J. Virol.* **66:** 235.

Neda, H., C.H. Wu, and G.Y. Wu. 1991. Chemical modification of an ecotropic murine leukemia virus results in redirection of its target cell specificity. *J. Biol. Chem.* **266:** 11176.

O'Hara, B., S.V. Johann, H.P. Klinger, D.G. Blair, H. Rubinson, K.J. Dunn, P. Sass, S.M. Vitek, and T. Robbins. 1990. Characterization of a human gene conferring sensitivity to infection by gibbon ape leukemia virus. *Cell Growth Differ.* **1:** 119.

Patience, C., A. McKnight, P.R. Clapham, M.T. Boyd, R.A. Weiss, and T.F. Schulz. 1994. CD26 antigen and HIV fusion? *Science* **264:** 1159.

Pollard, S.R., M.D. Rosa, J.J. Rosa, and D.C. Wiley. 1992. Truncated variants of gp120 bind CD4 with high affinity and suggest a minimum CD4 binding region. *EMBO J.* **11:** 585.

Poulin, L., L.A. Evans, S. Tang, A. Barboza, H. Legg, D.R. Littman, and J.A. Levy. 1991. Several CD4 domains can play a role in human immunodeficiency virus infection of cells. *J. Virol.* **65:** 4893.

Qureshi, N.M., D.H. Coy, R.F. Garry, and L.A. Henderson. 1990. Characterization of a putative cellular receptor for HIV-1 transmembrane glycoprotein using synthetic peptides. *AIDS* **4:** 553.

Sattentau, Q.J., P.R. Clapham, R.A. Weiss, P.C.L. Beverley, L. Montagnier, M.F. Al-halabi, J.-C. Gluckman, and D. Klatzmann. 1988. The human and simian immunodeficiency viruses HIV-1, HIV-2 and SIV interact with similar epitopes on their cellular receptor, the CD4 molecule. *AIDS* **2:** 101.

Schuitemaker, H., M. Koot, N.A. Kootstra, M.W. Dercksen, R.E.Y. de Goede, R.P. van Steenwijk, J.M.A. Lange, J.K.M. Eeftink Schattenkerk, F. Miedema, and M. Tersmette. 1992. Biological phenotype of human immunodeficiency virus type 1 clones at different stages of infection: Progression of disease is associated with a shift from monocytotropic to T-cell-tropic virus populations. *J. Virol.* **66:** 1354.

Schulz, T.F., J.D. Reeves, J.G. Hoad, C. Tailor, P. Stephens, G. Clements, S. Ortlepp, K.A. Page, J.P. Moore, and R.A. Weiss. 1993. Effect of mutations in the V3 loop of HIV-1 gp120 on infectivity and susceptibility to proteolytic cleavage. *AIDS Res. Hum. Retroviruses* **9:** 159.

Shioda, T., J.A. Levy, and C. Cheng-Mayer. 1991. Macrophage and T cell-line tropisms of HIV-1 are determined by specific regions of the envelope gp120 gene. *Nature* **349:** 167.

Signoret, N., P. Poignard, D. Blanc, and Q.J. Sattentau. 1993. Human and simian immunodeficiency viruses: Virus-receptor interactions. *Trends Microbiol.* **1:** 328.

Simon, J.H.M., C. Somoza, G.A. Schockmel, M. Collin, S.J. Davis, A.F. Williams, and W. James. 1993. A rat CD4 mutant containing the gp120-binding site mediates human immunodeficiency virus type 1 infection. *J. Exp. Med.* **177:** 949.

Smallheer, J.M., M.J. Otto, C.A. Amaral-Ly, R.A. Earl, M.J. Myers, P. Penner, D.C. Montefiori, and M.A. Wuonola. 1993. Synthesis and anti-HIV activity of a series of 2-

indolinones and related analogues. *Antiviral Chem. Chemother.* **4:** 27.

Sommerfelt, M.A. and R.A. Weiss. 1990. Receptor interference groups among 20 retroviruses plating on human cells. *Virology* **176:** 58.

Sommerfelt, M.A., B.P. Williams, A. McKnight, P.N. Goodfellow, and R.A. Weiss. 1990, Localization of the receptor gene for type D simian retroviruses on human chromosome 19. *J. Virol.* **64:** 6214.

Sommerfelt, M.A., B.P. Williams, P.R. Clapham, E. Solomon, P.N. Goodfellow, and R.A. Weiss. 1988. Human T cell leukemia viruses use a receptor determined by human chromosome 17. *Science* **242:** 1557.

Tailor, C.S., Y. Takeuchi, B. O'Hara, S.V. Johann, R.A. Weiss, and M.K.L. Collins. 1993. Mutation of amino acids within the gibbon ape leukemia virus (GALV) receptor differentially affects feline leukemia virus subgroup B, simian sarcoma-associated virus, and GALV infections. *J. Virol.* **67:** 6737.

Takeuchi, Y., M. Akutsu, K. Murayama, N. Shimuzu, and H. Hoshino. 1991. Host-range mutant of human immunodeficiency virus type 1: Modification of cell tropism by a single point mutation at the neutralization epitope in the *env* gene. *J. Virol.* **65:** 1710.

Takeuchi, Y., F.-L. Cosset, P.J. Lachmann, H. Okada, R.A. Weiss, and M.K.L. Collins. 1994. C-type retroviral inactivation by human complement is determined by both the viral genome and the producer cell. *J. Virol.* (in press).

Takeuchi, Y., R.G. Vile, G. Simpson, B. O'Hara, M.K.L. Collins, and R.A. Weiss. 1992. Feline leukemia virus subgroup B uses the same cell surface receptor as gibbon ape leukemia virus. *J. Virol.* **66:** 1219.

Tersmette, M., J.J.M. van Dongen, P.R. Clapham, R.E.Y. De Goede, I.L.M. Wolvers-Tettero, G.A. van Kessel, J.G. Huisman, R.A. Weiss, and F. Miedema. 1989. Human immunodeficiency virus infection studied in CD4-expressing human-murine T-cell hybrids. *Virology* **168:** 267.

Thali, M., C. Furman, E. Helseth, H. Repke, and J. Sodroski. 1992. Lack of correlation between soluble CD4-induced shedding of the human immunodeficiency virus type 1 exterior envelope glycoprotein and subsequent membrane fusion events. *J. Virol.* **66:** 5516.

Toggas, S.M., E. Masliah, E.M. Rockenstein, G.F. Rall, C.R. Abraham, and L. Mucke. 1994. Central nervous system damage produced by expression of the HIV-1 coat protein gp120 in transgenic mice. *Nature* **367:** 188.

Weiss, R.A. 1993. Viral glycoproteins and cellular receptors involved in retrovirus infection. In *Retroviridae* (ed. J.A. Levy), vol. 2, p.1. Plenum Press, New York.

3

CD4: The Receptor for HIV

Stephen C. Harrison
Howard Hughes Medical Institute and
Department of Molecular and Cellular Biology
Harvard University
Cambridge, Massachusetts 02138

CD4, the human immunodeficiency virus (HIV) receptor, is a T-cell surface glycoprotein (Reinherz et al. 1979, 1980). Its normal function is to participate as a coreceptor in the antigen- and class II major histocompatibility complex (MHC)-dependent interactions that initiate T-cell activation (for review, see Janeway et al. 1989). It is believed to form a complex with the T-cell receptor and a peptide-bearing class II molecule, as shown schematically in Figure 1. HIV infection requires CD4 expression, and attachment to CD4 is the initial step in viral entry (Dalgleish et al. 1984; Klatzmann et al. 1984; Maddon et al. 1985). It is likely that CD4 also has a second role—to trigger a conformational change in the HIV envelope glycoprotein and thereby to potentiate the fusion of viral and cellular membranes (Moore et al. 1991; Sattentau et al. 1991). HIV can attach only to CD4 from humans and closely related species (McClure et al. 1987). The extent and essential characteristics of the HIV-binding site on human CD4 have been thoroughly characterized by a combination of structural and mutational studies (Moebius et al. 1992a). The HIV-gp120 side of this contact is less well understood, because a crystal structure of the envelope glycoprotein is still lacking.

STRUCTURE OF CD4

The amino acid sequence of CD4, derived from initial cDNA cloning, revealed a 372-residue extracellular domain linked by a hydrophobic transmembrane segment to a 41-residue cytoplasmic tail (Fig. 2) (Maddon et al. 1985). More detailed analysis, based on additional sequences, suggested that the extracellular part contains four concatenated immunoglobulin (Ig)-like domains (Clark et al. 1987). Crystallographic studies of two fragments, designated D1D2 and D3D4, have confirmed this inference (Ryu et al. 1990; Wang et al. 1990; Brady et al. 1993).

A representation of the folded structure of D1D2 (residues 1–178 in

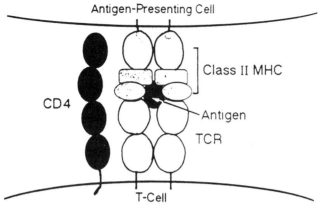

Figure 1 Diagram showing the molecules thought to be contacted by CD4 in the interaction between a T cell and an antigen-presenting cell. The antigen, a peptide, is bound in a groove of a class II MHC glycoprotein. It is recognized by the T-cell receptor (TCR). CD4 contacts one or more class II molecules, and it may also make lateral contacts with the TCR.

human CD4) appears in Figure 3a. The two domains form a rod-like unit. D1 is quite similar to an Ig Vκ domain. One β sheet, containing strands AGFCCC'C", packs against another containing strands BED. (For a guide to strand nomenclature, see the legend to Fig. 3). The residues at the core of the domain are the same as those found at homologous positions in antibody structures: a pair of disulfide-bridged cysteines linking strands B and F, a tryptophan in strand C packed against them, and other conserved hydrophobic residues (Lesk and Chothia 1982). There are also some special features characteristic of light-chain variable domains, such as a glycine in the AB loop and an Arg-Asp salt bridge between the D strand and the EF corner (Hunkapiller and Hood 1989; Williams et al. 1989). There are two key departures in D1 from standard Vκ architecture. First, the features of an Ig domain responsible for variable module dimerization are missing. These include extended CC' and FG loops and a bulge in the G strand (Colman 1988). Second, the C'C" and DE loops contain special elaborations. In particular, the DE loop contains a short, irregular helix that underlies the C'C" turn. The side chain of Trp-62, in

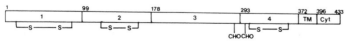

Figure 2 Relationship between the primary structure of the CD4 molecule and its various domains. Disulfide bridges are shown as S—S; CHO denotes sites of glycosylation in human CD4; TM indicates transmembrane segment; Cyt labels the cytoplasmic tail.

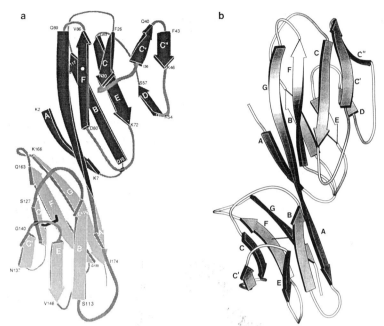

Figure 3 (*a*) Folded structure of human D1D2 (Ryu et al. 1990; Wang et al. 1990). The polypeptide chain is shown as a ribbon in β sheets and as a thin tube in inter-strand loops. Capital letters label the β strands, in the order in which they appear in each domain. Small numbers indicate first and last residues in a strand. (*b*) A similar representation of D3D4, derived from the rat D3D4 fragment (Brady et al. 1993). Coordinates of D3D4 courtesy of L. Brady (University of York).

the middle of this helix, lies beneath the C'C" turn and causes it to project away from the body of the domain. The C'C" loop, which corresponds to the CDR2 of a light chain IgV domain, is also longer than in most antibody molecules, so the C'C" edge of the domain has a strongly protruding character.

D2 is like a truncated IgV unit, in which the C" and D strands have been removed and replaced by a short connection between C' and E. The disulfide bond links strands C and F within a sheet, rather than two strands across the barrel. The two sheets can therefore lie at a somewhat greater separation. The C-strand cysteine occupies the position in the sequence usually held by the conserved tryptophan in Ig molecules, in register with the F-strand cysteine. The disulfide geometry is somewhat strained. A continuous β strand connects the two domains. This sort of rigid link is quite different from the V-to-C "switch" segment in Ig light or heavy chains. The amino acid sequence of CD4 contains six consecutive nonpolar residues at the domain boundary, and the side chains point alternately into the hydrophobic cores of D1 and D2. The two domains have a significant overlap, which stabilizes the conformation of the fragment. The BC and FG loops at the top of D2 splay apart to form a cradle for the bottom of D1. Any significant hinge motion at this "lap joint" is unlikely (Garrett et al. 1993).

A representation of D3D4, derived from crystallographic analysis of a recombinant fragment from rat CD4, appears in Figure 3b (Brady et al. 1993). The two domains are linked, as in D1D2, by a continuous β strand, and the relationship between D3 and D4 closely resembles the D1/D2 contact. D3 has an IgV-like fold, but no disulfide. The sheets are, as in D2, at a somewhat greater separation than in D1 (or in an Ig molecule), but the fundamental IgV design is preserved despite complete lack of conservation in the so-called "pin" of the domain (Lesk and Chothia 1982). D4 resembles D2, but within a truncated AB loop, conferring a rather blunt aspect on the membrane-proximal end.

A number of crystal forms have been obtained from recombinant, four-domain soluble CD4 (D1-D4), but none have yet afforded a structure. Electron microscopy and hydrodynamic measurements indicate that the D1-D4 fragment is monomeric and rod-like, approximately 125 Å in length (Kwong et al. 1990; T. Kirchhausen and S.C. Harrison, unpubl.). A comparative packing analysis of some of the crystal forms is consistent with this conclusion. The amino acid sequence at the D2/D3 boundary resembles those at the D1/D2 and D3/D4 boundaries, suggesting a similar continuous β-strand connector (Garrett et al. 1993). Moreover, a hydrophobic patch at the bottom of D2, formed by residues 108, 109, and 151, is likely to be in contact with a complementary patch at the top of D3, provided by its BC and FG loops. As on D2, these loops can provide a "cradle" for the preceding domain. It is possible to model the D2/D3 boundary so that the position of D3 with respect to D2 is similar to the position of D2 with respect to D1 (Fig. 4). Detailed analysis suggests that the axial separation of the D1D2 and D3D4 subfragments is likely to be somewhat greater than the separation at the D1/D2 or D3/D4 boundaries, diminishing the extent of overlap between D2 and D3 but still providing significant contact (Brady et al. 1993). There may thus be some flexibility at the D2/D3 junction, but the relative ease with which the D1-D4 fragment can be crystallized suggests that such flexibility is not likely to be substantial.

STEPS IN VIRAL ENTRY

Contact Surface on CD4 for HIV gp120

Mutational analysis has been used in a number of laboratories to map the surface of CD4 that interacts with the HIV envelope glycoprotein (see

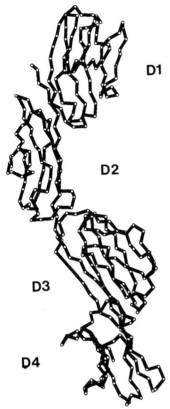

Figure 4 Model for the four-domain extracellular region of CD4, based on the structures of human D1D2 (Wang et al. 1990) and rat D3D4 (Brady et al. 1993). The D2/D3 connection has been modeled by examining the D1/D2 and D3/D4 interfaces and docking exposed hydrophobic residues on the "bottom" of D2 into a hydrophobic "cradle" on the "top" of D3. Some adjustment of loops has been made to avoid collisions.

Moebius et al. 1992a and references cited therein). The affinity of HIV for CD4 varies dramatically, depending on the source of virus. Virions from fresh patient isolates have, in general, a much lower affinity for CD4 than virions from extensively passaged stocks (Daar et al. 1990), but the affinity of free gp120 varies much less (Ashkenazi et al. 1991; Brighty et al. 1991; Turner et al. 1992). That is, tertiary or quaternary structural aspects of the organization of the gp120/gp41 oligomer on the surface of the virion significantly affect binding to CD4 (see below). Moreover, there is direct evidence that CD4 binding triggers a conformational change in the envelope glycoprotein from a "resting," low-affinity state to a fusion-competent, high-affinity state (Moore et al. 1991; Sattentau and Moore 1991). Quantitative measurements of affinity have therefore been carried out with free gp120, rather than with the envelope oligomer or with virions (Moebius et al. 1992a).

The gp120/CD4 interaction is essentially irreversible at low temperature, but it is readily reversible at 37°C. By carrying out binding experiments with soluble gp120 and CD4-expressing cells at physiological temperature, it is possible to obtain a proper equilibrium constant (Moebius et al. 1992a). The results of such studies are summarized in Figure 5. Most of the positions where mutation of a residue affects affinity lie along the C′ and C″ Strands in domain 1. This part of the domain that corresponds to the CDR2 of an IgV module has been called the "C′C″ ridge," because of the way it projects from the body of the protein (Wang et al. 1990). Phe-43, at the "top" of the C″ strand, is particularly critical. It is unusual in that its side chain is completely exposed. Various changes in this residue produce a graded series of effects ranging from a twofold decrease in affinity for Leu-43 to complete loss of

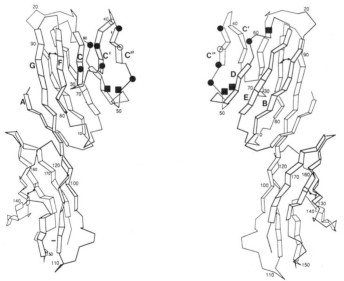

Figure 5 Diagram of D1D2 showing location of residues in which mutations affect gp120 binding (Moebius et al. 1992a). The position of each α carbon corresponds to the joint between segments of the folded ribbon that represents the polypeptide chain. Every tenth residue is numbered. Circles show residues with side chains that project away from the protein surface; squares show residues with buried side chains. Open circles show positions where certain changes can lead to increased affinity. (*Right*) View as in Fig. 2a; (*left*) view from the opposite surface.

detectable binding for Ile-43 and Ala-43 (Moebius et al. 1992a). Tyrosine and tryptophan yield intermediate affinities. These results suggest that gp120 contains a hydrophobic pocket complementary to the phenylalanyl side chain, and that the pocket can accommodate leucine, tyrosine, and tryptophan with varying degrees of strain, but not a β-branched residue such as isoleucine. Several positively charged residues in the C'C" ridge are also important for gp120 binding: Lys-35, Lys-46, and Arg-59. It is possible that conserved negative charges surround the gp120 hydrophobic pocket. The overall shape of the C'C" ridge is also critical for correct docking. Changes in two buried residues—Trp-62 near the "top" of the ridge and Ser-49 near the "bottom"—reduce affinity. The total interacting surface on CD4 is about 900 $Å^2$. The effects of the mutations shown in Figure 5 are quantitatively similar for at least two different HIV isolates, suggesting that the complementary surface on gp120 is conserved (Moebius et al. 1992a).

Various groups have proposed an additional role for the GH ("CDR3-like") loop of domain 1, either in binding gp120 or in a subsequent fusion event (Eiden and Lifson 1992). Recent experiments appear to rule out a specific role for this region, however (Broder and Berger 1993; Moore 1993), consistent with the absence of any prominent or unusual structural feature.

The HIV Envelope Glycoprotein

The HIV envelope glycoprotein is an oligomer—probably a tetramer (Pinter et al. 1989; Schawaller et al. 1989; Doms et al. 1990). It is synthesized as a heavily glycosylated gp160 precursor (about 850 amino acid residues) and cleaved (by a cellular protease) to gp120 and gp41 (Allan et al. 1983; Robey et al. 1985). Only gp41 is anchored in the viral membrane, and the absence of disulfide linkages between the two fragments permits some spontaneous dissociation of gp120 ("shedding"). The shed gp120 is a monomer (Moore et al. 1990, 1991). There is significant variation in the gp120 sequence from one isolate to another, but a conserved pattern of disulfide bonds (Leonard et al. 1990) and an evident clustering of hypervariable and constant amino acid residues (Starcich et al. 1986; Modrow et al. 1987) has led to a conventional subdivision of the protein into constant segments (C1–C5) and five variable regions (V1–V5) (Fig. 6). Mutations that affect CD4 binding map to a distributed set of locations in several of the constant regions. Extensive deletion analysis shows that a minimal, 287-residue structure (ENV59) derived by elimination of V1, V2, and V3, as well as removal of significant amino- and carboxy-terminal "tails," can still bind CD4 with

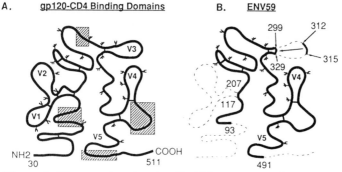

Figure 6 Diagram showing the disulfide structure of gp120 as diagrammed by Leonard et al. (1990). The amino acid backbone is represented by a heavy line, with crossbars showing S—S bridges. Glycosylation sites are shown by branched symbols. (*A*) Hatched areas show where mutations affect CD4 binding. (*B*) Fine, dashed lines show deletions leading to a minimal CD4-binding molecule. (Adapted, with permission, from Pollard et al. 1992 [copyright Oxford University Press]).

full affinity (Fig. 6) (Pollard et al. 1992).

The binding of CD4 to gp120 is modified by oligomerization, in a way that depends on the viral isolate. Laboratory strains of HIV bind monomeric CD4 with high affinity, whereas fresh patient isolates have a significantly weaker interaction (Daar et al. 1990). Free gp120, released from virions or expressed as a recombinant molecule, binds tightly, regardless of its source (Ashkenazi et al. 1991; Brighty et al. 1991; Turner et al. 1992). Passage in culture of a weakly binding fresh isolate, which is resistant to neutralization by soluble CD4, can convert it to a more tightly binding, CD4-sensitive strain. The minor sequence changes that occur in gp120 are not correlated from experiment to experiment, and the CD4 affinity of the free gp120 is not altered (Turner et al. 1992). Thus, it is plausible to conclude that some characteristic of the envelope oligomer is different, rather than the CD4-binding site on gp120 itself. Related observations suggest that a key difference is the relative ease with which the oligomer undergoes a CD4-triggered conformational change. Direct evidence that such a change occurs comes from antibody reactivity and protease sensitivity (Sattentau and Moore 1991). Moreover, CD4 binding induces gp120 shedding, and the patient isolates resistant to CD4 neutralization also release their gp120 less readily (Moore et al. 1990, 1991, 1992; Hart et al. 1991); that is, the CD4-induced conformational change appears to weaken the association of gp120 and gp41. The model in Figure 7 shows one way to account for these features of the virus-receptor interaction (Harrison et al. 1992).

$$[gp120/gp41]_4 \xrightarrow[\text{CD4}]{} [gp120/gp41]_4 (CD4)x \longrightarrow \{gp120\cdot gp41\}_4 (CD4)x \longrightarrow \begin{array}{l} x\,gp120\cdot CD4 \\ + (4-x)\,gp120 \\ + \{gp41\}_4 \end{array}$$

(1)	(2)	(3)	(4)
unbound state of env tetramer	binding of one or more CD4 (x≤4)	conformational change in env tetramer	dissociation of gp120 (with bound CD4 if occupied)
low affinity for CD4		high affinity for CD4	

Figure 7 Scheme for events accompanying the binding of CD4 to the HIV oligomeric envelope glycoprotein (here assumed to be a tetramer). State *3* might be the fusion-active configuration in actual viral infection (or formation), and state *4* might actually be a side reaction. Triggering of dissociation, state *4*, when virus is not bound to a cell surface, is believed to be a key mechanism for neutralization of laboratory strains by soluble CD4 (Moore et al. 1991, 1992). For simplicity, it is assumed that the proposed cooperative conformational change in the tetramer (from state *2* to *3*), which is triggered by binding of *x* CD4 ligands, leads to dissociation in state *4* of all gp120, whether liganded or not. The dotted line between gp120 and gp41 in the high-affinity state of the tetramer (braces) is meant to indicate weakened interaction between the two chains of the envelope glycoprotein.

CD4 binding is assumed to induce both tertiary and quaternary structural changes in gp120/gp41. The affinity of CD4 is necessarily lower for the unbound gp120/gp41 conformation. This statement is just a thermodynamic consequence of the assumption that CD4 binding triggers the change. Strains with gp120/gp41 oligomers that very readily undergo the transition bind CD4 more tightly than those that do not, because less free energy is "used up" in promoting the change in the one case than in the other.

It is useful to point out an analogy with the low-pH conformational change of influenza virus hemagglutinin (Wiley and Skehel 1987). In that case, the trigger is not receptor binding itself, but proton binding after passage into a low-pH compartment. Various mutants of influenza undergo the conformational change at a higher threshold pH (lower proton concentration); many of the corresponding amino acid changes in the hemagglutinin appear to affect the conformational change itself and the relative stability of the high- and low-pH forms, rather than proton binding as such (Daniels et al. 1985; Wiley and Skehel 1987). The fusion mutants of influenza are thus analogous to the laboratory-passaged strains of HIV; they undergo a conformational change more readily and bind protons more tightly. There are further apparent parallels. The low-pH conformational change in the influenza hemagglutinin involves spreading apart of the "top" receptor-binding domains of HA1 (Godley et al. 1992) and a coil-helix transition in HA2 (Carr and Kim 1993), possibly analogous to release of gp120 and a transition in gp41, respectively.

This discussion bears directly on possible CD4-based strategies for inhibiting HIV infection (Deen et al. 1988; Fisher et al. 1988; Hussey et al. 1988; Traunecker et al. 1988). Soluble CD4 is not a suitable drug, because the concentrations that would be required to neutralize patient strains are too high (Kahn et al. 1990; Schooley et al. 1990). What features of the low-affinity gp120-gp41 conformation lead to reduced CD4 binding? One possibility is simple steric hindrance. Intact CD4 is a relatively large ligand, and the position of its binding sites on the surface of a gp120/gp41 oligomer might be such that rearrangement would be necessary in order to avoid collision with a neighboring gp120. In this case, a small-molecule mimic of the CD4 C'C'' ridge might actually bind tightly to all strains of HIV. Another possibility is that the binding pocket on gp120 must change shape in order to accommodate CD4 properly, and that this shape change is in turn coupled to the gp120/gp41 interface and to the quaternary structure of the oligomer. In this case, it might be possible to find a drug that would be complementary to the initial shape of the pocket, by optimizing affinity for uncleaved gp160, in which both the quaternary structure and (presumably) the binding pocket would be constrained from conformational rearrangement.

Post-binding Events and Fusion

CD4 binding by HIV is not sufficient to ensure viral entry. HIV binds to murine cells expressing human CD4 but fails to fuse and infect (Maddon et al. 1986). The additional cofactor(s) present in human cells has not yet been identified. Because soluble human CD4 can trigger the envelope-glycoprotein conformational change, it is reasonable to suppose that these cofactors interact with the altered, "fusion-active" form. Entry is not pH-dependent (Stein et al. 1987; McClure et al. 1988), and fusion of viral and cellular membranes is believed to occur at the cell surface (Maddon et al. 1988).

OTHER CD4 INTERACTIONS

Contacts of CD4 with Class II MHC Proteins

The normal function of CD4 is to form a complex with class II MHC molecules and with the T-cell receptor (Fig. 1) (Biddison et al. 1982; Krensky et al. 1982; Meuer et al. 1982; Eichmann et al. 1987). The CD4/class II interaction cannot readily be detected by formation of a soluble complex or by binding of a soluble fragment of one glycoprotein to a cell bearing the other. Cell-cell adhesion assays have therefore been used to study the influence of mutations in CD4 (Doyle and Strominger 1987). The complexities of the experimental system have led to somewhat different interpretations in different groups, but examination of the data actually shows significant agreement (Fleury et al. 1991; Moebius et al. 1992b, 1993). Parts of both domains 1 and 2 affect the interaction, including most of the lateral surfaces of domain 1 (but not the tip) and the "upper" part of domain 2 (Fig. 8). Changes in Phe-43 produce graded effects similar to their effects on gp120 binding, indicating that the C'C" ridge is an important part of the contact. Residues on both faces of domain 1 contribute to the cell adhesion interaction, and it seems unlikely that contacts to a single class II molecule could create this pattern. It has therefore been proposed that more than one class II protein interacts with a CD4 molecule when the cells adhere (Moebius et al. 1993). Recent structural results raise the possibility that class II MHC proteins form dimers on the cell surface (Brown et al. 1993). CD4 may bind in the notch between the two partners of a class II dimer.

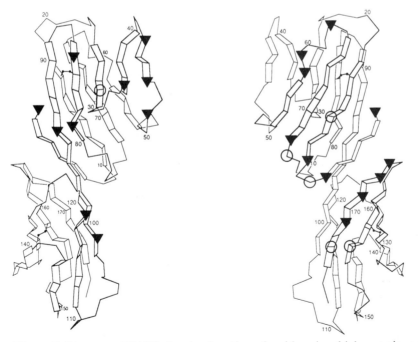

Figure 8 Diagram of D1D2 showing location of residues in which mutations affect the class II MHC interaction (Moebius et al. 1992b, 1993). Triangles show positions of strong observed effects on cell adhesion; open circles show positions of weaker effects. Views as in Fig. 5.

Cytoplasmic Contact of CD4

The cytoplasmic tail of CD4 associates with a *src*-family tyrosine kinase known as $p56^{lck}$ (Lck) (Rudd et al. 1988; Veillette et al. 1988). Two cysteines in CD4 and two in the amino-terminal region of Lck are essential for the interaction, and a metal ion (perhaps Zn^{++}) is a likely component (Shaw et al. 1989; Turner et al. 1990). Association with Lck is not required for CD4 to function as the primary HIV receptor (Bedinger et al. 1988), but Lck does inhibit the otherwise rapid endocytosis of CD4 (Pelchen-Matthews et al. 1991).

ACKNOWLEDGMENTS

I thank many colleagues and co-workers in my laboratory whose research is represented here, and I particularly acknowledge an on-going collaboration with Ellis L. Reinherz (Dana-Farber Cancer Institute, Boston). The work was supported in part by National Institutes of Health grants AI-30361 (to S.C.H.) and AI-27336 (to E.L. Reinherz).

REFERENCES

Allan, J., T.H. Lee, M.F. McLane, J. Sodroski, W.A. Haseltine, and M.Essex. 1983. Identification of the major envelope glycoprotein product of HTLV-III. *Science* **228:** 1091.

Ashkenazi, A., D.H. Smith, S.A. Marsters, L. Riddle, T.J. Gregory, D.D. Ho, and D.J. Capon. 1991. Resistance of primary isolates of human immunodeficiency virus type 1 to soluble CD4 is independent of CD4-gp120 binding affinity. *Proc. Natl. Acad. Sci.* **88:** 7056.

Bedinger, P., A. Moriarty, R.C. van Borstel II, N.J. Donovan, K.S. Steimer, and D.R. Littman. 1988. Internalization of the human immunodeficiency virus does not require the cytoplasmic domain of CD4. *Nature* **334:** 162.

Biddison, W.E., P. Rao, M. Thalle, G. Goldstein, and S. Shaw. 1982. Possible involvement of the IKT4 molecule in T cell recognition of class II HLA antigens: Evidence from studies of cytotoxic T lymphocytes specific for SB antigens. *J. Exp. Med.* **156:** 1065.

Brady, R.L., E.J. Dodson, G.G. Dodson, G. Lange, S.J. Davis, A.F. Williams, and A.N. Barclay. 1993. Crystal structure of domains 3 and 4 of rat CD4: Relation to NH2-terminal domains. *Science* **260:** 979.

Brighty, D.W., M. Rosenberg, I.S.Y. Chen, and M. Ivey-Hoyle. 1991. Envelope proteins from clinical isolates of human immunodeficiency virus type 1 that are refractory to neutralization by soluble CD4 possess high affinity for the CD4 receptor. *Proc. Natl. Acad. Sci.* **88:** 7802.

Broder, C.C. and E.A. Berger. 1993. CD4 molecules with a diversity of mutations encompassing the CDR3 region efficiently support HIV-1 envelope glycoprotein-mediated cell fusion. *J. Virol.* **67:** 913.

Brown, J.H., T.S. Jardetzky, J.C. Gorga, L.J. Stern, R.G. Urban, J.L. Strominger, and D.C. Wiley. 1993. The three-dimensional structure of the human class II histocompatibility antigen HLA-DR1. *Nature* **364**: 33.

Carr, C.M. and P.S. Kim. 1993. A spring-loaded mechanism for the conformational change of influenza hemagglutinin. *Cell* **73**: 823.

Clark, S.J., W.A. Jeffries, A.N. Barclay, and J. Gagnon. 1987. Peptide and nucleotide sequence of rat CD4 (W3/25) antigen: Evidence for derivation from a structure with four immunoglobulin-related domains. *Proc. Natl. Acad. Sci.* **84**: 1649.

Colman, P.M. 1988. Structure of antibody-antigen complexes: Implications for immune recognition. *Adv. Immunol.* **43**: 99.

Daar, E.S., X.L. Li, T. Moudgil, and D.D. Ho. 1990. High concentrations of recombinant soluble CD4 are required to neutralize primary human immunodeficiency virus type 1 isolates. *Proc. Natl. Acad. Sci.* **87**: 6574.

Dalgleish, A.G., P.C. Beverley, P.R. Clapham, D.H. Crawford, M.F. Greaves, and R. A. Weiss. 1984. The CD4 (T4) antigen is an essential component of the receptor for the AIDS retrovirus. *Nature* **312**: 763.

Daniels, R.S., J.C. Downie, A.J. Hay, M. Knossow, J.J. Skehel, M.L. Wang, and D.C. Wiley. 1985. Fusion mutants of the influenza virus haemagglutinin glycoprotein. *Cell* **40**: 431.

Deen, K.C., J.S. McDougal, R. Inacker, G. Folena-Wasserman, J. Arthos, J.Rosenberg, P.J. Maddon, R. Axel, and R.W. Sweet. 1988. A soluble form of CD4 (T4) protein inhibits AIDS virus infection. *Nature* **331**: 82.

Doms, R.W., P.L. Earl, S. Chakrabarti, and B. Moss. 1990. Human immunodeficiency virus types 1 and 2 and simian immunodeficiency virus *env* proteins possess a functionally conserved assembly domain. *J. Virol.* **64**: 3537.

Doyle, C. and J.L. Strominger. 1987. Interaction between CD4 and class II MHC molecules mediates cell adhesion. *Nature* **330**: 256.

Eichmann, K., J.-I. Jönsson, I. Falk, and F. Emmrich. 1987. Effective activation of resting mouse T lymphocytes by crosslinking submitogenic concentrations of the T cell antigen receptor with either Lyt-2 or L3T4. *Eur. J. Immunol.* **17**: 643.

Eiden, L. and J.D. Lifson. 1992. HIV interactions with CD4: A continuum of conformations and consequences. *Immunol. Today* **13**: 201.

Fisher, R.A., J.M. Bertonis, W. Meier, V.A. Johnson, D.S. Costopoulos, T.Liu, R. Tizard, B.D. Walker, M.S. Hirsch, R.T. Schooley, and R.A. Flavell. 1988. HIV infection is blocked *in vitro* by recombinant soluble CD4. *Nature* **331**: 76.

Fleury, S., D. Lamarre, S. Meloche, S.-E. Ryu, C. Cantin, W.A. Hendrickson, and R. P. Sekaly. 1991. Mutational analysis of the interaction between CD4 and class II MHC: Class II antigens contact CD4 on a surface opposite the gp120-binding site. *Cell* **66**: 1037.

Garrett, T.P., J. Wang, J. Liu, Y. Yan, and S.C. Harrison. 1993. Refinement and analysis of the structure of the first two domains of human CD4. *J. Mol. Biol.* **234**: 763.

Godley, L., J. Pfeifer, D. Steinhauer, B. Ely, G. Shaw, R. Kaufmann, E. Suchanek, C. Pabo, J.J. Skehel, D.C. Wiley, and S. Wharton. 1992. Introduction of intersubunit disulfide bonds in the membrane-distal region of the influenza hemagglutinin abolishes membrane fusion activity. *Cell* **68**: 635.

Harrison, S.C., J. Wang, Y. Yan, T. Garrett, J. Liu, U. Moebius, and E.L. Reinherz. 1992. Structure and interactions of CD4. *Cold Spring Harbor Symp. Quant. Biol.* **57**: 541.

Hart, T.K., R. Kirsh, H. Ellens, R.W. Sweet, D.M. Lambert, S.R. Petteway, Jr., J. Leary, and P.J. Bugelski. 1991. Binding of soluble CD4 proteins to human immunodeficiency virus type 1 and infected cells induces release of envelope glycoprotein gp120. *Proc. Natl. Acad. Sci.* **88**: 2189.

Hunkapiller, T. and L. Hood. 1989. Diversity of the immunoglobulin gene superfamily.

Adv. Immunol. **44**: 1.

Hussey, R.E., N.E. Richardson, M. Kowalski, N.R. Brown, H.-C. Chang, R.F. Siliciano, T. Dorfman, B. Walker, J. Sodroski, and E.L. Reinherz. 1988. A soluble CD4 protein selectively inhibits HIV replication and syncytium formation. *Nature* **331**: 252.

Janeway, C.A., Jr., J. Rojo, K. Saizawa, U. Dianzani, P. Portoles, J. Tite, S. Haque, B. Jones. 1989. The co-receptor of murine CD4. *Immunol. Rev.* **109**: 77.

Kahn, J.O., J.D. Allan, T.L. Hedges, L.D. Kaplan, C.J. Arri, H.F. Fitch, A. E. Izu, J. Mordenti, S.A. Sherwin, J.E. Groopman, and P.A. Volberding. 1990. The safety and pharmacokinetics of recombinant soluble CD4 (rCD4) in subjects with the acquired immunodeficiency syndrome (AIDS) and AIDS-related complex. *Ann. Intern. Med.* **112**: 247.

Klatzmann, D., E. Champagne, S. Chamaret, J. Gruest, D. Guetard, T. Hercend, J.-C. Gluckman, and L. Montagnier. 1984. T lymphocyte T4 molecule behaves as the receptor for human retrovirus LAV. *Nature* **312**: 767.

Krensky, A.M., S.C. Reiss, J.W. Mier, J.L. Strominger, and S.J. Burakoff. 1982. Long-term human cytolytic T cell lines allospecific for HLA-DR6 antigen are OKT4[+]. *Proc. Natl. Acad. Sci.* **79**: 2365.

Kwong, P.D., S.-E. Ryu, W.A. Hendrickson, R. Axel, R.M. Sweet, G. Folena-Wasserman, P. Hensley, and R.W. Sweet. 1990. Molecular characteristics of recombinant human CD4 as deduced from polymorphic crystals. *Proc. Natl. Acad. Sci.* **87**: 6423.

Leonard, C.K., M.W. Spellman, L. Riddle, R.J. Harris, J.N. Thomas, and T.J. Gregory. 1990. Assignment of intrachain disulfide bonds and characterization of potential glycosylation sites of the type 1 recombinant human immunodeficiency virus envelope glycoprotein (gp120) expressed in Chinese hamster ovary cells. *J. Biol. Chem.* **265**: 10373.

Lesk, A.M. and C.J. Chothia. 1982. Evolution of proteins formed by β-sheets. II. The core of the immunoglobulin domains. *J. Mol. Biol.* **160**: 325.

Maddon, P.J., A.G. Dalgleish, J.S. McDougal, P.R. Clapham, R.A. Weiss, and R. Axel. 1986. The T4 gene encodes the AIDS virus receptor and is expressed in the immune system and the brain. *Cell* **47**: 333.

Maddon, P.J., D.R. Littman, M. Godfrey, D.E. Maddon, L. Chess, and R. Axel. 1985. The isolation and nucleotide sequence of a cDNA encoding the lymphocyte protein T4: A new member of the immunoglobulin family. *Cell* **42**: 93.

Maddon, P.J., J.S. McDougal, P.R. Clapham, A.G. Dalgleish, S. Jamal, R.A. Weiss, and R. Axel. 1988. HIV infection does not require endocytosis of its receptor, CD4. *Cell* **54**: 865.

McClure, M.O., M. Marsh, and R.A. Weiss. 1988. Human immunodeficiency virus infection of CD4-bearing cells occurs by a pH-independent mechanism. *EMBO J.* **7**: 513.

McClure, M.O., Q.J. Sattentau, P.C.L. Beverley, J.P. Hern, A.K. Fitzgerald, A.J. Zuckerman, and R.A. Weiss. 1987. HIV infection of primate lymphocytes and conservation of the CD4 receptor. *Nature* **330**: 487.

Meuer, S.C., S.F. Schlossman, and E.L. Reinherz. 1982. Clonal analysis of human cytotoxic T lymphocytes: T4[+] and T8[+] effector T cells recognize products of different major histocompatibility complex regions. *Proc. Natl. Acad. Sci.* **79**: 4395.

Modrow, S., B.H. Hahn, G.M. Shaw, R.C. Gallo, F. Wong-Staal, and H. Wolf. 1987. Computer assisted analysis of envelope protein sequences of seven human immunodeficiency virus isolates: Prediction of antigenic epitopes in conserved and variable domains. *J. Virol.* **61**: 570.

Moebius, U., P. Pallai, S.C. Harrison, and E.L. Reinherz. 1993. Delineation of an extended surface contact area on human CD4 involved in class II MHC binding. *Proc. Natl. Acad. Sci.* **90:** 8259.

Moebius, U., L.K. Clayton, S. Abraham, S.C. Harrison, and E.L. Reinherz. 1992a. The HIV gp120 binding site on CD4: Delineation by quantitative equilibrium and kinetic binding studies of mutants in conjunction with a high resolution CD4 atomic structure. *J. Exp. Med.* **176:** 507.

Moebius, U., L.K. Clayton, S. Abraham, A. Diener, J.J. Yunis, S.C. Harrison, and E. L. Reinherz. 1992b. The HIV-gp120 binding C'C" ridge of CD4 domain 1 is also involved in interaction with class II MHC molecules. *Proc. Natl. Acad. Sci.* **89:** 12008.

Moore, J.P. 1993. A monoclonal antibody to the CDR-3 region of CD4 inhibits soluble CD4 binding to virions of human immunodeficiency virus type 1. *J. Virol.* **67:** 3656.

Moore, J.P., J.A. McKeating, W.A. Norton, and Q.J. Sattentau. 1991. Direct measurement of soluble CD4 binding to human immunodeficiency virus type 1 virions: gp120 dissociation and its implications for virus-cell binding and fusion reactions and their neutralization by soluble CD4. *J. Virol.* **65:** 1133.

Moore, J.P., J.A. McKeating, Y. Huang, A. Ashkenazi, and D.D. Ho. 1992. Virions of primary human immunodeficiency virus type 1 isolates resistant to soluble CD4 (sCD4) neutralization differ in sCD4 binding and glycoprotein gp120 retention from sCD4-sensitive isolates. *J. Virol.* **66:** 235.

Moore, J.P., J.A. McKeating, R.A. Weiss, Q.J. Sattentau, M.K. Gorny, and S. Zolla-Pazner. 1990. Dissociation of gp120 from HIV-1 virions induced by soluble CD4. *Science* **250:** 1139.

Pelchen-Matthews, A., J.E. Armes, G. Griffiths, and M. Marsh. 1991. Differential endocytosis of CD4 in lymphocytic cells. *J. Exp. Med.* **173:** 575.

Pinter, A., W.J. Honnen, S.A. Tilley, C. Bona, H. Zaghouani, M.K. Gorny, and S. Zolla-Pazner. 1989. Oligomeric structure of gp41, the transmembrane protein of human immunodeficiency virus type 1. *J. Virol.* **63:** 2674.

Pollard, S.R., M.D. Rosa, J.J. Rosa, and D.C. Wiley. 1992. Truncated variants of gp120 bind CD4 with high affinity and suggest a minimum CD4 binding region. *EMBO J.* **11:** 585.

Reinherz, E.L., P.C. Kung, G. Goldstein, and S.F. Schlossman. 1979. A separation of functional subsets of human T cells by a monoclonal antibody. *Proc. Natl. Acad. Sci.* **76:** 4061.

Reinherz, E.L., P. Kung, G. Goldstein, R.H. Levey, and S. Schlossman. 1980. Discrete stages of intrathymic differentiation: Analysis of normal thymocytes and leukemic lymphoblasts of T lineage. *Proc. Natl. Acad. Sci.* **77:** 1588.

Robey, W.G., B. Safai, S. Oroszlan, L. Arthur, M. Gonda, R. Gallo, and P.J. Fischinger. 1985. Characterization of envelope and core structural gene products of HTLV-III with sera from AIDS patients. *Science* **228:** 593.

Rudd, C.E., J.M. Trevillyan, J.D. Dasgupta, L.L. Wong, and S.F. Schlossman. 1988. The CD4 receptor is complexed in detergent lysates to a protein-tyrosine kinase (pp58) from human T lymphocytes. *Proc. Natl. Acad. Sci.* **85:** 5190.

Ryu, S.-E., P.D. Kwong, A. Truneh, T.G. Porter, J. Arthos, M. Rosenberg, X. Dai, N. Xuong, R. Axel, R.W. Sweet, and W.A. Henrickson. 1990. Crystal structure of HIV-binding recombinant fragment of CD4. *Nature* **348:** 419.

Sattentau, Q. and J.P. Moore. 1991. Conformational changes induced in the human immunodeficiency virus envelope glycoprotein by soluble CD4 binding. *J. Exp. Med.* **174:** 407.

Schawaller, M., G.E. Smith, J.J. Skehel, and D.C. Wiley. 1989. Studies with crosslinking reagents on the oligomeric structure of the *env* glycoprotein of HIV. *Virology* **172:** 367.

Schooley, R.T., T.C. Merigan, P. Gaut, M.S. Hirsch, M. Holodniy, T. Flynn, S. Liu, R.E. Byington, S. Henochowicz, E. Gushish, D. Spriggs, D. Kufe, J. Schindler, A. Dawson, D. Thomas, D.G. Hanson, B. Letwin, T. Liu, J. Gulinello, S. Kennedy, R. Fisher, and D.D. Ho. 1990. Recombinant soluble CD4 therapy in patients with the acquired immunodeficiency syndrome (AIDS) and AIDS-related complex. *Ann. Intern. Med.* **112:** 247.

Shaw, A.S., K.E. Amrein, C. Hammond, D.F. Stern, B.M. Sefton, and J.K. Rose. 1989. The lck tyrosine protein kinase interacts with the cytoplasmic tail of the CD4 glycoprotein through its unique amino-terminal domain. *Cell* **59:** 627.

Starcich, B.R., B.H. Hahn, G.M. Shaw, P.D. NcNeely, S. Modrow, H. Wolf, W.P. Parks, S.F. Josephs, R.C. Gallo, and F. Wong-Staal. 1986. Identification and characterization of conserved and variable regions in the envelope gene of HTLV-III/LAV, the retrovirus of AIDS. *Cell* **45:** 637.

Stein, B.S., S.D. Gowda, J.D. Lifson, R.C. Penhallow, K.G. Bensch, and E.G. Engelman. 1987. pH-independent HIV entry into CD4-positive T cells via virus envelope fusion to the plasma membrane. *Cell* **49:** 659.

Traunecker, A., W. Luke, and K. Karjalainen. 1988. Soluble CD4 molecules neutralize human immunodeficiency virus type 1. *Nature* **331:** 84.

Turner, J.M., M.H. Brodsky, B.A. Irving, S.D. Levin, R.M. Perlmutter, and D.R. Littman. 1990. Interaction of the unique N-terminal region of tyrosine kinase p56(lck) with cytoplasmic domains of CD4 and CD8 is mediated by cysteine motifs. *Cell* **60:** 755.

Turner, S., R. Tizard, J. DeMarinis, R.B. Pepinsky, J. Zullo, R. Schooley, and R. Fisher. 1992. Resistance of primary isolates of human immuno-deficiency virus type 1 to neutralization by soluble CD4 is not due to lower affinity with the viral envelope glycoprotein gp120. *Proc. Natl. Acad. Sci.* **89:** 1335.

Veillette, A., M.A. Bookman, E.M. Horak, and J.B. Bolen. 1988. The CD4 and CD8 T cell surface antigen are associated with the internal membrane tyrosine-protein kinase p56lck. *Cell* **56:** 301.

Wang, J., T. Garrett, Y. Yan, J. Liu, D. Rodgers, R.L. Garlick, G.E. Tarr, Y. Husain, E.L. Reinherz, and S.C. Harrison. 1990. Atomic structure of a fragment of human CD4 containing two immunoglobulin-like domains. *Nature* **348:** 411.

Wiley, D.C. and J.J. Skehel. 1987. The structure and function of the haemagglutinin membrane protein of influenza virus. *Annu. Rev. Biochem.* **56:** 365.

Williams, A.F., S.J. Davis, Q. He, and A.N. Barclay. 1989. Structural diversity in domains of the immunoglobulin superfamily. *Cold Spring Harbor Symp. Quant. Biol.* **54:** 637.

4

Cellular Receptors for Type C Retroviruses

James M. Cunningham and Jung Woo Kim
Department of Medicine and Howard Hughes Medical Institute
Brigham and Women's Hospital
Boston, Massachusetts 02115

HOST RANGE OF MAMMALIAN TYPE C RETROVIRUSES IS DETERMINED BY RECEPTOR EXPRESSION

Studies in mice have identified inbred strains that inherit proviruses encoding type C retroviruses which are expressed during fetal development, resulting in persistent viremia. These mice develop leukemia within 8–12 months after birth as a consequence of virus-induced changes in the expression of host genes that regulate cell growth. An important step in the pathogenesis of virus-induced leukemia is the appearance of recombinant retroviruses that carry alterations in envelope and long terminal repeat (LTR) sequences which enhance virus replication in hematopoietic cells (Elder et al. 1977; Cloyd et al. 1980). These viruses were initially identified because they infect mink fibroblasts (Chattopadhyay et al. 1981, 1982), a property that distinguishes them from the ecotropic parent virus, which infects only rodent cells (DeLarco and Todaro 1976). In addition, two other groups of type C viruses (amphotropic [Hartley et al. 1976; Rasheed et al. 1976]; xenotropic [Levy 1973]) have been identified in mice that also infect cells of other mammals. Comparison of mouse type C retroviral (murine leukemia virus [MuLV]) proteins identified differences in their envelope proteins that correlated with the pattern of infection of mammalian cells (Battini et al. 1992), a finding confirmed by pseudotyping experiments. In studies in mouse NIH-3T3 fibroblasts, Rein and Schultz (1984) correlated this property with the capacity of MuLVs to establish superinfection interference. Previous studies had suggested that the block to superinfection results from loss of sites for virus attachment caused by binding of newly synthesized envelope protein to host cell receptors (Steck and Rubin 1966). If true, these findings suggest that viruses within each group of type C MuLVs bind to a common receptor. Using interference assays, the existence of as many as six different receptors for type C retroviruses that infect human cells has been demonstrated (Sommerfelt et al. 1990). Groups of type C retroviruses that share host range and interference have also been identified in cats and in birds (Hunter and Swanstrom 1990).

Genetic determinants of MuLV infection were localized on specific mouse chromosomes by correlating susceptibility to infection with the chromosome content of hybrid cell lines formed by fusing permissive mouse fibroblasts to nonpermissive Chinese hamster lung fibroblasts. Hybrid cells that retained mouse chromosome 5 were susceptible to ecotropic MuLV infection (Oie et al. 1978). Likewise, susceptibility to amphotropic MuLV infection segregated with mouse chromosome 8 (Garcia et al. 1991), and polytropic and xenotropic MuLV infection required mouse chromosome 1 (Kozak 1983, 1985). Binding of ecotropic envelope surface protein, gp70, to a single class of saturable binding sites correlated with infection of these cell lines (Johnson and Rosner 1986), suggesting that a mouse gene encoding the receptor for ecotropic MuLV must reside on chromosome 5. The existence of distinct genes encoding receptors for each subgroup of avian type C retroviruses has also been suggested by genetic studies in chickens (Coffin 1984).

IDENTIFICATION OF MAMMALIAN TYPE C RETROVIRUS RECEPTORS

Several years ago, cDNA clones encoding putative receptors for ecotropic MuLV (Albritton et al. 1989) and a related type C retrovirus that causes leukemia in gibbon apes (GaLV) (O'Hara et al. 1990) were identified. They were recovered from cell lines that had acquired susceptibility to infection after transfer of DNA from permissive cells. These cell lines were identified by selection using cytotoxic drugs after exposure to recombinant retroviruses that carried genes which encoded for drug resistance. Analysis of the deduced amino acid sequence revealed they are hydrophobic proteins that contain a series of membrane-spanning domains connected by short hydrophilic loops. Computer-based sequence comparisons identified several domains in the core of the ecotropic MuLV receptor that are similiar in two yeast proteins, HIP1 (Tanaka and Fink 1985) and CAN1 (Hoffman 1985), which function as transporters of amino acids. Subsequent expression of the ecotropic MuLV receptor in *Xenopus* oocytes demonstrated its function as a transporter of the cationic amino acids, arginine, lysine, and ornithine (Kim et al. 1991; Wang et al. 1991). This protein has now been renamed MCAT-1 (mouse cationic amino acid transporter) to reflect its cellular function. Similiar analysis of the GaLV receptor (GaLVR) identified similarity with pho4, a phosphate permease in *Neurospora* (Johann et al. 1992).

Recent studies have directly demonstrated its function as a sodium-dependent phosphate transporter (Kavanaugh et al. 1994).

RELATED PROTEINS ARE RECEPTORS FOR OTHER
TYPE C RETROVIRUSES

Recently, infection by subgroup B of the feline leukemia viruses (FeLV) was found to interfere with GaLV infection of human fibroblasts (Takeuchi et al. 1992). Subsequent experiments confirmed that expression of GaLVR in nonpermissive cells was sufficient for infection by either virus. In addition, a second phosphate transporter that is related to the GaLVR has been identified in rat (RAM; Miller et al. 1994) and human (GaLVR2; van Ziejl et al. 1994) cells which determines infection by amphotropic MuLV. These findings suggest that a small number of related proteins may serve as receptors for many of the mammalian type C retroviruses. If true, this raises the possibility that some type C viruses may bind to closely related receptors. This hypothesis has been proposed as an explanation for the nonreciprocal interference observed upon infection with amphotropic MuLV and its MCF-like recombinant, 10A1 (Ott et al. 1990). The tissue-specific expression of an additional receptor(s) that permits infection of brain microglial or endothelial cells in rodents has been proposed to explain the tropism of ecotropic MuLVs that cause spastic paralysis (Paquette et al. 1989; Lynch et al. 1991; Masuda et al. 1993). Alternatively, tissue-specific posttranslational modifications of MCAT-1 in brain could explain these observations. Two other transporters of cationic amino acids that are related to MCAT-1 have been identified (Closs et al. 1993a,b), but to date, viruses that utilize these proteins as receptors have not been identified.

The weight of current evidence is most consistent with the existence of a single ecotropic MuLV receptor. Mapping studies have localized MCAT-1 on mouse chromosome 5, the chromosome required for infection of hybrid Chinese hamster cell lines (Kozak et al. 1990). In addition, the role of the rat counterpart of MCAT-1 (RCAT-1) in ecotropic MuLV infection of this species has been established (Wu et al. 1994). The ability of ecotropic MuLV vectors to infect mouse hepatocytes in primary culture, but not in vivo, has been correlated with MCAT-1 expression (Closs et al. 1993c). The ability of Moloney murine leukemia virus to infect fibroblasts from *Mus musculus,* but not *Mus dunni,* has been explained by differences in two residues in the envelope-binding domain of their CAT-1 proteins (Eiden et al. 1994). In addition, the resistance of Chinese hamster fibroblasts to infection with ecotropic MuLV is likely to be the result of glycosylation of hamster CAT, a finding that explains how exposure to tunicamycin, an inhibitor of N-glycosylation, can transiently overcome resistance to infection (Wilson and Eiden 1991). Introduction of MCAT-1 is sufficient for infection of human, monkey, Chinese hamster, canine, porcine, and avian cells. The relative efficiency of infection of these cell types is 10- to 50-fold lower than mouse fibroblasts, suggesting that additional host factors may influence virus infectivity. However, once infected, each of these cell lines produces replication-competent ecotropic MuLV that spreads throughout the culture (Albritton et al. 1989). Therefore, no additional barriers to ecotropic MuLV infection of mammalian or avian cell lines have been identified.

ROLE OF TRANSPORTERS IN ENVELOPE BINDING

The hydrophilic loops on the exofacial surface that connect the membrane-spanning domains of MCAT-1 and GaLVR are much shorter than the ectodomain of CD4, the type I membrane protein that binds the HIV envelope, gp120 (Dalgleish et al. 1984; Maddon et al. 1986). This structural difference raised the possibility that MCAT-1 and GaLVR might mediate a step in virus entry distinct binding to the envelope surface protein, gp70. Studies of chimeric CAT proteins identified a hydrophilic stretch of 29 residues that connects the third and fourth membrane-spanning domains of MCAT-1 which determined infection when introduced into the equivalent position of the nonpermissive human cationic amino acid transporter, HCAT-1 (Fig. 1) (Albritton et al. 1993). The presence of two glycosylated asparagine residues in this domain established its location on the exofacial surface of the plasma membrane (Kim and Cunningham 1993). In addition, expression of CAT proteins containing this domain in *Xenopus* oocytes was sufficient for binding of purified envelope surface protein, gp70. Replacement of only three residues, in HCAT-1 (PGV_{233-35}) by the equivalent residues (YGE_{235-37}) from this domain in MCAT-1 was sufficient for infection, suggesting these residues may directly interact with gp70. However, the existence of other proteins that interact with MCAT-1 has been proposed (Wells and Hediger 1992) and therefore, the possibility this domain determines infection by an allosteric effect cannot be excluded until a direct interaction with gp70 is demonstrated. Experiments of similiar design also identified a single hydrophilic domain connecting the fourth and fifth membrane-spanning domains of the human GaLVR protein, which is required for GaLV infection (Johann et al. 1992). Molecular models of GaLVR place this domain on the exofacial surface of the membrane (Fig. 1), but as yet, this location and role in envelope binding have not been determined experimentally.

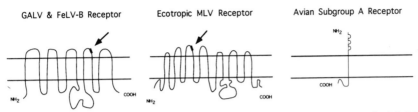

Figure 1 Schematic demonstrating probable orientation of ecotropic MuLV, gibbon ape/feline leukemia virus B, and avian subgroup A receptors with respect to the plasma membrane.

Expression of the amino-terminal 246 residues of the ecotropic MuLV gp70 is sufficient to establish interference, strongly suggesting this segment contains an MCAT-1-binding domain (Heard and Danos 1991). Computer-based comparison of the amino acid sequence of this portion of gp70 from seven mammalian type C retroviruses identified two variable regions, VRA and VRB (Battini et al. 1992), which are embedded in otherwise highly conserved residues. Chimeric viruses containing these domains from different type C MuLV envelope proteins demonstrate that VRA is dominant in specifying host range, suggesting it may interact directly with the receptor (Morgan et al. 1993). Additional evidence for the importance of VRA is suggested by the amino acid substitutions within this region that contribute to the pathogenicity of both FeLV 61C (Donahue et al. 1991) and MuLV PVC-211 (Masuda et al. 1993), two viruses suspected of altered receptor interaction. Recently, the pattern of disulfide bond formation between cysteine residues in the Friend MuLV gp70 has been determined (Linder et al. 1992). Identification of cysteine residues conserved in other mammalian type C envelope proteins may aid in the identification of receptor-binding domains. The relationships between VRA and VRB and the disulfide loops in the ecotropic and amphotropic MuLV are shown in Figure 2. Although the carboxy-terminal portion of gp70 is highly conserved among type C viruses, it has been suggested that this portion of the MCF gp70 may contribute to receptor binding and subgroup specificity (Ott and Rein 1992).

POSSIBLE ROLE OF TRANSPORTERS IN FUSION

Cleavage of 16 residues from the carboxyl terminus of the envelope transmembrane protein, p15e, occurs during the assembly of mammalian type C viruses (Green et al. 1981). Amino acid substitutions that prevented p15e cleavage abrogated virus infection, and premature expres-

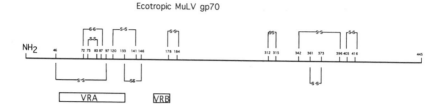

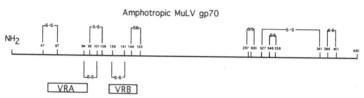

Figure 2 Relative positions of variable regions A and B (VRA and VRB) with respect to disulfide-bonded loops in the ecotropic (known) and amphotropic MuLV envelope surface proteins.

sion of the truncated TM protein (p12e) in infected NIH-3T3 fibroblasts resulted in massive syncytium formation by fusion of adjacent cells (Rein et al. 1994). Together, these observations suggest the cleavage of p15e may activate virions to fuse to the target cell membrane upon receptor binding. At present, an understanding of how cleavage of p15e within the nascent virion might promote fusion is unclear, but one report has demonstrated that small deletions in the membrane-spanning domain of p15e prevented establishment of interference (Granowitz et al. 1991), suggesting a possible remote effect on gp70 binding to MCAT-1. This suggests the possibility that MCAT-1 and GaLVR might also participate in fusion, perhaps coupled to the conformational changes that occur during translocation of cationic amino acids or phosphate across the membrane. Recently, a chicken protein related to the low density lipoprotein receptor has been identified as a receptor for avian subgroup A viruses (Bates et al. 1993; Young et al. 1993). Expression of this protein is sufficient for infection of mouse fibroblasts by Rous sarcoma virus, and antibodies directed against its ectodomain block virus infection. Although its cellular function is not known, the avian subgroup A receptor is a type I membrane protein that is unlikely on structural grounds to participate in transport of small solutes like MCAT-1 and GaLVR. However, postassembly processing of the transmembrane protein in avian retroviruses has also not been observed (Hunter and Swanstrom 1990), and therefore, there may be substantial differences in the mechanism of avian and mammalian type C virus infection.

RECEPTOR FUNCTION IN INFECTED CELLS

In MuLV-infected cells, the mobility of MCAT-1 on SDS/PAGE increased as a consequence of altered glycosylation of two asparagine residues in the envelope-binding domain (Kim and Cunningham 1993). Coexpression of the ecotropic, but not the MCF, envelope was sufficient to alter the glycosylation of MCAT-1, consistent with intracellular binding. Pulse-chase labeling experiments suggested that gp70 binding to MCAT-1 occurred in the endoplasmic reticulum, perhaps preventing transit of MCAT-1 to the Golgi. In HIV-infected cells, gp160 binding results in trapping of CD4 in the endoplasmic reticulum and eventual degradation targeted by the viral proteins, nef and vpu. However, MCAT-1 turnover was not changed in MuLV-infected cells. Indeed, MCAT-1-mediated uptake of arginine by cells was reduced only slightly by envelope expression sufficient to completely block detectable binding of exogenous gp70. These findings suggest that in MuLV-infected cells, the newly synthesized receptor protein is transported to the plasma membrane while bound to gp70 in a way that alters glycosylation, but not transport activity. Previous experiments demonstrated that exposure of MuLV-infected cells to tunicamycin, an inhibitor of N-glycosylation (Rein et al. 1982), could transiently reverse interference, raising the possibility that altered glycosylation of the envelope-binding domain of MCAT-1 might diminish virus binding. However, the function of an MCAT-1 protein carrying substitutions that prevented glycosylation was not detectably impaired in assays of arginine uptake, envelope binding, and virus infectivity. In addition, MuLV infection of cells that expressed the unglycosylated receptor resulted in superinfection interference that remained sensitive to tunicamycin. Therefore, tunicamycin-induced changes in the glycosylation of the virus envelope, perhaps at Asn-302 in Friend MuLV gp70 (Kayman et al. 1991), provide the probable molecular basis for glycosylation-dependent binding.

IDENTIFICATION OF ADDITIONAL RECEPTORS

Among the type C retroviruses in mammals, the receptors for the polytropic and xenotropic murine leukemia viruses, feline subgroups A and C, and human T-cell leukemia virus-1 (HTLV-1) have not been identified. The major experimental barrier to identification of these genes by transfer to nonpermissive cells is the preparation of recombinant retroviruses of sufficient titer to permit identification of permissive cell clones. Packaging lines that may be suitable for production of these viruses have been created (Danos and Mulligan 1988; Pear et al. 1993). Several published reports have identified alternative approaches to receptor identification that may also be fruitful. For example, antibodies prepared against the membranes of human B lymphocytes have been reported to block HTLV-1 infection by binding to an 80-kD glycoprotein expressed only on susceptible cells (Agadjanyan et al. 1994). This approach has been previously applied successfully to identify receptors for murine coronaviruses (Williams et al. 1991). Alternatively, positional cloning on chromosome 17q (Sommerfelt and Weiss 1990) may identify the gene encoding the HTLV-1 receptor. The identification and ordering of genetic markers on this chromosome is currently an area of intense interest by several laboratories in search of a breast cancer susceptibility gene. Fine mapping of genes on mouse chromosome 1 has already identified polymorphic markers in close linkage with the gene encoding the receptor for polytropic and xenotropic MuLVs (Hunter et al. 1993), which may be allelic. Finally, partial purification of the FeLVA receptor monitored by binding of purified gp70 has been reported (Ghosh et al. 1992). In this report, the investigators were able to covalently cross-link gp70 to the putative receptor protein.

REFERENCES

Agadjanyan, M.G., K.E. Ugen, B. Wang, W.V. Williams, and D.B. Weiner. 1994. Identification of an 80-kilodalton membrane glycoprotein important for human T-cell leukemia virus type I and type II syncytium formation and infection. *J. Virol.* **68**: 485.

Albritton, L.M., J.W. Kim, L. Tseng, and J. Cunningham. 1993. Envelope binding domain in the cationic amino acid transporter determines the host range of ecotropic murine retroviruses. *J. Virol.* **67**: 2091.

Albritton, L.M., L. Tseng, D. Scadden, and J.M. Cunningham. 1989. A putative murine ecotropic retrovirus receptor gene encodes a multiple membrane-spanning protein and confers susceptibility to virus infection. *Cell* **57**: 659.

Bates, P., J. Young, and H. Varmus. 1993. A receptor for subgroup A Rous sarcoma virus is related to the low density lipoprotein receptor. *Cell* **74**: 1043.

Battini, J-L., J.M. Heard, and O. Danos. 1992. Receptor choice determinants in the envelope glycoproteins of amphotropic, xenotropic and polytropic murine leukemia viruses. *J. Virol.* **66**: 1468.

Chattopadhyay, S.K., M.R. Lander, S. Gupta, E. Rands, and D.R. Lowy. 1981. Origin of mink cytopathic focus-forming (MCF) viruses: Comparison with ecotropic and xenotropic murine leukemia virus genomes. *Virology* **113**: 465.

Chattopadhyay, S.K., M.W. Cloyd, D.R. Linemeyer, M.R. Lander, E. Rands, and D.R. Lowy. 1982. Cellular origin and role of mink cell focus-forming viruses in murine thymic lymphomas. *Nature* **295**: 25.

Closs, E.I., L.M. Albritton, J.W. Kim, and J.M. Cunningham. 1993a. Identification of a low affinity, high capacity transporter of cationic amino acids in mouse liver. *J. Biol. Chem.* **268**: 7538.

Closs, E.I., R. Lyons, C. Kelly, and J.M. Cunningham. 1993b. Characterization of the third member of the MCAT family of cationic amino acid transporters. *J. Biol. Chem.* **268**: 20796.

Closs, E.I., I.H.B. Rinkes, A. Bader, M.L. Yarmush, and J.M. Cunningham. 1993c. Retroviral infection and expression of cationic amino acid transporters in rodent hepatocytes. *J. Virol.* **67:** 2097.

Cloyd, M.W., J.W. Hartley, and W.P. Rowe. 1980. Lymphomagenicity of recombinant mink cell focus-inducing virus. *J. Exp. Med.* **151:** 542.

Coffin, J.M. 1984. Endogenous viruses. In *Molecular biology of tumor viruses,* 2nd edition: *RNA tumor viruses 1/Text* (ed. R. Weiss et al.), p. 1109. Cold Spring Harbor Laboratory, Cold Spring Harbor, New York.

Dalgleish, A.C., P.C.L. Beverly, P.R. Clapham, D.H. Crawford, M.F. Greaves, and R.A. Weiss. 1984. The CD4 (T4) antigen is an essential component of the receptor for the AIDS retrovirus. *Nature* **312:** 763.

Danos, O. and R.C. Mulligan. 1988. Safe and efficient generation of recombinant retroviruses with amphotropic and ecotropic host ranges. *Proc. Natl. Acad. Sci.* **85:** 6460.

DeLarco, J. and G.J. Todaro. 1976. Membrane receptors for murine leukemia viruses: Characterization using purified viral envelope glycoprotein, gp71. *Cell* **8:** 365.

Donahue, P.T., S.L. Quackenbush, M.V. Gallo, C.M.C. deNoronha, E.A. Hoover, and J.I. Mullins. 1991. Viral genetic determinants of T-cell killing and immunodeficiency disease induction by the feline leukemia virus FeLV-FAIDS. *J. Virol.* **65:** 4461.

Eiden, M.V., D. Farrell, and C.A. Wilson. 1994. Glycosylation-dependent inactivation of the ecotropic murine leukemia virus receptor. *J. Virol.* **68:** 626.

Elder, J.H., J.W. Gatutsch, F.C. Jensen, R.A. Lerner, J.W. Hartley, and W.P. Rowe. 1977. Biochemical evidence that MCF murine leukemia viruses are envelope (env) gene recombinants. *Proc. Natl. Acad. Sci.* **74:** 4676.

Garcia, J.V., C. Jones, and A.D. Miller. 1991. Localization of the amphotropic murine leukemia virus receptor gene to the pericentromeric region of human chromosome 8. *J. Virol.* **65:** 6316.

Ghosh, A.K., M.H. Bachmann, E.A. Hoover, and J.I. Mullins. 1992. Identification of a putative receptor for subgroup A feline leukemia virus on feline T cells. *J. Virol.* **66:** 3707.

Granowitz, C., J. Colicelli, and S.P. Goff. 1991. Analysis of mutations in the envelope gene of moloney murine leukemia virus: Separation of infectivity from superinfection resistance. *Virology* **183:** 545.

Green, N., T.M. Shinnick, O. Witte, A. Ponticelli, J.G. Sutcliffe, and R.A. Lerner. 1981. Sequence-specific antibodies show that maturation of Moloney leukemia virus envelope polyprotein involves removal of a COOH-terminal peptide. *Proc. Natl. Acad. Sci.* **78:** 6023.

Hartley, J.W., W.P. Rowe, and R.J. Huebner. 1976. Naturally occurring murine leukemia viruses in wild mice: Characterization of a new "amphotropic" class. *J. Virol.* **5:** 221.

Heard, J.M. and O. Danos. 1991. An amino-terminal fragment of the Friend murine leukemia virus envelope glycoprotein binds the ecotropic receptor. *J. Virol.* **65:** 4026.

Hoffman, W. 1985. Molecular characterization of the CAN1 locus in *Saccharomyces cerevisiae. J. Biol. Chem.* **260:** 11831.

Hunter, E. and R. Swanstrom. 1990. Retrovirus envelope glycoproteins. *Curr. Top. Microbiol. Immunol.* **157:** 188.

Hunter, K.W., M.L. Watson, J. Rochelle, S. Ontiveros, D. Munroe, M.F. Seldin, and D.E. Housman. 1993. Single-strand conformational polymorphism (SSCP) mapping of the mouse genome: Integration of the SSCP, microsatellite, and gene maps of mouse chromosome 1. *Genomics* **18:** 510.

Johann, S.V., J.J. Gibbons, and B. O'Hara. 1992. GLVR1, a receptor for gibbon ape leukemia virus, is homologous to a phosphate permease of *Neurospora crassa* and is expressed at high levels in the brain and thymus. *J. Virol.* **66:** 1635.

Johnson, P.A. and M.R. Rosner. 1986. Characterization of murine-specific leukemia virus receptor from L cells. *J. Virol.* **58:** 900.

Kavanaugh, M.P., D.G. Miller, W. Zhang, W. Law, S.L. Kozak, D.K. Kabat, and A.D. Miller. 1994. Cell-surface receptors for gibbon ape leukemia virus and amphotropic murine retrovirus are inducible sodium-dependent phosphate symporters. *Proc. Natl. Acad. Sci.* **91:** 7071.

Kayman, S., R. Kopelman, S. Projan, D.M. Kinney, and A. Pinter. 1991. Mutational analysis of N-linked glycosylation sites of Friend murine leukemia virus envelope protein. *J. Virol.* **65:** 5323.

Kim, J.W. and J.M. Cunningham. 1993. N-linked glycosylation of the receptor for murine ecotropic retroviruses is altered in virus-infected cells. *J. Biol. Chem.* **268:** 16316.

Kim, J.W., E.I. Closs, L.M. Albritton, and J.M. Cunningham. 1991. Transport of cationic amino acids by the mouse ecotropic retrovirus receptor. *Nature* **352:** 725.

Kozak, C.A. 1983. Genetic mapping of a mouse chromosomal locus required for mink cell focus-forming virus replication. *J. Virol.* **48:** 300.

———. 1985. Susceptibility of wild mouse cells to exogenous infection with xenotropic leukemia viruses: control by a single dominant locus on chromosome 1. *J. Virol.* **55:** 690.

Kozak, C.A., L.M. Albritton, and J. Cunningham. 1990. Genetic mapping of a cloned sequence responsible for susceptibility to ecotropic murine leukemia viruses. *J. Virol.* **64:** 3119.

Levy, J.A. 1973. Xenotropic viruses: Murine leukemia viruses associated with NIH Swiss, NZB, and other mouse strains. *Science* **182:** 1151.

Linder, M., D. Linder, J. Hahnen, H.-H. Schott, and S. Stirm. 1992. Localization of the intrachain disulfide bonds of the envelope glycoprotein 71 from Friend leukemia virus. *Eur. J. Biochem.* **203:** 65.

Lynch, W.P., S. Czub, F.J. McAtee, S.F. Hayes, and J.L. Portis. 1991. Murine retrovirus-induced spongiform encephalopathy: Productive infection of microglia and cerebellar neurons in accelerated CNS disease. *Neuron* **7:** 365.

Maddon, P.J., A.G. Dalgleish, J.S. McDougal, P.R. Clapham, R.A. Weiss, and R. Axel. 1986. The T4 gene encodes the AIDS virus receptor and is expressed in the immune system and the brain. *Cell* **47:** 333.

Masuda, M., P.M. Hoffman, and S.K. Ruscetti. 1993. Viral determinants that control the neuropathogenicity of PVC-211 murine leukemia virus in vivo determine brain capillary endothelial cell tropism of the virus in vitro. *J. Virol.* **67:** 4580.

Miller, D.G., R.H. Edwards, and A.D. Miller. 1994. Cloning of the cellular receptor for amphotropic murine retroviruses reveals homology to that for gibbon ape leukemia virus. *Proc. Natl. Acad. Sci.* **91:** 78.

Morgan, R.A., O. Nussbaum, D.D. Muenchau, L. Shu, L. Couture, and F. Anderson. 1993. Analysis of the functional and host range-determining regions of the murine ecotropic and amphotropic retrovirus envelope proteins. *J. Virol.* **67:** 4712.

O'Hara, B., S.V. Johann, H.P. Klinger, D.G. Blair, H. Rubinson, K.J. Dunne, P. Sass, S.M. Vitek, and T. Robins. 1990. Characterization of a human gene conferring sensitivity to infection by gibbon ape leukemia virus. *Cell Growth Differ.* **3:** 199.

Oie, H.K., A.F. Gazdar, P.A. Lalley, E.K. Russell, J.D. Minna, J. DeLarco, G.J. Todaro, and U. Francke. 1978. Mouse chromosome 5 codes for ecotropic murine leukaemia virus cell-surface receptor. *Nature* **274:** 60.

Ott, D. and A. Rein. 1992. Basis for receptor specificity of nonecotropic murine leukemia virus surface glycoprotein gp70SU. *J. Virol.* **66:** 4632.

Ott, D., R. Friedrich, and A. Rein. 1990. Sequence analysis of amphotropic and 10A1 murine leukemia viruses: Close relationship to mink cell focus-inducing viruses. *J. Virol.* **64:** 757.

Paquette, Y., Z. Hanna, P. Savard, R. Brousseau, Y. Robitaille, and P. Jolicoeur. 1989. Retrovirus-induced murine motor neuron disease: Mapping the determinant of spongiform degeneration within the envelope gene. *Proc. Natl. Acad. Sci* **86:** 3896.

Pear, W.S., G.P. Nolan, M.L. Scott, and D. Baltimore. 1993. Production of high-titer helper-free retroviruses by transient transfection. *Proc. Natl. Acad. Sci.* **90:** 8392.

Rasheed, S., M.B. Gardner, and E. Chan. 1976. Amphotropic host range of naturally occuring wild mouse leukemia virus. *J. Virol.* **19:** 13.

Rein, A. and A. Schultz. 1984. Different recombinant murine leukemia viruses use different cell surface receptors. *Virology* **136:** 144.

Rein, A., A.M. Schultz, J.P. Bader, and R.H. Bassin. 1982. Short communications: Inhibitors of glycosylation reverse retroviral interference. *Virology* **119:** 185.

Rein, A., J. Mirro, J.G. Haynes, S.M. Ernst, and K. Nagashima. 1994. Function of the cytoplasmic domain of a retroviral transmembrane protein: p15E-p2E cleavage activates the membrane fusion capability of the murine leukemia virus Env protein. *J. Virol.* **68:** 1773.

Sommerfelt, M.A. and R.A. Weiss. 1990. Receptor interference groups of 20 retroviruses plating on human cells. *Virology* **176:** 58.

Steck, F.T. and H. Rubin. 1966. The mechanism of interference between an avian leukosis virus and Rous sarcoma virus. I. Establishment of interference. *Virology* **29:** 628.

Takeuchi, Y., R.G. Vile, G. Simpson, B. O'Hara, M.K.L. Collins, and R.A. Weiss. 1992. Feline leukemia virus subgroup B uses the same cell surface receptor as gibbon ape leukemia virus. *J. Virol.* **66:** 1219.

Tanaka, J. and G.R. Fink. 1985. The histidine permease gene (HIPI) of *Saccharomyces cerevisiae*. *Gene* **38:** 205.

Taylor, C.S., Y. Takeuchi, B. O'Hara, S.V. Johann, R.A. Weiss, and M.K. Collins. 1993. Mutation of amino acids within the gibbon ape leukemia virus (GALV) receptor differentially affects feline leukemia virus subgroup B, simian sarcoma-associated virus, and GALV infections. *J. Virol.* **67:** 6737.

van Zeijl, M., S.V. Johann, E.I Closs, and J.M. Cunningham. 1994. An amphotropic retrovirus receptor is the second member of the gibbon ape leukemia virus receptor family. *Proc. Natl. Acad. Sci.* **91:** 1168.

Wang, H., M.P. Kavanaugh, R.A. North, and D. Kabat. 1991. Cell surface receptor for ecotropic murine retroviruses is a basic amino-acid transporter. *Nature* **352:** 729.

Wells, R.G. and M.A. Hediger. 1992. Cloning of a rat kidney cDNA that stimulates dibasic and neutral amino acid transport and has sequence similarity to glucosidases. *Proc. Natl. Acad. Sci.* **89:** 5596.

Williams, R.K., G.S. Jiang, and K.V. Holmes. 1991. Receptor for mouse hepatitis virus is a member of the carcinoembryonic antigen family of glycoproteins. *Proc. Natl. Acad. Sci.* **88:** 5533.

Wilson, C.A. and M.V. Eiden. 1991. Viral and cellular factors governing hamster cell infection by murine and gibbon ape leukemia viruses. *J. Virol.* **65:** 5975.

Wu, J.Y., D. Robinson, H.J. Kung, and M. Hatzoglou. 1994. Hormonal regulation of the gene for the type C ecotropic retrovirus receptor in rat liver cells. *J. Virol.* **68:** 1615.

Young, J.A., P. Bates, and H. Varmus. 1993. Isolation of a chicken gene that confers susceptibility to infection by subgroup A avian leukosis and sarcoma viruses. *J. Virol.* **67:** 1811.

5

A Protein Related to the LDL Receptor Is a Cellular Receptor Specific for Subgroup A Avian Leukosis and Sarcoma Viruses

John A.T. Young[1,3] and Harold E. Varmus[1,2]
[1]Department of Microbiology and Immunology
[2]Department of Biochemistry and Biophysics
University of California School of Medicine
San Francisco, California 94143

[3]Gladstone Institute of Virology and Immunology
San Francisco General Hospital
San Francisco, California 94141-9100

Paul F. Bates
Department of Microbiology
University of Pennsylvania School of Medicine
Philadelphia, Pennsylvania 19104-6076

Retrovirus entry into cells requires the binding of viral envelope (Env) glycoproteins to specific host cell-surface receptors. Such interactions presumably activate the fusogenic potential of Env, leading to fusion of virus and cell membranes and entry of viral nucleoprotein core particles into the target cell cytoplasm. Despite the critical importance of these steps in virus infection, the early events in the retrovirus replication cycle are not well understood.

The Env proteins of retroviruses comprise two subunits, surface (SU) and transmembrane (TM) proteins, that are arranged as oligomeric complexes on the viral surface lipid bilayer (Einfeld and Hunter 1988; Pinter et al. 1989; Weiss et al. 1990). The receptor-binding determinants on the virus are commonly found in the SU Env protein (for review, see Weiss 1992). The TM viral Env protein contains the transmembrane and cytoplasmic tail domains that anchor Env at the virus surface, as well as a hydrophobic domain, designated the fusion peptide, that is required for membrane fusion (White 1990).

Since retrovirus envelope proteins resemble the HA1 and HA2 hemagglutinin proteins of influenza virus, it has been suggested that there may be a similar mechanism of membrane fusion mediated by these different viral surface proteins (White 1990). The pH-dependent entry of influenza virus into cells is relatively well understood. After influenza virus binds cell-surface sialic acid, it is taken up by receptor-mediated endocytosis and transported to late endosomes. The low pH within late endosomes drives structural changes in HA1 and HA2, leading to exposure of the hydrophobic fusion peptide domain at the amino terminus of HA2 and membrane fusion (White 1990). Although this system provides a useful framework for considering what might be important for retrovirus entry, it is clearly of limited application, since most retroviruses enter cells in a pH-independent manner, consistent with direct fusion between viral and host cell-surface membranes (Stein et al. 1987; McClure et al. 1988, 1990; Gilbert et al. 1990). Presumably, conformational changes that activate the fusogenic potential of retroviral Env proteins are driven by interactions between Env and specific host cell-surface factor(s), but this remains to be determined.

AVIAN LEUKOSIS AND SARCOMA VIRUS RECEPTORS

The interactions between avian leukosis and sarcoma viruses (ALSV) and their cellular receptors represent a useful model system for understanding how retroviruses recognize and infect target cells. First, like most other retroviruses, ALSV infect target cells in a pH-independent manner (Gilbert et al. 1990). Second, different subgroups of ALSV interact with distinct cellular receptors, raising the possibility that this system might reveal some common principles required for retrovirus infection.

There are five major subgroups of ALSV (A–E) that infect chickens. Viruses within each subgroup use the same cellular receptor, have immunologically related Env glycoproteins, and demonstrate cross-interference (Payne and Biggs 1964; Hanafusa 1965; Vogt 1965; Vogt and Ishizaki 1965; Ishizaki and Vogt 1966; Duff and Vogt 1969; Vogt and Friis 1971). Cross-interference is due to blocking of subgroup-specific ALSV receptors, presumably as a consequence of viral Env expression in infected cells, and this prevents superinfection of infected cells by viruses of the same subgroup. The subgroup specificity of ALSV operates at the level of virus entry and is determined by three non-contiguous variable regions of the viral SU Env protein (Dorner and Coffin 1986; Bova et al. 1988). These variable Env domains might therefore constitute the site(s) of receptor interaction.

Studies in chickens have identified susceptibility genes that presumably encode subgroup-specific virus receptors. Three autosomal chicken loci, designated *tv-a*, *tv-b*, and *tv-c*, govern susceptibility to infection by viral subgroups A, B, and C, respectively (Payne and Biggs 1964, 1966; Rubin 1965; Crittenden et al. 1967; Payne and Pani 1971). Interestingly, there are different alleles of each gene that determine either susceptibility or resistance to infection by the respective virus subgroups (for review, see Weiss 1992). Susceptibility alleles at each locus (e.g., tv-a^s) are dominant over those that determine resistance (e.g., tv-a^r): The tv-a and tv-c loci appear to be genetically linked, raising the possibility that these susceptibility genes might be related by a gene duplication event (Payne and Pani 1971). The receptors for ALSV subgroups B, D, and E appear to be related to each other, since these viruses exhibit varying degrees of cross-interference (for review, see Weiss 1992).

To gain insight into the mechanism of ALSV entry into cells, we have isolated and characterized an avian gene that encodes an ALSV susceptibility factor. Expression of this factor in mammalian cells is sufficient to confer susceptibility to specific infection by subgroup A-ALSV (ALSV-A), consistent with the tentative identification of the cloned gene as tv-a^s. At least two protein products of the gene function as ALSV-A susceptibility factors. These small membrane-associated proteins contain an extracellular domain related to the ligand-binding domains of the low-density lipoprotein (LDL) receptor.

RESULTS

A Gene Transfer Strategy Used to Generate Transfected Cells That Express an ALSV-A Susceptibility Factor

A gene transfer approach was used in an attempt to isolate the avian gene that confers susceptibility to specific infection by ALSV-A. Chicken genomic DNA was transfected into monkey COS-7 cells along with plasmid pMPneo DNA, conferring resistance to G418 (Young et al. 1993). Monkey COS-7 cells were used as recipients for transfection since they are normally resistant to ALSV-A but have no apparent intracellular block to ALSV replication up to the point of virus gene expression (Bova et al. 1988). To identify those transfected cells that express ALSV-A susceptibility factors, the G418-resistant colonies that arose were split onto duplicate plates and challenged with an ALSV-A vector containing a gene that confers resistance to hygromycin B (Fig. 1). In this approach, cells expressing ALSV-A susceptibility factors would give rise to multiple hygromycin-B-resistant colonies on duplicate plates. In contrast, nonspecific ALSV-A infection, which occurs at a very low efficiency in monkey cells (Bova et al. 1988), would give rise only to one or two hygromycin-B-resistant colonies (Fig. 1).

These experiments generated two independent pairs of duplicate

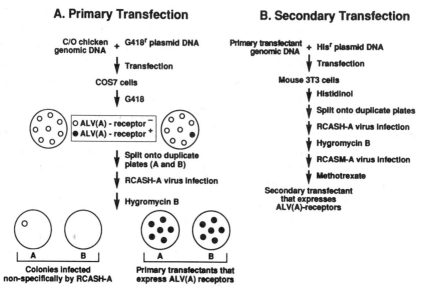

Figure 1 A genetic strategy to isolate the chicken ALSV-A susceptibility gene. (RCASH-A and RCASM-A) ALSV-A vectors containing genes conferring resistance to hygromycin B and methotrexate, respectively. (Reprinted, with permission, from Young et al. 1993.)

plates containing multiple hygromycin-B-resistant colonies. These cells were most probably derived from two independent primary transfectant colonies that express susceptibility factor(s) for ALSV-A (Fig.1). This notion was confirmed by Southern blot analysis, which demonstrated that colonies that arose on duplicate plates contained the same transfected chicken and plasmid DNA sequences (Young et al. 1993). Consistent with expression of an ALSV-A susceptibility factor in these cells, each of these colonies had been infected multiple times by virus (Young et al. 1993). Furthermore, these cells were also susceptible to infection by other subgroup-A-specific viruses (Young et al. 1993).

To segregate the ALSV-A susceptibility gene from other chicken DNA sequences in the primary transfectants, a second round of transfection and selection was performed. Genomic DNA from one of the primary transfectants was transfected into mouse BALB/3T3 cells along with plasmid pMPHis DNA, conferring resistance to histidinol (Fig.1). Histidinol-resistant cells that had taken up DNA were split onto duplicate plates and challenged with the subgroup A virus containing the hygromycin-B-resistance gene as before. In this protocol, cells could become drug-resistant as a consequence of expression of the ALSV-A susceptibility factor and infection by ALSV-A. Alternatively, cells that had taken up the ALSV-A vector proviral DNA from the primary transfectant would also be resistant to hygromycin B. To exclude this latter possibility, hygromycin-B-resistant colonies that arose were challenged with an ALSV-A vector containing a gene conferring resistance to methotrexate (Fig.1). This led to identification of a single secondary transfectant that expresses a susceptibility factor(s) for ALSV-A (Young et al. 1993).

Molecular Cloning of the Locus That Encodes a Susceptibility Factor Specific for ALSV-A

Southern blot analysis revealed that a single copy of pMPneo plasmid DNA used in the primary transfection had segregated with the ALSV-A susceptibility gene in the secondary transfectant (Young et al. 1993). Indeed, the plasmid DNA sequences served as a molecular tag to isolate this gene; chicken DNA sequences linked to the plasmid were found in both independent primary transfectants, cosegregating with the activity of the ALSV-A susceptibility factor (Young et al. 1993). Restriction enzyme mapping localized the susceptibility locus to a 7-kb fragment contained on two overlapping genomic DNA fragments that were cloned using a bacteriophage vector (λ1 and λ2, Fig. 2).

To test whether λ1 or λ2 encodes the ALSV-A susceptibility factor, these genomic clones were introduced into mouse 3T3 cells, and transfected cells were challenged with ALSV vectors containing a hygromycin-B-resistance gene. Cells transfected with λ1 were infected by subgroup-A, but not subgroup-B, virus (Young et al. 1993). In contrast, cells transfected with λ2 were not infected by ALSV. Therefore, the λ1 genomic clone encodes a susceptibility factor that is specific for ALSV-A.

Isolation of a Quail ALSV-A Susceptibility Gene

Conventional molecular approaches failed to identify exons of the cloned chicken gene (Young et al. 1993; Bates et al. 1993). An alternative approach used to identify putative coding regions of the gene was to compare the DNA sequence of the cloned chicken gene with that of the homolog from a different avian species. For this purpose, a related 5.5-kb quail genomic clone, encoding a subgroup-A-specific ALSV susceptibility factor, was isolated and characterized (Bates et al. 1993). Putative exons of the quail and chicken genes were identified as those regions of DNA sequence that are highly conserved between both species, flanked by consensus exon/intron boundaries. However, when these DNA frag-

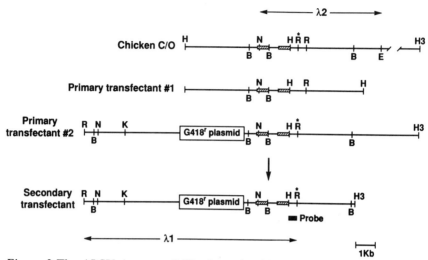

Figure 2 The ALSV-A susceptibility locus in chicken cells and in transfected cells. A 12-kb *Eco*RI fragment (λ1; bottom) which contained both plasmid and linked chicken DNA sequences was cloned from the secondary transfectant. An overlapping 7-kb *Eag*I fragment (λ2; top) was subsequently cloned from chicken cells by cross-hybridization to the λ1 probe indicated by the solid box. Hatched boxes represent CR1 chicken repeat DNA sequences (Stumph et al. 1981). Restriction enzymes: (B) *Bam*HI; (N) *Not*I; (H) *Hin*cII; (R) *Eco*RI (asterisk indicates polymorphic *Eco*RI site); (E) *Eag*I; (H3) *Hin*dIII. The ALSV-A susceptibility gene contains at least three other *Eag*I sites not indicated here. (Reprinted, with permission, from Young et al. 1993.)

ments were used as radioactively labeled probes for Northern blot analysis, they did not detect any related mRNA transcripts from avian cells. Furthermore, because of the high content of GC nucleotides in these regions, it was not possible to unambiguously assign the open reading frame of the susceptibility factor.

Exon-trapping Experiments Reveal That the ALSV-A Susceptibility Factor Is a Member of the LDL Receptor Family

Given the difficulties in defining the coding potential of the avian gene by conventional techniques, a retrovirus-based exon-trapping protocol was used to identify the susceptibility factor open reading frame (Bates et al. 1993). The quail susceptibility gene was introduced into a murine leukemia virus (MLV)-based vector, which also contains a gene conferring resistance to G418. This recombinant viral genome was introduced into mouse cells that express MLV Gag, Pol, and Env products. Viruses generated by this protocol contain MLV vector RNA in which introns of the quail susceptibility gene have been removed by RNA splicing (Bates et al. 1993). These viruses were used to infect mouse 3T3 cells, and infected cells were selected in G418. To identify those cells that had taken up a functional copy of the processed susceptibility gene, the G418-resistant cells were challenged by infection with an ALSV-A vector containing a gene conferring resistance to hygromycin B. In this way, two different classes of processed susceptibility gene that support ALSV-A infection were identified (Fig. 3): an 819-bp clone (pg800) and a 968-bp clone (pg950).

The pg800 and pg950 processed genes are predicted to encode similar protein products that share a putative 19-amino-acid signal peptide and an 83-amino-acid extracellular domain. However, these products differ at their carboxyl termini: The pg950 protein has a 23-amino-acid trans-membrane region and 32-amino-acid cytoplasmic tail; the pg800 protein has 15 hydrophobic amino acids and three hydrophilic amino acids that presumably suffice for cell-surface membrane attachment (Bates et al. 1993).

A search of the Genbank database revealed that the amino-terminal half of the extracellular domain of the putative pg800 and pg950 protein products is related to the ligand-binding repeat domains of the low-density lipoprotein receptor (LDLR; Fig. 4). This motif comprises six cysteines in addition to eleven other highly conserved amino acid residues (Sudhof et al. 1985). Similar domains are also found in several components of the complement cascade (Stanley et al. 1988), the α_2-macroglobulin receptor/LDL receptor-related protein (Strickland et al. 1990), and the human heparan sulfate proteoglycan, Perlecan (Murdoch et al. 1992).

An Antiserum Specific for the ALSV-A Susceptibility Factor Blocks ALSV-A Infection of Avian Cells

To characterize the expression and function of the ALSV-A susceptibility factor, a polyclonal rabbit antiserum was raised against a bacterially produced glutathione-S-transferase (GST)-susceptibility factor fusion protein. Western blot analysis using this antiserum revealed polypeptides of 27, 29, and 33–36 kD, encoded by pg950 in transfected mouse cells (Bates et al. 1993). However, this antiserum did not detect any specific proteins in quail QT6 cells. This observation, coupled with our inability to detect related mRNA transcripts in these cells and in primary chicken embryo fibroblasts, suggests that the susceptibility gene is probably expressed at low levels.

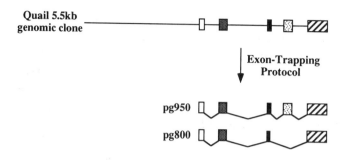

Quail 5.5kb
genomic clone

Exon-Trapping
Protocol

pg950

pg800

☐ Signal peptide exon (24 amino acids)

■ LDLR-related domain exon (59 amino acids)

▌ Membrane-proximal domain exon (26 amino acids)

▨ Transmembrane domain and cytoplasmic tail exon (pg950: 48 amino acids)

▨▨ Membrane anchor (pg800: 11 amino acids) and 3'untranslated region exon

Figure 3 An exon-trapping protocol generates two functional processed ALSV-A susceptibility genes (pg950 and pg800) from the quail 5.5-kb quail genomic clone.

Given the fact that the susceptibility factor protein could not be detected in avian cells, it was important to demonstrate that this product normally mediates ALSV-A infection. Therefore, the susceptibility factor-specific antiserum was tested for its ability to block ALSV infection of chicken embryo fibroblasts and quail QT6 cells. The antiserum blocked infection of chicken cells by ALSV-A, but had no effect on infection by ALSV-B, ALSV-C, or ALSV-D. Similarly, the antiserum blocked infection of QT6 cells by ALSV-A (Bates et al. 1993). These results clearly demonstrate that the cloned susceptibility factor gene encodes a product that is necessary for subgroup A virus infection of avian cells.

DISCUSSION

An avian gene encoding a susceptibility factor specific for ALSV-A has been isolated. This gene encodes LDL receptor-related proteins, which are sufficient to confer susceptibility to virus infection and have an extracellular domain of only 83 amino acids. The susceptibility factor proteins presumably mediate virus entry at the host cell surface. This idea is supported by the cell-surface localization of the processed gene protein products in transfected cells, as detected by immunofluorescence experiments (H. Wang et al., in prep.). Furthermore, a soluble form of

```
                        *       *         *     *     *   **  *
LDLR-Family Consensus   C    F C        G CI   W CD   DC D SDE  C
Quail ALVA-R            CPPGQFRCSEPPGAHGECYPQDWLCDGHPDCDDGRDEWGC
Chick ALVA-R            CSPEQFHCSEPRDPQTDCYPLEWLCDGHPDCDDGRDEWGC
```

Figure 4 Alignment of ALSV-A receptor amino acid residues with other LDL receptor-related protein sequences. Amino acid residues 11–50 of the quail ALSV-A receptor proteins encoded by pg800 and pg950 were compared to the 7 ligand-binding repeats of the human LDL receptor (Yamamoto et al. 1984), 8 domains of the rabbit very low density lipoprotein receptor (Takahashi et al. 1992), 11 domains of the α_2-macroglobulin receptor (Strickland et al. 1990), Perlecan (Murdoch et al. 1992), and complement components C8α and β and C9 (Stanley 1988). The consensus represents amino acids found at a frequency of more than 50% at these positions, but does not reflect minor spacing differences due to amino acid insertions/deletions between different family members. Asterisks indicate amino acids that are absolutely conserved between these family members.

the susceptibility factor blocks infection and binds specifically to ALSV-A (Connolly et al. 1994). These results, coupled with the ability of the susceptibility factor-specific antiserum to block virus infection, strongly suggest that the cloned gene encodes a receptor for ALSV-A.

Several lines of evidence suggest that the cloned ALSV-A susceptibility gene might be a susceptibility allele of *tv-a*, the genetically defined receptor locus for ALSV-A. First, transfected mouse cells that express this receptor can be infected by subgroup-A virus, and not by viruses of other ALSV subgroups. Second, a receptor-specific antiserum blocks infection of avian cells by ALSV-A, but has no effect on infection by virus subgroups B, C, and D (Bates et al. 1993). Indeed, restriction fragment length polymorphism studies have confirmed that the cloned gene maps to the *tv-a* locus (L. Crittenden et al., unpubl.).

Since the Env proteins of different retroviruses are similar to each other, it seems reasonable to expect that the entry processes used by these viruses share some common features. However, the cell-surface proteins used as retrovirus receptors do not share any obvious structural or sequence similarities to suggest a common function in virus entry. The heterogeneity of proteins that are used as retrovirus receptors indicates that these molecules might only play a passive role in virus cell membrane fusion; they might only serve to activate the fusogenic potential of viral Env proteins. Like the ALSV-A receptor, the CD4 receptor for human and simian immunodeficiency viruses (HIV-1, HIV-2, and SIV) and the receptor for bovine leukemia viruses (BLV) have a single transmembrane domain and a cytoplasmic tail domain (Maddon et al. 1986;

Ban et al. 1993). However, the extracellular domains of these proteins are totally unrelated; the ALSV-A receptor is a member of the LDL receptor family, CD4 is a member of the immunoglobulin superfamily (Maddon et al. 1986), and the BLV receptor is not related to any protein known to date (Ban et al. 1993). It should be noted that the ALSV-A receptor proteins described in this chapter are encoded by processed genes that were generated by an exon-trapping protocol. Therefore, it is possible that the susceptibility factor proteins expressed in avian cells have a different structure because of alternative splicing of the corresponding mRNA transcripts. In contrast with the virus receptors described above, the receptor for ecotropic murine leukemia viruses (MLV-E) and the receptors for gibbon ape leukemia virus (GALV) and subgroup-B feline leukemia virus (FeLV-B) are proteins that possess multiple membrane-spanning domains (Albritton et al. 1989; O' Hara et al. 1990; Takeuchi et al. 1992).

In addition to the structural variability of retrovirus receptors, these proteins do not share any common physiological function that might indicate a common role in virus entry; CD4 is known to participate in T-cell signaling events (Maddon et al. 1986), whereas the MLV-E receptor is a cationic amino acid transporter (Kim et al. 1991; Wang et al. 1991) and the GALV/FeLV-B receptor is related to a phosphate transporter of *Neurospora crassa* (Johann et al. 1992). Despite the fact that the ALSV-A receptor has a motif related to the ligand-binding repeats of the LDL receptor, this motif is also found in other proteins with diverse functions. Therefore, we cannot at present speculate on the physiological function of the ALSV-A receptor protein.

It is clear from studies on the best-understood retrovirus-receptor system, HIV-1/CD4 interactions, that retrovirus entry is a complicated process. CD4, although necessary for infection of CD4-positive human T cells and macrophages, is not sufficient to confer susceptibility to virus infection on other cell types (Maddon et al. 1986; Dragic et al. 1992). Indeed, it seems likely that CD4 functions to bind virus at the cell surface and that another unidentified cell-surface factor(s) is required to mediate postbinding steps in virus entry (Dragic et al. 1992).

ALSV-A receptor interactions provide an excellent model system for understanding how retrovirus Env/receptor interactions lead to virus entry. In contrast to CD4, the ALSV-A receptor confers susceptibility to virus infection upon cells derived from several diverse species, raising the possibility that this protein may be the only factor required for virus infection. The small ALSV-A receptor protein is well suited for future studies that will establish its role in binding and/or postbinding events of retrovirus entry.

REFERENCES

Albritton, L.M., L. Tseng, D. Scadden, and J.M. Cunningham. 1989. A putative murine ecotropic retrovirus receptor gene encodes a multiple membrane-spanning protein and confers susceptibility to virus infection. *Cell* **57:** 659.

Ban, J., D. Portetelle, C. Altaner, B. Horion, D. Milan, V. Krchnak, A. Burny, and R. Kettman. 1993. Isolation and characterization of a 2.3-kilobase-pair cDNA fragment encoding the binding domain of the bovine leukemia virus cell receptor. *J. Virol.* **67:** 1050.

Bates, P., J.A.T. Young, and H.E. Varmus. 1993. A receptor for subgroup A Rous sarcoma virus is related to the LDL receptor. *Cell* **74:** 1043.

Bova, C.A., J.C. Olsen, and R. Swanstrom. 1988. The avian retrovirus *env* gene family: Molecular analysis of host range and antigenic variants. *J. Virol.* **62:** 75.

Connolly, L., K. Zingler, and J.A.T. Young. 1994. A soluble form of a receptor for subgroup A avian leukosis and sarcoma viruses (ALSV-A) blocks infection and binds directly to ALSV-A. *J. Virol.* **68:** 2760.

Crittenden, L.B., H.A. Stone, R.H. Reamer, and W. Okazaki. 1967. Two loci controlling genetic cellular resistance to avian leukosis-sarcoma viruses. *J. Virol.* **1:** 898.

Dorner, A.J. and J.M. Coffin. 1986. Determinants for receptor interaction and cell killing on the avian retrovirus glycoprotein gp85. *Cell* **45:** 365.

Dragic, T., P. Charneau, F. Clavel, and M. Alizon. 1992. Complementation of murine cells for human immunodeficiency virus envelope/CD4-mediated fusion in human/murine heterokaryons. *J. Virol.* **66:** 4794.

Duff, R.G. and P.K. Vogt. 1969. Characteristics of two new avian tumor virus subgroups. *Virology* **39:** 18.

Einfeld, D. and E. Hunter. 1988. Oligomeric structure of a prototype retrovirus glycoprotein. *Proc. Natl. Acad. Sci.* **85:** 8688.

Gilbert, J.M., D. Mason, and J.M. White. 1990. Fusion of Rous sarcoma virus with host cells does not require exposure to low pH. *J. Virol.* **64:** 5106.

Hanafusa, H. 1965. Analysis of the defectiveness of Rous sarcoma virus. III. Determining influence of a new helper virus on the host range and susceptibility to interference of RSV. *Virology* **25:** 248.

Ishizaki, R. and P.K. Vogt. 1966. Immunological relationships among envelope antigens of avian tumor viruses. *Virology* **30:** 375.

Johann, S.V., J.J. Gibbons, and B. O'Hara. 1992. GLVR1, a receptor for gibbon ape leukemia virus, is homologous to a phosphate permease of *Neurospora crassa* and is expressed at high levels in the brain and thymus. *J. Virol.* **66:** 1635.

Kim, J.W., E.I. Closs, L.M. Albritton, and J.M. Cunningham. 1991. Transport of cationic amino acids by the mouse ecotropic retrovirus receptor. *Nature* **352:** 725.

McClure, M.O., M. Marsh, and R.A. Weiss. 1988. Human immunodeficiency virus infection of CD4-bearing cells occurs by a pH-independent mechanism. *EMBO J.* **7:** 513.

McClure, M.O., M.A. Sommerfelt, M. Marsh, and R.A. Weiss. 1990. The pH independence of mammalian retrovirus infection. *J. Gen. Virol.* **71:** 767.

Maddon, P.J., A.G. Dalgleish, J.S. McDougal, P.R. Clapham, R.A. Weiss, and R.Axel. 1986. The T4 gene encodes the AIDS virus receptor and is expressed in the immune system and the brain. *Cell* **47:** 333.

Murdoch, A.D., G.R. Dodge, I. Cohen, R.S. Tuan, and R.V. Iozzo. 1992. Primary structure of the human heparin sulfate proteoglycan from basement membrane (HSPG2/Perlecan). *J. Biol. Chem.* **267:** 8544.

O'Hara, B., S.V. Johann, H.P. Klinger, D.G. Blair, H. Rubinson, K.J. Dunn, P. Sass, S.

M. Vitek, and T. Robins. 1990. Characterization of a human gene conferring sensitivity to infection by gibbon ape leukemia virus. *Cell Growth Differ.* **1:** 119.

Payne, L.N. and P.M. Biggs. 1964. Differences between highly inbred lines of chickens in the response to Rous sarcoma virus of the chorioallantoic membrane and of embryonic cells in tissue culture. *Virology* **24:** 610.

————. 1966. Genetic basis of cellular susceptibility to the Schmidt-Ruppin and Harris strains of Rous sarcoma virus. *Virology* **29:** 190.

Payne, L.N. and P.K. Pani. 1971. Evidence for linkage between genetic loci controlling response of fowl to subgroup A and subgroup C sarcoma viruses. *J. Gen. Virol.* **13:** 253.

Pinter, A., W.J. Honnen, S.A. Tilley, C. Bona, H. Zaghouani, M.K. Gorny, and S. Zolla-Pazner. 1989. Oligomeric structure of gp41, the transmembrane protein of human immunodeficiency virus type 1. *J. Virol.* **63:** 2674.

Rubin, H. 1965. Genetic control of cellular susceptibility to pseudotypes of Rous sarcoma virus. *Virology* **26:** 270.

Stanley, K.K. 1988. The molecular mechanism of complement C9 insertion and polymerisation in biological membranes. *Curr. Top. Microbiol. Immunol.* **140:** 49.

Stein, B.S., S.D. Gowda, J.D. Lifson, R.C. Penhallow, K.G. Bensch, and E.G. Engleman. 1987. pH-independent HIV entry into CD4-positive T cells via virus envelope fusion to the plasma membrane. *Cell* **49:** 659.

Strickland, D.K., J.D. Ashcom, S. Williams, W.H. Burgess, M. Migliorini, and W.S. Argraves. 1990. Sequence identity between the α-2 macroglobulin receptor and low density lipoprotein receptor-related protein suggests that this molecule is a multifunctional receptor. *J. Biol. Chem.* **265:** 17401.

Stumph, W.E., P. Kristo, M.J. Tsai, and B.W. O'Malley. 1981. A chicken middle-repetitive DNA sequence which shares homology with mammalian ubiquitous repeats. *Nucleic Acids Res.* **9:** 5383.

Sudhof, T.C., J.L. Goldstein, M.S. Brown, and D.W. Russell. 1985. The LDL receptor gene: A mosaic of exons shared with different proteins. *Science* **228:** 815.

Takahashi, S., Y. Kawarabayasi, T. Nakai, J. Sakai, and T. Yamamoto. 1992. Rabbit very low density lipoprotein receptor: A low density lipoprotein receptor-like protein with distinct ligand specificity. *Proc. Natl. Acad. Sci.* **89:** 9252.

Takeuchi, Y., R.G. Vile, G. Simpson, B. O'Hara, M.K. Collins, and R.A. Weiss. 1992. Feline leukemia virus subgroup B uses the same cell surface receptor as gibbon ape leukemia virus. *J. Virol.* **66:** 1219.

Vogt, P.K. 1965. A heterogeneity of Rous sarcoma virus revealed by selectively resistant chick embryo cells. *Virology* **25:** 237.

Vogt, P.K. and R.R. Friis. 1971. An avian leukosis virus related to RSV(O). Properties and evidence for helper activity. *Virology* **43:** 223.

Vogt, P. and R. Ishizaki. 1965. Reciprocal patterns of genetic resistance to avian tumor viruses in two lines of chickens. *Virology* **26:** 664.

Wang, H., M.P. Kavanaugh, R.A. North, and D. Kabat. 1991. Cell surface receptor for ecotropic murine retroviruses is a basic amino acid transporter. *Nature* **352:** 729.

Weiss, C.D., J.A. Levy, and J.M. White. 1990. Oligomeric organization of gp120 on infectious human immunodeficiency virus type 1 particles. *J. Virol.* **64:** 5674.

Weiss, R.A. 1992. Cellular receptors and viral glycoproteins involved in retrovirus entry. In *The retroviridae* (ed. J.A. Levy), p. 1. Plenum Press, New York.

White, J.M. 1990. Viral and cellular membrane fusion proteins. *Annu. Rev. Physiol.* **52:** 675.

Yamamoto, T., C.G. Davis, M.S. Brown, W.J. Schneider, M.L. Casey, J.L. Goldstein, and D.W. Russel. 1984. The human LDL receptor: A cysteine-rich protein with multiple Alu sequences in its mRNA. *Cell* **39:** 27

Young, J.A.T., P. Bates, and H.E. Varmus. 1993. Isolation of a chicken gene that confers susceptibility to infection by subgroup A avian leukosis and sarcoma viruses. *J. Virol.* **67:** 1811.

6

Receptors for Picornaviruses

Richard L. Crowell and Richard P. Tomko
Department of Microbiology and Immunology
Hahnemann University School of Medicine
Philadelphia, Pennsylvania 19102

Infection of specific host cells by picornaviruses is initiated by the attachment of virions to host cells (for reviews, see Crowell and Landau 1983; Colonno 1987, 1992; Crowell 1987; Flore et al. 1990; Lentz 1990; Stanway 1990; Koike et al. 1992b; Racaniello 1992). This event is usually a specific one, in that susceptible cells possess membrane-associated molecules, called receptors (R), which virions recognize in a specific way. The receptors generally are plasma membrane glycoproteins, which are embedded in the membrane lipid bilayer of the cell by the transmembrane region of the molecule, with the amino-terminal amino acid chain extending away from the cell and the carboxy-terminal region extending into the cytoplasm. It is presumed that picornaviruses have evolved differentiated regions in their symmetrical capsid structure, referred to as virion attachment sites (VAS), which recognize specific features of selected cellular membrane proteins for binding. The receptors for virus attachment also serve the cell for other functions, which are just becoming known for some picornaviruses (Greve at al. 1989; Staunton et al. 1989; Tomassini et al. 1989b; Bergelson et al. 1992, 1994; Huber 1994).

Interest in the early events of infection of cells by picornaviruses was ushered in by the early studies of poliovirus attachment to mammalian cells (McLaren et al. 1959; Holland 1961). These studies revealed the importance of the presence of specific cellular receptors to initiate infection. Only primate cells possessed specific receptors and were permissive to poliovirus infection, whereas nonprimate cells were devoid of specific receptors for polioviruses and, therefore, were refractory to infection. This observation was verified by the finding that infectious poliovirus RNA would replicate in nonprimate cells as well as in primate cells, since infectious viral RNA was taken up by the cells by a non-receptor-mediated mechanism (Holland et al. 1959). Thus, nonprimate cells were capable of replicating virus even in the absence of a specific receptor, and the resistance of nonprimate cells to poliovirus was considered solely

to be a receptor-mediated resistance. This observation has been confirmed by the transfection of a receptor gene into receptor-negative cells
(Mendelsohn et al. 1989). The transfected cells that expressed the receptor protein acquired the capacity to bind virus and thereby became susceptible to infection. These studies were extended by the development of
transgenic mice (Ren et al. 1990; Koike et al. 1991b), which received the
gene for the human poliovirus receptor and thereby acquired the capacity
to be infected with wild-type polioviruses with the development of
paralytic disease not unlike that found in poliovirus-infected humans and
monkeys (Ren and Racaniello 1992a). Thus, mice that were resistant to
infection by wild-type polioviruses were converted to susceptible hosts
by the introduction of only one human gene, which permitted the expression of the human receptor protein. These studies have provided con-
firmation of the central role of specific cellular receptors as determinants
of virus tropism in the pathogenesis of poliovirus infection.

The members of the picornavirus group, which infect humans and
animals, were classified according to the types of diseases produced and
the histopathology observed in infected hosts, as reviewed by Melnick
(1990). It was unexpected to find that the receptor specificity of the different species of picornaviruses grouped many of these viruses according
to their original species classification (Crowell 1976; Lonberg-Holm et
al. 1976a). That is, the three types of polioviruses competed for a common receptor on cells, which was different from the receptor used by the
six serotypes of the group B coxsackieviruses (Crowell and Syverton
1961; Quersin-Thiry and Nihoul 1961; Crowell 1963; 1966). Further
receptor families are identified in Table 1. Because the assignment of all
of the newer isolated picornaviruses could not be definitively placed in
the existing species, newer members have been assigned numbers, instead of species (Melnick 1974). It will be of interest to learn whether
these viruses are related to any of the original species, as based on their
receptor specificity. As discussed below, the specificity of virus/receptor
interaction is based on virus and receptor structures, both of which are
subject to variation by mutation. Furthermore, it has been found that a
given virus may utilize more than one receptor specificity for infection of
host cells (Reagan et al. 1984; Mohanty and Crowell 1993).

PICORNAVIRUSES AND VAS

The picornaviruses are small, nonenveloped, single-stranded RNA
viruses that replicate in the cytoplasm of infected cells. The RNA has a
low-molecular-weight protein (VPg) covalently bonded to the 5' end and
a polyadenylated tract at the 3' end. The genome is translated into a large

Table 1 Cellular receptor families for picornavirus species that serve as cellular adhesion molecules or have an unknown function

Virus	Receptor function and size	References
HRV (major group, 90 serotypes)	ICAM-1, 90 kD	Greve et al. (1989); Staunton et al. (1989); Tomassini et al. (1989b)
HRV (minor group, 10 serotypes)	LDLR, 120 kD	Mischak et al. (1988); Hofer et al. (1994)
Polio 1-3	NCAM (?) 67 and 80 kD	Mendelsohn et al. (1989); Bernhardt et al. (1994)
	CD44, 100 kD	Shepley et al. (1988); Shepley and Racaniello (1994)
Echo 1 and 8	VLA-2 (α-2 chain), 145 kD	Bergelson et al. (1992, 1993)
Echo 3,6,7, 11,12,20,21	CD55 (DAF), 70 kD	Bergelson et al. (1994)
Coxsackie B 1-6	(?), 46–49 kD	Mapoles et al. (1985)
Coxsackie B3-RD	CD55 (DAF),60 kD	Mohanty and Crowell (1993); Paglini and Crowell (1992); R.L. Crowell and R.W. Finberg (unpubl.)
Coxsackie A2 and A5	(?), ——	Schultz and Crowell (1980)
Coxsackie A13,15,18,21	ICAM-1, 90 kD	Colonno et al. (1986); Lonberg-Holm et al. (1976a)
Coxsackie A9	integrin (RGD blocks)	Roivainen et al. (1991)
FMDV (8 subtypes)	integrin (RGD blocks)	Baxt and Becker (1990); Fox et al. (1989); Mason et al. (1994)
Encephalomyocarditis	glycophorin A (erythrocyte) VCAM-1	Allaway and Burness (1986); Huber (1994)
Theiler	(?), 34 kD	Kilpatrick and Lipton (1991)
Hepatitis A	α_2-macroglobulin	Zajac et al. (1991)

Determined by virus competition and/or by blockade of receptors by receptor-specific monoclonal antibody (Crowell 1976; Lonberg-Holm et al. 1976a; Sekiguchi et al. 1982; Minor et al. 1984; Nobis et al. 1985; Hsu et al. 1988).

polyprotein, which is cleaved into functional proteins by proteases encoded in the genome. Some of the viral proteins (VP1–4) are the four capsid proteins which surround the RNA genome upon maturation of the viral particle. The capsid proteins are found in equimolar ratios, 60 monomeres of each, which associate to form a lipid- and carbohydrate-free icosahedral-shaped particle (for review, see Rueckert 1990).

The atomic structure of the capsid of a number of picornaviruses has been determined by X-ray crystallographic analyses (Hogle et al. 1985; Rossmann et al. 1985; Acharya et al. 1989; Luo et al. 1987; Filman et al. 1989; Kim et al. 1989; Yeates et al. 1991; Grant et al. 1992; Li et al. 1992; Luo et al. 1992) to reveal some unique features that are distinctive for some of the species. These features are primarily those regions on the virion surface that combine with specific cellular receptors (Chapman and Rossmann 1993). The rhinovirus 14 and poliovirus TI have marked depressions (canyons) encircling the vertices of the icosahedrons, which have been shown to bind to specific cellular receptors (Hogle et al. 1985; Rossmann et al. 1985; Olson et al. 1993). On the other hand, the foot-and-mouth-disease virus (FMDV) appears to lack this type of depression (Acharya et al. 1989) and is believed to bind to receptors through a loop, containing an arginine-glycine-aspartic acid (RGD) sequence, on the virion surface between residues 135 and 158 of its largest polypeptide, VP1 (Fox et al. 1989; Acharya et al. 1990). Mengovirus and Theiler murine encephalomyelitis virus have only a concave region (pit) in place of a canyon for binding (Luo et al. 1987, 1992; Grant et al. 1992). Regardless of the architecture, the respective regions that serve to bind cell receptors on each of these picornaviruses are considered to be the VAS. These recessed regions of the respective virions are of such dimensions or of such special amino acid configurations as to preclude the binding of antibody molecules at these sites (Rossmann 1989), although antibodies with specificity for the rim of the canyon can block virus binding (Colonno et al. 1989; Smith et al. 1993). Because the VAS is secluded from reacting with antibodies, the use of anti-idiotypic antibodies prepared against antiviral antiserum has been of limited value in identifying picornavirus receptors (Baxt and Morgan 1986; McClintock et al. 1986). Furthermore, a recent report (Davis et al. 1992) suggests that the use of anti-idiotypic antibodies is unlikely to lead to the discovery of a new receptor.

Virions have evolved, evidently, with their VAS sequestered from the potential inhibitory activity of antibodies, to ensure that viral infection can be initiated without interference from preexisting antibodies that might be circulating in a host. For example, the VAS of the virions are less likely to mutate (Rossmann and Palmenberg 1988) than those virion surface regions that bind neutralizing antibodies (Minor et al. 1986; Sherry et al. 1986). Mutations in the VAS can occur, however, and influence the affinity or avidity of the binding of virus to the receptors. Analysis of the canyon floor of human rhinovirus 14 (HRV-14) by site-specific mutagenesis of four amino acid residues with side chains that protrude upward from the canyon floor illustrate such effects on virion attachment (Colonno et al. 1988). It also is possible that mutations within the VAS could lead to host-range viral variants, although in some cases, host-range viral mutants may emerge as a consequence of mutational changes in other sites of the virion, providing the virion with a second specificity for binding to a different receptor (Lindberg et al. 1992).

Smith et al. (1986) and Pevear et al. (1989) have shown by X-ray crystallography that relatively small chemical compounds can be inserted into a hydrophobic pocket underneath the canyon floor. These compounds altered the canyon structure by displacing regions of VP1 and causing a shift in the β sheet under the floor, which reduced virus attachment to receptors. Thus, VAS/receptor interactions have provided a focus for the development of antiviral compounds (Zhang et al. 1992; Shepard et al. 1993), although virus escape mutants have become a major concern (Heinz et al. 1989).

CELLULAR RECEPTORS: DEFINITION AND ACTIVITIES

The surfaces of mammalian cells are studded with a multitude of membrane glycoproteins (Roesing et al. 1975; Mannweiler et al. 1990; Springer 1990; Hynes 1992; Singer 1992), providing the cell with a variety of cellular functions. It is likely that picornaviruses have evolved to take advantage of some of these different cell-surface proteins as receptors, to enable them to initiate infection. Early studies established that the receptors for polioviruses and coxsackieviruses are proteins, which are limited to the cell surface and not part of the intracellular milieu (Zajac and Crowell 1965). This observation has been substantiated, since the poliovirus receptor gene has been cloned and expressed as a glycoprotein (Zibert and Wimmer 1992) that may take multiple forms, pending the amount of glycosylations added by different cell types (Rademacher et al. 1988). The genes for the receptors for polioviruses (Miller et al. 1974; Couillin et al. 1987; Shepley et al. 1988; Siddique et al. 1988; Schonk et al. 1989; Koike et al. 1991a; Racaniello 1992), the major group of human rhinoviruses (Greve et al. 1989), and some echoviruses and coxsackievirus B3 (Couillin et al. 1987) all have been localized on human chromosome 19. The significance of the location of these genes within one region of the same chromosome for the different receptor proteins is not known, and their specific transcription and translation control mechanisms remain to be determined (Koike et al. 1990; Ren and Racaniello 1992a).

The early events in picornavirus infections have become the focus of an increasing amount of interest, following the demonstration of the solubilization of functional membrane receptor proteins (Crowell and Siak 1978) and also of the development of methodologies for the molecular cloning of receptor genes (Greve et al. 1989; Mendelsohn et al. 1989; Bergelson et al. 1992). The significance of this renewed interest is based on the realization that the early events in the virus life cycle play pivotal roles in determining virus tropisms in the pathogenesis of infection.

The definition of the early events in the life cycle of picornaviruses has not changed significantly during the past 10 years (Crowell and Landau 1983), although a number of studies have provided new insights into the mechanisms leading to the uncoating of the viral genomes (Flore et al. 1990; Gromeier and Wetz 1990; Greve et al. 1991; Wetz and Kucinski 1991; Koike et al. 1992b; Hoover-Litty and Greve 1993; Mason et al. 1993). The virion first approaches a susceptible cell and becomes oriented toward binding to specific receptors through some long-range electrostatic forces (Leckband et al. 1992). The appropriate charges arranged on the two interacting surfaces of the molecules must play a major role in the binding of virions to their receptors, since those conditions that modify these interactions also cause changes in the surface charges, e.g., low pH and removal of divalent or monovalent cations (Crowell 1976). Subsequent firm binding of virions results through hydrophobic and other short-range forces, which in large measure are determined by the three-dimensional conformation of the two interacting surfaces (Flore et al. 1990; Bibb et al. 1994).

At 37°C, the virus/receptor complex starts changing; the virion loses its internal capsid proteins, VP4 (Crowell and Philipson 1971), and the "A" (altered) particle is formed. This process is termed virus eclipse, which is an irreversible event from which no infectious virus particles can be recovered following detergent disruption of the cells (Crowell and Landau 1979). In studies of virus inactivation by diverse environmental conditions, e.g., heat, high pH, urea, the virion disassembles along a pathway not unlike that mediated by receptors (Roesing et al. 1975; Crowell and Siak 1978). It also has been shown that this major conformational change in the virion structure (eclipse) can be brought about by solubilized receptor proteins, independent of the live cell (Crowell and Siak 1978; Kaplan et al. 1990; Koike et al. 1992b; Hoover-Litty and

Greve 1993; Martin et al. 1993). Thus, receptors are considered to possess two functions; first, to attach virions and second, to eclipse virus infectivity (Zajac and Crowell 1969; Crowell and Siak 1978).

"A" particles contain their viral RNA, still sequestered from the action of applied ribonucleases, but in some cases, they have lost their capacity to combine with their specific receptors (Crowell and Philipson 1971), which probably accounts for their lack of infectivity. For those "A" particles that bind to cells (Fricks and Hogle 1990; Moscufo et al. 1993), no evidence has been provided that they still bind to their original receptor, which is specific for virions. The "A" particles can be stabilized by a HeLa cell plasma membrane extract (McGeady and Crowell 1979), and they have been shown to be more lipophilic than their virions (Lonberg-Holm et al. 1976b). The 30 amino acids located at the amino terminus of VP1 serve to interact with the hydrophobic regions of the cell membrane during penetration of the plasma membrane (Flore et al. 1990). One could imagine that the "A" particle functions as a fusion protein (Crowell et al. 1983) to accomplish virus transport across the cell membrane in a manner corresponding to that proposed for the hemagglutinin protein of influenza virus (White 1992). Although the "A" particle acquires sensitivity to proteolytic enzymes, in contrast to virions, proteolytic cleavage of viral proteins does not appear to mediate coxsackievirus B3 uncoating by HeLa cells (McGeady and Crowell 1981). The role of the smallest viral capsid protein, VP4, in virus uncoating remains unknown, but a mutation in VP4 has rendered virus noninfectious (Muscufo et al. 1993). It has been suggested that the reconstitution of purified receptor proteins into artificial membranes (liposomes) should provide a system to determine the capacity of purified receptors, in the absence of cofactors, to completely disassemble the virion's capsid structure to release the viral genome (Crowell and Landau 1983).

It has been proposed that picornaviruses enter cells by a mechanism of receptor-mediated endocytosis, where the virion encounters the lower pH of the endosome. The lower pH is thought to aid the uncoating process (Madshus et al. 1984a,b; Carrillo et al. 1984; Zeichhardt et al. 1985); however, in the case of enteroviruses, which are acid-pH-resistant, this putative role of the endosome may not be essential (Gromeier and Wetz 1990; Wetz and Kucinski 1991; Mason et al. 1993; Perez and Carrasco 1993). Those picornaviruses which are acid labile, like rhinoviruses and the FMDV, may indeed be uncoated in the endosome (Carrillo et al. 1984; Mason et al. 1993). It is becoming evident that it is difficult to propose a uniform mechanism for the uncoating (disassembly) of all picornaviruses; additional studies are needed to define the mechanism for each species.

CELLULAR RECEPTOR SPECIFICITIES

The first determination of receptor specificity for picornaviruses was made independently by Quersin-Thiry and Nihoul (1961) and by Crowell and Syverton (1961). It was found that the saturation of cellular receptors with one virus blocked the binding of the same or closely related virus, without inhibiting the binding of an unrelated virus. This type of experiment was extended to a number of picornavirus species and to unrelated viruses (Crowell 1966, 1976; Lonberg-Holm et al. 1976a) to result in the establishment of receptor families (Table 1). It was unexpected to find that certain unrelated viruses shared a common receptor; e.g., adenovirus T2 shared a receptor with coxsackievirus B3, and HRV-14 shared a receptor with some of the coxsackieviruses of group A (Lonberg-Holm et al. 1976a). No good explanation for these shared specificities has been forthcoming, other than to suggest that related receptor specificities parallel the similar diseases caused by the respective viruses. Nevertheless, the observation that adenoviruses can serve as vectors for delivery of genes by attaching them to the surface of the virions (Curiel et al. 1992) provides renewed interest in cloning the gene for the adenovirus T2 and T5 receptor. It is likely that this gene is highly conserved with that for the group B coxsackieviruses and provides additional impetus to clone this latter gene.

Conclusive evidence for determining the specificity of virus attachment to specific receptors is based on demonstrating saturation of receptors (Crowell 1966; Lonberg-Holm and Philipson 1981). This evidence is of fundamental importance to exclude binding of virus to nonspecific surfaces (which are nonsaturable), which might be confused with specific receptors (Harter and Choppin 1965). A large number of environmental factors, e.g., pH, temperature, ions, viscosity, cell and virus concentrations, influence rates of virus attachment and should be controlled to obtain accurate measurements of virus attachment rates (Crowell 1976; Crowell and Landau 1983). In addition, virus stability under the conditions of the experiment must be taken into account. The rates of binding of different picornaviruses to specific receptors may be vastly different (Crowell 1976; McClintock et al. 1980). We know that all picornaviruses do not share a similar type of cellular receptor and that the configuration of the VAS on the virions is different for the different viruses. We also recognize that a given virus may utilize more than one receptor specificity for infecting cells (Reagan et al. 1984; Lindberg et al. 1992; Mohanty and Crowell 1993). Therefore, the definition of each of the reactants at the molecular level in the early events of virus infection has become more demanding. Caution in reaching conclusions about receptor specificity of viruses is prudent.

The development of monoclonal antibodies against receptors for different picornaviruses (Campbell and Cords 1983; Minor et al. 1984; Nobis et al. 1985; Colonno et al. 1986; Crowell et al. 1986; Hsu et al. 1988; Shepley et al. 1988; Bergelson et al. 1992) as an extension of antireceptor polyclonal antisera (Axler and Crowell 1968) has confirmed the identity of specific receptor families, e.g., a monoclonal antibody prepared against the receptor for poliovirus T1 blocked the binding of all three poliovirus serotypes to cells pretreated with the monoclonal antibody without blocking attachment of unrelated viruses (Minor et al. 1984; Nobis et al. 1985). Thus, receptor specificity is established by virus competition as well as by competition with receptor-specific monoclonal antibody experiments. In a similar way, the number of receptor sites on cells is determined by the addition of increasing amounts of virus or of a corresponding receptor-specific monoclonal antibody until saturation is obtained (Hsu et al. 1988). This latter measurement reveals the presence of approximately three- to tenfold more receptors per cell due to the bivalency of antibodies and their smaller size than virions, which are multivalent. Regardless, it is evident that different cell types may have different numbers of receptors for a given virus (Hsu et al. 1988) and that the regulation of expression of some cellular receptors is controlled by differentiation and by cytokines (Dustin et al. 1988; Tomassini et al. 1989b).

The significance of the number of receptors per cell is speculative, since the expression of receptors on cells does not guarantee that they are susceptible to infection (Schultz and Crowell 1983). Some factors associated with cellular differentiation are required for making the cells permissive to virus infection (Landau et al. 1972; Schultz and Crowell 1980, 1983), and these remain to be determined. However, it is well known that higher levels of receptors result in proportionally faster rates of virus attachment to cells (Crowell 1976). Although high numbers of receptors per cell might facilitate a more rapid rate of virus infection, nevertheless, unless the environment is detrimental to virus survival, it only takes a few receptors on cells to permit virus infection. This is an important consideration for those who design experiments to inhibit virus infection by blocking the availability of receptors as an approach to viral chemotherapy or prophylaxis (Colonno and Tomassini 1987; Hayden et al. 1988). It is unlikely that one could develop a reagent with sufficient capacity to block 100% of receptors, and such an approach seems doomed to failure. On the other hand, where one hopes only to reduce the rate of virus infection to permit the immune responses to combat the infecting virus, this approach to viral chemotherapy may have some value. To date, no practical application of receptor blockade has been developed which is effective in the prevention of virus infection, although this strategy may prove useful in combination therapies.

PURIFICATION, CHARACTERIZATION, AND GENE CLONING OF RECEPTORS

Specific cellular receptors for picornaviruses have been purified only with great difficulty; consequently, there is very little information about the characteristics of purified preparations. The relatively limited number of receptors per cell ($\sim 2 \times 10^3$ to 1×10^5) has been a major obstacle in obtaining sufficient quantities of receptor protein for detailed biochemical analysis. A quantitative chemiluminescence assay was developed recently for monitoring the recovery of receptor protein at different stages of receptor purification (Mohanty and Crowell 1993). When applied to the purification of a cellular receptor for coxsackievirus B3-RD, it was found that 98% of the total receptor protein was lost during the early steps of purification. Thus, this assay should help to improve the purification protocol in order to obtain yields sufficient for characterization.

Affinity chromatography using receptor-specific monoclonal antibodies has permitted the purification of amounts of receptors sufficient for amino acid sequencing (Colonno et al. 1989; Greve et al 1989) to provide information for the generation of oligonucleotides used for cloning of receptor genes. In the absence of purified receptor preparations, many studies have focused on the use of cells, cell plasma membrane preparations, or detergent-solubilized cell membranes to obtain information about the biochemical characteristics of receptors (Crowell and Landau 1983; Krah and Crowell 1985; Colonno 1987). In general, all of the picornavirus receptors are glycoproteins, which can be blocked by lectins or recovered on lectin columns. They are all sensitive to cleavage by proteolytic enzymes, a few are sensitive to neuraminidase, e.g., HRV-87 (Uncapher et al. 1991), cardioviruses (McClintock et al. 1980), or FMDV (Baxt and Morgan 1986), and they range in size from 34 kD to more than 100 kD. Their molecular arrangement in the plasma membrane is not known, although they may be arranged in clusters of pentameric design to accommodate the fivefold axis of symmetry of the canyons encircling the vertices of the icosahedral-shaped virions (Crowell 1987). Gel filtration of detergent-solubilized receptors for coxsackievirus B3 (Krah and Crowell 1985) and HRV-14 (Tomassini and Colonno 1986) revealed multimeric forms that closely resembled the size of pentameric equivalents. Recent evidence has been provided that each HRV virion is capable of binding 60 molecules of ICAM-1 receptor protein (Olson et al. 1993), with 5 molecules of receptor bound to each vertex, thereby making the above hypothesis feasible.

The picornavirus receptors are glycoproteins and, consequently, there has been a certain amount of interest in determining their carbohydrate composition and its function in recognition of virions (Tomassini et al. 1989a). There appears to be consensus that the amino-terminal loop is devoid of glycosylation sites and that this disulfide-bonded loop contains the specific virus recognition site for ICAM-1 (Lineberger et al. 1990, 1992; Staunton et al. 1990; McClelland et al. 1991; Register et al. 1991) and for the poliovirus receptor (PVR) (Freistadt and Racaniello 1991; Koike et al. 1991a, 1992a; Selinka et al. 1991; Racaniello 1992; Zibert and Wimmer 1992). Thus, it would appear that the carbohydrate component of the ICAM-1 molecule and of the PVR molecule is not required for the recognition of virions. However, the absence of carbohydrate in the other domains of ICAM-1 resulted in a lack of virus binding by ICAM-1 (Lineberger et al. 1990), which suggests that glycosylations of the receptor molecule provide some essential conformational structure or participate in the formation of a multimeric receptor structure (Tomassini and Colonno 1986) that is essential for virus recognition. The majority of the sugar molecules are N-linked, as determined by the inhibition of glycosylation when cells are grown in the presence of tunicamycin or swainsonine (Greve et al. 1989; Kaplan et al. 1990). On the other hand, Krah and Crowell (1985) did not find that tunicamycin inhibited the synthesis of the receptor for the group B coxsackieviruses, and Fotiadis et al. (1991) found that O-glycanase treatment of cells reduced the binding of Theiler virus (BeAn strain), suggesting that the carbohydrate was O-linked. The relevance of these observations to the foregoing remains to be determined.

Further evidence that the amino-terminal loops of ICAM-1 and PVR, immunoglobulin-like molecules, provide the virion recognition site is found in reports of the creation of chimeric receptor molecules between human-murine ICAM-1 (Staunton et al. 1990; McClelland et al. 1991; Register et al. 1991) and human-mouse homolog PVR (Morrison and Racaniello 1992), and between the PVR-ICAM-1 molecules (Selinka et al. 1991). Most notable about these experiments is that non-virus reactive molecules were converted to virus-binding receptors by the transfer of the amino-terminal loop of the functional receptor to the nonreactive molecule by recombinant DNA technology. Receptor-negative cells that were transfected were converted to virus susceptibility, as governed by the specificity of the amino-terminal loop of the specific receptor, which was combined with the remaining portion of the heterologous immuno-globulin-like molecule. In contrast, structural alterations in the carboxyl half of the receptor molecules appeared to have no effect on virus infection (Koike et al. 1991a; Staunton et al. 1992).

The cloning of the cellular receptor genes for the major group of HRV and for polioviruses has permitted the preparation of soluble forms of receptors (Kaplan et al. 1990; Marlin et al. 1990; Greve et al. 1991; Koike et al. 1991a; Hoover-Litty and Greve 1993) for ease of purification, characterization, and potential application for antiviral therapy (Martin et al. 1993). It has been found that these receptors in their soluble form are capable of "neutralizing" virus infectivity in an irreversible manner, i.e., "A" particle formation. The uncoating of viral RNA, however, may require additional factors, even though the transfection of only one receptor gene into receptor-negative cells converts those cells to a state of susceptibility to virus infection. Studies have shown also that the cytoplasmic tail of the receptor molecule for rhinovirus (Staunton et al. 1992) or poliovirus (Koike et al. 1991a) is not essential for virus infection. In fact, it is likely that the essential feature of receptors for initiating infection by acid-pH-labile viruses is to bring the virion sufficiently close to the cell for internalization into endosomes, where the lower-pH environment aids the disassembly of the virion (Mason et al. 1993). In this example, antibody-complexed FMDV, but not poliovirus, can infect normally insusceptible cells via the Fc receptor. Future studies are needed to explain the signals that are generated to result in the receptor-mediated endocytosis of viruses that have different degrees of stability to acid pH (Skern et al. 1991; Hoover-Litty and Greve 1993).

The numerous studies of the receptors for polioviruses and human rhinoviruses have dominated the recent picornavirus literature, as several research groups have confirmed each other's results. The ability to obtain molecular clones of the receptor genes was the key that facilitated these studies. Studies of the receptors for other picornaviruses (Mapoles et al. 1985; Hsu and Crowell 1989; Baxt and Becker 1990; Kilpatrick and Lipton 1991; Roivainen et al. 1991; Mbida et al. 1992; Mohanty and Crowell 1993) have not led to the determination of their respective genes, with the exception of those of Allaway and Burness (1986), who identified the erythrocyte receptor as glycophorin A and VCAM-1 on endothelial cells (Huber 1994) for the encephalomyocarditis (EMC) virus and those of Bergelson et al. (1992, 1993), who recently identified the integrin VLA-2 (very late antigen-2) molecule as the receptor for echoviruses 1 and 8. In this latter study, monoclonal antibodies capable of inhibiting attachment of echoviruses 1 and 8 to HeLa cells immunoprecipitated proteins that were similar to those associated with $\beta 1$ integrins. Antibodies to VLA-2, the $\alpha 2$ and $\beta 1$ subunits, identified the same proteins as those which blocked echovirus 1 attachment. Evidence that the $\alpha2$ subunit of VLA-2 was responsible for virus attachment was obtained by transfection of rhabdomyosarcoma (RD) cells, which normally expressed the $\beta1$ subunit, but lacked $\alpha2$ expression. The transfected cells expressed $\alpha2$ and thereby became susceptible to infection by echoviruses 1 and 8.

It is anticipated that the molecular cloning of the genes for the receptors for the other picornavirus members will be forthcoming during the next few years. The application of this information to studies of viral pathogenesis will permit a better understanding of the role of receptors in viral tropism and in the production of diseases by these viruses.

RECEPTORS IN PICORNAVIRUS PATHOGENESIS

The study of the pathogenesis of infection is the most important and yet the most difficult portion of classical picornavirology remaining to be solved. That is because the study of the entire gene products of each virus that permits infection at the cellular level, the mode of virus spread in the host, the different cell types that become infected, together with all of the host responses to the infecting virus, is very complex. The minireview by Morrison and Fields (1991), who have compared the pathogenesis of polioviruses and reoviruses as enteric viruses that produce neurological diseases, is particularly informative. The portion of viral pathogenesis that is influenced by specific cellular receptors for picornaviruses is a more limited aspect of pathogenesis and is the focus of the next part of this discussion.

The early finding that the receptor specificity of the different species of picornaviruses assorted them into their respective species, according to the way in which they were originally classified by disease and tissue pathology, as mentioned above, suggested that cellular receptors play an important role in the tropism of picornavirus infections in the pathogenesis of disease production (Crowell and Syverton 1961; Quersin-Thiry and Nihoul 1961; Crowell 1966, 1976; Lonberg-Holm et al. 1976a). In addition, it is likely that host-range virus mutants emerge following extensive passage of large virus populations in unnatural hosts (or in different cell types) or by different routes of inoculation (Armstrong 1939; Pappenheimer et al. 1951; Vizozo and Sanders 1964). These virus variants probably acquired an additional receptor specificity to account for their capacity to replicate in different cell types, as found for the coxsackievirus B3-RD variant (Reagan et al. 1984; Hsu et al. 1990). A second receptor specificity for mouse-adapted polioviruses remains to be identified (Martin et al. 1988; Murray et al. 1988).

The molecular cloning of the PVR gene has made possible the search for those cell types in human and animal tissues that express mRNA for the receptor gene (Freistadt et al. 1990). When these results were correlated with the production of receptor protein and susceptibility to virus infection, cell types that normally are considered resistant to poliovirus infection (Bodian 1955) expressed receptor-specific mRNA and receptor protein. These results led the authors to conclude that poliovirus-specific tissue tropism cannot be explained solely by a limited distribution of receptor protein. These findings question the need to evaluate the second function associated with receptors, namely, the capacity of receptors to eclipse and uncoat the viral RNA (Schultz and Crowell 1983; Crowell et al. 1985). Thus, unless this second receptor function can be assayed in situ, the true role of receptors as determinants of virus tropism remains open.

The elegant studies of Ren and Racaniello (1992a,b) and of Koike et al. (1991b) of the pathogenesis of poliovirus in a transgenic mouse model constructed to express the human PVR (Ren et al. 1990; Koike et al. 1991b) have shown the progression of disease following inoculation of wild-type poliovirus by different routes. Intracerebral, intraperitoneal, and intravenous injections of PV resulted in the production of paralytic poliomyelitis with tremors and death, not unlike that found in human poliomyelitis. However, the normal route of infection of humans, the oral route, failed to produce infection in transgenic mice, which suggests that these mice have some limitation as a model of human disease. Nevertheless, these mice have permitted detailed studies of poliovirus pathogenesis, employing molecular and immunological probes that previously were only applicable to studies of primates.

The intramuscular inoculation of poliovirus into the hind limb of transgenic mice expressing the human PVR revealed extensive poliovirus replication in skeletal muscle (Ren and Racaniello 1992b). Furthermore, virus was found to spread from the site of inoculation to the inferior and superior spinal cord and then to the brain via retrograde neuronal transport. Transection of the sciatic nerve abrogated lethal disease, to verify this finding. Thus, although poliovirus may spread to the central nervous system (CNS) via the blood (Bodian 1955; Freistadt et al. 1993), this study provides convincing evidence for the role of skeletal muscle and neuronal spread of poliovirus in the pathogenesis of CNS disease.

It is unlikely that the strategy for the development of transgenic mice can be used to study viral pathogenesis of human rhinovirus disease, since mouse cells have a defect, in addition to the lack of a specific receptor, which makes them nonpermissive to HRV replication (Lomax and Yin 1989). Since the coxsackieviruses, cardioviruses, and the viruses of foot-and-mouth disease all replicate in mice, it is obvious that transgenic mice are not needed for studies of pathogenesis of these picornaviruses. However, since only echovirus 9 will produce disease in mice, the application of transgenic mice bearing human receptor proteins for the other echoviruses would seem appropriate.

The introduction of "knockout" mice to the study of the functions of cellular receptors, like those for polioviruses, remains to be developed (Capecchi 1989). The removal of the gene that controls the production of the mouse homolog to the human PVR (Morisson and Racaniello 1992) should provide information as to the function of the PVR protein in the mouse, provided the defect produced is not lethal. The receptor protein described by Shepley and colleagues (1988), which is of a larger molecular size (100 kD) than that reported for the PVR (67–80 kD), remains to be defined in relation to its role in poliovirus pathogenesis. This molecule, now known to be CD44, a lymphocyte homing receptor (Shepley and Racaniello 1994) and not a specific PVR, could be a helper molecule, when present, to facilitate poliovirus infection. Further studies are needed to clarify this possible relationship. Certainly there is evidence that picornaviruses may use more than one receptor specificity for infection of cells (Armstrong 1939; Reagan et al. 1984; Martin et al. 1988; Murray et al. 1988; Hsu et al. 1990; Mohanty and Crowell 1993). Thus, further study of the role of different receptors in the pathogenesis of host-range variant viruses is in order (Crowell et al. 1985; Hsu et al. 1990).

PERSPECTIVES AND CONCLUSIONS

The specificity of cellular receptors for the separate species of picornaviruses suggests that receptors are important determinants of virus tropism in the pathogenesis of infection. Only relatively recently have we come to recognize that more than one receptor specificity may permit infection of certain cell types by host-range variants of picornaviruses. Accordingly, the contribution to viral pathogenesis of the many different receptor specificities, excluding ICAM-1 for the major group of human rhinoviruses, has not been elucidated. It is reasonably clear that viruses have evolved to utilize specific cellular molecules for receptors, thus, viruses have adapted to their environment in a clever way that allows these molecules to retain their cellular functions, while permitting viruses the freedom to initiate infection. The molecular cloning of the genes for some of the picornavirus receptors has had a dramatic impact on our understanding of receptor distribution in animal and human tissues. It has been found that receptor distribution in transgenic mice that express the poliovirus receptor alone cannot account for the selective nature of polioviruses for infection of certain cell types. However, since receptors are known to have dual functions, to both bind and eclipse virus infectivity, methods must be developed to assess the capacity of receptors to carry out *both* functions, before we can conclude that their distribution in the animal or human is not of importance to viral pathogenesis. The capacity of receptors to eclipse virus infectivity may be concentration-dependent and influenced by cellular differentiation and cytokine modulation. Additional work is needed to clarify the regulatory events that control the eclipse and uncoating activities of receptors.

The major advances in our understanding of picornavirus architecture, through X-ray crystallographic methods, have permitted the rational design of drugs that can bind near the virion attachment site and influence receptor activities for binding and eclipsing virus infectivity. The future holds promise for more innovations in drug design to prevent virus/receptor interaction leading to infection. The molecular constructs of soluble receptors to serve as decoys for viruses also should continue to hold promise for the reduction in virus replication rates, to permit the immune responses of the host to gain the upper hand in controlling virus infection. Thus, we have come a long way in understanding virus/receptor interactions, but there are many more exciting discoveries to be developed as our current knowledge is applied to the understanding of receptors in picornavirus pathogenesis.

ACKNOWLEDGMENTS

The senior author (R.L.C.) is grateful to the National Institute of Allergy and Infectious Diseases of the U.S. Public Health Service for continuous research support on the study of viral receptors over the past 32 years (AI-03771). The senior author also is appreciative of the extensive effort and stimulating discussions by the many graduate students, postdoctorates, research associates, colleagues, and technician Barbara Goldberg Alstein, who, over the many years, helped to advance our knowledge of virus/receptor interactions.

REFERENCES

Acharya, R., E. Fry, D. Stuart, G. Fox, D. Rowlands, and F. Brown 1989. The three-dimensional structure of foot-and-mouth disease virus at 2.9 Å resolution. *Nature* **337:** 709.

Acharya, R., E. Fry, D. Logan, D. Stuart, F. Brown, G. Fox, and D. Rowlands. 1990. The three-dimensional structure of foot-and-mouth disease virus. In *New aspects of positive-strand RNA viruses* (ed. M.A. Brinton and F.X. Heinz), p. 211. ASM Press, Washington, D.C.

Allaway, G.P. and A.T.H. Burness. 1986. Site of attachment of encephalomyocarditis virus on human erythrocytes. *J. Virol.* **59**: 768.

Armstrong, C. 1939. Successful transfer of the Lansing strain of poliomyelitis virus to the white mouse. *Pub. Health Rep.* **54**: 2302.

Axler, D.A. and R.L. Crowell. 1968. The effect of anticellular serum on the attachment of enteroviruses to HeLa cells. *J. Virol.* **2**: 813.

Baxt, B. and Y. Becker. 1990. The effect of peptides containing the arginine-glycine-aspartic acid (RGD) sequence on the adsorption of foot-and-mouth disease virus to tissue culture cells. *Virus Genes* **1**: 73.

Baxt, B. and D.O. Morgan. 1986. Nature of the interaction between foot-and-mouth disease virus and cultured cells. In *Virus attachment and entry into cells* (ed. R.L. Crowell and K. Lonberg-Holm), p. 126. American Society for Microbiology Press, Washington, D.C.

Bergelson, J.M., M.P. Shepley, B.M.C. Chan, M.E. Hemler, and R.W. Finberg. 1992. Identification of the integrin VLA-2 as a receptor for echovirus 1. *Science* **255**: 1718.

Bergelson, J.M., M. Chan, K. Solomon, N.F. St. John, H. Lin, and R.W. Finberg. 1994. Decay-accelerating factor (CD55), a glycosylphosphotidylinositol-anchored complement regulatory protein, is a receptor for many echoviruses. *Proc. Natl. Acad. Sci.* **91**: 6245.

Bergelson, J.M., N. St. John, S. Kawaguchi, M. Chan, H. Stubdal, J. Modlin, and R.W. Finberg. 1993. Infection by echoviruses 1 and 8 depends on the alpha 2 subunit of human VLA-2. *J. Virol.* **67**: 6847.

Bernhardt, G., J.A. Bibb, J. Bradley, and E. Wimmer. 1994. Molecular characterization of the cellular receptor for poliovirus. *Virology* **199**: 105.

Bibb, J.A., G. Witherell, G. Bernhardt, and E. Wimmer. 1994. Interaction of poliovirus with its cell surface binding site. *Virology* **201**: 107.

Bodian, D. 1955. Emerging concept of poliomyelitis infection. *Science* **122**: 105.

Campbell, E.A. and C.E. Cords. 1983. Monoclonal antibodies that inhibit attachment of group B coxsackieviruses. *J. Virol.* **48**: 561.

Capecchi, M.R. 1989. Altering the genome by homologous recombination. *Science* **244**: 1288.

Carrillo, E.C., C. Giachetti, and R.H. Campos. 1984. Effect of lysosomotropic agents on foot-and-mouth disease virus replication. *Virology* **135**: 542.

Chapman, M.S. and M.G. Rossmann. 1993. Comparison of surface properties of picornaviruses: Strategies for hiding the receptor site from immune surveillance. *Virology* **195**: 745.

Colonno, R.J. 1987. Cell surface receptors for picornaviruses. *BioEssays* **5**: 270.

———. 1992. Molecular interactions between human rhinoviruses and their cellular receptors. *Semin. Virol.* **3**: 101.

Colonno, R.J. and J. E. Tomassini. 1987. Viral receptors: A novel approach for the prevention of human rhinovirus infection. In *Proceedings of the Sixth International Symposium on Medical Virology* (ed. L.M. de la Maza and E.M. Peterson), p. 331. Elsevier, Amsterdam.

Colonno, R.J., P.L. Callahan, and W.J. Long. 1986. Isolation of a monoclonal antibody that blocks attachment of the major group of human rhinoviruses. *J. Virol.* **57**: 7.

Colonno, R.J., P.L. Callahan, D.M. Leippe, R.R. Rueckert, and J.E. Tomassini. 1989. Inhibition of rhinovirus attachment by neutralizing monoclonal antibodies and their Fab fragments. *J. Virol.* **63**: 36.

Colonno, R.J., J.H. Condra, S. Mizutani, P.L. Callahan, M.E. Davies, and M.A. Murcko 1988. Evidence for the direct involvement of the rhinovirus canyon in receptor binding.

Proc. Natl. Acad. Sci. **85:** 5449.

Couillin, P., F. Huyghe, M.C. Grisard, N. Van Cong, M.F. Louis, H. Hofmann-Radvanyi, and A. Boue. 1987. Echovirus 6, 11, 19; coxsackievirus B3 sensitivities and poliovirus I, II, III sensitivities are on chromosome 19 respectively on 19pter-q133 and 19q131-q133. *Cytogenet. Cell. Genet.* **46:** 599.

Crowell, R.L. 1963. Specific viral interference in HeLa cell cultures chronically infected with Coxsackie B5 virus. *J. Bacteriol.* **86:** 517.

————. 1966. Specific cell surface alteration by enteroviruses as reflected by viral attachment interference. *J. Bacteriol.* **91:** 198.

————. 1976. Comparative generic characteristics of picornavirus-receptor interactions. In *Ninth Miles International Symposium. Cell membrane receptors for viruses, antigens and antibodies, polypeptide hormones and small molecules* (ed. R.F. Beers and E.G. Bassett), p. 179. Raven Press, New York.

————. 1987. Cellular receptors in virus infections. *ASM News* **53:** 422.

Crowell, R.L. and B.J. Landau. 1979. Receptors as determinants of cellular tropism in picornavirus infections. In *Receptors and human diseases* (ed. A.G. Bearn and P.W. Choppin), p.1. Independent Publications Group, Port Washington, New York.

————. 1983. Receptors in the initiation of picornavirus infections. In *Comprehensive virology* (ed. H. Fraenkel-Conrat and R.R. Wagner), vol. 18, p. 1. Plenum Press, New York.

Crowell, R.L. and L. Philipson 1971. Specific alterations of coxsackievirus B3 eluted from Hela cells. *J. Virol.* **8:** 509.

Crowell, R.L. and J.S. Siak. 1978. Receptors for Group B coxsackieviruses: Characterization and extraction from HeLa cell plasma membranes. *Perspect. Virol.* **10:** 39.

Crowell, R.L. and J.T. Syverton. 1961. The mammalian cell-virus relationship. VI. Sustained infection of HeLa cells by Coxsackie B3 virus and effect on superinfection. *J. Exp. Med.* **113:** 419.

Crowell, R.L., D.L. Krah, J.E. Mapoles, and B.J. Landau. 1983. Methods for assay of cellular receptors for picornaviruses. *Meth. Enzymol.* **96:** 443.

Crowell, R.L., K.J. Reagan, M. Schultz, J.E. Mapoles, J.B. Grun, and B.J. Landau. 1985. Cellular receptors as determinants of viral tropism. *Banbury Rep.* **22:** 147.

Crowell, R.L., K.A. Field, W. Schleif, W. Long, R.J. Colonno, and J.E. Mapoles, E.A. Emini. 1986. Monoclonal antibody that inhibits infection of HeLa cells and rhabdomyosarcoma cells by selected enteroviruses through receptor blockade *J. Virol.* **57:** 438.

Curiel, D.T., E. Wagner, M. Cotten, M.L. Birnstiel, S. Agarwal, C.M. Li, S. Loechel, and P.C. Hu. 1992. High-efficiency gene transfer mediated by adenovirus coupled to DNA-polylysine complexes. *Human Gene Ther.* **3:** 147.

Davis, S.J., G.A. Schockmel, C. Somoza, D.W. Buck, D.G. Healey, E.P. Rieber, C. Reiter, and A.F. Williams. 1992. Antibody and HIV-1 gp120 recognition of CD4 undermines the concept of mimicry between antibodies and receptors. *Nature* **358:** 76.

Dustin, M.L., D.E. Staunton, and T.A. Springer. 1988. Supergene families meet in the immune system. *Immunol. Today* **9:** 213.

Filman, D.J., R. Syed, M. Chow, A.J. Macadam, P.D. Minor, and J.M. Hogle. 1989. Structural factors that control conformational transitions and serotype specificity in type 3 poliovirus. *EMBO J.* **8:** 1567.

Flore, O., C.E. Fricks, D.J. Filman, and J.M. Hogle. 1990. Conformational changes in poliovirus assembly and cell entry. *Semin. Virol.* **1:** 429.

Fotiadis, C., D.R. Kilpatrick, and H.L. Lipton. 1991. Comparison of the binding characteristics to BHK-21 cells of viruses representing the two Theiler's virus neurovirulence groups. *Virology* **182**: 365.

Fox, G., N.R. Parry, P.V. Barnett, B. McGinn, D.J. Rowlands, and F. Brown. 1989. The cell attachment site on foot-and-mouth disease virus includes the amino acid sequence RGD (arginine-glycine-aspartic acid). *J. Gen. Virol.* **70**: 625.

Freistadt, M.S. and V.R. Racaniello. 1991. Mutational analysis of the cellular receptor for poliovirus. *J. Virol.* **65**: 3873.

Freistadt, M.S., H.B. Fleit, and E. Wimmer. 1993. Poliovirus receptor on human blood cells: A possible extraneural site of poliovirus replication. *Virology* **195**: 7898.

Freistadt, M.S., G. Kaplan, and V.R. Racaniello. 1990. Heterogeneous expression of poliovirus receptor-related proteins in human cells and tissues. *Mol. Cell. Biol.* **10**: 5700.

Fricks, C.E. and J.M. Hogle. 1990. Cell-induced conformational change of poliovirus: Externalization of the amino terminus of VP1 is responsible for liposome binding. *J. Virol.* **64**: 1934.

Grant, R.A., D.J. Filman, R.S. Fujinami, J.P. Icenogle, and J.M. Hogle. 1992. Three-dimensional structure of Theiler virus. *Proc. Natl. Acad. Sci.* **89**: 2061.

Greve, J.M., C.P. Forte, C.W. Marlor, A.M. Meyer, H. Hoover-Litty, D. Wunderlich, and A. McClelland. 1991. Mechanisms of receptor-mediated rhinovirus neutralization defined by two soluble forms of ICAM-1. *J. Virol.* **65**: 6015.

Greve, J.M., G. Davis, A.M. Meyer, C.P. Forte, S.C. Yost, C.W. Marlow, M.E. Kamarck, and A. McClelland. 1989. The major human rhinovirus receptor is ICAM-1. *Cell* **56**: 839.

Gromeier, M. and K. Wetz. 1990. Kinetics of poliovirus uncoating in HeLa cells in a nonacidic environment. *J. Virol.* **64**: 3590.

Harter, D.H. and P.W. Choppin. 1965. Adsorption of attenuated and neurovirulent poliovirus strains to central nervous system tissues of primates. *J. Immunol.* **95**: 730.

Hayden, F.G., J.M. Gwaltney, and R.J. Colonno. 1988. Modification of experimental rhinovirus colds by receptor blockade. *Antiviral Res.* **9**: 233.

Heinz, B.A., R.R. Rueckert, D.A. Shepard, F.J. Dutko, M.A. McKinlay, M. Fancher, M.G. Rossmann, J. Badger, and T.J. Smith. 1989. Genetic and molecular analysis of spontaneous mutants of human rhinovirus 14 resistant to an antiviral compound. *J. Virol.* **63**: 2476.

Hofer, F., M. Gruenberger, H. Kowalski, H. Machat, M. Huettinger, E. Kuechler, and D. Blaas. 1994. Members of the low density lipoprotein receptor family mediate cell entry of a minor-group common cold virus. *Proc. Natl. Acad. Sci.* **91**: 1839.

Hogle, J.M., M. Chow, and D.J. Filman. 1985. Three-dimensional structure of poliovirus at 2.9 Å resolution. *Science* **229**: 1358.

Holland, J.J. 1961. Receptor affinities as major determinants of enterovirus tissue tropisms in humans. *Virology* **15**: 312.

Holland, J.J., L.C. McLaren, and J.T. Syverton. 1959. The mammalian cell-virus relationship. IV. Infection of naturally insusceptible cells with enterovirus nucleic acid. *J. Exp. Med.* **110**: 65.

Hoover-Litty, H. and J.M. Greve. 1993. Formation of rhinovirus-soluble ICAM-1 complexes and conformational changes in the virion. *J. Virol.* **67**: 390.

Hsu, K.-H. and R.L. Crowell. 1989. Characterization of a YAC-1 mouse cell receptor for group B coxsackieviruses. *J. Virol.* **63**: 3105.

Hsu, K.-H.L., K. Lonberg-Holm, B. Alstein, and R.L. Crowell. 1988. A monclonal antibody specific for the cellular receptor for the group B coxsackieviruses. *J. Virol.* **62**: 1647.

Hsu, K.-H.L., S. Paglini, B. Alstein, and R.L. Crowell. 1990. Identification of a second cellular receptor for a coxsackievirus B3 variant (CB3-RD). In *New aspects of positive-strand RNA viruses* (ed. M.A. Brinton and F.X. Heinz), p. 271. ASM Press, Washington, D.C.

Huber, S.A. 1994. VCAM-1 is a receptor for encephalomyocarditis virus on murine vascular endothelial cells. *J. Virol.* **68:** 3453.

Hynes, R.O. 1992. Integrins: Versatility, modulation, and signaling in cell adhesion. *Cell* **69:** 11.

Kaplan, G.M., M.S. Freistadt, and V.R. Racaneillo. 1990. Neutralization of poliovirus by cell receptors expressed in insect cells. *J. Virol.* **64:** 4697.

Kilpatrick, D.R. and H.L. Lipton. 1991. Predominant binding of Theiler's viruses to a 34-kilodalton receptor protein on susceptible cell lines. *J. Virol.* **65:** 5244.

Kim, S., T.J. Smith, M.S. Chapman, D.C. Pevear, F.J. Dukto, P.J. Felock, G.D. Diana, and M.A. McKinlay. 1989. Crystal structure of human rhinovirus serotype 1A (HRV1A). *J. Mol. Biol.* **210:** 91.

Koike, S., I. Ise, and A. Nomoto. 1991a. Functional domains of the poliovirus receptor. *Proc. Natl. Acad. Sci.* **88:** 4104.

Koike, S., I. Ise, Y. Sato, H. Yonekawa, O. Gotoh, and A. Nomoto. 1992a. A second gene for the African Green Monkey poliovirus receptor that has no putative N-glycosylation site in the functional N-terminal immunoglobulin-like domain. *J. Virol.* **66:** 7059.

Koike, S., I. Ise, Y. Sato, K. Mitsui, H. Horie, H. Umeyama, and A. Nomoto. 1992b. Early events in poliovirus infection. *Semin. Virol.* **3:** 109.

Koike, S., C. Toya, T. Kurata, S. Abe, I. Ise, H. Yonekawa, and A. Nomoto. 1991b. Transgenic mice susceptible to poliovirus. *Proc. Natl. Acad. Sci.* **88:** 951.

Koike, S., H. Horie, I. Ise, A. Okitsu, M. Yoshida, N. Iizuka, K. Takeuchi, T. Takegami, and A. Nomoto. 1990. The poliovirus receptor protein is produced both as membrane-bound and secreted forms. *EMBO J.* **9:** 3217.

Krah, D.L. and R.L. Crowell. 1985. Properties of the deoxycholate-solubilized HeLa cell plasma membrane receptor for binding group B coxsackieviruses. *J. Virol.* **53:** 867.

Landau, B.J., R.L. Crowell, W. Boclair, and B.A. Zajac. 1972. The permissiveness of differentiating mouse muscle cell cultures to infection by group A coxsackieviruses types 1 and 5. *Proc. Soc. Exp. Biol. Med.* **141:** 753.

Leckband, D.E., J.N. Israelachvili, F.-J. Schmitt, and W. Knoll. 1992. Long-range attraction and molecular rearrangements in receptor-ligand interactions. *Science* **255:** 1419.

Lentz, T.L. 1990. The recognition event between virus and host cell receptor: A target for antiviral agents. *J. Gen. Virol.* **71:** 751.

Li, T., A.Q. Zhang, N. Iizuka, A. Nomoto, and E. Arnold. 1992. Crystallization and preliminary x-ray diffraction studies of coxsackievirus B1. *J. Mol. Biol.* **223:** 1171.

Lindberg, M.A., R.L. Crowell, R. Zell, R. Kandolf, and U. Pettersson. 1992. Mapping of the RD phenotype of the Nancy strain of Coxsackievirus B3. *Virus Res.* **24:** 187.

Lineberger, D.W., D.J. Graham, J.E. Tomassini, and R.J. Colonno. 1990. Antibodies that block rhinovirus attachment map to domain 1 of the major group receptor. *J. Virol.* **64:** 2582.

Lineberger, D.W., C.R. Uncapher, D.J. Graham, and R.J. Colonno. 1992. Human-murine chimeras of ICAM-1 identify amino acid residues critical for rhinovirus and antibody binding. *J. Virol.* **65:** 6589.

Lomax, N.B. and F.H. Yin. 1989. Evidence for the role of the P2 protein of human rhinovirus in its host range change. *J. Virol.* **63:** 2396.

Lonberg-Holm, K. and L. Philipson, eds. 1981. *Virus receptors*, Part 2. *Receptors and recogniton* series B, vol. 8. Chapman and Hall, London.

Lonberg-Holm, K., R.L. Crowell, and L. Philipson. 1976a. Unrelated animal viruses share receptors. *Nature* **259:** 679.

Lonberg-Holm, K., L.B. Gosser, and E.J. Shimshick. 1976b. Interaction of liposomes with subviral particles of poliovirus type 2 and rhinovirus type 2. *J. Virol.* **19:** 746.

Luo, M., C. He, K.S. Toth, C.X. Zhang, and H.L. Lipton. 1992. Three-dimensional structure of Theiler murine encephalomyelitis virus (BeAn strain). *Proc. Natl. Acad. Sci.* **89:** 2409.

Luo, M., G. Vriend, G. Kamer, P. Minor, E. Arnold, M.G. Rossmann, U. Boege, D.G. Scraba, G.M. Duke, and A.C. Palmenberg. 1987. The atomic structure of mengo virus at 3.0 Å resolution. *Science* **235:** 182.

Madshus, I.H., S. Olsnes, and K. Sandvig. 1984a. Requirements for entry of poliovirus RNA into cells at low pH. *EMBO J.* **3:** 1945.

————. 1984b. Mechanism of entry into the cytosol of poliovirus type 1: Requirement for low pH. *J. Cell Biol.* **98:** 1194.

Mannweiler, K., P. Nobis, H. Hohenberg, and W. Bohn. 1990. Immunoelectron microscopy on the topographical distribution of the poliovirus receptor. *J. Gen. Virol.* **71:** 2737.

Mapoles, J.E., D.L. Krah, and R.L. Crowell. 1985. Purification and identification of a receptor protein from HeLa cells which binds group B coxsackieviruses. *J. Virol.* **55:** 560.

Marlin, S.D., D.E. Staunton, T.A. Springer, C. Stratowa, W. Sommergruber, and V.J. Merluzzi. 1990. A soluble form of intercellular adhesion molecule-1 inhibits rhinovirus infection. *Nature* **344:** 70.

Martin, A., C. Wychowski, T. Couderc, R. Crainic, J. Hogle, and M. Girard. 1988. Engineering a poliovirus type 2 antigenic site on a type 1 capsid results in a chimeric virus which is neurovirulent for mice. *EMBO J.* **7:** 2839.

Martin, S., J.M. Casasnovas, D.E. Staunton, and T.A. Springer. 1993. Efficient neutralization and disruption of rhinovirus by chimeric ICAM-1/immunoglobulin molecules. *J. Virol.* **67:** 3561.

Mason, P.W., E. Reider, and B. Baxt. 1994. RGD sequence of foot-and-mouth disease virus is essential for infecting cells via the natural receptor but can be bypassed by an antibody-dependent enhancement pathway. *Proc. Natl. Acad. Sci.* **91:** 1932.

Mason, P.W., B. Baxt, F. Brown, J. Harber, A. Murdin, and E. Wimmer. 1993. Antibody complexed foot-and-mouth disease virus, but not poliovirus, can infect normally insusceptible cells via the Fc receptor. *Virology* **192:** 568.

Mbida, A.D., B. Pozzetto, O.G. Gaudin, F. Grattard, J.-C. LeBihan, Y. Akono, and A. Ros. 1992. A 44,000 glycoprotein is involved in the attachment of echovirus-11 onto susceptible cells. *Virology* **189:** 350.

McClelland, A., J. de Bear, S. Connolly-Yost, A.M. Meyer, C.W. Marlor, and J.M. Greve 1991. Identification of monoclonal antibody epitopes and critical residues for rhinovirus binding in domain 1 of intercellular adhesion molecule 1. *Proc. Natl. Acad. Sci.* **88:** 7993.

McClintock, P.R., L.C. Billups, and A.L. Notkins. 1980. Receptors for encephalomyocarditis virus on murine and human cells. *Virology* **196:** 261.

McClintock, P.R., B.S. Prabhakar, and A.L. Notkins. 1986. Anti-idiotypic antibodies to monoclonal antibodies that neutralize coxsackievirus B4 do not recognize viral receptors. *Virology* **150:** 352.

McGeady, M.L. and R.L. Crowell. 1979. Stabilization of "A" particles of coxsackievirus B3 by a HeLa cell plasma membrane extract. *J. Virol.* **32:** 790.

————. 1981. Proteolytic cleavage of VP1 in "A" particles of coxsackievirus B3 does not appear to mediate virus uncoating by HeLa cells. *J. Gen. Virol.* **55:** 439.

McLaren, L.C., J.J. Holland, and J.T. Syverton. 1959. The mammalian cell-virus relationship. I. Attachment of poliovirus to cultivated cells of primate and non-primate origin. *J. Exp. Med.* **109:** 475.

Melnick, J.L. 1974. Picornaviridae. *Intervirology* **4:** 303.

———. 1990. Enteroviruses: Polioviruses, coxsackieviruses, echoviruses and newer enteroviruses. In *Virology*, 2nd edition, (ed. B.N. Fields and D.M. Knipe), p. 549. Raven Press, New York.

Mendelsohn, C.L., E. Wimmer, and V.R. Racaniello. 1989. Cellular receptor for poliovirus: Molecular cloning, nucleotide sequence, and expression of a new member of the immunoglobulin super family. *Cell* **56:** 855.

Miller, D.A., O.J. Miller, V.G. Dev, S. Hashmi, R. Tantravahi, L. Medrano, and H. Green. 1974. Human chromosome 19 carries a poliovirus receptor gene. *Cell* **1:** 167.

Minor, P.D., M. Ferguson, D.M.A. Evans, J.W. Almond, and J.P. Icenogle. 1986. Antigenic structure of polioviruses of serotypes 1, 2 and 3. *J. Gen. Virol.* **67:** 1283.

Minor, P.D., P.A. Pipkin, D. Hockley, G.C. Schild, and J.W. Almond. 1984. Monoclonal antibodies which block cellular receptors of poliovirus. *Virus Res.* **1:** 203.

Mischak, H., C. Neubauer, B. Berger, E. Kuechler, and D. Blaas. 1988. Detection of the human rhinovirus minor group receptor on renaturing Western blots. *J. Gen. Virol.* **69:** 2653.

Mohanty, J.G. and R.L. Crowell. 1993. Attempts to purify a second cellular receptor for a coxsackievirus B3 variant, CB3-RD, from HeLa cells. *Virus Res.* **29:** 305.

Morrison, L.A. and B.N. Fields. 1991. Parallel mechanisms in neuropathogenesis of enteric virus infections. *J. Virol.* **65:** 2767.

Morrison, M. and V.R. Racaniello. 1992. Molecular cloning and expression of a murine homolog of the human poliovirus receptor gene. *J. Virol.* **66:** 2807.

Moscufo, N., A.G. Yafal, A. Rogove, J. Hogel and M. Chow. 1993. A mutation in VP4 defines a new step in the late stages of cell entry by poliovirus. *J. Virol.* **67:** 5075.

Murray, M.G., J. Bradley, X.-F. Yang, E. Wimmer, E.G. Moss, and V.R. Racaniello. 1988. Poliovirus host range is determined by a short amino acid sequence in neutralization antigenic site I. *Science* **241:** 213.

Nobis, P., R. Zibirre, G. Meyer, J. Kuhne, G. Warnecke, and G. Koch. 1985. Production of a monoclonal antibody against an epitope on HeLa cells that is the functional poliovirus binding site. *J. Gen. Virol.* **66:** 561.

Olson, N.H., P.R. Kolatkar, M.A. Oliveira, R.H. Cheng, J.M. Greve, A. McClelland, T. S. Baker, and M.G. Rossmann. 1993. Structure of a human rhinovirus complexed with its receptor molecule. *Proc. Natl. Acad. Sci.* **90:** 507.

Paglini, S. and R.L. Crowell. 1992. Receptor presente en eritrocitos humanos para la variante RD del virus coxsackie B3. *Acta Bioquim. Clin. Latinoam.* **26:** 85.

Pappenheimer, A.M., L.J. Kunz, and S. Richardson. 1951. Passage of coxsackievirus (Connecticut-5 strain) in adult mice with production of pancreatic disease. *J. Exp. Med.* **94:** 45.

Peaver, D.C., M.J. Fancher, P.J. Felock, M.G. Rossmann, M.S. Miller, G. Diana, A.M. Trasurywala, M.A. McKinlay, and F.J. Dutko. 1989. Conformational change in the floor of the human rhinovirus canyon blocks adsorption to HeLa cell receptors. *J. Virol.* **63:** 2002.

Perez, L. and L. Carrasco. 1993. Entry of poliovirus into cells does not require a low pH step. *J. Virol.* **67:** 4543.

Quersin-Thiry, L. and E. Nihoul. 1961. Interaction between cellular extracts and animal viruses. II. Evidence for the presence of different inactivators corresponding to different viruses. *Acta Virol.* **5:** 283.

Racaniello, V.R. 1992. Interaction of poliovirus with its cell receptor. *Semin. Virol.* **3:** 473–481.

Rademacher, T.W., R.B. Parekh, and R.A. Dwek. 1988. Glycobiology. *Annu. Rev. Biochem.* **57:** 785.

Reagan, K.J., B. Goldberg, and R.L. Crowell. 1984. Altered receptor specificity of coxsackievirus B3 variants following growth in rhabdomyosarcoma cells. *J. Virology* **49:** 635.

Register, R.B., C.R. Uncapher, A.M. Naylor, D.W. Lineberger, and R.J. Colonno. 1991. Human-murine chimeras of ICAM-1 identify amino acid residues critical for rhinovirus and antibody binding. *J. Virol.* **65:** 6589.

Ren, R. and V.R. Racaniello. 1992a. Human poliovirus receptor gene expression and poliovirus tissue tropism in transgenic mice. *J. Virol.* **66:** 296.

———. 1992b. Poliovirus spreads from muscle to the central nervous system by neural pathways. *J. Infect. Dis.* **166:** 747.

Ren, R., F.C. Costantini, E.J. Gorgacz, J.J. Lee, and V.R. Racaniello. 1990. Transgenic mice expressing a human poliovirus receptor: A new model for poliomyelitis. *Cell* **63:** 353.

Roesing, T.G., P.A. Toselli, and R.L. Crowell. 1975. Elution and uncoating of coxsackievirus B3 by isolated HeLa cell plasma membranes. *J. Virol.* **15:** 654.

Roivainen, M., T. Hyypia, L. Piirainen, N. Kalkkinen, G. Stanway, and T. Hovi. 1991. RGD-dependent entry of coxsackievirus A9 into host cells and its bypass after cleavage of VP1 protein by intestinal proteases. *J. Virol.* **65:** 4735.

Rossmann, M.G. 1989. The canyon hypothesis. Hiding the host cell receptor attachment site on a viral surface from immune surveillance. *J. Biol. Chem.* **263:** 14587.

Rossmann, M.G. and A.C. Palmenberg. 1988. Conservation of the putative receptor attachment site in picornaviruses. *Virology* **164:** 373–382.

Rossmann, M.G., A.E. Erickson, E.A. Frankenberger, J.P. Griffith, H.-J. Hecht, J.E. Johnson, G. Kamer, M. Luo, A.G. Mosser, R.R. Rueckert, B. Sherry, and G. Vriend. 1985. Structure of a human common cold virus and functional relationship to other picornaviruses. *Nature* **317:** 145.

Rueckert, R.R. 1990. Picornaviridae and their replication. In *Virology*, 2nd edition (ed. B.N. Fields and D.M. Knipe), p. 507. Raven Press, New York.

Schonk, D., P. Van Dijk, P. Riegmann, J. Trapman, C. Holm, T.C. Willcocks, P. Sillekens, W. Van Venrooij, E. Wimmer, A.G. Van Kessel, H.H. Ropers, and B. Wieringa. 1989. Assignment of seven genes to distinct intervals on the mid-portion of human chromosome 19q surrounding the myotonic dystrophy gene region. *Cytogenet. Cell Genet.* **54:** 15.

Schultz, M. and R.L. Crowell. 1980. Acquisition of susceptibility to coxsackievirus A2 by the rat L8 cell line during myogenic differentiation. *J. Gen. Virol.* **46:** 39.

———. 1983. Eclipse of coxsackievirus infectivity: The restrictive event for a nonfusing myogenic cell line. *J. Gen. Virology,* **64:** 1725.

Sekiguchi, K., A.J. Franke, and B. Baxt. 1982. Competition for cellular receptor sites among selected aphthoviruses. *Arch. Virol.* **74:** 53.

Selinka, H.-C., A. Zibert, and E. Wimmer. 1991. Poliovirus can enter and infect mammalian cells by way of an intercellular adhesion molecule 1 pathway. *Proc. Natl. Acad. Sci.* **88:** 3598.

Shepard, D.A., B.A.Heinz, and R.R. Rueckert. 1993. WIN 52035-2 inhibits both attachment and eclipse of human rhinovirus 14. *J. Virol.* **67:** 2245.

Shepley, M.P. and V.R. Racaniello. 1994. A monoclonal antibody that blocks poliovirus attachment recognizes the lymphocyte homing receptor CD4. *J. Virol.* **68:** 1301.

Shepley, M.P., B. Sherry, and H.L. Weiner. 1988. Monoclonal antibody identification of a 100-kDa membrane protein in HeLa cells and human spinal cord involved in poliovirus attachment. *Proc. Nat. Acad. Sci.* **85:** 7743.

Sherry, B., A.G. Mosser, R.J. Colonno, and R.R. Rueckert. 1986. Use of monoclonal antibodies to identify four neutralization immunogens on a common cold picornavirus, human rhinovirus 14. *J. Virol.* **57:** 246.

Siddique, T., R. McKinney, W. Hung, R.J. Bartlett, G. Burns, T.K. Mohandas, H. Ropers, C. Wilfert, and A.D. Poses. 1988. The poliovirus sensitivity (PVS) gene is on chromosome 19q12-q13.2. *Genomics* **3:** 156.

Singer, S.J. 1992. Intercellular communication and cell-cell adhesion. *Science* **255:** 1671.

Skern, T., H. Torgersen, H. Auer, E. Kuechler, and D. Blaas. 1991. Human rhinovirus mutants resistant to low pH. *Virology* **183:** 757.

Smith, T.J., M.J. Kremer, M. Luo, G. Vriend, E. Arnold, G. Kamer, M.G. Rossmann, M.A. McKinlay, G.D. Diana, and M.J. Otto. 1986. The site of attachment in human rhinovirus 14 for antiviral agents that inhibit uncoating. *Science* **233:** 1286.

Smith, T.J., N.H. Olson, R.H. Cheng, H. Liu, E.S. Chase, W.M. Lee, D.M. Lippe, A.G. Mosser, R.R. Rueckert, and T.S. Smith. 1993. Structure of human rhinovirus complexed with Fab fragments from a neutralizing antibody. *J. Virol.* **67:** 1148.

Springer, T.A. 1990. Adhesion receptors of the immune system. *Nature* **346:** 425.

Stanway, G. 1990. Structure, function and evolution of picornaviruses. *J. Gen. Virol.* **71:** 2483.

Staunton, D.E., M.L. Dustin, H.P. Erickson, and T.A. Springer. 1990. The arrangement of the immunoglobulin-like domains of ICAM-1 and the binding sites for LFA-1 and rhinovirus. *Cell* **61:** 243.

Staunton, D.E., A. Gaur, P-Y. Chan, and T. Springer. 1992. Internalization of a major group human rhinovirus does not require cytoplasmic or transmembrane domains of ICAM-1. *J. Immunol.* **148:** 3271.

Staunton, D.E., V.J. Merluzzi, R. Rothlein, R. Barton, S.D. Marlin, and T.A. Springer. 1989. A cell adhesion molecule, ICAM-1, is the major surface receptor for rhinoviruses. *Cell* **56:** 849.

Tomassini, J.E. and R.J. Colonno. 1986. Isolation of a receptor protein involved in attachment of human rhinoviruses. *J. Virol.* **58:** 290.

Tomassini, J.E., T.R. Maxson, and R.J. Colonno. 1989a. Biochemical characterization of a glycoprotein required for rhinovirus attachment. *J. Biol. Chem.* **264:** 1656.

Tomassini, J.E., D. Graham, C.M. DeWitt, D.W. Lineberger, J.A. Rodkey, and R.J. Colonno. 1989b. cDNA cloning reveals that the major group rhinovirus receptor on HeLa cells is intercellular adhesion molecule 1. *Proc. Natl. Acad. Sci* **86:** 4907.

Uncapher, C.R., C.M. DeWitt, and R.J. Colonno. 1991. The major and minor group receptor families contain all but one human rhinovirus serotype. *Virology* **180:** 814.

Vizozo, A.D. and F.K. Sanders. 1964. Alteration of the pathogenicity of some group B coxsackie viruses under different conditions of passage. I. Virus type 4. *Acta Virol.* **8:** 38.

Wetz, K. and T. Kucinski. 1991. Influence of different ionic and pH environments on structural alterations of poliovirus and their possible relation to virus uncoating. *J. Gen. Virol.* **72:** 2541.

White, J.M. 1992. Membrane fusion. *Science* **258:** 917.

Yeates, T.O., D.H. Jacobson, A. Martin, C. Wychowski, M. Girard, D.J. Filman, and J.M. Hogle. 1991. Three-dimensional structure of a mouse-adapted type 2/type 1 poliovirus chimera. *EMBO J.* **10:** 2331.

Zajac, A.J., E.M. Amphlett, D.J. Rowlands, and D.V. Sangar. 1991. Parameters influencing the attachment of hepatitis A virus to a variety of continuous cell lines. *J. Gen. Virol.* **72:** 1667.

Zajac, I. and R.L. Crowell. 1965. Location and regeneration of enterovirus receptors of HeLa cells. *J. Bacteriol.* **89:** 1097.

————. 1969. Differential inhibition of attachment and eclipse activities of HeLa cells for enteroviruses. *J. Virol.* **3:** 422.

Zeichhardt, H., K. Wetz, P. Willingmann, and K.O. Habermehl. 1985. Entry of poliovirus type 1 and Mouse Elberfeld (ME) virus into Hep 2 cells: Receptor-mediated endocytosis and endosomal or lysosomal uncoating. *J. Gen. Virol.* **66:** 483.

Zhang, A., R.G. Nanni, D.A. Oren, E.J. Rozhon, and E. Arnold. 1992. Three-dimensional structure-activity relationships for antiviral agents that interact with picornavirus capsids. *Semin. Virol.* **3:** 453.

Zibert, A. and E. Wimmer. 1992. N glycosylation of the virus binding domain is not essential for function of the human poliovirus receptor. *J. Virol.* **66:** 7368.

7

Poliovirus Receptors

Eckard Wimmer, James J. Harber,[1]
James A. Bibb,[2] Matthias Gromeier,
Hui-Hua Lu, and Günter Bernhardt[3]
Department of Molecular Genetics and Microbiology
SUNY at Stony Brook
Stony Brook, New York 11794-8621

Poliovirus (PV) is the etiological agent of poliomyelitis, an acute human disease of the central nervous system (CNS). Invasion of PV into the CNS results in the destruction predominantly of motor neurons, leading to paralysis. Poliomyelitis, however, is a rare complication of PV infections of humans. The virus proliferates mainly in cells of the oropharyngeal and enteric tract, from where it can spread to the CNS. Neither the precise nature of cells in which the virus primarily replicates in the natural host, nor the route by which the virus enters the CNS has been elucidated. Viremia is frequent and can lead to infection of monocytes (Freistadt et al. 1993). It is likely that invasion of the CNS occurs both by overcoming the blood/brain barrier (Freistadt et al. 1993) and by retrograde axonal migration in neurons (Ren and Racaniello 1992a).

Only humans are known natural hosts of the virus, although monkeys can be infected orally with high doses of PV leading to poliomyelitis (Wenner et al. 1959). Whereas the tissue tropism of PV is predominantly governed by the presence of a cellular receptor (Holland 1961), it is likely that other factors, such as auxiliary proteins (Barnert et al. 1992; Shepley and Racaniello 1994; Shepley, this volume) or intracellular restrictions, influence the susceptibility of tissue cells to viral infection. Available evidence all but rules out the possibility that PV can make use of more than one receptor entity, the human poliovirus receptor (hPVR), to enter cells of human origin.

PV is a small RNA virus belonging to the family of Picornaviridae, genus Enterovirus. It is a nonenveloped particle consisting of only five

Present addresses: [1]Department of Biology, California Institute of Technology, Pasadena, California; [2]Laboratory of Molecular and Cellular Neuroscience, Rockefeller University, New York, New York 10021-6399; [3]Max-Delbrück-Centrum für Molekulare Medizin, Robert-Rössle-Strasse 10, 13122 Berlin, Germany.

species of macromolecules: a single-stranded RNA genome surrounded by 60 copies each of the capsid proteins VP1, VP2, VP3, and VP4 (Rueckert 1976; Kitamura et al. 1981) forming the shell of the virion. The building block of the shell is the protomer consisting of one copy of each of the four capsid proteins (Fig. 1). The folding patterns of the large capsid proteins (VP1, 2, and 3) are nearly identical in that they form eight-stranded antiparallel β barrels, whereas the small myristoylated VP4 lines part of the interior (Hogle et al. 1985; Rossmann and Johnson 1989).

The surface of the virion, although appearing smooth in images of electron micrographs (Mannweiler et al. 1990), is in fact characterized by pronounced indentations and protrusions (Fig. 1a) (Hogle et al. 1985). The β strands of the capsid proteins forming the β barrel are connected by amino acid loops which are characteristic for each of the three capsid proteins and "decorate" the outer surface of the virion. Some of these loop sequences elicit neutralizing antibodies and, consequently, they are neutralizing antigenic sites (N-Ags). PV has four major N-Ags (Hogle and Filman 1989; Murdin et al. 1992 and reference therein). However, PV expresses only three unique sets of the four antigenic sites and, hence, it exists in only three serotypes (PV1, PV2, and PV3). The molecular basis of this peculiar restriction is not understood (Wimmer et al. 1993). One of the antigenic sites is formed by the BC loop of VP1 (N-AgIa), an amino acid sequence 10 residues in length that is located in the

Figure 1 (*a*) Surface topography of PV1(M). The picture, kindly provided by J.-Y. Sgro and A. Palmenberg, was generated using the "grasp" program (Nichols et al. 1991) based on coordinates deposited by J. Hogle in the protein database (entry number 2plv). Five threefold axes (3x) define an open pentagon, the pentamer, at the center of which the fivefold axis (5x) of symmetry is located. Each pentamer is composed of five copies of the protomer, the biologically relevant building unit of the capsid. The protomer is composed of a copy each of the capsid proteins VP1, VP2, VP3 (designated as VP3[i]), and VP4 (not seen). The pseudoprotomer also consists of the four capsid proteins but includes VP3(ii) of the neighboring protomer instead of VP3(i). This arrangement is usually chosen as the representative unit of the virion surface. Ia, Ib, II, and III indicate the locations of the neutralizing antigenic sites. The canyon, the depression surrounding the 5x axis, is shaded dark (region B). A points at the north rim, and C at the south rim of the canyon. (*b*) A view of the canyon defined by the geometric array A, B, C as given in *a*. The eight-stranded antiparallel structure of VP1, VP2, and VP3 is apparent in this ribbon model (VP4 is not shown). VP1 and VP2 build up the side walls where the BC loop (position A) and the GH loop (position C) of VP1 are shaded dark, whereas the back wall given by VP3 is shaded only lightly. This illustration was generated by M. deCrombrugghe using the program "Molscript" (Kraulis 1991).

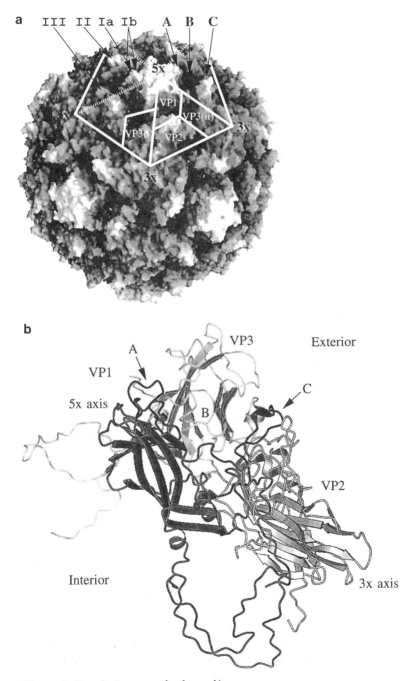

Figure 1 (See facing page for legend.)

vicinity of the apex at the fivefold axis (see Fig. 1b). Immediately below N-AgIa is the "canyon," a cleft that encircles the apexes of the virion forming a structural feature found not only in PV, but also in other picornaviruses such as rhinoviruses. By analogy to major group rhinoviruses, it was assumed that the PV canyon is likely to be the binding site for the hPVR (Fig. 1) (Rossmann 1989; Chapman and Rossmann 1993) and, fittingly, monoclonal antibodies binding to N-AgIa can block PV binding to host cells (see below).

GENETICS OF THE PV RECEPTOR

No known rodent cell line can be infected with PV. However, transfection of rodent cells with virion RNA leads to one round of viral replication (Holland et al. 1959), even in enucleated mouse L cells (Morgan-Detjen et al. 1978). Since mouse cells cannot significantly bind PV (McLaren et al. 1959; Bibb et al. 1994c), it was reasoned that the barrier to infection of rodent cells with PV is the absence of a suitable virus receptor and that this receptor must be encoded in the genome of primates (Holland 1961).

Somatic cell genetics has proven this hypothesis and shown that the sensitivity to PV infection is an autosomal trait, specific for primate cells. Hybridization of human cells with mouse cells led to the isolation of cell lines susceptible to PV infection (Medrano and Green 1973). The phenotype of PV sensitivity was then mapped to human chromosome 19 (Miller et al. 1974), specifically to position 19q13.1-13.2 (Siddique et al. 1988; Schonk et al. 1989; Koike et al. 1990).

On the basis of these observations, a genetic strategy was designed to identify hPVR and its gene by cotransformation of suitable mouse cells (L aprt⁻/tk⁻) with human genomic DNA from HeLa cells and a vector expressing the thymidine kinase gene. This was followed by HAT selection and screening of surviving cells for expression of a PV-specific receptor with monoclonal antibody (MAb) D171 (Mendelsohn et al. 1986, 1989). MAb D171 was isolated by Nobis et al. (1985) by immunization of mice with HeLa cells and screening of hybridoma fluids for their ability to protect HeLa cells against infection with PV1. Indeed, MAb D171 protected all human and monkey cells that were tested against PV1, PV2, and PV3 infection, which immediately suggested that the receptor may reside in a single molecular entity. hPVR-specific monoclonal antibodies with similar properties were also isolated by Minor et al. (1984) using Hep-2C cells, by Koike et al. (1992a) using recombinant hPVR expressed in baculovirus, and by Lionetti and Wimmer (described by Mendelsohn et al. 1986), using HeLa cells, as immunogens.

The identification and cloning of hPVR[+] L cells were carried out by "rosetting" with MAb D171 and red-blood-cell conjugated anti-mouse Ig antibodies (Littman et al. 1985) and "panning" (Mendelsohn et al. 1986). Secondary hPVR[+] transformants were then used to isolate hPVR-specific cDNAs via protocols essentially following those developed for identifying cDNA of oncogenes (see, e.g., Shih et al. 1981). Two groups reported on the isolation and characterization of cDNAs encoding cell-surface polypeptides belonging to the Ig superfamily (see below) whose transient expression in mouse L cells rendered the cells susceptible to PV infection (Mendelsohn et al. 1989; Koike et al. 1990).

Koike et al. (1990), using cosmid clones, determined that the human gene encoding hPVR contains 8 exons distributed over 20 kbp of chromosomal DNA (Fig. 2). The complete genomic organization, however, remains to be determined since neither transcriptional start sites nor the promoter region was identified. Nevertheless, some of the genomic clones of hPVR appeared to contain a complete set of genetic information, since they could be used to generate transgenic mice which, upon infection with PV, developed poliomyelitis (Ren et al. 1990; Koike et al. 1991b and this volume; Ren and Racaniello 1992b; Horie et al. 1994). Similarly, a complete hPVR gene was used to generate a transformed mouse L-cell line (JA-1) that expressed, under the control of its own promoter, the expected splice variants of hPVR (Bernhardt et al. 1994a). Accordingly, JA-1 cells are susceptible to PV infection. The results of these studies showed that the hPVR gene is expressed in the form of four splice variants, of which two (hPVRα and hPVRδ) encode membrane-bound proteins, whereas the other two splice variants (hPVRβ and hPVRγ) lack all or part of the exon specifying the membrane-spanning domain (Fig. 2) (Mendelsohn et al. 1989; Koike et al. 1990). hPVRβ and hPVRγ are therefore excreted forms of the receptor (Koike et al. 1990). A similar study by Koike et al. (1992a) on the gene for monkey PVR (mPVR) revealed interesting differences. These authors identified two separate loci encoding mPVR-specific sequences. Two splice variants, AGMα1 (mPVRα1) and AGMδ1 (mPVRδ1), are encoded by the first locus (Fig. 3). These isoforms are homologous to hPVR isoforms α and δ. With respect to the α1 isotype, two sequences were reproducibly obtained (referred to as AGMα1 and AGMα1′), which differ in only one amino acid and, therefore, are likely to be alleles. The second genetic locus encodes the single splice variant AGMα2 (mPVRα2), which is related to AGMα1 (mPVRα1). On the basis of the extent of the sequence divergence between AGMα2 (mPVRα2) and AGMα1 (mPVRα1) (2.6% synonymous changes), it is likely that a duplication of the PVR gene occurred after species differentiation between the human and monkey

a
Genomic structure

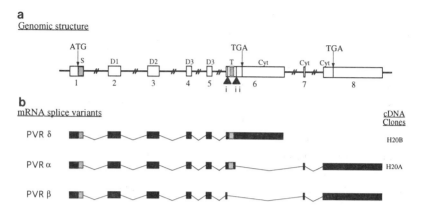

b
mRNA splice variants

Figure 2 Genetic organization of hPVR. (*a*) The exon-intron structure of the gene. ATG and TGA determine the open reading frames for the hPVR proteins. Open boxes represent the eight exons specifying the three extracellular domains D1, D2, and D3, as well as those harboring the coding sequences for the signal peptide (S), the transmembrane region (T), and the cytoplasmic tails (Cyt). Black triangles indicate splice donor sites used to generate hPVRβ mRNA (i) and hPVRα mRNA (ii), respectively. (*b*) The composition of the different hPVR proteins (hPVRδ, hPVRα, hPVRβ, hPVRγ) in the form of the mRNA splice variants coding them (Koike et al. 1990). The hPVR isoforms δ and α are also encoded by the cDNA clones H20B and H20A, isolated by Mendelsohn et al. (1989).

lineages (Koike et al. 1992a). cDNAs encoding soluble (excreted) forms of mPVR have not been detected in monkey primary or secondary cell lines, but they could occur in specific tissues or during specific stages of development of the animals (Koike et al. 1992a).

Morrison and Racaniello (1992) have characterized the gene for the murine homolog to hPVR (murine PVR homolog, MPH), which appears to be expressed in the form of two splice variants (yielding 2-kb and 3-kb transcripts as determined by Northern blot analysis). Only the exon-intron structure of the open reading frame of the 2-kb transcript was reported in detail by these authors; it revealed a coding sequence of an immunoglobulin-like cell-surface protein with the same general domains as hPVR (Fig. 3). MPH cannot function as a receptor for PV, as expected. Somewhat surprisingly, however, MPH is also not the receptor for mouse-adapted PV strains, such as PV2 (Lansing). MPH was also analyzed by Aoki et al. (1994) who found that the 3-kb MPH transcript encodes a variant lacking the *trans*-membrane domain, an observation suggesting that a soluble form of MPH is also produced in the mouse.

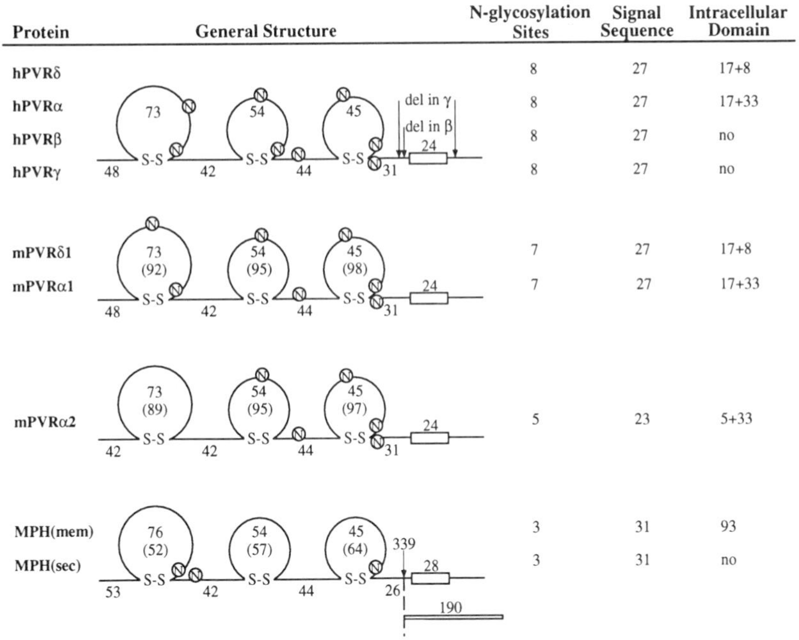

Protein	General Structure	N-glycosylation Sites	Signal Sequence	Intracellular Domain
hPVRδ		8	27	17+8
hPVRα	73 / 54 / 45 / del in γ	8	27	17+33
hPVRβ	/ del in β / 24	8	27	no
hPVRγ	48 / 42 / 44 / 31	8	27	no
mPVRδ1	73 (92) / 54 (95) / 45 (98)	7	27	17+8
mPVRα1	48 / 42 / 44 / 31 / 24	7	27	17+33
mPVRα2	73 (89) / 54 (95) / 45 (97) / 42 / 42 / 44 / 31 / 24	5	23	5+33
MPH(mem)	76 (52) / 54 (57) / 45 (64) / 339	3	31	93
MPH(sec)	53 / 42 / 44 / 26 / 28 / 190	3	31	no

Figure 3 Schematic representation of the species-specific PVR molecules. Given are the lengths of the extracellular polypeptides subdivided by the cysteine disulfide bonds characteristic for the Ig-like domains, the lengths of the transmembrane regions (*open boxes*), and, as columns, the number of potential extracellular glycosylation sites, as well as the lengths of the signal sequences and intracellular domains (the intracellular domains of hPVRα and hPVRδ share 17 amino acid residues; this is the same for mPVRα1 and mPVRδ1). The homologies of the extracellular domains of the PVR-related proteins compared to the corresponding hPVR domains are calculated in percentage and shown as the numbers in parentheses inside each circle representing a domain.

Unpublished data referred to in Morrison and Racaniello (1992) and Aoki et al. (1994) suggest that the MPH gene maps to mouse chromosome 7, which is known to be syntenic with human chromosome 19. Thus, hPVR, mPVR, and MPH polypeptides are likely to have similar, albeit as yet obscure function(s).

PROPERTIES OF PVR-RELATED PROTEINS

Inspection of the amino acid sequences predicted from cDNA sequences revealed that hPVR is a type Ia single-pass *trans*-membrane glycoprotein with three extracellular immunoglobulin-like domains, designated V-C2-C2 (Mendelsohn et al. 1989; Koike et al. 1990). All hPVR molecules possess eight potential *N*-glycosylation sites and, depending on the character of the splice variant, a *trans*-membrane domain of 24 residues and a cytoplasmic carboxy-terminal domain of 25 or 50 residues (Fig. 3).

The extracellular domains of the mPVRs are closely related to hPVR, with the exception of the number and location of *N*-glycosylation sites (Fig. 3) (Koike et al. 1992a). Since the virus binds exclusively to the V domain, this observation implies that the carbohydrate chains of the receptor molecules are not directly involved in viral attachment.

The mouse homolog of hPVR, which carries only three potential *N*-glycosylation sites, is closely related to hPVR in structure, but not in the predicted sequence (see Fig. 3 for domain-specific homologies) (Morrison and Racaniello 1992). Neither mPVR nor MPH has been characterized at the protein level.

The molecular masses of the mature core polypeptides (i.e., without signal peptide, see below) of hPVRα and hPVRδ are 42.5 kD and 40 kD, respectively. Expression of hPVRα with a vaccinia virus expression vector in HeLa cells (Zibert et al. 1991), or of hPVRδ with a baculovirus expression vector in insect cells (Kaplan et al. 1990a), yielded functional receptor molecules with apparent molecular masses of approximately 67 kD. In vitro translation of synthetic mRNA transcribed from hPVRα cDNA in the presence of dog pancreas microsomes also yielded a polypeptide of 67 kD (Zibert et al. 1991). However, recent evidence has shown that the 67-kD hPVR-related proteins are glycosylation intermediates and artifacts of the expression systems used (Bernhardt et al. 1994a). By applying hPVR-specific monoclonal antibodies isolated in Nomoto's laboratory (Koike et al. 1992a), Bernhardt et al. (1994a) identified in metabolically labeled cell lysates membrane-bound glycoforms of hPVR with molecular masses of 80–85 kD. If HeLa cells, infected with vaccinia virus expressing hPVRα, were labeled early in the infectious cycle, both the 67-kD and 80- to 85-kD species were observed. However, when labeling was started late in infection, only the 67-kD glycoform could be detected. Furthermore, inhibitors of the glycosylation pathway have allowed the monitoring of the modification of the hPVR core proteins when passing through the processing pathway of uninfected cells. Only a 67-kD receptor species is observed if cells are labeled in the presence of the inhibitor deoxymannojirimycin (Bernhardt et al. 1994a). It was concluded that the 67-kD molecule is an intermediate glycoform probably located in the endoplasmic reticulum (ER) or *cis*-Golgi whose further modification is blocked in response to the infection with vaccinia virus (Bernhardt et al. 1994a). This was supported by the finding that despite the expression of both glycoforms, only the 80- to 85-kD hPVR proteins could be identified by surface iodination of cells infected with hPVRα recombinant vaccinia virus (Bernhardt et al. 1994a).

Deglycosylation using the enzyme N-glycanase converted all of the 80- to 85-kD hPVR proteins detected in various tissue culture cell lines to 45-kD and 43-kD molecules corresponding approximately to the predicted molecular weight of the core proteins of the splice variants α and δ. The small difference in the predicted molecular weights may be due to incomplete deglycosylation, as observed frequently when N-glycanase is used. More likely, it is an artifact due to aberrant gel migration. The relative expression levels of hPVRα and hPVRδ varied considerably with respect to each other, depending on the cell line (Bernhardt et al. 1994a).

Taken together, these results show that hPVRs are glycoproteins bearing sialylated complex-type oligosaccharides with a molecular mass of 80–85 kD (Bernhardt et al. 1994a). This is important for analyses of the distribution of hPVR in human tissues; reports of hPVR molecules with larger or smaller molecular masses than 80–85 kD are probably artifacts of the assay procedures employed (for discussion, see Freistadt, this volume).

Amino-terminal signal peptides serving to direct a nascent polypeptide chain to the ER are on the average 18–20 residues long (von Heinje 1985). Sequence analysis of the 80- to 85-kD and 67-kD species of hPVR revealed an aspartic acid at the amino terminus, suggesting that the cleavage of the signal peptide from pre-hPVR occurred at a Gly*Asp amino acid pair (Bibb et al. 1994a). The signal peptide of pre-hPVR, therefore, consists of 27 amino acids. Although this is significantly above the average size, all known features of a typical signal peptide could be identified by computer analysis (Bibb et al. 1994a). (For discussions of the corresponding elements in pre-mPVR and pre-MPH, see Bibb et al. [1994a].)

The carboxy-terminal, intracellular regions of hPVRα and hPVRδ are 50 and 25 residues long, respectively. Metabolic labeling of cells with [^{32}P]orthophosphate revealed that one or more serine residues of hPVRα, but not of hPVRδ, are phosphorylated (Bibb et al. 1994b). Preliminary studies employing kinase inhibitors suggested that the multifunctional kinase CaMK II may be involved in this modification. Since the cellular function(s) of hPVR is obscure, the significance of the phosphorylation of one of the splice variants remains unknown. On the other hand, it seems unlikely that phosphorylation affects the ability of hPVRα to mediate PV infection (Bibb et al. 1994b). That the intracellular domain(s) of hPVR is not essential for PV uptake was already suggested by the findings that carboxy-terminally truncated hPVRs (Koike et al. 1991b) or hybrid hPVR/hICAM-1 (see Fig. 4D) and CD4 receptors mediate PV infectivity (Selinka et al. 1991, 1992; Bernhardt et al. 1994b).

INTERACTION OF THE POLIOVIRION WITH THE RECEPTOR

The Canyon Hypothesis

A remarkable surface feature of both polioviruses and rhinoviruses is a deep cleft, called the canyon, between the broad plateau of the threefold axis and the star-shaped mesa of the fivefold axis (Fig. 1) (Hogle et al. 1985; Rossmann et al. 1985). As generally recognized for proteins whose three-dimensional structures have been solved, clefts of such magnitude may serve a special function. Rossmann and his colleagues, after having elucidated the crystal structure of human rhinovirus type 14 (HRV-14), immediately suggested an important function for the viral canyon as the receptacle for the viral receptor (Rossmann et al. 1985; Rossmann 1989). Furthermore, the canyon hypothesis postulates that by using a narrow cleft for receptor binding, this site is inaccessible to antibodies and, hence, escapes immunosurveillance (Rossmann 1989; Chapman and Rossmann 1993). The evidence supporting the hypothesis that the canyon is the binding site of the hICAM-1 receptor for major receptor group rhinoviruses (e.g., HRV-14) is compelling (see Greve and Rossmann,

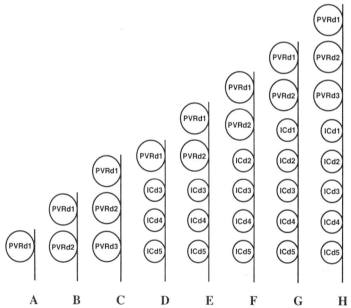

A   B   C   D   E   F   G   H

Figure 4 Schematic representation of the truncated or hybrid hPVR molecules used to identify hPVR regions important for the function as poliovirus receptor. The larger circles denote hPVR domains and the smaller circles domains of hICAM-1. All hybrid molecules possess the hICAM-1 transmembrane and cytoplasmic region (for details, see Bernhardt et al. 1994b).

this volume). For PV, however, the case for the canyon as binding site for hPVR is only circumstantial at best. Nevertheless, considering the similarity of the rhinovirus and poliovirus structures, and the observations that (1) the amino-terminal domains of the Ig-like receptors interact with rhino- and polioviruses (see below), (2) N-AgIa-specific MAbs inhibit PV from binding to HeLa cells (Altmeyer et al. 1991) (see below), (3) several of the mutations inhibiting the binding of PV to a soluble receptor map to the rim of the PV canyon (Colston and Racaniello 1992), and (4) mutations constructed to fall inside the canyon yield a virus-binding phenotype (J.J. Harber et al., in prep.; see below), it is likely that binding of PV to hPVR involves the canyon.

Domains of hPVR Involved in Virus Binding and Uptake

A cell-surface molecule with the general organization shown in Figure 3 is likely to interact with a ligand as large as the poliovirion via its amino-terminal region. Indeed, deletion of different portions of the receptor molecule provided evidence that the V domain of hPVR is necessary and sufficient for virus binding, uncoating, and infection (Fig. 4A) (Koike et al. 1991a; Selinka et al. 1991, 1992). Molecular models of the V domain have recently been presented by Aoki et al. (1994), Morrison et al. (1994), and Bernhardt et al. (1994b). These models rely on the observation that hPVR is an Ig-like molecule. Features characterizing and identifying members of this family of proteins were taken as a guideline to assign domain borders and to predict the folding pattern of the first V-like domain of hPVR. The V-domain model by Bernhardt et al. (1994b) is used for discussion. This model predicts that the V domain embraces residues 28–140 (Fig. 5). Deletions within these borders are likely to inactivate the domain, which serves to explain why removal of amino acids 137–256 from hPVR has been reported to abolish receptor function (Freistadt and Racaniello 1991; Morrison et al. 1994; see also below).

Although the V domain alone can function as a PVR, this single domain is impaired not only with respect to PV and antibody binding, but also in its ability to promote infection. "Spacing" of the V domain from the cell surface and its proper folding have been considered to play a role in the deficiencies of this artificial single-domain receptor (Koike et al. 1991a; Selinka et al. 1991). Indeed, if the V domain (residues 1–143) was fused to domains 3–5 of ICAM-1 (Fig. 4D) (Selinka et al. 1991) or to domains 3–4 of the T-cell receptor CD4 (Selinka et al. 1992), the function of the V domain improved, but it did not reach wild-type efficiency. Experiments using a variety of hPVR/ICAM-1 fusion molecules (see Fig. 4) were performed to investigate the requirement for

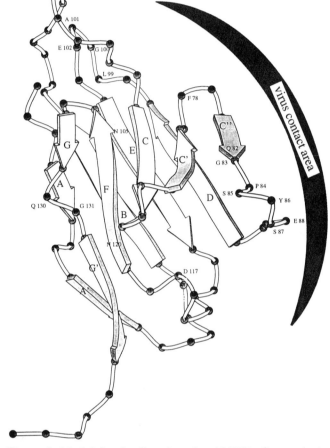

Figure 5 Model for the first domain of hPVR. β strands A–G′ are shown by ribbons with the arrowheads indicating the amino- to carboxy-terminal direction. Loops are characterized by a "pearls on a string" presentation. The dark circles represent amino acids; those probably involved in virus binding or uptake (see text) are identified by number and the single-letter code. The region of the first domain believed to contact the surface of PV1(M) is indicated (for details, see Bernhardt et al. 1994b).

spacing and the possible contribution of the C-like hPVR domains in receptor function in more detail. The results have indicated that spacing appears to play a minor role, if any (Bernhardt et al. 1994b). Specifically, only a hybrid receptor with a complete set of hPVR domains (Fig. 4H) functioned with an efficiency comparable to that of wild-type hPVR (Fig. 4C) (Bernhardt et al. 1994b). Since it is unlikely that either domain 2 or domain 3 participates directly in virus-binding reactions, it appears that these domains provide a "scaffold" for maintaining a precise conformation for the V domain. This specific conformation is characterized by a distinct three-dimensional distribution of discontinuous binding epitopes for PV, on the one hand, and for different monoclonal antibodies, on the other hand. Virus binding then depends on the correct presentation of these epitopes (Bernhardt et al. 1994b).

Hybrid receptors have also been constructed between hPVR and the mouse homolog MPH (Aoki et al. 1994; Morrison and Racaniello 1992; Morrison et al. 1994). Results obtained with these constructs agree with the above-mentioned conclusion of the pivotal role of the V domain in virus binding. In general, domains 2 and 3 of MPH (both C2 domains) appear to provide better scaffolding for the hPVR V domain than the C domains of hICAM-1. Considering the degree of sequence homologies, this may not be surprising. An interesting hPVR/MPH hybrid (referred to as E2) was analyzed by Morrison et al. (1994) that consisted (amino- to carboxy-terminal) of the hPVR (residues 1–131) and MPH (mouse residue homolog to hPVR amino acid 132 to carboxyl terminus). It was found that the hybrid molecule was normal in virus binding but impaired in the destabilization of the virion (A-particle formation) and promotion of infection. Morrison et al. (1994) concluded that the second domain of hPVR was involved in steps following adsorption. This is difficult to comprehend in view of the V-domain activity either as a single entity or in context of ICAM and CD4 hybrid receptors (Koike et al. 1991a; Selinka et al. 1991, 1992). An alternative explanation is that splicing of the MPH sequence to the hPVR V domain inside the G' strand (Fig. 5) distorted some structural elements of the V domain and, thus, impaired the uncoating function of this domain (see above). This explanation is supported by two observations. First, mutational analysis has suggested that the G' and A strands (see Fig. 5) are in contact (Aoki et al. 1994). Since the MPH-specific segment that replaced, in part, the hPVR G strand in E2 is heterologous in amino acid sequence, distortion of this region may be possible. Second, replacement of two amino acids immediately upstream of the G' strand in hPVR (Q130G/GD) resulted in an interesting phenotype of the mutant receptor (containing all three domains). PV3 (Sabin) was able to bind to, but not infect, cell lines expressing the mutant receptor (J.J. Harber et al., in prep.). This result led to the suggestion that the region including the G strands is involved in uncoating (J.J. Harber et al., in prep.) (see below).

Mutational Analysis and Model of the V Domain

Once the role of the amino-terminal domain of hPVR in PV infection was established, three groups subjected the V domain to extensive mutational analysis. One strategy made use of the known sequence of the murine homolog MPH of hPVR, which is receptor-inactive. It was assumed that amino acids that differed in the respective V domains might be involved in virus binding (homolog scanning mutagenesis) (Aoki et al. 1994; Morrison et al. 1994). A different approach was taken by Bernhardt et al. (1994b), who modeled the V domain and targeted mutagenesis to exposed regions likely to interact with virus. The best assessment of mutant phenotypes was obtained when the expression of mutant receptors was measured by fluorescence-activated cell sorting (FACS) analyses using a panel of monoclonal antibodies. Moreover, these antibodies (all isolated on the basis of blocking PV attachment) allowed the identification of antibody-binding epitopes and the measurement of the effect of a given mutation on virus and antibody binding. Most receptor variants retained the binding of several monoclonal antibodies, which suggested that the effects of the mutations were specific to receptor/virus interaction and not to an overall change of domain structure (Bernhardt et al. 1994b).

In the study by Bernhardt et al. (1994b), 44 mutations (single and multiple amino acid exchanges; removal of existing, or introduction of new, N-glycosylation sites) were analyzed for virus binding, binding of different monoclonal antibodies, and viral proliferation, either in transient receptor expression assays, or in cell lines expressing the receptor construct. Some mutations were carried out in the context of a hybrid receptor (containing all domains of hPVR and hICAM-1, see above; Fig. 4H), a construct that expressed nearly wild-type function and was stably expressed in cell lines. Since all available anti-hPVR monoclonal antibodies appeared to possess binding epitopes in the first hPVR domain, the expression of receptor mutants in this domain was monitored using two hICAM-1-specific monoclonal antibodies to separate antibody-binding from virus-binding epitopes.

Aoki et al. (1994) performed an extensive "homolog scanning" between hPVR and MPH (30 mutants), and they also exchanged segments between the two domains. Although these authors used only transient expression of the mutant receptor, they have monitored expression with a panel of monoclonal antibodies. Morrison et al. (1994), also following the homolog scanning approach, have analyzed 9 receptor mutants, all of which were expressed in cell lines for further analysis.

The most surprising result of the mutational analysis of the V domain of hPVR was that the tip of the structure, particularly the well-exposed BC loop (Fig. 5), is not involved in virus (poliovirus type 1, Mahoney; PV1[M]) binding. In that regard, the interactions between PV and hPVR, on the one hand, and between major group HRV and ICAM-1 (see Greve and Rossman, this volume), appear to differ. On the other hand, mutations in regions C'C", C"D, DE, EF, and GG' exerted an influence on the function of the receptor molecule. Of these, the GG' may be involved in uncoating, as discussed below. The mutations in the EF loop with drastic effects on receptor function appear to result from extensive structural rearrangement, since binding of most monoclonal antibodies was abrogated also. The mutations in C'C", C"D, and DE, on the other hand, interfere directly with PV1(M) binding (Aoki et al. 1994; Bernhardt et al. 1994b; Morrison et al. 1994). It is concluded, therefore, that PV binds at the "right side" of the V domain (Fig. 5) to regions most distal to the putative carboxyl terminus of the first domain. Surprisingly, mutational analysis, together with model building of the V domain of hPVR, revealed structural and functional homology with the T-cell receptor CD4, whose C'C", C"D, and DE regions play an important role in ligand binding (Peterson and Seed 1988; Arthos et al. 1989; Ashkenazi et al. 1990; Moebius et al. 1992a,b, 1993).

Absence of the two N-glycosylation sites in the V domain of hPVR does not abrogate receptor function (Koike et al. 1992a; Zibert and Wimmer 1992). This result was not unexpected, since the monkey homolog mPVRα2, which lacks N-glycosylation sites in the V domain, is active as a PV receptor (Koike et al. 1992a). Surprisingly, removal of four N-glycosylation sites (two in the V domain and two in the adjacent C2 domain) by site-directed mutagenesis enhanced virus binding and receptor activity significantly (Bernhardt et al. 1994b), which suggests that the carbohydrate chains in these outer domains present a steric hindrance for viral attachment. It was found that the sugar moiety attached to Asn-105 of the first domain is mainly responsible for this phenomenon (Bernhardt et al. 1994b).

VIRAL VARIANTS AND THE INTERACTION BETWEEN THE POLIOVIRION AND hPVR

Antigenic Hybrid Viruses and Receptor Binding

The 10-residue-long BC loop of capsid protein VP1 is a surface protrusion of the virion located near the north rim of the canyon (Fig. 1). As mentioned before, this structure elicits neutralizing antibodies (Minor 1990) and is therefore a (continuous) neutralization antigenic site referred to as N-AgIa. Exchange of this loop with heterologous sequences by cartridge mutagenesis (Murray et al. 1988b) has generated new antigenic sites (for references, see Lu et al. 1994), some of which conferred to the viral variant novel biological properties, such as an extended host range (Martin et al. 1988; Murray et al. 1988a; see below). In

a special case, 8 amino acids of the VP1 BC loop of PV1(M) were replaced with 12 amino acids of an equivalent structure of HRV-14,
referred to as neutralizing immunogenic site IA (NImIA). This PV
variant was neutralized by antisera specific for both PV1(M) and HRV-
14, and it was able to elicit neutralizing antibodies to PV1(M) and HRV-
14. It is, thus, an antigenic hybrid virus (referred to as W1/HRV-14; Altmeyer et al. 1991).

W1/HRV-14 grew to nearly wild-type titers in HeLa cells; it expressed a small-plaque phenotype, but it was not temperature sensitive.
hPVR-specific MAb D171 completely blocked growth of W1/HRV-14,
and so did neutralizing monoclonal antibodies (MAb20 and MAb1)
specific for NImAI of HRV-14. Similarly, Fab fragments prepared from
MAb20 and MAb1 were also able to inhibit binding of W1/HRV-14,
ruling out the possibility that neutralization was significantly affected by
viral aggregation (Altmeyer et al. 1991). These results suggested (1) that
W1/HRV-14 cannot use hICAM-1 as an alternative receptor for infection
(which is not surprising) and (2) that, in analogy with studies with HRV-
14 (Colonno et al. 1989), binding of an immunoglobulin to the altered
BC loop may neutralize the hybrid virus by preventing W1/HRV-14
from binding to hPVR. This was found to be true: Both MAb20 and
MAb1 inhibited binding of W1/HRV-14 to HeLa cells; similarly,
MAb95, a monoclonal antibody elicited against N-AgIa of PV1(M)
(Wiegers and Dernick 1987), was found to block binding of PV1(M) to
HeLa cells. These results strongly support the notion that the interaction
between PV and hPVR is similar to that between HRV-14 and ICAM-1;
that is, by interaction with the canyon (Altmeyer et al. 1991).

Formation of PV A Particles, and Soluble
Receptor-resistant PV Mutants

Binding of PV, sedimenting in sucrose gradients at 160S, to cells expressing hPVR or mPVR at 37°C leads to an irreversible alteration of the
particle: All copies of the small capsid protein VP4 are released, resulting in the formation of 135S "A particles" ($[VP1-3]_{60}$RNA) (for earlier
references, see Crowell and Landau 1983; see below). A particles have
undergone extensive structural transitions: They express C-reactive
antigenicity (which means they do not bind neutralizing antibodies), can
no longer bind to permissive cells, and are sensitive to protease and
strong detergent (SDS) but resistant to RNase (Holland and Hoyer 1963;
McLaren et al. 1968; Chan and Black 1970; Crowell and Philipson 1971;
Roesing et al. 1975; DeSena and Mandel 1976, 1977; Guttman and Baltimore 1977 and references therein). In addition, they are more hydro-

phobic than the 160S poliovirion (Lonberg-Holm et al. 1976; Fricks and Hogle 1990). Since A particles are not infectious, incubation of poliovirions with receptor-containing entities (intact cells or membrane fractions) "neutralizes" viral infectivity. It is currently thought that the formation of A particles is the earliest step in uncoating.

Kaplan et al. (1990a) and Gomez-Yafal et al. (1993) have shown that a solubilized membrane fraction of insect cells that expressed the 67-kD version of hPVRδ was able to induce conversion of poliovirions to A particles, a result that confirmed the role of hPVR in this reaction. Generation of PV A particles was also achieved with a soluble form of the two amino-terminal domains (V-C2) of hPVR (Zibert et al. 1992). In neither of these experiments was the hPVR protein purified, leaving open the possibility that additional cellular molecule(s) play a role in this step of uncoating. This possibility was eliminated by Koike et al. (1992b), who purified a hPVR-Ig fusion protein (V-C2-C2-hinge-Fc domain) to homogeneity by affinity chromatography. The purified hPVR-Ig fraction was able to quantitatively convert purified poliovirions (sedimenting at 160S) to A particles (135S). However, the mechanism by which the extrusion of VP4 is triggered remains unknown.

On incubation of poliovirions with detergent-solubilized hPVRδ, Kaplan et al. (1990b) observed that not all infectivity of the original inoculum could be "neutralized." This was due to the selection of PV mutants (already present in the inoculum, as is common in a population of RNA viruses; [Wimmer et al. 1993]) that apparently resisted conversion to A particles under the conditions of the reaction. These soluble receptor-resistant (srr) PV mutants readily infect HeLa cells; that is, the resistance phenotype is "leaky," as would be expected. Apparently, the mutations in different srr variants map to regions interior or exterior to the capsid (Colston and Racaniello 1992), but their identity has not been published. Nevertheless, srr mutants will provide useful information on how to generate viral variants with which it may be possible to dissect individual steps in uncoating.

Serotype Polymorphism of the Receptor-binding Site

Studies with the three PV serotypes and with several viral capsid mutants have revealed differences in receptor binding, uptake, and replication. For these experiments, cell lines were used that expressed hybrid receptors (Fig. 4H) with specific mutations in the V-like domain of hPVR (Bernhardt et al. 1994b). Interestingly, one of these cell lines (Q130G/GD) was capable of binding but not replicating type-3 polioviruses (PV3[S] and PV3[L]), even if the viruses were administered at high moi, whereas type-1 and type-2 polioviruses did not bind at all. Further analyses showed that the type-3 particles, although they bound to the mutant receptor Q130G/GD, were not converted into A particles, suggesting that this mutation in the GG' strand of the first domain (Fig. 5) abrogated the earliest step in uncoating. Whether this region is directly involved in altering the conformation of the bound virions remains to be seen.

Another receptor mutation (P84SYS/HYSA) in the proposed attachment region for PV1(M), mapping to the C"D region of the first domain (Fig. 5), showed different binding phenotypes for the three serotypes. Specifically, the binding and uptake (measured at 25°C) of PV2(S) and PV3(S) mediated by the hybrid receptor P84SYS/HYSA was significantly more efficient when compared to type-1 polioviruses (J.J. Harber et al., in prep.). It should be noted that binding affinities and binding on-rates of two different PV strains (PV1[M] and PV3[S]) to cells expressing the wild-type receptor (HeLa) have revealed no differences between the two serotypes (Bibb et al. 1994c). Thus, whereas wild-type receptor binds these virions with an efficiency that is indistinguishable by the assays used, subtle differences in the interaction between receptor and serotypes become apparent as the structure of the receptors is slightly altered by mutation.

Characterization of PV1(M) Mutants

Mutations in the receptor that weaken the interaction with wild-type PV1(M) were also used to assay for effects of mutations introduced throughout the canyon region of PV1(M) by site-directed mutagenesis (J.J. Harber et al., in prep.). A PV1(M) mutant located at the southern rim of the canyon (GH loop of VP1) showed reduced binding to wild-type hPVR but replicated without delays in eclipse and grew to titers comparable to wild-type virus, thus displaying an attachment phenotype. When this mutant virus was grown on a receptor cell line defective for wild-type virus binding, such as P84SYS/HYSA, a large reduction in burst size was evident when compared to wild-type virus growth. This indicated that the combination of defects in the binding site of the virus and of hPVR caused further inefficiency in the early steps of infection. Therefore, mutant receptors may provide a more sensitive tool than the wild-type receptor to detect influences of viral mutations in standard binding assays and one-step growth curves. In the case of HRV-14, it was shown previously that canyon-bottom mutations defective in binding to hICAM-1 were also delayed in the timing of the eclipse (Colonno et al. 1988). Our PV1(M) mutants mapping to the canyon bottom have a similar phenotype of both binding and delay of eclipse (J.J. Harber et al., in prep.).

POLIOVIRUS NEUROVIRULENCE IN WILD-TYPE MICE

As pointed out before, PV can infect only primates, among whom humans are the only natural host. The narrow host range for mammalian cells of primate origin is, for the most part, determined by the PVR expressed by these cells (see Freistadt, this volume). The mouse homolog to PVR (Morrison and Racaniello 1992; Aoki et al. 1994) cannot serve as surrogate receptor for PV as it lacks the ability to bind any of the PV strains tested.

Early efforts to develop animal models for the study of poliomyelitis led to the selection of mouse-adapted PV strains. The first was a 1937 field isolate from a fatal case in Lansing, Michigan, which upon intracerebral passage, first in cotton rats and subsequently in white mice, caused a syndrome in these rodents termed "polioencephalitis" (Armstrong 1939). It was later determined that the virus was a type-2 PV (PV2[L]). Most of the early PV strains displaying the mouse neurovirulent (*mn*) phenotype where of the same serotype. Interestingly, some field isolates of type-2 polioviruses were found to possess the *mn* phenotype without adaptation, as, for example, PV2(MEF-1) isolated in 1941 in Cairo, Egypt (Schlesinger et al. 1943), or PV2(IND) isolated in 1992 in India (O. Kew, pers. comm.). Adaptation of type-1 and type-3 viruses to mouse neurovirulence appeared difficult in the 1930s and 1940s, when methods like plaque assay and PV propagation in nonneuronal tissue cultures had not yet been developed. However, Li and Schaeffer (1954) reported the isolation of a *mn* derivative of PV1(M), termed PV1(LS-a). The parental strain was passaged 14 times in monkey testicular and kidney tissue cells and 60 times through the mouse CNS, after which it had accumulated 54 point mutations (Li and Schaeffer 1954; Lu et al. 1994b). More recently, the passage of PV1(M) in mouse CNS yielded PV variants with the potential of being *mn*. The resulting viruses had one or very few mutations mapping to the capsid proteins (Moss and Racaniello 1991; Couderc et al. 1993).

What is the molecular basis of the *mn* phenotype of PV strains in wild-type mice? Neither the dissection of the genotypes of *mn* viruses in terms of transplanting different parts of the *mn* genome back into a wild-type virus, nor an analysis of the pathology of the disease syndrome caused by mouse-adapted PV strains, has yielded an answer.

1. None of the known *mn* strains can infect mouse tissue culture cells. Thus, the ability to bind to, and penetrate, mouse cell membranes appears to be restricted to cells in the mouse CNS.

2. Mouse cells expressing MPH are not permissive to infection with a *mn* PV strain such as PV2(L) (Racaniello 1992). MPH by itself, therefore, may not play a role in PV mouse neurovirulence.

3. Genetic alterations of PV1(M), leading to the *mn* phenotype, can be of very different nature: (a) a change of very few amino acids in the VP1 BC loop (N-AgIa; see above), a structure well exposed at the surface of the virion, as determined through the construction of a PV1(M) mutant whose VP1 loop was replaced by that of PV2(L) (Martin et al. 1988; Murray et al. 1988); (b) mutations in capsid protein VP1 in combination with mutations in the coding region for the nonstructural protein 2A^{pro} as in PV1(LS-a) (Lu et al. 1994b), and (c) point mutations leading to one or a few amino acid exchanges of capsid proteins VP1 or VP2, located on the inner surface of the capsid protein shell (Moss and Racaniello 1991; Couderc et al. 1993). Clearly, capsid mutations, whether located inside the capsid or on the outside of the shell, play a major role in the expression of the *mn* phenotype, but the involvement of the coding region of 2A^{pro} in *mn* of PV1(LS-a) was surprising. Nevertheless, except for the Mahoney/Lansing antigenic hybrid, most capsid mutations are able to affect capsid stability (Moss and Racaniello 1991; Couderc et al. 1993; Lu et al. 1994b).

4. Whereas infection of transgenic mice expressing the hPVR with wild-type PV consistently yields a syndrome reminiscent of primate poliomyelitis (as given by the exclusive eradication of anterior horn motor neurons), infection of wild-type mice with *mn* PV strains produced highly variable appearances of neurological syndromes that differed dramatically depending on the *mn* strain applied to infect the animals (M. Gromeier et al., in prep.). Accordingly, none of the *mn* strains studied by Gromeier et al. (in prep.) produced poliomyelitis (as seen in primates) in wild-type mice. This is not surprising, since the progression of the neurological disease leading to primate poliomyelitis depends on the specific expression of the PVR (see Koike et al., this volume). Since the mouse homolog MPH of hPVR cannot function as a PV receptor, *mn* strains must use unknown pathways of cell entry independent of MPH. Whatever the nature of receptor(s) for the *mn* PV strains in wild-type mice is, the receptors may not be distributed like the hPVR in humans or hPVR transgenic mice; this may explain the development of different disease syndromes caused by *mn* PV strains in mice (M. Gromeier et al., in prep.).

CONCLUSION

Entry of PV into primate cells is mediated by cell-surface glycoproteins that belong to the immunoglobulin superfamily. Of these, the hPVR-related proteins have been characterized in great detail, but the regulation of expression of the cognate hPVR gene in different tissues, possibly by alternative splicing, is poorly understood. Moreover, the function(s) of the hPVR-related proteins, either of the membrane-associated or of the excreted splice variants, is obscure.

Available evidence suggests that hPVRα and hPVRδ are the only proteins that PV can use as receptor in human tissue culture cells. This does not exclude the possibility that other proteins, such as the 100-kD polypeptide described by Shepley (this volume), play a role in early steps of the infection. Some field isolates of PV2 and several mouse-adapted PV1 and PV2 strains, on the other hand, are able to infect cells of the mouse CNS. Since the mouse homolog (MPH) of hPVR cannot function as a PV receptor, these *mn* polioviruses must infect the target mouse cells via a mechanism that appears to bypass hPVR-like polypeptides. Not surprisingly, polioviruses expressing the mn phenotype do not cause poliomyelitis in wild-type mice but, depending on the viral isolate, cause a whole spectrum of neurological syndromes. Whether PV variants can enter a similar, hPVR-unrelated pathway of cell invasion in the human CNS, thereby producing neurological disease other than poliomyelitis, such as meningitis, remains a fascinating, but unanswered question.

Mutational analysis of hPVR has shown that the amino-terminal V domain of the three-domain Ig-like glycoprotein is necessary and sufficient to function as a PV receptor. The other two C2 domains, however, are involved in providing a scaffold for the normal folding of the V domain to occur. Surprisingly, removal of four *N*-glycosylation sites (two in each of the V domains and adjacent C2 domains) increases virus binding.

Computer-aided modeling has revealed that the V domain of hPVR may assume a conformation related to that of the amino-terminal V domain of the lymphocyte T4 receptor CD4 (Harrison, this volume). The V domain appears to interact with PV1(M) not by insertion of its tip into the canyon, but through interactions of regions mapping to the side of the Ig-like fold. This is different from the results obtained with the major receptor group of rhinoviruses, but it resembles the interaction between CD4 and gp120 of HIV (Harrison, this volume). Studies with viral capsid mutants suggest that the PV canyon is involved in the virus/receptor interaction.

The interaction of purified hPVR with poliovirions at 37°C destabilizes the virion and leads to the loss of VP4 and the formation of A particles, a reaction that is likely to be the first step in uncoating. This process can be completed before uptake into the host cell and, as a consequence, A particles may be "sloughed off" the cell surface. Since A particles are not infectious, conversion of virions to the subviral entity before uptake leads to an abortion of infection. Whether this plays a role in the pathology of human PV infections remains unknown. One could envision, however, that efficient excretion of soluble hPVR molecules, leading to high local concentrations of the receptor molecules in specific tissues, may protect cells from PV invasion. Apart from the interferon response and antibody-mediated neutralization, this may be a very clever mechanism of host defense against an otherwise very stable and highly virulent infectious agent.

ACKNOWLEDGMENTS

Work in the laboratory of E.W. was supported by grants provided by the National Institutes of Health, the National Cancer Institute, the World Health Organization, and the Human Frontier Science Program. G.B. and M.G. are recipients of fellowships of the Stipendiumprogramm "Infektionsforschung," Heidelberg, Germany. J.J.H. and J.A.B. were members of the graduate training programs in Genetics and in Molecular and Cellular Biology at SUNY, Stony Brook, respectively.

REFERENCES

Altmeyer, R., A.D. Murdin, J.J. Harber, and E. Wimmer. 1991. Construction and characterization of a poliovirus/rhinovirus antigenic hybrid. *Virology.* **184:** 636.

Aoki, J., S. Koike, I. Ise, Y. Sato-Yoshida, and A. Nomoto. 1994. Amino acid residues on human poliovirus receptor involved in interaction with poliovirus. *J. Biol. Chem.* **269:** 8431.

Armstrong, C. 1939. Successful transfer of the Lansing strain of poliomyelitis virus from the cotton rat to the white mouse. *Public Health Rep.* **54:** 2302.

Arthos, J., K.C. Deen, M.A. Chaikin, J.A. Fornwald, G. Sathe, Q. Sattentau, P.R. Clapham, R.A. Weiss, J.S. McDougal, C. Pietropaolo, R. Axel, A. Truneh, P.J. Maddon, and R.W. Sweet. 1989. Identification of the residues in human CD4 critical for the binding of HIV. *Cell* **57:** 469.

Ashkenazi, A., L.G. Presta, S.A. Marsters, T.R. Camerato, K.A. Rosenthal, B.M. Fendly, and D.J. Capon. 1990. Mapping the CD4 binding site for human immunodeficiency virus by alanine scanning mutagenesis. *Proc. Natl. Acad. Sci.* **87:** 7150.

Barnert, R.H., H. Zeichhardt, and K.O. Habermehl. 1992. Identification of 50- and 23-25-kDa HeLa cell membrane glycoproteins involved in poliovirus infection: Occurrence of poliovirus specific binding sites on susceptible and nonsusceptible cells. *Virology* **186:** 533.

Bernhardt, G., J.A. Bibb, J. Bradley, and E. Wimmer. 1994a. Molecular characterization of the cellular receptor for poliovirus. *Virology* **199:** 105.

Bernhardt, G., J.J. Harber, A. Zibert, M. deCrombrugghe, and E. Wimmer. 1994b. The poliovirus receptor: Identification of domains and amino acid residues critical for virus binding. *Virology* **203**: 344.

Bibb, J.A., G. Bernhardt, and E. Wimmer. 1994a. Cleavage site of the signal sequence of the poliovirus receptor. *J. Gen. Virol.* **75**: 1875.

————. 1994b. The human poliovirus receptor alpha is a serine phosphoprotein. *J. Virol.* **68**: 6111.

Bibb, J.A., G. Witherell, G. Bernhardt, and E. Wimmer. 1994c. Interaction of poliovirus with its cell surface binding site. *Virology.* **201**: 107.

Chan, V.F. and F.L. Black. 1970. Uncoating of poliovirus by isolated membranes. *J. Virol.* **5**: 309.

Chapman, M.S. and M.G. Rossmann. 1993. Comparison of surface properties of picornaviruses: Strategies for hiding the receptor site from immune surveillance. *Virology.* **195**: 745.

Colonno, R.J., P.L. Callahan, D.M. Leippe, R.R. Rueckert, and J.E. Tomassisi. 1989. Inhibition of rhinovirus attachment by neutralizing monoclonal antibodies and their Fab fragments. *J. Virol.* **63**: 36.

Colonno, R.J., J.H. Condra, S. Mizutani, P.L. Callahan, M.E. Davies, and M.A. Murcko. 1988. Evidence for the direct involvement of the rhinovirus canyon in receptor binding. *Proc. Natl. Acad. Sci.* **85**: 5449.

Colston, E.M. and V.R. Racaniello. 1992. Capsid residues that control structural transitions in poliovirus during cell entry. *J. Cell. Biochem. Suppl.* **16C**: 116. (Abstr.)

Couderc, T., J. Hogle, H. LeBlay, F. Horaud, and B. Blondel. 1993. Molecular characterization of mouse-virulent poliovirus type 1 Mahoney mutants: Involvement of residues of polypeptides VP1 and VP2 located on the inner surface of the capsid protein shell. *J. Virol.* **67**: 3808.

Crowell, R.L. and B.J. Landau. 1983. Receptors in the initiation of picornavirus infections. In *Comprehensive virology* (ed. H. Fraenkel-Conrat and R.R. Wagner), p. 1. Plenum Press, New York.

Crowell, R.L. and L. Philipson. 1971. Specific alterations of Coxsackie virus B3 eluted from HeLa cells. *J. Virol.* **8**: 509.

DeSena, J. and B. Mandel. 1976. Studies on the in vitro uncoating of poliovirus 1. Characterization of the modifying factor and the modifying reaction. *Virology* **70**: 470.

————. 1977. Studies on the in vitro uncoating of poliovirus 1. Characterization of the membrane-modified particle. *Virology.* **78**: 554.

Freistadt, M.S. and V.R. Racaniello. 1991. Mutational analysis of the cellular receptor for poliovirus. *J. Virol.* **65**: 3873.

Freistadt, M., H.B. Fleit, and E. Wimmer. 1993. Poliovirus receptor on human blood cells: A possible extraneural site of poliovirus replication. *Virology.* **195**: 798.

Fricks, C.E. and J.M. Hogle. 1990. Cell-induced conformational change of poliovirus: Externalization of the amino terminus of VP1 is responsible for liposome binding. *J. Virol.* **64**: 1934.

Gomez-Yafal, A., G. Kaplan, V.R. Racaniello, and J.M. Hogle. 1993. Characterization of poliovirus conformational alteration mediated by soluble cell receptors. *Virology* **197**: 501.

Guttman, N. and D. Baltimore. 1977. A plasma membrane component able to bind and alter virions of poliovirus type 1: Studies on cell free alteration using a simplified assay. *Virology.* **82**: 25.

Hogle, J.M. and D.J. Filman. 1989. The antigenic structure of poliovirus. *Philos. Trans. R. Soc. Lond. B Biol. Sci.* **323**: 467.

Hogle, J.M., M. Chow, and D.J. Filman. 1985. The three dimensional structure of poliovirus at 2.9 Å resolution. *Science* **229**: 1358.

Holland, J.J. 1961. Receptor affinities as major determinants of enterovirus tissue tropism in humans. *Virology* **15**: 312.

Holland, J.J. and B.H. Hoyer. 1963. Early stages of enterovirus infection. *Cold Spring Harbor Symp. Quant. Biol.* **27**: 101.

Holland, J.J., L.C. McLaren, and J.T. Syverton. 1959. Mammalian cell-virus relationship. III. Poliovirus production by non-primate cells exposed to poliovirus ribonucleic acid. *Proc. Soc. Exp. Biol. Med.* **100**: 843.

Horie, H., S. Koike, T. Kurata, Y. Sato-Yoshida, I. Ise, Y. Ota, S. Abe, K. Hioki, H. Kato, C. Taya, T. Nomura, S. Hashizume, H. Yonekawa, and A. Nomoto. 1994. Transgenic mice carrying the human poliovirus receptor: New animal model for study of poliovirus neurovirulence. *J. Virol.* **68**: 681.

Kaplan, G., M.S. Freistadt, and V.R. Racaniello. 1990a. Neutralization of poliovirus by cell receptors expressed in insect cells. *J. Virol.* **64**: 4697.

Kaplan, G., D. Peters, and V.R. Racaniello. 1990b. Poliovirus mutants resistant to neutralization with soluble cell receptors. *Science* **250**: 1596.

Kitamura, N., B.L. Semler, P.G. Rothberg, G.R. Larsen, C.J. Adler, A.J. Dorner, E.A. Emini, R. Hanecak, J. Lee, S. van der Werf, C.W. Anderson, and E. Wimmer. 1981. Primary structure, gene organization and polypeptide expression of poliovirus RNA. *Nature* **291**: 547.

Koike, S., I. Ise, and A. Nomoto. 1991a. Functional domains of the poliovirus receptor. *Proc. Natl. Acad. Sci.* **88**: 4104.

Koike, S., I. Ise, Y. Sato, H. Yonekawa, O. Gotoh, and A. Nomoto. 1992a. A second gene for the African green monkey poliovirus receptor that has no putative N-glycosylation site in the functional N-terminal immunoglobulin-like domain. *J. Virol.* **66**: 7059.

Koike, S., I. Ise, Y. Sato, K. Mitsui, H. Horie, H. Umeyama, and A. Nomoto. 1992b. Early events of poliovirus infection. *Semin. Virol.* **3**: 109.

Koike, S., C. Taya, T. Kurata, S. Abe, I. Ise, H. Yonekawa, and A. Nomoto. 1991b. Transgenic mice susceptible to poliovirus. *Proc. Natl. Acad. Sci.* **88**: 951.

Koike, S., H. Horie, I. Ise, A. Okitsu, M. Yoshida, N. Iizuka, K. Takeuchi, T. Takegami, and A. Nomoto. 1990. The poliovirus receptor protein is produced both as membrane-bound and secreted forms. *EMBO J.* **9**: 3217.

Kraulis, P.J. 1991. MOLSCRIPT: A program to produce both detailed and schematic plots of protein structures. *J. Appl. Crystallogr.* **24**: 946.

Li, C.P. and M. Schaeffer. 1954. Isolation of a non-neurotropic variant of type 1 poliomyelitis virus. *Proc. Soc. Exp. Biol. Med.* **87**: 148.

Littman, D.R., Y. Thomas, P.J. Maddon, L. Chess, and R. Axel. 1985. The isolation and sequence of the gene encoding T8: A molecule defining functional classes of T lymphocytes. *Cell* **40**: 237.

Lonberg-Holm, K., L.B. Gosser, and E.J. Shimshick. 1976. Interaction of liposomes with subviral particles of poliovirus type 2 and rhinovirus type 2. *J. Virol.* **19**: 746.

Lu, H.-H., L. Alexander, and E. Wimmer. 1994a. Antigenic and dicistronic poliovirus hybrids as a novel delivery system for foreign antigens. In *Novel delivery systems for oral vaccines* (ed. D.T. O'Hagan), p. 129. CRC Press, Boca Raton, Florida.

Lu, H.-H., C.-F. Yang, A.D. Murdin, J.J. Harber, O.M. Kew, and E. Wimmer. 1994b. Mouse-neurovirulence determinants of poliovirus type 1 strain LS—A map to the coding regions of capsid protein VP1 and proteinase 2A^{pro}. *J. Virol.* (in press).

Mannweiler, K., P. Nobis, H. Hohenberg, and W. Bohn. 1990. Immunoelectron microscopy on the topographical distribution of the poliovirus receptor. *J. Gen. Virol.* **71**:

2737.

Martin, A., C. Wychowski, T. Couderc, R. Crainic, J. Hogle, and M. Girard. 1988. Engineering a poliovirus type 2 antigenic site on a type 1 capsid results in a chimaeric virus which is neurovirulent for mice. *EMBO J.* **7:** 2839.

McLaren, L.C., J.J. Holland, and J.T. Syverton. 1959. The mammalian cell-virus relationship. I. Attachment of poliovirus to cultivated cells of primate and non-primate origin. *J. Exp. Med.* **109:** 475.

McLaren, L.C., J.V. Scaletti, and C.G. James. 1968. Isolation and properties of enterovirus receptors. In *Biological properties of the mammalian surface membrane* (ed. L.A. Manson), p. 123. Wistar Institute, Philadelphia.

Medrano, L. and H. Green. 1973. Picornavirus receptors and picornavirus multiplication in human mouse hybrid cell lines. *Virology.* **54:** 515.

Mendelsohn, C.L., E. Wimmer, and V.R. Racaniello. 1989. Cellular receptor for poliovirus: Molecular cloning, nucleotide sequence, and expression of a new member of the immunoglobulin superfamily. *Cell* **56:** 855.

Mendelsohn, C., B. Johnson, K.A. Lionetti, P. Nobis, E. Wimmer, and V.R. Racaniello. 1986. Transformation of a human poliovirus receptor gene into mouse cells. *Proc. Natl. Acad. Sci.* **83:** 7845.

Miller, D.A., O.J. Miller, V.G. Dev, S. Hashmi, R. Tantravahi, L. Medrano, and H. Green. 1974. Human chromosome 19 carries a poliovirus receptor gene. *Cell* **1:** 167.

Minor, P.D. 1990. Antigenic structure of picornaviruses. *Curr. Top. Microbiol. Immunol.* **161:** 121.

Minor, P.D., P.A. Pipkin, D. Hockley, G.C. Schild, and J.W. Almond. 1984. Monoclonal antibodies which block cellular receptors of poliovirus. *Virus Res.* **1:** 203.

Moebius, U., P. Pallai, C.H. Harrison, and E.L. Reinherz. 1993. Delineation of an extended surface contact area on human CD4 involved in class II major histocompatibility complex binding. *Proc. Natl. Acad. Sci.* **90:** 8259.

Moebius, U., L.K. Clayton, S. Abraham, S.C. Harrison, and E.L. Reinherz. 1992a. The human immunodeficiency virus gp120 binding site on CD4: Delineation by quantitative equilibrium and kinetic binding studies of mutants in conjunction with a high-resolution CD4 atomic structure. *J. Exp. Med.* **176:** 507.

Moebius, U., L.K. Clayton, S. Abraham, A. Diener, J.J. Yunis, S.C. Harrison, and E.L. Reinherz. 1992b. Human immunodeficiency virus gp120 binding C'C'' ridge of CD4 domain 1 is also involved in interaction with class II major histocompatibility complex molecules. *Proc. Natl. Acad. Sci.* **89:** 12008.

Morgan-Detjen, B., J. Lucas, and E. Wimmer. 1978. Poliovirus single-stranded and double-stranded RNA: Differential infectivity in enucleated cells. *J. Virol.* **27:** 582.

Morrison, M.E. and V.R. Racaniello. 1992. Molecular cloning and expression of a murine homolog of the human poliovirus receptor gene. *J. Virol.* **66:** 2807.

Morrison, M.E., Y.-J. He, M.W. Wien, J.M. Hogle, and V.R. Racaniello. 1994. Homolog-scanning mutagenesis reveals poliovirus receptor residues important for virus binding and replication. *J. Virol.* **68:** 2578.

Moss, E. and V.R. Racaniello. 1991. Host range determinants located on the interior of the poliovirus capsid. *EMBO J.* **10:** 1067.

Murdin, A.D., H.H. Lu, M.G. Murray, and E. Wimmer. 1992. Poliovirus antigenic hybrids simultaneously expressing antigenic determinants from all three serotypes. *J. Gen. Virol.* **73:** 607.

Murray, M.G., J. Bradley, X.-F. Yang, E. Wimmer, E.G. Moss, and V.R. Racaniello. 1988a. Poliovirus host range is determined by a short amino acid sequence in neutralization antigenic site I. *Science* **241:** 213.

Murray, M.G., R.J. Kuhn, M. Arita, N. Kawamura, A. Nomoto, and E. Wimmer. 1988b. Poliovirus type 1/type 3 antigenic hybrid virus constructed in vitro elicits type 1 and type 3 neutralizing antibodies in rabbits and monkeys. *Proc. Natl. Acad. Sci.* **85:** 3203.

Nichols, A., K.A. Sharp, and B. Honig. 1991. Protein folding and association: Insights from the interfacial and thermodynamic properties of hydrocarbons. *Proteins Struct. Funct. Genet.* **11:** 281.

Nobis, P., R. Zibirre, G. Meyer, J. Kühne, G. Warnecke, and G. Koch. 1985. Production of a monoclonal antibody against an epitope on HeLa cells that is the functional poliovirus binding site. *J. Gen. Virol.* **66:** 2563.

Peterson, A. and B. Seed. 1988. Genetic analysis for monoclonal antibody and HIV binding sites on the human lymphocyte antigen CD4. *Cell* **54:** 66.

Racaniello, V.R. 1992. Interaction of poliovirus with its cell receptor. *Semin. Virol.* **3:** 473.

Ren, R. and V.R. Racaniello. 1992a. Poliovirus spreads from muscle to the central nervous system by neural pathways. *J. Infect. Dis.* **166:** 747.

———. 1992b. Human poliovirus receptor gene expression and poliovirus tissue tropism in transgenic mice. *J. Virol.* **66:** 296.

Ren, R., F. Costantini, E.J. Gorgacz, J.J. Lee, and V.R. Racaniello. 1990. Transgenic mice expressing a human poliovirus receptor: A new model for poliomyelitis. *Cell* **63:** 353.

Roesing, T.G., P.A. Toselli, and R.L. Crowell. 1975. Elution and uncoating of coxsackievirus B3 by isolated HeLa cell plasma membranes. *J. Virol.* **15:** 654.

Rossmann, M.G. 1989. The canyon hypothesis. Hiding the host cell receptor attachment site on a viral surface from immune surveillance. *J. Biol. Chem.* **264:** 14587.

Rossmann, M.G. and J.E. Johnson. 1989. Icosahedral RNA virus structure. *Annu. Rev. Biochem.* **58:** 533.

Rossmann, M.G., E. Arnold, J.W. Erickson, E.A. Frankenberger, J.P. Griffith, H.J. Hecht, J.E. Johnson, G. Kamer, M. Luo, A.G. Mosser, R.R. Rueckert, B. Sherry, and G. Vriend. 1985. Structure of a human common cold virus and functional relationship to other picornaviruses. *Nature* **317:** 145.

Rueckert, R.R. 1976. On the structure and morphogenesis of picornaviruses. In *Comprehensive virology* (ed. H. Fraenkel-Conrat and R.R. Wagner), vol. 6, p. 131. Plenum Press, New York.

Schlesinger, R.W., J.M. Morgan, and P.K. Olitsky. 1943. Transmission to rodents of Lansing type poliomyelitis virus originating in the Middle East. *Science* **98:** 452.

Schonk, D., P. van Dijk, P. Riegmann, J. Trapman, C. Holm, T.C. Willcocks, P. Sillekens, W. van Venrooij, E. Wimmer, A. Geurts van Kessel, H.-H. Ropers, and B. Wieringa. 1989. Assignment of seven genes to distinct intervals on the midportion of human chromosome 19q surrounding the myotonic dystrophy gene region. *Cytogenet. Cell Genet.* **54:** 15.

Selinka, H.C., A. Zibert, and E. Wimmer. 1991. Poliovirus can enter and infect mammalian cells by way of an intercellular adhesion molecule 1 pathway. *Proc. Natl. Acad. Sci.* **88:** 3598.

———. 1992. A chimeric poliovirus/CD4 receptor confers susceptibility to poliovirus on mouse cells. *J. Virol.* **66:** 2523.

Shepley, M.P. and V.R. Racaniello. 1994. A monoclonal antibody that blocks poliovirus attachment recognizes the lymphocyte homing receptor CD44. *J. Virol.* **68:** 1301.

Shih, C., L.C. Padhy, M. Murray, and R.A. Weinberg. 1981. Transforming genes of carcinomas and neuroblastomas introduced into mouse fibroblasts. *Nature* **290:** 261.

Siddique, T., R. McKinney, W.-Y. Hung, R.J. Bartlett, G. Bruns, T.K. Mohandas, H.-H.

Ropers, C. Wilfert, and A.D. Roses. 1988. The poliovirus sensitivity (PVS) gene is on chromosome 19q12-q13.2. *Genomics* **3:** 156.

von Heinje, G. 1985. Signal sequences. The limits of variation. *J. Mol. Biol.* **184:** 99.

Wenner, H.A., P. Kamitsuka, M. Lenahan, and I. Archetti. 1959. The pathogenesis of poliomyelitis. Sites of multiplication of poliovirus in cynomolgus monkeys after alimentary infection. *Arch. Gesamte Virusforsch.* **9:** 558.

Wiegers, K.J. and R. Dernick. 1987. Binding site of neutralizing monoclonal antibodies obtained after in vivo priming with purified VP1 of poliovirus type 1 is located between amino acid residues 93 and 104 of VP1. *Virology* **157:** 248.

Wimmer, E., C.U.T. Hellen, and X.M. Cao. 1993. Genetics of poliovirus. *Annu. Rev. Genet.* **27:** 353.

Zibert, A. and E. Wimmer. 1992. N-glycosylation of the virus binding domain is not essential for function of the human poliovirus receptor. *J. Virol.* **66:** 7368.

Zibert, A., H.C. Selinka, O. Elroy-Stein, and E. Wimmer. 1992. The soluble form of two N-terminal domains of the poliovirus receptor are sufficient for blocking viral infection. *Virus Res.* **25:** 51.

Zibert, A., H.C. Selinka, O. Elroy-Stein, B. Moss, and E. Wimmer. 1991. Vaccinia virus-mediated expression and identification of the human poliovirus receptor. *Virology* **182:** 250.

8

Entry of Minor Group Human Rhinoviruses into the Cell

Dieter Blaas, Franz Hofer,
Martin Gruenberger, Heinrich Kowalski,
Herwig Machat, and Ernst Kuechler
Institute of Biochemistry
Medical Faculty, University of Vienna
A-1030 Vienna, Austria

Manfred Huettinger
Institute of Medical Chemistry
Medical Faculty, University of Vienna
A-1090 Vienna, Austria

So far, there are 102 immunologically characterized serotypes of human rhinoviruses (HRVs), the main pathogens of the common cold (Uncapher et al. 1991). HRVs belong to the large family of picornaviridae, characterized by an icosahedral protein shell assembled of 60 protomers which in turn contain one copy of the viral capsid proteins VP1 through VP4 (for review, see Stanway 1990). The RNA genome is of positive polarity and about 7500 nucleotides in length. Following entry into the cytoplasm, it is translated into a polyprotein, which is cotranslationally cleaved into the structural and nonstructural proteins by two virus-encoded proteinases (see, e.g., Kuechler et al. 1993). Concomitantly with RNA encapsidation, a maturation cleavage of VP0 to VP2 and VP4 takes place. This is carried out by a proteinase which has not yet been identified.

The majority (91 serotypes) of the HRVs gain access to the cell via the intercellular adhesion molecule 1 (ICAM-1). How this protein manages the rapid delivery of the virus into the cell is not clear, since it is devoid of an internalization signal in its cytoplasmic carboxy-terminal region (Greve et al. 1989; Staunton et al. 1989; Tomassini et al. 1989). Only one serotype (HRV-87) attaches to a sialylated membrane protein of unknown function. However, the remainder of 10 serotypes, the minor receptor group, is internalized via membrane proteins which for a long time escaped identification. Whereas major group viruses exclusively bind to cells of human or primate origin, minor group viruses attach to cells of a large variety of species; nevertheless, in most cases no replication takes place. Since receptor-negative cells are therefore not available, the common strategy of transfection and screening for the gain of binding activity or for the appearance of viral replication was not applicable. Thus, classic protein purification methodology was employed to enrich and characterize the minor group receptor. Fortunately, this protein withstands mild denaturation conditions as used for polyacrylamide gel electrophoresis in the absence of reducing agents and transfer to nitrocellulose membranes (Mischak et al. 1988b). Therefore, ligand blots could be used to follow the enrichment of the binding activity during the various purification steps. This technique enabled us to purify a soluble form of the minor group receptor from the supernatant of HeLa cells grown in suspension (Hofer et al. 1992). The material thus obtained was proteolytically cleaved, and selected peptides were subjected to amino-terminal protein sequencing. The peptides showed identity with the sequence of the human low-density lipoprotein receptor (LDLR). Moreover, use of ligand blotting also indicated that the α_2-macroglobulin receptor/LDLR-related protein (α_2MR/LRP) was recognized by minor receptor group viruses as well. HRVs of the minor receptor group type therefore bind to LDLR, to α_2MR/LRP, and probably to other members of the LDLR family (Hofer et al. 1994).

A RHINOVIRUS MINOR GROUP BINDING PROTEIN IS RELEASED INTO THE CELL SUPERNATANT

In the course of experiments aimed to purify the rhinovirus minor group receptor from HeLa cell membranes (Mischak et al. 1988a), we reasoned that this membrane protein could possibly be released from the cell surface as a soluble fragment by treatment with various hydrolytic enzymes. This would make the use of detergents for the solubilization of the membrane-bound receptor unnecessary. Therefore, cells were incubated with trypsin, papain, and phospholipase C, respectively. The supernatants were concentrated and applied onto polyacrylamide gels, and the polypeptides were separated under nonreducing conditions. The proteins were transferred onto immobilon membranes, which were then probed for virus-binding activity with ^{35}S-labeled HRV-2, a prototype of the minor receptor group (Mischak et al. 1988b). Although the material obtained from the incubations with the enzymes lacked any binding activity, HRV-2 attached to two proteins of apparent molecular weights of about 85 kD and 100 kD present in the supernatant of the control incubations carried out in the absence of any enzymes (Hofer et al. 1992). Further experiments established that these proteins were indeed of cellular origin and not serum components trapped onto the cell surface. More-over, the 85-kD polypeptide turned out to be a degradation product of the larger protein. When the incubation of cells was performed in the presence of metal chelators such as EDTA, EGTA, or o-phenanthroline, no binding activity could be recovered. From these experiments, it was concluded that the HRV-binding protein was released by a Ca^{++}-dependent process (Hofer et al. 1992).

IDENTIFICATION OF THE HRV-BINDING PROTEIN AS HUMAN LDLR

As we had shown that a protein with binding activity for minor receptor group HRVs was released from HeLa cells upon mere incubation with buffer, we reasoned that this protein might also be shed into the medium upon growing the cells under normal tissue culture conditions. Applying a purification scheme, comprising chromatography on an anion ex-changer, on *Lens culinaris* lectin, ammonium sulfate precipitation, chro-matography on *Jacalin* agarose, and MonoQ ion-exchange chromatog-raphy (Mischak et al. 1988a; Hofer et al. 1994), the binding protein was isolated from 200 liters of HeLa cell culture supernatant. A homo-geneous preparation was obtained by preparative polyacrylamide gel electro-phoresis. The material was subjected to tryptic digestion and resolved by reversed-phase HPLC, and six selected peptides were sub-jected to amino-terminal protein sequencing. When the amino acid se-quences thus obtained were compared to the SwissProt databank, it turned out that they all were derived from the LDLR (Yamamoto et al. 1984). Moreover, the presence of a valine at position 612 unequivocally identified the isolated protein as a fragment of the human LDLR, since the bovine protein contains an isoleucine at the equivalent position (Rus-sell et al. 1984). This excluded the possibility of the isolated protein's being a component of the cell culture medium.

HRVs OF THE MINOR RECEPTOR GROUP ATTACH TO THE CELLS VIA THE LDLR

To examine whether the LDLR was also responsible for the attachment and internalization of HRVs by living cells, [^{35}S]methionine-labeled HRV-2 was incubated with normal human fibroblasts and fibroblasts from a patient with familial hypercholesteremia (FH), which are deficient in the LDLR, respectively. The expression level of the LDLR is subject to regulation by the serum concentration of sterols. Therefore, both cell types were grown either in delipidated serum or in the presence of cholesterol/25-hydroxy cholesterol preceding the binding experiment (Davis et al. 1987). As shown in Figure 1A, FH cells internalized only 5% of the amount of HRV-2 internalized into normal human fibroblasts under conditions of LDLR up-regulation. If the LDLR was down-regulated (i.e., in presence of the sterols), however, internalization into normal fibroblasts was reduced to about 7%. Binding of HRV-2 was abolished by heating of the virus to 56°C, a treatment which destroys the ability of HRVs to bind to their receptors (Lonberg-Holm and Yin 1973). Binding was also reduced to background levels by the presence of a thousandfold excess of cold HRV-2 during incubation. As expected, FH cells grown under both tissue culture conditions (i.e., up- or down-regulation of the LDLR) showed no significant difference in virus internalization. The same amount of ^{35}S-labeled HRV-14 associated with both normal human fibroblasts and FH fibroblasts regardless of the growth conditions employed in this experiment.

LDL and HRV-2 mutually competed for the binding sites on the cell surface (Fig. 1B). When unlabeled purified HRV-2 was present during

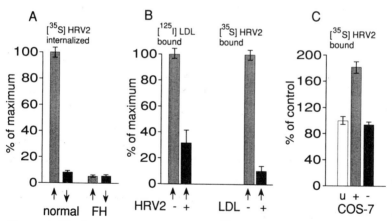

Figure 1 Binding and internalization of ^{35}S-labeled HRV-2 to cells under various conditions. (A) Normal human fibroblasts or FH cells were grown either in the absence (↑) or in the presence (↓) of sterols and incubated with labeled HRV-2. Internalized virus was measured after removal of surface-bound HRV with trypsin and EDTA. (B) Fibroblasts were grown as in A in the absence of sterols; ^{35}S-labeled virus or ^{125}I-labeled LDL binding was determined in the presence or in the absence of an excess of the respective unlabeled competitor. (C) COS-7 cells were transfected with pSVL-LDLr $^+$ (+) or pSVL-LDLr $^-$ ($-$) respectively, and grown in the presence of the sterols to suppress expression of endogenous LDLR. Binding of ^{35}S-labeled HRV-2 was determined 36 hr post-transfection as in B. Radioactivity bound to untransfected cells (u) was set to 100%.

the incubation of the cells with ^{125}I-labeled LDL (Huettinger et al. 1992), binding was reduced to about one third. Likewise, unlabeled LDL decreased the binding of ^{35}S-labeled HRV-2 to about 10%. Similar to the results of Beisiegel et al. (1982) who found only partial inhibition of LDL binding by the LDLR-specific monoclonal antibody IgG-C7, incubation of the cells with this particular antibody prior to challenge with HRV-2 reduced virus binding to about 50%.

OVEREXPRESSION OF THE LDLR IS CORRELATED WITH INCREASED HRV BINDING

COS-7 cells were transfected with the eukaryotic expression vector pSVL carrying the entire coding sequence of the human LDLR in the sense (pSVL-LDLr$^+$) or in the antisense (pSVL-LDLr$^-$) orientation and were tested for virus binding. When the cells were grown in the presence of cholesterol/25-hydroxy cholesterol in order to suppress the production of endogenous LDLRs, twice as much HRV-2 was attached to those cells which carried the sense construction when compared to cells with the antisense construction or to untransfected cells (Fig. 1C).

LDLR-DEFICIENT HUMAN FIBROBLASTS CAN BE INFECTED WITH HRV-2

Since the attachment of HRV-2 to normal fibroblasts was clearly dependent on the amount of LDLR present on the cells, one would have expected that cells deficient in this receptor would not allow virus to enter and would therefore be refractive to infection. Nevertheless, the small amount of virus that was found to associate to FH fibroblasts suggested the existence of an additional binding protein(s) different from the LDLR. Therefore, it was not surprising that the FH cells could be infected with HRV-2. However, despite the considerable difference in the amount of virus bound to FH cells and to normal fibroblasts, respectively, both cell types showed similar cytopathic effects after infection. Virus yields from normal human fibroblasts grown in LDL-free medium exceeded those from cells with down-regulated LDLR by a factor of about 100, whereas FH cells gave intermediate yields. As a control, cells were infected with the major group virus HRV-14 under the same conditions; as expected, the virus yield varied only marginally as a function of up- or down-regulation of the LDLR.

α_2MR/LRP ALSO BINDS HRVs OF THE MINOR RECEPTOR GROUP

The latter results indeed indicated the presence of an additional receptor(s) which permitted HRV-2 to infect cells — although with a somewhat lower yield—in the absence of a functional LDLR. A potential candidate for such a receptor is another member of the LDLR family, α_2MR/LRP (Herz et al. 1988; Kowal et al. 1989; Strickland et al. 1990). This large polypeptide is synthesized as a 600-kD precursor. It is cleaved into a 515-kD and an 85-kD subunit in the *trans* Golgi, which remain non-covalently associated (Herz et al. 1990). In contrast to the 7 cysteine-rich repeats present in the LDLR, the large subunit of the α_2MR/LRP contains 31 such repeats which are thought to be involved in binding the various ligands of this multifunctional protein (Herz et al. 1988).

Plasma membrane extracts were prepared from normal fibroblasts and from FH cells, respectively, and the material was applied onto gradient SDS polyacrylamide gels that permit large polypeptides to be resolved (Fig. 2). The separated proteins were transferred onto nitrocellulose paper and probed with ^{35}S-labeled HRV-2. In the extract obtained from normal fibroblasts (lane 1), as well as from FH cells (lane 3), HRV-2 bound to a protein with an approximate molecular mass of 500 kD. Identity of this protein with α_2MR/LRP was revealed with a specific antiserum (lanes 2 and 4), which not only recognizes the high-molecular-

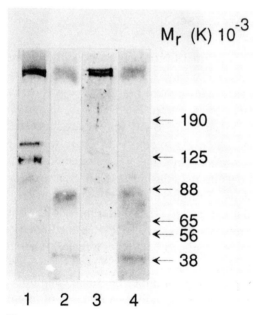

M_r (K) 10^{-3}

← 190

← 125

← 88

← 65
← 56

← 38

1   2   3   4

Figure 2   HRV-2 binds to the LDLR and to α_2MR/LRP on ligand blots. Membrane proteins from normal fibroblasts (lanes *1* and *2*) and from FH cells (lanes *3* and *4*) were electrophoresed under nonreducing conditions, transferred to nitrocellulose, and probed with ^{35}S-labeled HRV-2 (lanes *1* and *3*) or with an antiserum against α_2MR/LRP (lanes *2* and *4*).

weight component, but also the noncovalently associated 84-kD subunit and the 39-kD receptor-associated protein (Moestrup and Gliemann 1991). Binding of HRV-2 to a protein of apparent molecular mass of about 120 kD was evident only in the extracts made from normal fibroblasts (lane 1). Comigration of this protein with the LDLR was verified with the monoclonal antibody IgG-C7 (Beisiegel et al. 1981); extracts made from FH cells lacked the band corresponding to the LDLR (data not shown).

RECEPTOR-ASSOCIATED PROTEIN INHIBITS INFECTION OF LDLR-DEFICIENT HUMAN FIBROBLASTS

A protein of an approximate molecular mass of 39 kD was identified in preparations of α_2MR/LRP (Herz et al. 1991) and was termed receptor-associated protein (RAP). It was shown to control the activity of the latter receptor, possibly by changing its conformation and thereby preventing the attachment of various ligands (Williams et al. 1992). Incubation of FH cells with recombinant RAP prior to infection with HRV-2 indeed reduced the cytopathic effect, whereas all cells were killed by HRV-14 under the same conditions. To more quantitatively investigate the inhibitory effect, the yield of HRV-2 as a function of the concentration of RAP was determined. As shown in Figure 3, there is indeed a relationship between the virus yield and the concentration of RAP present during infection, with a decrease to about 10% at the highest concentration tested. Again, no effect of RAP was seen in controls with HRV-14.

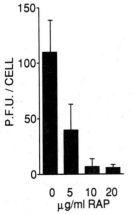

Figure 3   Virus yields obtained from FH cells infected with HRV-2 in the presence of various concentrations of recombinant RAP. Infectious virus was determined by plaque assays.

CONCLUSIONS

Human rhinoviruses of the minor group type attach to the LDLR and to α_2MR/LRP. Both proteins require the presence of Ca^{++} ions for their stability (Herz et al. 1988); removal of those ions with complexing agents might have destroyed the integrity of the LDLR or, indeed, activated a proteinase as originally suggested (Hofer et al. 1992).

There is a clear correlation between the amount of LDLR present on the cell surface and the amount of HRV-2 attaching to the cells. Furthermore, the virus yield obtained after infection depends on the number of LDLRs. However, cells lacking LDLR (FH fibroblasts) are capable of supporting HRV-2 replication. In these FH cells, virus production is reduced by preincubation with RAP, also clearly establishing the role of α_2MR/LRP in viral infection. However, it is not understood why cells deficient in the LDLR give rise to almost as much virus progeny as normal cells, despite attaching only less than 10% of the amount of HRV-2 bound to normal fibroblasts. Both the LDLR and α_2MR/LRP are designed for the internalization of various ligands and their ultimate delivery to lysosomes. This is in marked contrast to the poliovirus receptor (Mendelsohn et al. 1989) and to the rhinovirus major group receptor, which belong to the immunoglobulin superfamily and lack internalization signals. Nevertheless, both are highly efficient in delivering their respective viral ligands into the cell. Since monoclonal anti-ICAM-1 antibodies remain stably associated with the receptor for more than 48 hours and effectively block infection, major group HRV internalization is possibly triggered by multivalent attachment (Colonno et al. 1986).

Whether the comparably high virus yield of FH cells is due to transport of the HRV-2 to different cellular compartments via the α_2MR/LRP as compared to the LDLR, or whether the receptors differ in their efficiency of supporting RNA release, remains to be seen. It is conceivable that LDLR-bound virions might give rise to a higher proportion of abortive infection, whereas α_2MR/LRP delivers the RNA genome to the cytoplasm more effectively. This model, however, does not explain why the virus yield of normal cells with down-regulated LDLR is lower than that of FH cells. Nevertheless, our findings are in line with recent data of Choi and Cooper (1993), who have demonstrated that in cells expressing both the LDLR and α_2MR/LRP, the contribution of the latter is difficult to prove for ligands shared by both proteins.

The presence of at least two different receptors for minor group HRVs renders it much more difficult to completely interrupt the transport of the viruses into the cell; this even more so as mutual competition of the various ligands binding to the multifunctional receptor α_2MR/LRP is never complete. Since no human cells with a deficiency in both the

LDLR and α_2MR/LRP are available (and may never be because they are presumably not viable), it is not possible to experimentally exclude the presence of still another minor group receptor.

The three-dimensional structures of HRV-1A and HRV-14, members of the minor and of the major receptor group, respectively, are available (Rossmann et al. 1985; Kim et al. 1989). Both show a deep crevice, the canyon, encircling the axis of the fivefold symmetry of the icosahedric viral shell. For HRV-14, it has been shown that the site of interaction with the receptor is at the bottom of this canyon. By extrapolation, this is presumably also true for all other major group HRVs. Whereas the monomeric ICAM-1 is able to penetrate into this canyon, the tetrameric IgGs as well as dimeric Fab fragments are too large to interact with the amino acid residues in this region. This allows a certain conservation of amino acid clusters in the receptor-binding site, since they escape the immune surveillance (Rossmann 1989; Chapman and Rossmann 1993).

No structure is yet available for the LDLR or for α_2MR/LRP. One reason for this is the difficulty of obtaining sufficient amounts of purified protein. Moreover, the comparable large number of cysteines present in these proteins precludes the expression of the native proteins in bacteria due to misfolding. The question whether the interaction of minor group viruses with their receptor(s) also takes place at the bottom of the canyon is therefore still open. Site-directed mutagenesis of residues in HRV-2 equivalent to the ones involved in the interaction between HRV-14 and ICAM-1 have mostly led to inviable virus (Duechler et al. 1993). The only indication that the attachment site might be different between the two virus groups comes from the finding that a Pro:Gly mutation equivalent to the one leading to increased binding in HRV-14 was without effect in HRV-2. It is hoped that cryoelectron microscopy image reconstruction (Olson et al. 1993) of complexes between minor group HRVs with their receptors will yield indications about the site of interaction in the future.

Major group viruses as well as poliovirus are neutralized when incubated with their respective receptors at 37°C. The role of this catalytic effect for the viral life cycle is not understood, since mutants resistant to receptor-mediated neutralization are still viable (Kaplan et al. 1990a,b; Greve et al. 1991; Hooverlitty and Greve 1993). Due to lack of sufficient material, it has not yet been possible to examine the effect of LDLR or α_2MR/LRP on minor group HRVs.

Recently, another member of the LDLR family has been identified as a viral receptor by a transfection cloning strategy (Bates et al. 1993; Young et al. 1993). This membrane protein can serve as a receptor for the retrovirus subgroup A Rous sarcoma virus when expressed in mouse cells. Interestingly, in contrast to the rather low specificity of minor group HRVs which attach to at least two members of the LDLR family, these retroviruses have so far been shown to recognize only this small protein, apparently via a domain similar to the cysteine-rich repeats characteristic of all members of the family. Surprisingly, this protein has not been identified in normal avian cells susceptible to Rous sarcoma virus, although specific antisera inhibit infection. The characteristics necessary for recognition of the various members of the LDLR family by the different viruses will be the subject of further studies.

ACKNOWLEDGMENTS

This work was supported by the Austrian Ministry of Science, the Austrian Science Foundation, and by Boehringer Ingelheim.

REFERENCES

Bates, P., J.A.T. Young, and H.E. Varmus. 1993. A receptor for subgroup A Rous sarcoma virus is related to the low density lipoprotein receptor. *Cell* **74:** 1043.

Beisiegel, U., W.J. Schneider, M.S. Brown, and J.L. Goldstein. 1982. Immunoblot analysis of low density lipoprotein receptors in fibroblasts from subjects with familial hypercholesterolemia. *J. Biol. Chem.* **257:** 13150.

Beisiegel, U., W.J. Schneider, J.L. Goldstein, R.G.W. Anderson, and M.S. Brown. 1981. Monoclonal antibodies to the low density lipoprotein receptor as probes for study of receptor-mediated endocytosis and the genetics of familial hypercholesterolemia. *J. Biol. Chem.* **256:** 11923.

Chapman, M.S. and M.G. Rossmann. 1993. Comparison of surface properties of picornaviruses: Strategies of hiding the receptor site from immune surveillance. *Virology* **195:** 745.

Choi, S.Y. and A.D. Cooper. 1993. A comparison of the roles of the low density lipoprotein (LDL) receptor and the LDL receptor-related protein/α_2-macroglobulin receptor in chylomicron remnant removal in the mouse *in vivo. J. Biol. Chem.* **268:** 15804.

Colonno, R.J., P.L. Callahan, and W.J. Long. 1986. Isolation of a monoclonal antibody that blocks attachment of the major group of human rhinoviruses. *J. Virol.* **57:** 7.

Davis, C.G., J.L. Goldstein, T.C. Südhof, R.G.W. Anderson, D.W. Russell, and M.S. Brown. 1987. Acid-dependent ligand dissociation and recycling of LDL receptor mediated by growth factor homology region. *Nature* **326:** 760.

Duechler, M., S. Ketter, T. Skern. E. Kuechler, and D. Blaas. 1993. Rhinoviral receptor discrimination: The canyon regions of HRV14 and HRV2 have different sensitivities to mutational change. *J. Gen. Virol.* **74:** 2287.

Greve, J.M., C.P. Forte, C.W. Marlor, A.M. Meyer, H. Hooverlitty, D. Wunderlich, and A. McClelland. 1991. Mechanisms of receptor-mediated rhinovirus neutralization defined by two soluble forms of ICAM-1. *J. Virol.* **65:** 6015.

Greve, J.M., G. Davis, A.M. Meyer, C.P. Forte, S. Connolly-Yost, C.W. Marlor, M.E. Kamarck, and A. McClelland. 1989. The major human rhinovirus receptor is ICAM-1.

Cell **56**: 839.

Herz, J., R.C. Kowal, J.L. Goldstein, and M.S. Brown. 1990. Proteolytic processing of the 600 kd low density lipoprotein receptor-related protein (LRP) occurs in a *trans*-Golgi compartment. *EMBO J.* **9**: 1769.

Herz, J., J.L. Goldstein, D.K. Strickland, Y.K. Ho, and M.S. Brown. 1991. 39-kDa protein modulates binding of ligands to low density lipoprotein receptor-related protein/α_2-macroglobulin receptor. *J. Biol. Chem.* **266**: 21232.

Herz, J., U. Hamann, S. Rogne, O. Myklebost, H. Gausepohl, and K.K. Stanley. 1988. Surface location and affinity for calcium of a 500-kd liver membrane protein closely related to the LDL-receptor suggests a physiological role as lipoprotein receptor. *EMBO J.* **7**: 4119.

Hofer, F., M. Gruenberger, H. Kowalski, H. Machat, M. Huettinger, E. Kuechler, and D. Blaas. 1994. Members of the low density lipoprotein receptor family mediate cell entry of a minor group common cold virus. *Proc. Natl. Acad. Sci.* **91**: 1839.

Hofer, F., B. Berger, M. Gruenberger, H. Machat, R. Dernick, U. Tessmer, E. Kuechler, and D. Blaas. 1992. Shedding of a rhinovirus minor group binding protein: Evidence for a Ca^{++}-dependent process. *J. Gen. Virol.* **73**: 627.

Hooverlitty, H. and Greve, J.M. 1993. Formation of rhinovirus-soluble ICAM-1 complexes and conformational changes in the virion. *J. Virol.* **67**: 390.

Huettinger, M., H. Retzek, M. Hermann, and H. Goldenberg. 1992. Lactoferrin specifically inhibits endocytosis of chylomicron remnants but not alpha-macroglobulin. *J. Biol. Chem.* **267**: 18551.

Kaplan, G., M.S. Freistadt, and V.R. Racaniello. 1990a. Neutralization of poliovirus by cell receptors expressed in insect cells. *J. Virol.* **64**: 4697.

Kaplan, G., D. Peters, and V.R. Racaniello. 1990b. Poliovirus mutants resistant to neutralization with soluble cell receptors. *Science* **250**: 1596.

Kim, S., T.J. Smith, M.S. Chapman, M.G. Rossmann, D.C. Pevear, F.J. Dutko, P.J. Felock, G.D. Diana, and M.A. McKinlay. 1989. Crystal structure of human rhinovirus serotype 1A (HRV1A). *J. Mol. Biol.* **210**: 91.

Kowal, R.C., J. Herz, J.L. Goldstein, V. Esser, and M.S. Brown. 1989. Low density lipoprotein receptor-related protein mediates uptake of cholesterol esters derived from apoprotein E-enriched lipoproteins. *Proc. Natl. Acad. Sci.* **86**: 5810.

Kuechler, E., H.-D. Liebig, M. Luderer, H. Klump, D. Blaas, and T. Skern. 1993. Strategies of human rhinoviruses. In *Virus strategies, molecular biology and pathogenesis* (ed. W. Doerfler and P. Böhm), p. 97, VCH Verlagsgesellschaft mbH, Weinheim, Germany.

Lonberg-Holm, K. and F.H. Yin. 1973. Antigenic determinants of infective and inactivated human rhinovirus type 2. *J. Virol.* **12**: 114.

Mendelsohn, C.L., E. Wimmer, and V. Racaniello. 1989. Cellular receptor for poliovirus: Molecular cloning, nucleotide sequence, and expression of a new member of the immunoglobulin superfamily. *Cell* **56**: 855.

Mischak, H., C. Neubauer, E. Kuechler, and D. Blaas. 1988a. Characteristics of the minor group receptor of human rhinoviruses. *Virology* **163**: 19.

Mischak, H., C. Neubauer, B. Berger, E. Kuechler, and D. Blaas. 1988b. Detection of the human rhinovirus minor group receptor on renaturing western blots. *J. Gen. Virol.* **69**: 2653.

Moestrup, S.K. and J. Gliemann. 1991. Analysis of ligand recognition by purified α_2-macroglobulin receptor (low density lipoprotein receptor-related protein). *J. Biol. Chem.* **266**: 14011.

Olson, N.H., P.R. Kolatkar, M.A. Oliveira, R.H. Cheng, J.M. Greve, A. McClelland, T.S.

Baker, and M.G. Rossmann. 1993. Structure of a human rhinovirus complexed with its receptor molecule. *Proc. Natl. Acad. Sci.* **90:** 507.

Rossmann, M.G. 1989. The canyon hypothesis — Hiding the host cell receptor attachment site on a viral surface from immune surveillance. *J. Biol. Chem.* **264:** 14587.

Rossmann, M.G., E. Arnold, J.W. Erickson, E.A. Frankenburger, J.P. Griffith, H.-J. Hecht, J.E. Johnson, G. Kramer, M. Luo, A. G. Mosser, R.R. Rueckert, B. Sherry, and G. Vriend. 1985. Structure of a human common cold virus and functional relationship to other picornaviruses. *Nature* **317:** 145.

Russell, D.W., W.J. Schneider, T. Yamamoto, K.L. Luskey, M.S. Brown, and J.L. Goldstein. 1984. Domain map of the LDL receptor: Sequence homology with the epidermal growth factor precursor. *Cell* **37:** 577.

Stanway, G. 1990. Structure, function and evolution of picornaviruses. *J. Gen. Virol.* **71:** 2483.

Staunton, D.E., V.J. Merluzzi, R. Rothlein, R. Barton, S.D. Marlin, and T.A. Springer. 1989. A cell adhesion molecule, ICAM-1, is the major surface receptor for rhinoviruses. *Cell* **56:** 849.

Strickland, D.K., J.D. Ashcom, S. Williams, W.H. Burgess, M. Migliorini, and W.S. Argraves. 1990. Sequence identity between the α_2-macroglobulin receptor and low density lipoprotein receptor-related protein suggests that this molecule is a multifunctional receptor. *J. Biol. Chem.* **265:** 17401.

Tomassini, E., D. Graham, C. DeWitt, D. Lineberger, J. Rodkey, and R. Colonno. 1989. cDNA cloning reveals that the major group rhinovirus receptor on HeLa cells is intercellular adhesion molecule 1. *Proc. Natl. Acad. Sci.* **86:** 4907.

Uncapher, C.R., C.M. DeWitt, and R.J. Colonno. 1991. The major and minor group receptor families contain all but one human rhinovirus serotype. *Virology* **180:** 814.

Williams, S.E., J.D. Ashcom, W.S. Argraves, and D.K. Strickland. 1992. A novel mechanism for controlling the activity of α_2-macroglobulin receptor/low density lipoprotein receptor-related protein. *J. Biol. Chem.* **267:** 9035.

Yamamoto, T., C.G. Davis, M.S. Brown, W.J. Schneider, M.L. Casey, J.L. Goldstein, and D.W. Russell. 1984. The human LDL receptor: A cysteine-rich protein with multiple Alu sequences in its mRNA. *Cell* **39:** 27.

Young, J.A.T., P. Bates, and H.E. Varmus. 1993. Isolation of a chicken gene that confers susceptibility to infection by subgroup A avian leukosis and sarcoma viruses. *J. Virol.* **67:** 1811.

9

Cellular Receptors for Alphaviruses

James H. Strauss, Tillmann Rümenapf,[1]
Ronald C. Weir,[2] Richard J. Kuhn,[3]
Kang-Sheng Wang,[4] and Ellen G. Strauss
Division of Biology
California Institute of Technology
Pasadena, California 91125

Receptors on host cells that are used by viruses to enter cells and initiate infection have received a great deal of attention of late because of their obvious importance in determining in large part the host range, tissue tropism, and virulence of a virus. The alphaviruses represent an interesting and special situation. The members of this group have an enormous host range that comprises both invertebrate hosts and vertebrate hosts (Chamberlain 1980; Griffin 1986; Niklasson 1988; Peters and Dalrymple 1990). All alphaviruses are transmitted by arthropod vectors, in which the virus replicates. Mosquitoes are used as vectors by most alphaviruses, but Fort Morgan and Bijou Bridge viruses are vectored by swallow bugs, and several alphaviruses, including Sindbis virus (SIN) (Shah et al. 1960) and eastern equine encephalitis virus (EEE) (Scott and Weaver 1989), have been isolated from mites and other hematophagous arthropods as well as from mosquitoes. In the case of EEE, the major vector is the mosquito *Culiseta melanura*, but other mosquitoes can also transmit the virus and naturally infected chicken mites have been shown to be able to transmit the virus, albeit inefficiently. During the process of mosquito transmission, the virus must productively infect several tissues within the mosquito. The virus is ingested when the insect feeds on a viremic host and first infects cells of the midgut; later the infection must spread to the salivary glands in order for the mosquito to transmit the virus when it next feeds on a vertebrate. A wide variety of vertebrates, mainly birds and mammals but also amphibians and reptiles, serve as hosts for alphaviruses. Within vertebrates, alphaviruses replicate in a wide variety of

Present addresses: [1]Bundesforschungsanstalt für Viruskrankheiten der Tiere, Paul-Ehrlich Strasse 28, D-7400 Tübingen, Germany; [2]Biochemistry Department, Faculty of Science, Australian National University, GPO Box 4, Canberra, ACT, 2601, Australia; [3]Department of Biological Sciences, Purdue University, West Lafayette, Indiana 47907; [4]Chiron Corporation, 4560 Horton Street, Emeryville, California 94608.

cells, including neurons and glial cells, striate and smooth muscle cells, cells of lymphoid origin, synovial cells, and brown fat cells; for transmission they must cause a viremia sufficiently intense to infect a mosquito taking a blood meal. As examples of a broad vertebrate host range, birds serve as the primary vertebrate hosts for both SIN and EEE, but EEE causes encephalitis in man and strains of SIN cause polyarthritis in man. How do SIN and other alphaviruses achieve their enormous host range? Do they use a conserved receptor found throughout the animal kingdom, or have they evolved the ability to recognize more than one receptor, or both? All alphaviruses are closely related and share a minimum of 35% amino acid sequence identity in the glycoproteins that attach to the cell. Do all alphaviruses use the same receptor(s) or do different alphaviruses use different receptors? In this chapter, we describe a number of studies from our laboratory and from other laboratories that address these issues. These studies have shown that alphaviruses use protein receptors, that different alphaviruses may use the same or different receptors, that a given virus can use more than one receptor and may use different receptors in different cells, that the nature of the receptors used affects the virulence of the virus, and that one or a few amino acid changes in the envelope glycoproteins can lead to utilization of different sets of receptors.

STRUCTURE OF ALPHAVIRUSES

The alphaviruses contain a plus-strand RNA genome of about 12 kb (Strauss and Strauss 1986). The genomic RNA is translated to produce nonstructural proteins required for replication of the RNA and for transcription of a subgenomic messenger of about 4 kb called 26S RNA. The structural proteins that are assembled into progeny virions are translated from the subgenomic RNA. These consist of a basic nucleocapsid protein of about 30 kD and two envelope glycoproteins called E1 and E2. The capsid protein assembles with the viral genomic RNA in the cytoplasm to form a T = 4 icosahedral nucleocapsid, so that 240 molecules of capsid protein are present in the nucleocapsid (Paredes et al. 1993). The envelope proteins are transported to the cell plasma membrane and virions form when the nucleocapsid buds through the plasma membrane and acquires an envelope containing cell-derived lipids, but only viral glycoproteins. The glycoproteins are present in the virus in a T = 4 icosahedral lattice as 80 trimers of E1-E2 heterodimers (von Bonsdorff and Harrison 1975; Fuller 1987; Paredes et al. 1993). These trimers are called spikes, and it is the spikes that bind to receptors on the surface of a susceptible cell to initiate virus infection. The 1:1 molar ratio between glycoproteins and capsid protein is thought to arise in part from a specific interaction between the cytoplasmic domain of each E2 glycoprotein and a capsid protein subunit (Garoff and Simons 1974; Lopez et al. 1994).

EARLY STUDIES OF ALPHAVIRUS RECEPTORS

The number of alphavirus receptors on the surface of a cell has been examined by electron microscopy (Birdwell and Strauss 1974) and by quantitation of labeled virus bound to cells (Fries and Helenius 1979; Smith and Tignor 1980). The number of receptors varied between 4×10^4 and 4×10^6 per cell, depending on the virus, the cell line, and even the individual cell. The apparent binding constant for Semliki forest virus (SF) was 10^{10} to 10^{11} M^{-1}.

Early studies that examined the nature of the receptors for alphaviruses reached the conclusion that the receptors for SIN were proteins because treatment of cells with proteases, but not with phospholipases or neuraminidases, greatly reduced or abolished virus binding (Smith and Tignor 1980). These authors studied two strains of SIN, a neurovirulent strain AR86 isolated from South Africa and a nonvirulent strain AR339 isolated from Egypt. They found that the two strains did not compete with one another for binding and thus concluded that these viruses used completely different receptors. They also found that two different neuronal cell lines contained many more receptors for the neurovirulent strain than for the avirulent strain, and in fact contained more receptors for the neurovirulent strain than did nonneuronal cells for either strain. Thus, the nature of the receptors used appeared to determine at least in part the virulence of the virus. Finally, they found that SIN AR86 and EEE partially competed for binding and suggested that these two neurovirulent alphaviruses shared some of their receptors; the fact that the competition was only partial suggested that each virus can use more than one receptor.

Maassen and Terhorst (1981) attempted to identify receptors for SIN on lymphoblastic cell lines. They showed that the SIN glycoproteins could be cross-linked to a cell-surface protein of 90 kD and concluded that this protein must either be a SIN receptor or be found near the SIN receptor.

Helenius et al. (1978) suggested that antigens of the major histocompatibility complex (MHC), HLA-A and HLA-B in humans or H-2K and H-2D in mice, served as receptors for SF, based on their findings that these MHC antigens bound to SF glycoproteins. This binding was demonstrated in several different ways, including the isolation of specific complexes between the spike glycoproteins and MHC antigens. It is important to note, however, that MHC antigens are expressed in large amounts by the cells used and these cells, nevertheless, do not serve as efficient host cells. Subsequently, it was found that murine F9 and PCC4 teratoma cells that did not express H-2 MHC antigens, as well as H-2⁻ murine lymphoblastoid cells, were nonetheless sensitive to infection by SF, demonstrating that H-2 antigen expression is not required for infection by SF (Oldstone et al. 1980). Thus, it is unclear at present whether the binding of SF to MHC is functional for virus entry, but it is possible that MHC antigens serve as one of several possible receptors for SF.

ANTI-IDIOTYPIC ANTIBODIES AS ANTIRECEPTOR ANTIBODIES

We (Wang et al. 1991) and other workers (Ubol and Griffin 1991) have recently studied the use of anti-idiotypic antibodies as potential antireceptor antibodies for alphaviruses. At least some neutralizing monoclonal antibodies (MAbs) are thought to block virus binding to cells by binding to that domain of the virus that interacts with the receptor on the cell. Anti-idiotypic antibodies that express an internal image of the antibody idiotype may mimic the binding domain on the virus and thus serve as antireceptor antibodies (Gaulton and Greene 1986). For studies with alphaviruses, neutralizing monoclonal antibodies reactive with one of the glycoproteins of the virus, E1 or E2, were used to generate polyclonal anti-idiotypic antibodies in rabbits. Wang et al. (1991) found that three anti-idiotypic antibodies, all directed against glycoprotein E2, bound to chicken cells and blocked virus binding by about 50% (Fig. 1). One antibody, anti-Id 49 made to MAb 49, bound to chicken cells with the highest affinity and has been the most extensively characterized. Binding of this antibody to chicken cells as determined by fluorescence-activated cell sorting (FACS) assays is illustrated in Figure 2. Also shown in Figure 2 is the lack of reactivity of this antibody with BHK cells. The finding that an anti-idiotypic antibody made against a purified monoclonal antibody that was selected to be reactive with a virus would bind to the surface of uninfected chicken cells and block virus binding is strongly suggestive evidence that this antibody is an antireceptor antibody. Anti-Id 49 also immunoprecipitated a protein of about 63 kD from chicken membrane preparations that is a prospective receptor molecule (Fig. 3). Nothing is known about this protein at present other than its molecular weight and that it is expressed on the surface of chicken cells.

Further characterization of the effects of anti-Id 49 on infection of chicken cells suggested that there are at least two receptors in chicken cells and that the anti-idiotypic antibody recognizes only one of these.

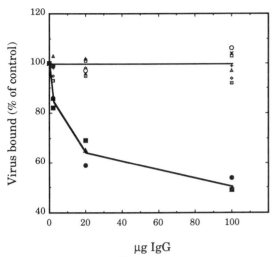

μg IgG

Figure 1 Binding of ³⁵S-labeled SIN to chicken cells in the presence of affinity-purified anti-idiotypic antibodies. Confluent monolayers of secondary chicken cells were incubated for 60 min at 0°C with affinity-purified anti-idiotypic antibody followed by incubation for 2 hr with purified ³⁵S-labeled SIN. The monolayers were washed and dissolved in 0.5% SDS, and the bound radioactivity was determined. Three anti-Ids blocked virus binding: (*filled box*) anti-Id 49; (*filled circle*) anti-Id 50; (*filled triangle*) anti-Id 23. Other anti-Ids and various control antisera indicated by other symbols did not interfere with virus binding. Reprinted, with permission, from Wang et al. (1991).

First, the antibody could only block virus binding by 50% (Fig. 1), suggesting that the virus can also bind to chicken cells by another receptor not recognized by the anti-idiotypic antibody. Second, a variant of SIN, called v49, was not blocked in its binding by anti-Id 49 (Fig. 4A). This variant was selected to be resistant to neutralization by MAb 49 and the amino acid difference that renders it resistant to MAb 49 is the change of Arg-214→Pro in glycoprotein E2. Thus, a single change in E2 renders v49 insensitive to the effects of the anti-idiotypic antibody, suggesting that it is no longer using the receptor recognized by anti-Id 49 to enter chicken cells. Presumably, v49 can utilize those receptors used by the 50% of the wild-type virus that are resistant to the effects of the anti-idiotypic antibody. The resistance of v49 to the effects of the antibody also makes it unlikely that the anti-idiotypic antibody simply interferes with the uptake of the virus in some nonspecific fashion and provides further evidence that anti-Id 49 is an internal image antibody.

Wang et al. (1991) also found that anti-Id 49 did not bind to BHK cells (Fig. 2) and had no effect on virus binding to BHK cells (Fig. 4B).

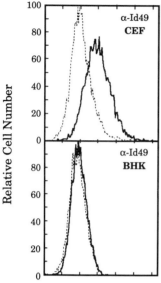

Figure 2   Binding of anti-idiotypic antibody 49 to chicken and BHK cells. Monolayers of chicken or BHK cells were washed, removed from the plate with EDTA, and treated with DNase. Affinity-purified anti-Id 49 (10 μg) was added to 10^6 cells in 250 μl and the cells were incubated for 40 min on ice. After washing, FITC-conjugated goat anti-rabbit IgG was added and the cells were incubated 30 min on ice. The cells were washed, filtered, and analyzed by FACS assay. Dashed lines indicate the distribution of cells reacted with preimmune serum and solid lines indicate cells reacted with the anti-idiotypic antiserum. Modified, with permission, from Wang et al. (1991).

This result indicates that the effect of the anti-Id on virus infectivity in chicken cells is not due to an inactivation of the virus by the antibody. Evidently, BHK cells do not express a homolog of the 63-kD chicken protein on their surface (or at least do not express a homolog which can be recognized by anti-Id 49), and thus the major receptors used by the virus to enter avian cells and hamster cells appear to be distinct.

Related results were reported by Ubol and Griffin (1991). These authors found that an anti-Id 209 bound to murine N18 neuroblastoma cells and blocked virus binding by 50%. This antibody immunoprecipitated proteins of 110 kD and 74 kD from N18 cells, suggesting that these proteins are receptors for SIN in neuronal cells. These proteins were present on mouse brain cells at birth as shown by the binding of anti-Id 209 to these cells, but by 4 days after birth, half of the cells had ceased expression of proteins reactive with the anti-Id. The temporal control of the expression of this protein may therefore be responsible for the age-

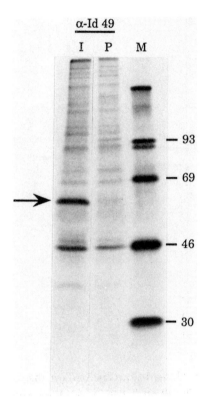

Figure 3 Precipitation of a chicken protein by anti-Id 49. A plasma membrane fraction was purified from secondary chicken fibroblasts labeled with [^{35}S]methionine and solubilized with Triton X-100. The extracts were precipitated with anti-Id 49 (I) or with preimmune serum (P) from the same rabbit. The lane marked M contains molecular-weight markers as indicated. A protein of 63 kD is specifically immunoprecipitated by the anti-Id 49 serum. Reprinted, with permission, from Wang et al. (1991).

dependent susceptibility of mice to fatal encephalitis caused by SIN (Griffin 1986). It is interesting that these authors also found only partial blocking by the anti-Id, suggesting that more than one receptor for the virus is also present on mouse neuronal cells.

LAMININ RECEPTOR AS A MAMMALIAN RECEPTOR

Wang et al. (1992), observing that their antireceptor antibody was effective for chicken cells but not for BHK cells, set out to obtain an antireceptor monoclonal antibody that would function for BHK cells. Mice were immunized with whole BHK cells, hybridoma supernatants were screened for virus-blocking activity, and a monoclonal antibody

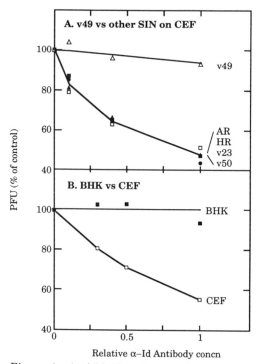

Figure 4   Anti-Id 49 antiserum does not block binding of SIN v49 to chicken cells nor SIN wild type to BHK cells. The ability of anti-Id 49 to block virus binding to chicken (CEF) or BHK cells was tested in a plaque assay. Confluent monolayers of secondary chicken cells were treated with the anti-Id for 90 min at room temperature; then an equal volume of buffer containing 200 pfu of SIN was added, and incubation continued for 60 min. The inoculum was removed and the monolayers overlaid with medium containing 1% agarose. After overnight incubation at 37°C, the plaques were visualized by staining with neutral red. In *A*, affinity-purified antiserum was used at a maximum concentration of 500 µg/ml. The different symbols indicate different strains of SIN, as indicated. (AR) Parental or wild-type strain. In *B*, unpurified antiserum was used at a maximum concentration of 10%. Modified, with permission, from Wang et al. (1991).

was isolated that blocked virus binding to BHK cells by up to 80% (Fig. 5). This monoclonal antibody, called 1C3, bound to BHK cells, as expected, and immunoprecipitated a protein of apparent molecular size 67 kD from membrane fractions of BHK cells. Screening of λgt11 libraries with MAb 1C3 revealed that it bound to the carboxy-terminal domain of a cell-surface protein referred to as the high-affinity laminin receptor. The nature of this protein is controversial at present. It was originally isolated as a 67-kD protein that bound to laminin with high affinity.

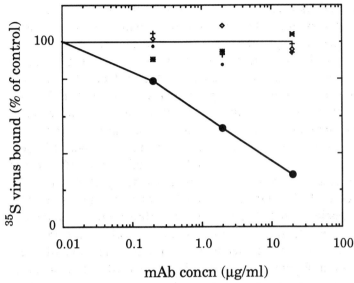

Figure 5   MAb 1C3 blocks SIN binding to BHK cells. BHK cells were in-cubated with affinity-purified MAb 1C3 at the indicated concentrations and the ability of ^{35}S-labeled SIN to bind to the treated cells was examined as in Fig. 1. (*Filled circle*) MAb 1C3. The other symbols indicate various control antibodies, including two MAbs, 2G8 (*open diamonds*) and 2B7 (*filled diamonds*) isolated during the search for 1C3 that bind to BHK cells but do not block virus binding. Modified, with permission, from Wang et al. (1992).

Screening of libraries with antibodies to this protein (Wewer et al. 1986; Grosso et al. 1991) identified an mRNA with an open reading frame (ORF) encoding a protein of only 295 amino acids; the same ORF was found by Wang et al. (1992) in their screening. There is no evidence for an mRNA encoding a longer ORF (Wewer et al. 1986; Rao et al. 1989; see also below), and considerable evidence has been presented that the 67-kD protein and the 295-amino-acid ORF possess amino acid sequence in common (Wewer et al. 1986, 1987; Castronovo et al. 1991a,b; K.-S. Wang et al., unpubl.). It has been proposed that the 295-residue protein is a precursor to the 67-kD form (for review, see Castronovo et al. 1991a). Glycosylation is not involved in the modification (Castronovo et al. 1991b; Grosso et al. 1991), and Castronovo et al. (1991a,b) have pro-posed that the 295-residue protein is covalently linked to another protein to produce the 67-kD form. Grosso et al. (1991), in contrast, have pro-posed that the 295-residue protein is unrelated to the laminin receptor and that the mRNA for the 67-kD protein is yet to be identified.

Castronovo et al. (1991a) found that antibodies made to synthetic peptides derived from the carboxy-terminal part of the 295-residue ORF (specifically, residues carboxy-terminal to position 107) would bind to intact cells, whereas antibodies to synthetic peptides from the region from 1 to 103 reacted only with permeabilized cells. This provides direct evidence that the 295-residue protein, or a protein sharing sequence identity with this protein, is expressed on the surface of cells. The antibody results together with a computer analysis (Rao et al. 1991) supported a model where the amino terminus is intracellular, residues 86–101 form a membrane-spanning domain, and the carboxyl terminus is extracellular. Castronovo et al. (1991a) also found that a synthetic peptide comprising residues 161–180 bound to laminin. MAb 1C3, which binds to the surface of BHK cells and blocks binding of SIN to BHK cells (Wang et al 1992), reacted with λgt11 clones containing residues 248–295, suggesting that SIN binds to this carboxy-terminal region of the protein. A schematic diagram showing how the 295-residue protein is thought to span the plasma membrane and illustrating the different regions is shown in Figure 6. If this protein is covalently bound to a second protein, it is unknown if the second protein also spans the membrane or is restricted to one side or the other of the membrane.

Transformation of hamster cells with vectors that overexpressed the

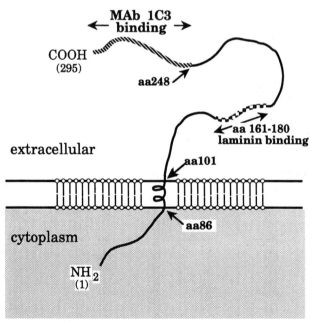

Figure 6 Schematic model for the orientation of the 295-residue protein of the high-affinity laminin receptor in the cell surface. The laminin-binding domain and the putative MAb 1C3-binding domain are indicated.

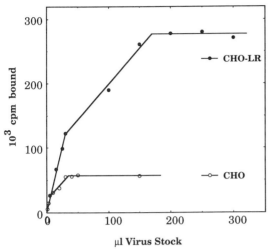

Figure 7 Overexpression of the 295-residue laminin receptor ORF results in increased binding of SIN to the surface of hamster cells. CHO cells were transformed with the 295-residue laminin receptor ORF in a high-efficiency mammalian expression vector (CHO-LR) or transformed with the vector only (CHO). Monolayers of each cell line were tested for their ability to bind ^{35}S-labeled SIN in a saturation binding assay. Conditions were similar to those in Fig. 1. Binding is saturable and the cells overexpressing the 295-residue ORF bind 4.6 times as much SIN at saturation. Reprinted, with permission, from Wang et al. (1992).

295-residue ORF gave rise to cells that bound up to four times as much radiolabeled virus, and the efficiency with which the virus formed plaques on such cells was increased by up to sevenfold. Binding of labeled virus to parental cells or to cells overexpressing the 295-residue protein was saturable (Fig. 7), suggesting that increased production of this protein leads to the presence of increased numbers of virus receptors on the cell surface. Expression of antisense RNA led to decreased sensitivity to the virus, suggesting that the antisense RNA interfered with the expression of this protein, and to the presence of fewer receptors on the cell surface. Cells transformed with the plus sense and antisense constructs were shown to bind more or less MAb 1C3, respectively, using FACS assays, directly demonstrating the presence of more or less protein reactive with 1C3 on the surface and consistent with the binding of more or less virus by these cells (Fig. 8). Quantitation of the amount of laminin receptor on the cell surface as assayed by the binding of 1C3, of the amount of radioactive virus bound, and of the sensitivity of the cell to virus infection as measured by a plaque assay, showed that binding of the virus varied linearly with the concentration of laminin receptor on the

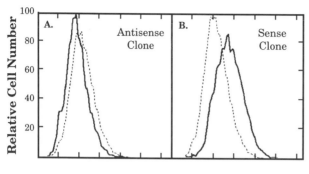

Fluorescent Intensity ⟶

Figure 8 Increased or decreased binding of MAb 1C3 to cells transformed with plus sense or minus sense cDNA encoding the 295-residue ORF. BHK cells were transformed with a high-efficiency mammalian vector expressing plus sense or minus sense 295-residue laminin receptor ORF. Transformed cells were tested for their ability to bind MAb 1C3 in a FACS assay as in Fig. 2. The dashed lines refer to cells transformed with vector only, the solid lines to cells transformed with antisense-expressing vector (*A*) or sense-expressing vector (*B*). Modified, with permission, from Wang et al. (1992).

cell surface, whereas the sensitivity to the virus measured by a plaque assay varied with the 1.4 power of the receptor concentration, suggesting that interaction with more than one receptor aids virus penetration (Fig. 9). Thus, the high-affinity laminin receptor as defined by the 295-residue protein is functionally a receptor or a part of a receptor for SIN in BHK cells.

MAb 1C3 was found to block virus binding to a number of other cultured mammalian cells tested, including murine, monkey, and human cells (Fig. 10). It thus appears that the high-affinity laminin receptor is a major receptor for Sindbis virus in all mammalian cells. This receptor, or at least the 295-residue ORF studied to date, is highly conserved among mammals. There are only two amino acid differences between the hamster sequence and a human sequence and between the hamster sequence and a bovine sequence; the hamster sequence was identical to a sequence obtained from mice (Wang et al. 1992). Because the laminin receptor is highly conserved in amino acid sequence among mammals and widely expressed, it appears that the ability of the virus to infect many different mammals and to infect many different tissues within mammals results at least in part from utilization by the virus of a highly conserved protein receptor. Wang et al. (1992) also found that 1C3 partially blocked binding of SIN to mosquito cells, suggesting that the laminin receptor is conserved in mosquito cells and serves as a receptor in these cells.

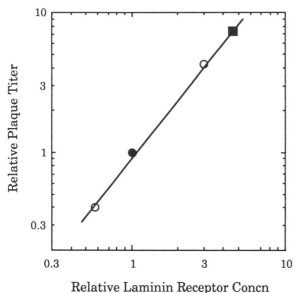

Figure 9   Plaque formation on hamster cells as a function of the number of laminin receptors expressed on their surface. Hamster cells were transformed with sense or antisense laminin receptor cDNA, and the ability of the cells to bind MAb 1C3 and/or labeled SIN was assayed. The cells were also tested for their ability to support formation of plaques by a defined number of virions under suboptimal conditions. The relative plaque titer varies as the 1.4 power of the number of receptor molecules expressed on the surface assayed by binding of 1C3 or of virus. (*Open circles*) BHK cells transformed with antisense or sense laminin receptor cDNA. (*Filled circle*) BHK or CHO cells transformed with vector only. (*Filled box*) CHO cells transformed with plus sense cDNA. Reprinted, with permission, from Wang et al. (1992).

CHICKEN LAMININ RECEPTOR

Although MAb 1C3 blocked virus binding to many different mammalian cells, it had only slight effects (~10%) on the binding of SIN to chicken cells (Fig. 10). This result complements those found with anti-Id 49, and the major receptor used by the virus to enter chicken cells must be different from that used to enter mammalian cells. The 63-kD chicken protein precipitated by anti-Id 49 is different from the chicken laminin receptor, because MAb 1C3 was found to precipitate a protein of 71 kD, presumably the chicken laminin receptor, from chicken membranes.

The reactivity of the apparent chicken laminin receptor with MAb 1C3 suggested that the chicken protein was closely related to the mammalian protein. This conclusion was strengthened by Northern blot analysis of chicken RNA using hamster cDNA encoding the 295-residue

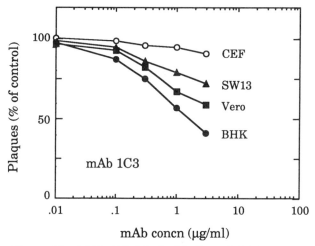

Figure 10 MAb 1C3 blocks binding of SIN to mammalian cells but not to chicken cells. Various mammalian cells (SW13 is a strain of human adenocarcinoma cells, Vero are green monkey kidney cells, BHK are baby hamster kidney cells) or chicken (CEF) cells were treated with MAb 1C3 at the indicated concentrations and tested for their ability to support plaque formation by SIN (see Fig. 4). Modified, with permission, from Wang et al. (1992).

ORF. Washing the blot at low stringency revealed a labeled 1.2-kb RNA band (Fig. 11); note that only one band is seen in RNA from any of the cell lines probed. The chicken gene therefore shares sufficient nucleotide sequence identity with the hamster gene to react with the hamster probe; the laminin receptor gene is single copy in birds but present in multiple copies in mammals (Bignon et al. 1992), and this seems to be reflected in the presence of smaller amounts of reactive mRNA in chicken than in hamster cells. Using this information, a chicken cDNA library was prepared and screened with the hamster probe. Several positive clones were identified and two clones containing the longest inserts were sequenced. The 1006-nucleotide sequence obtained is shown in Figure 12.

The chicken laminin receptor ORF is 296 residues in length. The protein encoded is very similar to the mammalian protein. There is one amino acid inserted in the chicken protein (Pro-241) relative to the mammalian proteins. In the remaining 295 residues, there are only 5 amino acid differences between chicken and hamster or mouse and 6 differences between chicken and man or cow (~98% amino acid sequence identity). The extraordinary conservation of this protein between birds and mammals, which diverged more than 200 million years ago, is remarkable. The high level of conservation is consistent with the finding

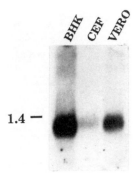

Figure 11 Northern blot of RNA reactive with cDNA for the 295-residue laminin receptor ORF. Total RNA (10 μg) from BHK cells, chicken embryo cells, or Vero cells was treated with 0.2 M glyoxal and separated on a denaturing 0.8% agarose gel. RNA was transferred to a filter, and the filter was hybridized at low stringency (48°C, 7% SDS, 0.5 M Na$_2$HPO$_4$) to a cDNA probe derived from a clone of the BHK laminin receptor (T. Rümenapf, unpubl.).

that MAb 1C3 reacts with mosquito cells and suggests that the mosquito protein may also share considerable sequence identity with the vertebrate proteins. The extreme conservation of the 295-residue protein suggests an ancient function for this protein that tolerates little change in sequence, consistent with its being a component of a receptor for laminin, as the interaction between cells and laminin in basement membranes has apparently changed little during the evolution of multicellular organisms.

The similarity in the sequence of the chicken and mammalian laminin receptors suggests that the chicken protein could be used by the virus as a receptor. Apparently, however, there is a virus receptor on chicken cells to which the virus binds with higher affinity and which is possibly present in greater amounts. The fact that alphaviruses utilize a different protein for a receptor on chicken cells, even when a homolog of the BHK receptor is available, is consistent with the hypothesis that the very broad host range of the virus is achieved in part by the ability to use more than one protein as a receptor.

A MOSQUITO RECEPTOR FOR VEE

G.V. Ludwig and J.V. Smith (pers. comm.) have recently developed a direct binding assay to search for mosquito cell receptors for alphaviruses. Proteins from plasma membrane preparations were separated on acrylamide gels and transferred to nitrocellulose, and the blot was probed with radiolabeled Venezuelan equine encephalitis virus (VEE). The virus bound to a protein of 32 kD that was expressed on the surface

```
  1 TCC CGC GAG GCC TCC ACA CGG CGT TGT CCA CGT TCC CTG TCG TCG CTT CCT AAG GGA AAC

 61 CCC ACG ATG TCC GGA GGT CTC GAT GTC CTG CAG ATG AAG GAG GAG GAT GTC CTC AAG TTT
  1         M   S   G   G   L   D   V   L   Q   M   K   E   E   D   V   L   K   F
                      *
121 CTT GCT GCC GGG ACC CAC CTG GGA GGC ACC AAC CTC GAC TTC CAG ATG GAG CAG TAT ATC
 19  L   A   A   G   T   H   L   G   G   T   N   L   D   F   Q   M   E   Q   Y   I

181 TAC AAG AGA AAG AGC GAT GGT ATT TAC ATC ATC AAT CTG AAG AGG ACC TGG GAG AAG CTC
 39  Y   K   R   K   S   D   G   I   Y   I   I   N   L   K   R   T   W   E   K   L

241 CTT TTG GCA GCC CGT GCT ATT GTG GCT ATT GAG AAT CCA GCT GAT GTG AGC GTC ATT TCT
 59  L   L   A   A   R   A   I   V   A   I   E   N   P   A   D   V   S   V   I   S

301 TCC AGG AAT ACC GGA CAG CGT GCT GTT CTG AAG TTT GCT GCT GCC ACT GGG GCT ACT CCT
 79  S   R   N   T   G   Q   R   A   V   L   K   F   A   A   A   T   G   A   T   P

361 ATT GCT GGA CGC TTC ACC CCT GGT ACC TTC ACA AAT CAG ATC CAG GCG GCT TTC CGT GAG
 99  I   A   G   R   F   T   P   G   T   F   T   N   Q   I   Q   A   A   F   R   E
                                          +
421 CCA CGA CTC CTG GTT GTT ACA GAT CCC CGA GCT GAT CAT CAG CCA CTG ACC GAG GCT TCT
119  P   R   L   L   V   V   T   D   P   R   A   D   H   Q   P   L   T   E   A   S

481 TAC GTC AAC ATC CCC ACC ATT GCG CTG TGC AAC ACC GAC TCC CCG CTG CGC TAT GTG GAT
139  Y   V   N   I   P   T   I   A   L   C   N   T   D   S   P   L   R   Y   V   D
                     *
541 ATT GCT ATC CCC TGC AAC AAC AAG GGA GCA CAT TCA GTG GGC CTG ATG TGG TGG ATG CTG
159  I   A   I   P   C   N   N   K   G   A   H   S   V   G   L   M   W   W   M   L

601 GCT CGG GAG GTC CTG CGC ATG CGT GGC ACC ATC TCC CGT GAA CAT CCA TGG GAA GTC ATG
179  A   R   E   V   L   R   M   R   G   T   I   S   R   E   H   P   W   E   V   M

661 CCT GAC TTG TAC TTC TAC AGG GAT CCT GAG GAG ATT GAG AAG GAG GAG CAG GCT GCT GCT
199  P   D   L   Y   F   Y   R   D   P   E   E   I   E   K   E   E   Q   A   A   A

721 GAG AAA GCA GTG ACA AAG GAG GAG TTC CAG ACC GAA TGG ACA GCC CCA GCT CCT GAA TTC
219  E   K   A   V   T   K   E   E   F   Q   T   E   W   T   A   P   A   P   E   F
                                              *
781 ACA GCT CCT CCT CAG CCT GAG GTT GCT GAT TGG TCT GAG GGA GTG CAG GTC CCA TCT GTG
239  T   A   P   P   Q   P   E   V   A   D   W   S   E   G   V   Q   V   P   S   V
                 Δ   ☐
841 CCA ATC CAG CAG TTC CCC ACA GAG GAC TGG AGT GCC CAG CCT GCC ACT GAG GAC TGG TCA
259  P   I   Q   Q   F   P   T   E   D   W   S   A   Q   P   A   T   E   D   W   S
                                                          +
901 GCA GCT CCC ACT GCC CAA GCA ACG GAG TGG GTT GGG ACT ACC ACG GAG TGG TCT TAA CTT
279  A   A   P   T   A   Q   A   T   E   W   V   G   T   T   T   E   W   S  Och
                                                  ◆   ☐
961 CAG CGC CGC TGT ACT ATC AAA AAT AAA GAC TGG TTT AAT ACC CAT CCT-Poly(A)
```

Figure 12 Translated sequence of cDNA encoding the chicken 296-residue laminin receptor ORF. The nine amino acid residues at which the chicken sequence differs from the published laminin receptor sequences for hamster (Wang et al. 1992), mouse (Makrides et al. 1988), human (Yow et al. 1988), or cow (Grosso et al. 1991) are shown in regular type. At three positions (∗) the chicken sequence differs from a residue conserved in all four mammalian sequences (residue 4 is Ala, residue 142 is Leu, and residue 229 is Gly in mammals). At two positions (+) the bovine sequence is different from all the others (Asn at 109 and Ser at 273). At position 242 (☐), the human sequence has Thr but hamster, mouse, and cow have Ala. The chicken sequence has a Pro inserted at residue -241 (Δ) that is not present in the mammalian sequences. At residue 291 the bovine amino acid is the same as the chicken, but hamster, mouse, and human are Ala (◆). The human sequence only has Asp at 293 (☐). (T. Rümenapf, unpubl.).

of mosquito cells. This 32-kD protein also bound laminin and cross-reacted immunologically with the high-affinity laminin receptor, consistent with the results of Wang et al. (1992) that a protein in mosquito cells reactive with MAb 1C3 acts as a receptor for some alphaviruses. The exact correspondence between the 32-kD protein expressed in mosquito cells, the product expressed from the 295-residue ORF, and the 67-kD high-affinity laminin receptor remains to be determined. G.V. Ludwig and J.F. Smith (pers. comm.) reported that VEE and SIN competed for binding, consistent with the hypothesis that they both bind to a protein related to the laminin receptor. They also found that higher molecular weight proteins from mosquito cells cross-reacted immunologically with the 32-kD protein and bound VEE and laminin, and that VEE bound to 32-kD and 67-kD proteins from BHK cells, consistent with the hypothesis that the 32-kD and 67-kD proteins share some sequence identity.

RECEPTOR-BINDING DOMAIN ON THE VIRUS

Evidence is developing that the constellation of cellular receptors that an alphavirus can use can be altered by relatively minor changes in E1 and E2. In one study, two strains of SIN that were identical except for a single amino acid difference in E2 (Gly-172→Arg) were examined for their ability to bind to cells of neuronal origin in culture; it was found that the more neurovirulent of the two strains, possessing Gly-172, bound more readily to neuronal cells than did the less virulent strain, although the two strains bound identically to BHK cells (Tucker and Griffin 1991). In other studies, variants of SIN that differed in their neurovirulence for mice were sequenced and used to construct recombinant viruses, and it was shown that amino acid substitutions in E1 and E2 affected the neurovirulence of the virus (Lustig et al. 1988; Tucker et al. 1993). In the case of at least some of these mutants, it was shown that the virus replicated less well in the brain if it was less virulent. Other studies by Johnston and colleagues (Davis et al. 1986; Polo et al. 1988; Polo and Johnston 1990, 1991) have also demonstrated that changes in E1 and E2 can alter the neurovirulence of SIN for mice. Although these studies, unlike the Tucker and Griffin study (1991), do not demonstrate a direct effect of changes in the glycoproteins on virus binding to neurons, it is suspected that at least some of these changes do affect the ability of the virus to bind to receptors expressed on neurons, although it is also possible that changes in E1 and E2 could affect other stages of the penetration process or affect the ability of the virus to replicate in neurons.

Changes in E2 of a second alphavirus, Ross River virus (RR), have also been shown directly to affect the ability of the virus to bind to and infect different cells. RR, in contrast to SIN, is maintained in nature in small marsupial mammals rather than birds, and the virus binds poorly to chicken cells in culture. Variants of the Nelson Bay strain of RR were selected for increased efficiency of infection of chicken cells by repeated passaging in chicken cells (Kerr et al. 1993). The passaged virus had single changes in E2: In two of three independent variants sequenced, the change was Asn-218→Lys, and in the third variant, the change was Glu-4→Lys. Acting on this information, R.C. Weir and R.J. Kuhn (unpubl.) examined the effect of changing E2 Asn-218 to threonine, lysine, or arginine in the T48 strain of RR. A full-length cDNA clone of RR T48 has been constructed, and the virus recovered from this cDNA clone has been characterized (Kuhn et al. 1991 and in prep.), making a study of such changes in RR feasible. The parental T48 virus recovered from the full-length clone was found to infect only about 2% of chicken cells in culture, using an immunofluorescence assay with antibodies directed against RR structural proteins to detect infected cells. Virus with Thr-218 or Lys-218 infected about 6% of chicken cells, but virus with Arg-218 infected about 40% of chicken cells. Thus, the single change Asn-218→Arg in E2 led to a 20-fold increase in the ability of RR T48 to infect chicken cells. Serial passage of the Arg-218 virus in chicken cells led to selection of a strain of RR that retained Arg-218 but had in addition two other changes, Cys-153→Arg in E2 and Asp-323→Tyr in E1. This strain infects almost all chicken cells in culture and will form plaques on chicken monolayers. The individual effects of these two additional changes are being tested, but it appears that changing two amino acids in E2 and one amino acid in E1 of RR changes the virus from one able to infect only 2% of cultured chicken cells to one that infects 100% of cultured chicken cells.

Suggestive supporting evidence for the importance of the domain of RR E2 near residue 218 for the host range of the virus comes from studies of RR isolated during an epidemic of RR in humans. Between April 1979 and February 1980, a large epidemic of RR polyarthritis swept through the Pacific region, infecting hundreds of thousands of people (Marshall and Miles 1984). The epidemic is believed to have been initiated by a single focus of infection in Nadi, Fiji from a viremic air traveler from Australia, where the virus is endemic; the epidemic then spread to Samoa, the Wallis Islands, New Caledonia, and, finally, the Cook Islands. In Australia the virus is maintained in small marsupials, but during this human epidemic the virus is believed to have been maintained by direct man-mosquito-man transmission. Sequence of E2 from virus isolated at the beginning of the epidemic and from virus isolated during and near the end of the epidemic showed that a single nucleotide change had occurred, which led to the amino acid substitution Thr-219→ Ala, suggesting that this change may have been selected because it adapted the virus to humans.

Finally, studies of the domains of E2 that interact with neutralizing monoclonal antibodies also indicate the importance of the E2 region near residue 200 for cell binding. The anti-idiotypic antibodies that function as antireceptor antibodies in chicken cells were made to neutralizing anti-E2 antibodies that bind to this domain, as shown by two different methods. First, variants resistant to these antibodies possessed changes at E2 residues 214 (MAb 49), 216 (MAb 23), or at 181, 190, and 205 (MAb 50) (Strauss et al. 1991). Second, MAb 23 was shown to bind to λgt11 clones expressing fusion proteins containing the E2 region between residues 173 and 220 (Wang and Strauss 1991). Thus, there is the presumption that this domain directly interacts with the cellular receptor (at least in chicken cells). This domain is hydrophilic and has attached a polysaccharide chain at Asn-196 in SIN, and thus would be predicted to be exposed to the solvent where it could interact with a receptor. A schematic diagram of the sequence of this region showing the various changes observed in different strains is shown in Figure 13.

CONCLUSIONS

The results from several lines of study suggest that the very wide host range of the alphaviruses results in part from the ability of the virus to use a receptor that is highly conserved (the high-affinity laminin receptor in the case of SIN and VEE viruses and perhaps other alphaviruses), and in part from the ability of the virus to use more than one receptor on the surface of the cell. The relationships between the various receptor proteins studied in the different laboratories are unknown. In most cases, only the protein molecular weights estimated from acrylamide gel electrophoresis were determined, and side-by-side comparisons of these proteins, including immunological studies, will be necessary to determine if they are all different. It also appears clear from competition experiments, antibody-blocking experiments, and host-range considerations that different alphaviruses can use different sets of receptors to enter cells.

It also seems clear that the alphaviruses are a fairly plastic system in terms of host range and potential virulence. Limited changes, primarily in E2 but also in E1, allow the virus to recognize new sets of receptors which can lead to an altered host range or altered disease-causing potential. The limits to this flexibility are unknown, but it is striking that al-

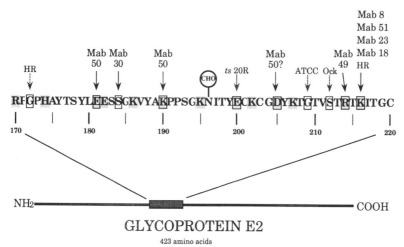

GLYCOPROTEIN E2

423 amino acids

Figure 13 Sequence of a region of SIN E2 important for binding to cells. The sequence of a region of 51 amino acids from SIN E2 is shown with amino acids numbered from the amino terminus of the protein. Charged amino acids are shaded. Boxed amino acids have been found to vary in different strains of virus as indicated. Residues that when altered render the virus resistant to various monoclonal antibodies are shown with the name of the antibody. HR is the heat-resistant strain of AR339 SIN. The position of an asparagine-linked carbohydrate chain is shown (CHO). The E2 proteins of SIN and RR are in register in this region, and Asn-218 changed in chicken-adapted virus corresponds to Thr-218 in SIN.

though RR T48 is virtually unable to infect chicken cells, two changes in E2 and one change in E1 enable it to do so efficiently. Presumably, the ecological constraints in terms of available insect vectors and suitable vertebrate hosts select for the virus best able to persist in a particular habitat. However, alphaviruses appear to be able to readily adapt to new sets of hosts if circumstances change.

The primary organ of attachment of the virus is the spike, a trimer of E1-E2 heterodimers. It is unknown whether there is only one binding site for a cellular receptor in the spike, and thus that all of the different receptors used by the virus share a common "epitope" that can be bound at this site, or whether there exist more than one site in the spike that can bind a receptor, in which case two or more unrelated receptors could in theory be utilized. The E2 domain from about residue 170 to residue 220 (SIN numbering) is particularly important for binding to at least some cells, but domains in E1 almost certainly participate in binding as well. Omar and Koblet (1988) found that proteinase treatment of SF virus under defined conditions resulted in virions that had lost E2 while retaining E1.

This virus retained infectivity, showing that virus containing only E1 is able to attach to cells and initiate infection. However, the conditions used to produce the E2-lacking particles included detergent treatment that resulted in inactivation of most of the virus infectivity (as shown by loss of infectivity by control virus not treated with proteinase), and efficiency of binding of treated virions relative to the binding of untreated virions is not clear.

The broad host range of alphaviruses contrasts with the narrow host range of viruses whose proteinaceous receptors have been characterized to date. Continuing studies, including structural studies, to define the nature and limits of variability of the interactions between alphavirus spikes and cellular receptors will be of interest for years to come.

ACKNOWLEDGMENTS

The work of the authors was supported by grants AI-20612 and AI-10793 from the National Institutes of Health. T.R. was supported by a fellowship from the Deutsche Forschungsgemeinschaft. R.C.W. was on sabbatical leave from the Australian National University in Canberra.

REFERENCES

Bignon, C., M. Roux-Dossteo, M.E. Zeigler, M.-G. Mattei, J.-C. Lissitzky, M.S. Wicha, and P.-M. Martin. 1992. Genomic analysis of the 67-kDa laminin receptor in normal and pathological tissues: Circumstantial evidence for retroposon features. *Genomics* **10**: 481.

Birdwell, C.R. and J.H. Strauss. 1974. Distribution of the receptor sites for Sindbis virus on the surface of chicken and BHK cells. *J. Virol.* **14**: 672.

Castronovo, V., G. Taraboletti, and M.E. Sobel. 1991a. Functional domains of the 67-kDa laminin receptor precursor. *J. Biol. Chem.* **266**: 20440.

Castronovo, V., A.P. Claysmith, K.T. Barker, V. Cioce, H.C. Krutzsch, and M.E. Sobel. 1991b. Biosynthesis of the 67 kDa high affinity laminin receptor. *Biochem. Biophys. Res. Commun.* **177**: 177.

Chamberlain, R.W. 1980. Epidemiology of arthropod-borne togaviruses: The role of arthropods as hosts and vectors and of vertebrate hosts in natural transmission cycles. In *The togaviruses* (ed. R.W. Schlesinger), p. 175. Academic Press, New York.

Davis, N.L., F.J. Fuller, W.G. Dougherty, R.A. Olmsted, and R.E. Johnston. 1986. A single nucleotide change in the E2 glycoprotein gene of Sindbis virus affects penetration rate in cell culture and virulence in neonatal mice. *Proc. Natl. Acad. Sci.* **83**: 6771.

Fries, E. and A. Helenius. 1979. Binding of Semliki Forest virus and its spike glycoprotein to cells. *Eur. J. Biochem.* **97**: 213.

Fuller, S.D. 1987. The T=4 envelope of Sindbis virus is organized by interactions with a complementary T=3 capsid. *Cell* **48**: 923.

Garoff, H. and K. Simons. 1974. Location of the spike glycoproteins in the Semliki Forest virus membrane. *Proc. Natl. Acad. Sci.* **71**: 3988.

Gaulton, G.N. and M.I. Greene. 1986. Idiotypic mimicry of biological receptors. *Annu. Rev. Immunol.* **4**: 253.

Griffin, D.E. 1986. Alphavirus pathogenesis and immunity. In *The togaviridae and flaviviridae* (ed. S. Schlesinger and M.J. Schlesinger), p. 209. Plenum Publishing, New York.

Grosso, L.E., P.W. Park, and R.P. Mecham. 1991. Characterization of a putative clone for the 67-kilodalton elastin/laminin receptor suggests that it encodes a cytoplasmic protein rather than a cell surface receptor. *Biochemistry* **30**: 3346.

Helenius, A., B. Morrein, E. Fries, K. Simons, P. Robinson, V. Schirrmacher, C. Terhorst, and J.L. Strominger. 1978. Human (HLA-A and -B) and murine (H2-K and -D) histocompatibility antigens are cell surface receptors for Semliki Forest virus. *Proc. Natl. Acad. Sci.* **75**: 3846.

Kerr, P.J., R.C. Weir, and L. Dalgarno. 1993. Ross River virus variants selected during passage in chick embryo fibroblasts: Serological, genetic, and biological changes. *Virology* **193**: 446.

Kuhn, R.J., H.G.M. Niesters, Z. Hong, and J.H. Strauss. 1991. Infectious RNA transcripts from Ross River virus cDNA clones and the construction and characterization of defined chimeras with Sindbis virus. *Virology* **182**: 430.

Lopez, S., J.-S. Yao, R.J. Kuhn, E.G. Strauss, and J.H. Strauss. 1994. Nucleocapsid-glycoprotein interactions required for alphavirus assembly. *J. Virol.* **68**: 1316.

Lustig, S., A. Jackson, C.S. Hahn, D.E. Griffin, E.G. Strauss, and J.H. Strauss. 1988. Molecular basis of Sindbis virus neurovirulence in mice. *J. Virol.* **62**: 2329.

Maassen, J.A. and C. Terhorst. 1981. Identification of a cell-surface protein involved in the binding site of Sindbis virus on human lymphoblastic cell lines using a heterobifunctional cross-linker. *Eur. J. Biochem.* **115**: 153.

Makrides, S., S.T. Chitpatima, R. Bandyopadhyay, and G. Brawerman. 1988. Nucleotide sequence for a major messenger RNA for a 40 kilodalton polypeptide that is under translational control in mouse tumor cells. *Nucleic Acids Res.* **16**: 2349.

Marshall, I.D. and J.A.R. Miles. 1984. Ross River virus and epidemic polyarthritis. *Curr. Top. Vector Res.* **2**: 31.

Niklasson, B. 1988. Sindbis and Sindbis-like viruses. In *The arboviruses, epidemiology and ecology* (ed. T.P. Monath), p. 167. CRC Press, Boca Raton, Florida.

Oldstone, M.B.A., A. Tishon, F. Dutko, S.I.T. Kennedy, J.J. Holland, and P.W. Lampert. 1980. Does the major histocompatibility complex serve as a specific receptor for Semliki Forest virus? *J. Virol.* **34**: 256.

Omar, A. and H. Koblet. 1988. Semliki Forest virus particles containing only the E1 envelope glycoprotein are infectious and can induce cell-cell fusion. *Virology* **166**: 17.

Paredes, A.M., D.T. Brown, R.B. Rothnagel, W. Chiu, R.J. Schoepp, R.E. Johnston, and B.V.V. Prasad. 1993. Three-dimensional structure of a membrane-containing virus. *Proc. Natl. Acad. Sci.* **90**: 9095.

Peters, C.J., and J.M. Dalrymple. 1990. Alphaviruses. In *Virology* (ed. B.N. Fields and D. M. Knipe), p.713. Raven Press, New York.

Polo, J.M. and R.E. Johnston. 1990. Attenuating mutations in glycoproteins E1 and E2 of Sindbis virus produce a highly attenuated strain when combined in vitro. *J. Virol.* **64**: 4438.

———. 1991. Mutational analysis of a virulence locus in the E2 glycoprotein gene of Sindbis virus. *J. Virol.* **65**: 6358.

Polo, J.M., N.L. Davis, C.M. Rice, H.V. Huang, and R.E. Johnston. 1988. Molecular analysis of Sindbis virus pathogenesis in neonatal mice using virus recombinants constructed in vitro. *J. Virol.* **62**: 2124.

Rao, C.N., V. Castronovo, C.M. Schmitt, U.M. Wewer, A.P. Claysmith, L.A. Liotta, and M.E. Sobel. 1989. Evidence for a precursor of the high-affinity metastasis-associated murine laminin receptor. *Biochemistry* **28:** 7476-7486.

Scott, T.W. and S.C. Weaver. 1989. Eastern equine encephalomyelitis virus: Epidemiology and evolution of mosquito transmission. *Adv. Virus Res.* **37:** 277.

Shah, K.V., H.N. Johnson, T.R. Rao, P.K. Rajagopalan, and B.S. Lamba. 1960. Isolation of five strains of Sindbis virus in India. *Indian J. Med. Res.* **48:** 300.

Smith, A.L. and G.H. Tignor. 1980. Host cell receptors for two strains of Sindbis virus. *Arch. Virol.* **66:** 11.

Strauss, E.G. and J.H. Strauss. 1986. Structure and replication of the alphavirus genome. In *The togaviridae and flaviviridae* (ed. S. Schlesinger and M.J. Schlesinger), p. 35. Plenum Publishing, New York.

Strauss, E.G., D.S. Stec, A.L. Schmaljohn, and J.H. Strauss. 1991. Identification of antigenically important domains in the glycoproteins of Sindbis virus by analysis of antibody escape variants. *J. Virol.* **65:** 4654.

Tucker, P.C. and D.E. Griffin. 1991. Mechanism of altered Sindbis virus neurovirulence associated with a single-amino-acid change in the E2 glycoprotein. *J. Virol.* **65:** 1551.

Tucker, P.C., E.G. Strauss, R.J. Kuhn, J.H. Strauss, and D.E. Griffin. 1993. Viral determinants of age-dependent virulence of Sindbis virus for mice. *J. Virol.* **67:** 4605.

Ubol, S. and D.E. Griffin. 1991. Identification of a putative alphavirus receptor on mouse neural cells. *J. Virol.* **65:** 6913.

von Bonsdorff, C.-H. and S.C. Harrison. 1975. Sindbis virus glycoproteins form a regular icosahedral surface lattice. *J. Virol.* **16:** 141.

Wang, K.-S. and J.H. Strauss. 1991. Use of a λgt11 expression library to localize a neutralizing antibody-binding site in glycoprotein E2 of Sindbis virus. *J. Virol.* **65:** 7037.

Wang, K.-S., A.L. Schmaljohn, R.J. Kuhn, and J.H. Strauss. 1991. Antiidiotypic antibodies as probes for the Sindbis virus receptor. *Virology* **181:** 694.

Wang, K.-S., R.J. Kuhn, E.G. Strauss, S. Ou, and J.H. Strauss. 1992. High affinity laminin receptor is a receptor for Sindbis virus in mammalian cells. *J. Virol.* **66:** 4992.

Wewer, U.M., G. Taraboletti, M.E. Sobel, R. Albrechtsen, and L.A. Liotta. 1987. Role of laminin receptor in tumor cell migration. *Cancer Res.* **47:** 5691.

Wewer, U.M., L.A. Liotta, M. Jaye, G.A. Ricca, W.A. Drohan, A.P. Claysmith, C.N. Rao, P. Wirth, J. Coligan, R. Albrechtsen, M. Mudry, and M.E. Sobel. 1986. Altered levels of laminin receptor mRNA in various human carcinoma cells that have different abilities to bind laminin. *Proc. Natl. Acad. Sci.* **83:** 7137.

Yow, H., J.M. Wong, H.S. Chen, C. Lee, G.D.S. Steele, and L.B. Chen. 1988. Increased mRNA expression of a laminin-binding protein in human colon carcinoma: Complete sequence of a full-length cDNA encoding the protein. *Proc. Natl. Acad. Sci.* **85:** 6394.

10

Membrane Cofactor Protein (CD46) Is a Receptor for Measles Virus That Determines Viral Host Specificity

Ruth E. Dörig,[1] Anne Marcil,[1] and Christopher D. Richardson [1,2,3]

[1]Biotechnology Research Institute
National Research Council of Canada
Montréal, Québec, Canada H4P 2R2
[2]Department of Microbiology and Immunology
McGill University
Montréal, Québec, Canada H3A 2M3

The symptoms induced by measles virus range from the acute childhood disease characterized by respiratory infection, fever, leukopenia, and rash to less common chronic infections affecting the nervous system (Norrby and Oxman 1990). The very rare persistent viral infections occur later in life; they include subacute sclerosing panencephalitis, measles inclusion body encephalitis, autoimmune chronic active hepatitis, and possibly Paget's bone disease (Billeter and Cattaneo 1991; Randall and Russell 1991). Acute infection by measles virus is still the major killer disease of children in impoverished nations. The virus infects 44 million individuals per year and kills 1.5 million of them (Weiss 1992). Recent failures in developing countries with the high-titer Edmonston/Zagreb vaccines have prompted the World Health Organization to reevaluate immunization procedures (Weiss 1992). Administration of the high-titer vaccine to infants prior to the age of 9 months is associated with 20–80% increased mortality (biased toward females) due to secondary gastrointestinal and respiratory infections (Garenne et al. 1991; Aaby et al. 1993; Holt et al. 1993). This could be due to the immunosuppressive nature of measles virus (Esolen et al. 1993; Griffin and Ward 1993; Hilleman 1994). The high-titer vaccine has subsequently been withdrawn from the world market. There is now an increased effort to develop a vaccine that will target children prior to the age of 9 months, decrease seroconversion failures, possess better thermostability, and be able to be administered to a

[3]Present address: Amgen and Ontario Cancer Institutes, 620 University Avenue, Suite 706, Toronto, Canada M5G 2C1.

Cellular Receptors for Animal Viruses
© 1994 Cold Spring Harbor Laboratory Press 0-87969-429-7/94 $5 + .00

wider proportion of the world population. Children in North America are normally immunized after 15 months using the standard Moraten vaccine after maternal antibodies have subsided. Despite the decreased incidence of measles in richer nations, a 10-fold increase in the number of reported cases in the United States and Canada occurred between 1988 and 1991. This was probably due to neglect in immunization and a 5% failure of some vaccinees to seroconvert (Rota et al. 1992; Weiss 1992). Genetic variation of vaccine strains in the laboratory and wild-type strains from recent epidemics throughout the world has been reported (Rota et al. 1992, 1994a,b). However, the contribution of these mutations to the disease process and vaccination is not known at this time.

Measles virus is a member of the Paramyxoviridae family and contains an RNA genome (15 kb) complementary to viral mRNA. The viral genomic RNA is associated with a nucleocapsid protein (NP), a phosphoprotein (P), and an RNA polymerase (L). Surrounding the nucleocapsid is an envelope that contains two glycoproteins: the hemagglutinin (H) (Alkhatib and Briedis 1986) and the membrane fusion (F) protein (Richardson et al. 1986). In addition, a nonglycosylated matrix protein (M) is situated at the inner surface of the envelope and maintains an association between the membrane glycoproteins and the nucleocapsid. The H protein is required for viral attachment to the host cell receptor; the F protein mediates viral penetration at the host plasma membrane and is also responsible for syncytium formation (for review, see Norrby and Oxman 1990; Kingsbury 1991).

MEASLES VIRUS NORMALLY INFECTS PRIMATES

Human beings and some monkey species are susceptible to measles virus infections via the respiratory route (Albrecht et al. 1980; Norrby and Oxman 1990). Rodents are not normally infected by this virus, and there is no satisfactory small animal model for this virus that yields the disease symptoms commonly produced in children. However, neurotropic variants can be generated by intracerebral injections of the virus into the brains of rats, hamsters, and mice (Carrigan 1986; Liebert and ter Meulen 1987). In the laboratory these viruses must usually be isolated by cocultivation of brain cells with Vero monkey kidney cells. In addition, measles virus can be attenuated and adapted to cells derived from chick embryos, dog kidneys, ferret kidneys, hamster embryos, and mouse L cells by repeated passage in culture (Matumoto 1966; Schumacher et al. 1972; Fraser and Martin 1978). Adaptation to nonprimate cells requires many passages in culture before cytopathic effects are observed, and extracellular viral titers are generally low. This process is often associated with accumulated mutations in the virus, but it is still not known whether these changes alter receptor interaction with the host cell or affect the replication and assembly of the virus (Calain and Roux 1988; Rota et al. 1994b).

PREVIOUS ATTEMPTS TO IDENTIFY THE MEASLES VIRUS RECEPTOR

The first receptor identified for a paramyxovirus was determined to be sialic acid for Sendai virus (Markwell et al. 1981). This moiety was found on either glycoproteins or glycolipids. Many other paramyxoviruses such as mumps, Newcastle disease virus, and human respiratory syncytial virus, as well as the influenza viruses, also bind specifically to sialic acid (Markwell 1991). Even though measles and canine distemper viruses are members of the morbillivirus subgroup of the Paramyxoviridae family, these pathogens do not appear to interact with sialic acid. Incubation of the host cells with neuraminidase, which removes sialic acid, does not prevent measles virus from binding to the host cell, but rather enhances agglutination of monkey red blood cells with measles virus (Tischer 1967; Howe and Lee 1972; Dore-Duffy and Howe 1978). On the other hand, treatment of cynomolgous monkey erythrocytes with trypsin (Norrby 1962; Periés and Chany 1962) or chymotrypsin (Tischer 1967) reduces or abolishes binding of measles virus. Taken together, this evidence suggests that measles virus employs a protein moiety for attachment rather than merely a carbohydrate residue.

One of the first attempts to isolate cellular receptor proteins for measles virus was reported in 1979. Solubilized proteins from erythrocytes were tested for their ability to inhibit measles virus binding to monkey red blood cells (Fenger and Howe 1979). Two glycoproteins of 48 kD and 90 kD were identified from the membranes of monkey cells as candidates for high-affinity viral receptors. However, other proteins from rabbit, human, and monkey erythrocytes also bound to the virus, making these experiments somewhat inconclusive. In another study, the production of mouse anti-idiotypic antibodies prepared against measles virus antisera yielded antibodies that recognized specific cellular proteins (Krah and Choppin 1988). These host-cell proteins were thought to contain the receptor pocket. However, the anti-idiotypic approach has recently been questioned, since binding pockets are often unavailable for interaction with the larger-sized antibodies; neutralizing antibodies blocking attachment are usually directed against the surface sites surrounding the pocket (Weis et al. 1988). Substance P receptor has also been implicated as a measles virus-binding protein (Schroeder 1986; Harrowe et al. 1990, 1992), but this claim warrants further exploration. Recently, more systematic approaches were initiated to identify the receptor for measles virus using monoclonal antibodies (Naniche et al. 1992, 1993b) and mouse/human hybrid cell lines (Dörig et al. 1993).

MEASLES VIRUS BINDS TO AND INFECTS PRIMATE CELL LINES

A wide variety of cell types in primates are susceptible to measles virus (Matumoto 1966; Fraser and Martin 1978; Norrby and Oxman 1990). In our laboratory we confirmed the primate specificity for measles virus using a variety of cultured cell lines (Dörig et al. 1993). Lymphocyte (B, T, and myeloid), epithelial, and fibroblast cell lines from primates, mice, and hamsters were infected with measles virus and incubated up to 1 week. Western immunoblot analysis indicated that only cell lines derived from primates could be infected. In addition to monkey kidney fibroblasts (Vero, CV1), all human cell lines supported infection, independent of their tissue of origin: premyeloid leukemia (HL60), myeloid leukemia (K562), B-cell lymphoma (Raji and Daudi), T-cell leukemia (P30 Ohkubo, MOLT-4, Jurkat, Peer, and RPMI 8402), and epitheloid cervical carcinoma (HeLa). Consequently, a receptor for measles virus would be expected to be widely distributed throughout different human tissues. It has been noted that monkey erythrocytes of several species (including cercopithecus, rhesus, cynomolgous, baboon) can be agglutinated by measles virus, whereas red blood cells from humans and chimpanzees lack this capability (Periés and Chany 1960; Norrby 1962; Fraser and Martin 1978; R.E. Dörig et al., unpubl.). This presence of a receptor for measles virus on African green monkey (cercopithecus) red blood cells is the basis of an assay to detect virus attachment to target host cells (i.e., monkey red blood cells adhere to a susceptible host cell in the presence of measles virus) (Valdimarsson et al. 1975; Dörig et al. 1993). On the other hand, human erythrocytes are one of the few cell types that do not bind measles virus, which suggests that they lack the receptor for this virus; consequently, human red blood cells will not form rosettes in the presence of measles virus.

Since direct binding assays with radioactively labeled virus are often inconsistent due to difficulties in obtaining large quantities of virus free of contaminating cellular debris, the rosette binding assay was used to investigate the distribution of receptors on human, monkey, mouse, and hamster cell lines. All primate cells, including HeLa, Vero, Jurkat, Daudi, Raji, Peer, MOLT-4, RPMI 8402, P30 Ohkubo, HL60, and K562, were capable of forming rosettes (Table 1). On the other hand, mouse cell lines, including psi 2, J558/L, SP2/0, GM0347 (or L), NS0, EL4.IL-2, BW5147.3, P388D1, and Chinese hamster ovary (CHO) cells did not bind red blood cells in the presence of virus (Table 1).

MOUSE/HUMAN HYBRID CELL LINES CONTAINING HUMAN
CHROMOSOME 1 BIND MEASLES VIRUS

As a preliminary step toward identifying the human gene responsible for specifying the receptor for measles virus, we assayed a number of hybrid

Table 1 Analysis of human and rodent cell lines with respect to measles virus binding, susceptibility to infection, and expression of CD46

Cell line (H synthesis)	Rosette formation[a]	Infection[b]	CD46 expression[c]
HeLa	++++++	++++	100++
Jurkat	++++	+++	100++
MOLT-4	+++	+++	100++
RPMI 8402	++	+	100++
P30 Ohkubo	++	++	100++
Peer	++	+++	100+
HL-60	++	+	100++
K562	+++	+	100++
Raji	+++	+++	100++
Daudi	+++	+	100+
Vero	++++	+++	0
psi2	–	–	0
L (GM0347)	–	–	0
CHO	–	–	0
J558/L	–	–	0
NS0	–	–	0
SP2/0	–	–	10
BW5147.3	–	–	0
P388D$_1$	–	–	0

(Reprinted, with permission, from Dörig et al. 1993.)

[a]Rosette formation between monkey red blood cells and measles virus absorbed to host cells was an indication of virus binding to a susceptible target cell. Each (+) indicates that at least 1–2 cells were bound to the majority of host cells. A (–) indicates the absence of rosette formation.

[b]Infectivity was measured by the production of measles H protein in cells inoculated with measles virus over 1 week. Cellular proteins were assayed by immunoblot with the monoclonal antibody 2B1-3 directed against H. Each (+) is indicative of the intensity of the H protein band. A (–) sign indicates the absence of infection.

[c]Expression of CD46 was monitored by FACS using a commercial monoclonal antibody (J4-48) specific for the human cell-surface antigen. The percentage of total cells that exhibited fluorescence for CD46 is indicated numerically. A (+) indicates that the mean fluorescence was 2–10x that of the IgG1 negative control; (++) indicates the signal was 10–100x the mean of the IgG1 control. A polyclonal antibody directed against human CD46 recognizes a protein on Vero cells (unlike monoclonal antibody J4-48) and other human cell lines but fails to interact with any protein on rodent cells (R.E. Dörig et al. unpubl.).

mouse cell lines that contained a variety of human chromosomes (Dörig et al. 1993). These cell lines were tested for their ability to form rosettes with monkey red blood cells in the presence of measles virus (Table 2; Fig. 1). The cells tested contained the human chromosomes indicated in parentheses (der, derivative; t, translocation): GM10880(1,3,14), GM07299(1,X), GM10660A(der[1]t[1;17][p34.3;q11.2],14), GM11130 (2,18,der[21]t[1;21][p31;q22],X),   GM09142(3,5,der[21]t[[X;21][p21; p12]),   GM07300(6,8,11,X),   GM10482(7,der[11]t[X;11][q26;   q23]), GM10792(12,19), GM10322(21,22). Every cell line that contained human chromosome 1, except GM11130, was capable of binding to measles virus. GM11130 and GM10660A cell lines each contained a rearranged chromosome resulting from translocations between chromosome 1;21 and 1;17, respectively. The GM11130 cell line contained a chromosome 21 derivative that consisted of most of the 1p arm, some of the 21q bands, the 21p arm, and the centromere of chromosome 21. This cell line did not support binding of measles virus. GM10660A cells also contained a translocated chromosome 1 that contained the 1q arm, some of the 1p bands, the 17p arm, and the centromere of chromosome 1. These cells were able to bind measles virus. Thus, the gene for the receptor appeared to be situated proximal to 1p31 or somewhere on the 1q arm. Measles virus readily infects all lymphocytes, and a survey of

Table 2 Analysis of mouse/human somatic hybrid cell lines for measles virus-binding activity and expression of CD46

Cell line	Human chromosome[a]	Rosette formation[b]	CD46 expression[c]
GM10880	1, 13, 14	+++	77+
GM07299	1, X	++++	100+
GM10660A	t(1, 17), 14	+++	80+
GM11130	t(1, 21), 2, 18, X	−	0
GM09142	3, 5, t(X, 21)	−	0
GM07300	6, 8, 11, X	−	0
GM10482	7, t(X,11)	−	0
GM10792	12, 19	−	0
GM10322	21, 22	−	0

(Reprinted, with permission, from Dörig et al. 1993.)

[a]Mouse/human hybrid cell lines that contained the indicated human chromosomes were tested for their ability to bind measles virus and for the presence of CD46 at their cell surface.

[b]Ability of cell lines to bind measles virus monitored by rosette formation between target host cell, virus, and monkey red blood cells. Each (+) indicates that at least 1–2 erythrocytes bound to most of the cells and a (−) shows that no rosettes were present.

[c]CD46 expression was assayed by FACS using the monoclonal antibody (J4-48). The percentage of total cells that were CD46$^+$ is indicated numerically. Fluorescence intensity is indicated with a (+) as described in Table 1.

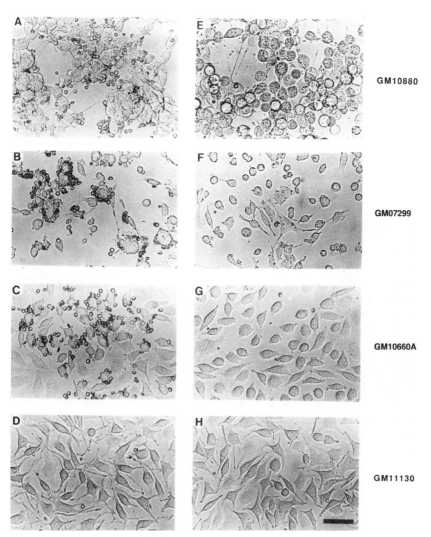

Figure 1 Measles virus-binding assays for mouse/human somatic cell hybrids using monkey red blood cells. Measles virus (20 pfu per cell) was added to mouse somatic hybrid cell lines that contained specific human chromosomes as described in the text. GM10880 (*A*), GM07299 (*B*), GM10660A (*C*), and GM11130 (*D*) cells were incubated with virus, washed, incubated with African green monkey red blood cells, and washed. Control cells were incubated with media that did not contain virus but were treated in the same way: GM10880 (*E*), GM07299 (*F*), GM 10660A (*G*), and GM11130 (*H*). Bar,   50 μm. (Reprinted, with permission, from Dörig et al. 1993.)

lymphocyte markers (Barclay et al. 1993) suggested that members from a group of antigens on part of chromosome 1 could function as a receptor. This group included CD2, CD53, CD58, CD48, CD62, CD1, Fc receptors, CD16, CDw32, L selectin, CD45, CD21, CD34, CD35, CD46, and CD55. In short, since only cells containing the 1q and part of the 1p arm bound virus, the gene for the receptor for measles virus was probably located on chromosome 1.

A MONOCLONAL ANTIBODY DIRECTED AGAINST A CELL-SURFACE PROTEIN INHIBITS MEASLES VIRUS BINDING AND INFECTIONS

Another laboratory (Naniche et al. 1992) demonstrated that a monoclonal antibody (MCI20.6) directed against a human cell-surface glycoprotein was capable of inhibiting measles virus binding to the host cell. This antibody recognized two polypeptides with molecular masses of 57 kD and/or 67 kD from HeLa, Raji, Jurkat, and Vero cells. From our search of lymphocyte markers on chromosome 1, only the CD46 (membrane cofactor protein, MCP) gene could produce proteins of this magnitude. CD46 also seemed an ideal candidate for the measles virus receptor, since it is expressed widely on the surface of most human tissues, including T cells, B cells, monocytes, normal kidney cells, endothelial cells, epithelial cells, placenta, and sperm. However, human erythrocytes do not express CD46, which correlates with the inability of the red blood cell to bind measles virus. We set out to prove that CD46 was indeed the receptor for measles virus by using polyclonal antibodies directed against CD46 to block binding and infection, and by expressing the coding sequence for CD46 in CHO cells in an attempt to render them susceptible to infection.

POLYCLONAL ANTIBODIES DIRECTED AGAINST CD46 INHIBIT MEASLES VIRUS BINDING AND INFECTION OF HELA CELLS

We reasoned that polyclonal antibodies and possibly some monoclonal antibodies directed against CD46 should interfere with virus binding and prevent infection (Dörig et al. 1993). Rabbit polyclonal antiserum prepared from highly purified CD46 and a monoclonal antibody (GB24) were obtained from John P. Atkinson (Seya et al. 1988; Cho et al. 1991). Another commercial CD46 monoclonal antibody (J4-48) was purchased from AMAC Inc. Preincubation of HeLa cells with polyclonal antibodies at dilutions of 1/8 to 1/500 completely abolished measles virus binding and infection, but the monoclonals had no effect, suggesting that they interact at sites distinct from those used in virus binding. In addition, we used these immunological reagents to screen primate, rodent, and mouse/human hybrid cell lines for the presence of CD46 using fluorescence-activated cell sorting (FACS) analysis. All cell lines susceptible to infection by measles virus reacted with the CD46 antisera (Table 1). Vero monkey kidney cells did not bind the CD46 monoclonal antibody (J4-48), but they were recognized by the CD46 polyclonal antisera (A. Marcil, unpubl.). The mouse/human cell lines containing the 1q arm of human chromosome 1 also expressed CD46 as expected. However, mouse and hamster cell lines which neither bound virus nor were infected did not express CD46 (Table 1). From these results, we were quite certain that human CD46 was indeed the receptor for measles virus.

A MONOCLONAL ANTIBODY THAT INHIBITS VIRUS BINDING AND INFECTION RECOGNIZES CD46

Independent of our studies, Denis Gerlier's laboratory (Naniche et al. 1993a) purified the 57-kD and 67-kD proteins that react with the monoclonal antibody (MCI20.6) by immunoaffinity chromatography and subjected them to amino-terminal sequencing. The first 15 amino acids of the two polypeptides corresponded to the amino-terminal sequence of mature CD46. Their data provided the first biochemical evidence that the protein recognized by their inhibitory monoclonal antibody was indeed CD46. This same laboratory demonstrated that newly synthesized H protein in the infected cell causes internalization or down-regulation of CD46 at the cell surface. The mechanism of down-regulation is not clear, but the two proteins may interact with each other inside the cell, interfering with their expression on the cell surface (Naniche et al. 1993b). CD46/hemagglutinin interaction was also shown to be important for uptake of measles virus antigens prior to major histocompatibility complex (MHC) class-II-restricted presentation of processed peptides to T cells (Gerlier et al. 1994).

STRUCTURE OF CD46

CD46, also known as membrane cofactor protein (MCP), belongs to a family of structurally, functionally, and genetically related proteins (RCA, regulators of complement activation), which are clustered at the 1q32 locus of human chromosome 1 (Liszewski et al. 1991; Liszewski and Atkinson 1992). Other members of this family are decay-accelerating factor (CD55), complement receptor 1 (CD35), complement receptor 2 (CD21), inhibitor of reactive lysis (CD59), C4b binding protein (C4bp), and factor H. These regulatory proteins are composed largely of short consensus repeats (SCRs), which are the sites for binding by C3 and C4 complement component derivatives. The CD46 gene spans more than 43 kb on the genomic DNA and encodes 14 exons (Post et al. 1991). Alternative splicing gives rise to a number of polyprotein isoforms (Post et al. 1991; Purcell et al. 1991). All of them possess a signal peptide of 34 amino acids, which is removed during maturation of the protein. The amino terminus of the mature protein consists of four short consensus repeats (SCR I–IV) and one to three (Ser/Thr/Pro)-rich domains (STP^A, STP^B, and STP^C), which vary depending on the exon used. Further toward the carboxyl terminus there are 13 amino acids of unknown significance (U) and 24 hydrophobic amino acids which form the transmembrane domain. One of two cytoplasmic domains (CYT1 or CYT2) can be chosen to form the carboxyl terminus. The isoforms are named according to the presence of the Ser/Thr/Pro-rich domains and cytoplasmic tails (e.g., MCP-ABC1 for a protein containing STP^A, STP^B, and STP^C and the cytoplasmic domain CYT1). Mainly four isoforms of CD46 are expressed in the majority of cells examined; the proteins fall into groups of two different apparent molecular masses: 51–58 kD and 59–68 kD. In addition, CD46 is highly glycosylated, and three potential N-glycosylation sites are present in the short consensus repeats I, II, and IV, whereas the STP domains carry 5–10 O-linked sugar chains. The structure of the protein is represented in Figure 2.

CD46 NORMALLY FUNCTIONS AS A COMPLEMENT REGULATORY PROTEIN

The complement system is one mechanism that vertebrates use to defend themselves against foreign organisms (Abbas et al. 1991). One consequence of complement binding is the activation of proteolytic cascades of serum proteins, which leads to the assembly of the membrane attack complex (MAC) on the surface of invading cells to form a pore that renders the cell sensitive to osmotic shock. Components of the complement system can also act as opsonins to stimulate phagocytosis of microbes by macrophages, initiate clearance of immune complexes deposited on erythrocytes, and stimulate anaphylaxis and neutrophil infiltration. There are two pathways that activate the complement system: One is the classic pathway that acts in the presence of antibodies directed against the foreign antigen, and the second is the alternative pathway, which is antibody-independent and is stimulated by complement binding to microbial surfaces and polysaccharides. Complement activation proceeds through a proteolytic cascade which forms first the C3 and subsequently the C5 convertase complexes. C3 convertases contain com-

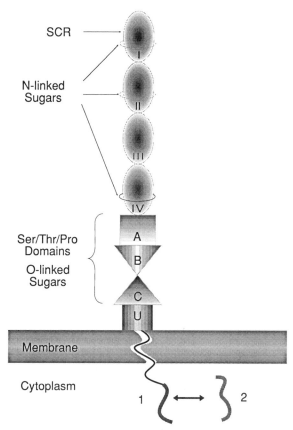

SCR

N-linked
Sugars

Ser/Thr/Pro
Domains

O-linked
Sugars

Membrane

Cytoplasm

Figure 2 Molecular structure of CD46 (MCP). CD46 is a complement-binding protein containing 4 SCR elements (I–IV) in the amino-terminal half of the protein. SCRI, II, and IV each contain one site for *N*-linked glycosylation. Following the SCRs, there are 1–3 Ser/Thr/Pro domains (represented by A, B, and C) which are *O*-linked to carbohydrate. Alternative splicing of A, B, and C exons gives rise to a number of isoforms. A short region of undefined function (U) is situated just above the membrane next to the hydrophobic membrane-spanning region. One of two different cytoplasmic domains (1 or 2) is chosen to form the carboxyl terminus. The isoforms are named according to the presence of specific Ser/Thr/Pro-rich domains and the cytoplasmic tail used. (Modified, with permission, from Liszewski and Atkinson 1992.)

ponent C3b in the alternative pathway and contain C4b in the classic pathway. Uncontrolled activation of complement can be detrimental, leading to formation of the MAC on self tissues, phagocytosis of healthy cells, and excessive production of inflammatory mediators. Consequently, the classic and alternative complement cascades are tightly regulated by several fluid-phase and membrane-associated proteins, which interact with specific components of the complement system.

There are several RCA that are also involved in the negative control of C3 convertase. These include complement receptor 1 (CD35), CD55, C4b binding protein (C4bp), factor H, and CD46 (MCP). CD46 is an integral membrane protein which is expressed on the surface of most human cells and serves as a cofactor for proteolytic inactivation of C3b and C4b by factor I, a serine protease in the plasma (for review, see Hourcade et al. 1989; Liszewski et al. 1991; Liszewski and Atkinson 1992). Since CD46 is present on virtually all human cells except erythrocytes and also has the ability to inactivate C3b/C4b, it plays an important role in discriminating self from non-self and helps to prevent destruction of the host cell via the MAC.

EXPRESSION OF CD46 PROTEIN IN RODENT CELL LINES MAKES THEM SUSCEPTIBLE TO INFECTION BY MEASLES VIRUS

To prove conclusively that CD46 was a receptor for measles virus, our laboratory generated stable hamster cell lines, which stably expressed this membrane glycoprotein (Dörig et al. 1993). The coding region for CD46 was isolated from a placenta cDNA library and cloned into two different expression vectors under control of either the ubiquitin or CMV early gene. In our laboratory, two different splicing variants (MCP-BC2 and MCP-C2) were expressed in CHO cells. Cells were selected in the presence of neomycin and assayed for expression by FACS analysis with monoclonal antibodies. As predicted, all CD46$^+$ cell lines produced rosettes in the presence of measles virus and monkey erythrocytes, whereas control cells did not (Fig. 3). In addition, when inoculated with measles virus, the CD46$^+$ CHO cells produced syncytia in a time-dependent manner between 48 hours and 96 hours postinfection. The giant cells increased in size between 72 hours and 96 hours postinfection. This fusion was not as extensive as that seen in Vero or HeLa cells, since only 15–20% of the CD46$^+$ CHO cells produced syncytia. However, higher levels of CD46 expression would probably have increased the level of syncytium formation. Finally, CD46$^+$ CHO cells produced virus-specific proteins following infection with measles virus. Cells were harvested at different times postinfection and analyzed by Western immunoblot analysis with antibodies specific for the H and F proteins of measles virus (Fig. 4). Again, these virus-specific glycoproteins were synthesized in a time-dependent fashion and paralleled syncytium formation. These experiments provided definitive proof that CD46 was a receptor for measles virus and rendered the cells susceptible to infection.

Very similar experiments were performed by Denis Gerlier's group in France using mouse fibroblast (Ltk$^-$) and mouse lymphoblastoma (M12)

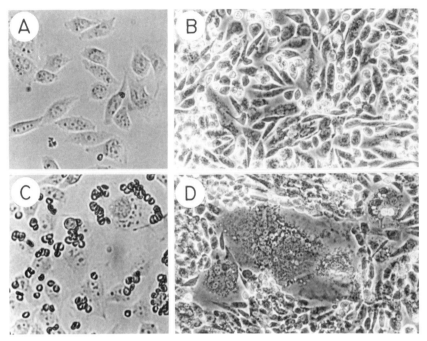

Figure 3 Measles virus-binding assays and infections of CHO cells expressing β-galactosidase or CD46. CHO cells producing β-galactosidase (*A, B*) or CD46 (isoform MCP-C2) (*C, D*) were assayed for their ability to bind measles virus (*A, C*) and for their susceptibility to infection by measles virus (*B, D*). (*A, C*) Measles virus was incubated with CHO cell lines. Nonadsorbed virus was removed by washing, and cells were subsequently incubated with African green monkey red blood cells. Rosettes were evident on cells expressing CD46. (*B, D*) Cells were inoculated with measles virus, incubated for 96 hr, and viewed by phase contrast microscopy. Cytopathic effect (syncytium formation) was obvious only on CD46$^+$ cells.

cell lines expressing CD46 (Naniche et al. 1993b). The presence of CD46 at the cell surface was verified by FACS and immunoprecipitation analysis. Measles virus binding was first established by FACS analysis using a monoclonal antibody specific for the H protein of measles virus; a shift in fluorescence indicated that binding occurred. The ability of CD46$^+$ cells to produce syncytia was assayed by infecting the cells with vaccinia recombinant virus expressing both measles virus H and F proteins (VV-H/F). Syncytium formation normally requires both the H and F proteins to be synthesized in addition to the presence of a specific receptor for the H protein; mouse cell lines do not normally fuse when infected with the vaccinia recombinant (Wild et al. 1991). The CD46$^+$

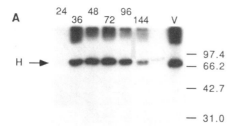

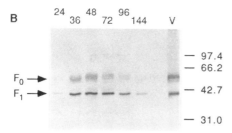

Figure 4 Immunoblots performed on lysates from CHO cells expressing CD46. CHO cells expressing the MCP-BC2 isoform of CD46 were infected with measles virus, and total cell lysates were collected at 24, 36, 48, 72, 96, and 144 hr postinfection. (*A*) The immunoblot was probed with a monoclonal antibody (2B1-3) directed against measles hemagglutinin (H) protein. (*B*) A duplicate immunoblot was probed with polyclonal antisera directed against a carboxy-terminal peptide of the measles virus fusion (F) protein. Both viral glycoproteins (H and F) were produced in a time-dependent manner, indicating that $CD46^+$ CHO cells are susceptible to infection by measles virus.

mouse cell lines produced syncytia when infected with VV-H/F much in the same way that HeLa and Jurkat cells did. Measles virus was shown to replicate only in the $CD46^+M12$ cells and not the $CD46^+Ltk^-$ cells, since syncytia, low titers of virus (4×10^4 pfu/ml), and H protein were obtained in the mouse lymphoblastoid cell line. The absence of replication in the mouse $CD46^+$ fibroblasts was attributed to the absence of some cell-specific factor which has still not been identified. However, taken together, the work from two independent laboratories has confirmed that CD46 is indeed a receptor for measles virus.

SUSCEPTIBILITY TO MEASLES VIRUS PARALLELS CD46 TISSUE DISTRIBUTION

Virtually all tested primate cells, including sperm and trophoblast, express CD46 (Seya et al. 1988; Holmes et al. 1992; Cervoni et al. 1993;

Johnson 1993), and CD46 expression appears to be of great importance for protection against complement-mediated damage. One prominent group of cells that do not express CD46 are the red blood cells from some higher primates. The erythrocytes of human and gorilla do not express CD46 on their surface, whereas orangutan red blood cells are recognized by an antibody directed against CD46 (Nickells and Atkinson 1990). Human and chimpanzee red blood cells do not hemagglutinate in the presence of measles virus (Periés and Chany 1960; Martin and Fraser 1978; R.E. Dörig et al., unpubl.); this appears to correlate with an absence of CD46 on their cell surface. On the other hand, erythrocytes from rhesus, cynomolgus, patas, cercopithecus, marmoset, and baboon do agglutinate in the presence of measles virus. Preliminary data in our laboratory demonstrate that these cells express CD46. In contrast, red blood cells from other mammals such as sheep, cow, horse, cat, rabbit, chicken, guinea pig, hamster, mouse, and rat do not bind measles virus (Periés and Chany 1960; Rosanoff 1961). Primate tissues appear to be the only target for normal measles virus capable of causing a generalized systemic infection.

The situation is somewhat more complex when one considers infections of the central nervous system in mice. Although mice are not susceptible to natural measles infections via the respiratory or intravenous route, an artificial infection can be achieved by injecting the virus directly into the brain (Liebert and ter Meulen 1987). A functional homolog of CD46/DAF has recently been shown to be expressed in a wide variety of mouse tissues (Li et al. 1993). However, its sequence is much closer to CD35 (complement receptor 1) than to CD46 (MCP) (Paul et al. 1990), which would explain its inability to interact with measles virus. On the other hand, primary rat and human brain astrocytes express a protein that is recognized by antibodies directed against CD46 (Gordon et al. 1992; Yang et al. 1993). Therefore, it seems realistic that the mouse brain cells may also express a protein with some sequence similarity to CD46. The presence of an astrocyte CD46-like protein could explain the susceptibility of mouse brain for measles virus following intracerebral injection.

SPECIFIC BINDING DOMAINS ON CD46 (MCP) REMAIN TO BE DETERMINED

The question arises whether measles virus uses the same binding domains on CD46 (MCP) as do the complement components. The CD46 domains that bind to C3b and C4b were previously mapped to SCR III–IV and SCR II–IV, respectively, using deletion mutants (Adams et al. 1991). In addition, a monoclonal antibody directed against CD46,

GB24, inhibits in vitro binding of C3b to CD46, as well as C3b proteolytic degradation (Adams et al. 1991; Cho et al. 1991). However, this antibody does not affect binding or infection by measles virus. In contrast, a polyclonal antiserum directed against CD46 completely prevents virus attachment, demonstrating that virus/CD46 interaction can be blocked with the appropriate antibody (Dörig et al. 1993). Taken together, these results suggest that the complement components and measles virus use distinct binding sites on CD46. In addition to the results discussed above, it is clear that at least the two Ser/Thr/Pro-rich domains A and B are dispensable for viral attachment, since a CD46 isoform that contains only the Ser/Thr/Pro-rich domain STP^C (MCP-C2) supports binding and infection (Dörig et al. 1993; Naniche et al. 1993b). Recently, it was also demonstrated that multiple isoforms of CD46 (C1, C2, BC1, and BC2) can function equally well as receptors for measles virus (Manchester et al. 1994). It is relevant to note that the receptor for Epstein-Barr virus (EBV) is CD21 (also known as CR2), which is also a member of the RCA family found on chromosome 1 (Tanner et al. 1987; Ahearn and Fearon 1989). However, CD21 contains 15 or 16 amino-terminal SCRs which are similar in structure but immunologically distinct from those found in CD46. SCR domains I–IV of CD21 bind the complement components C3d and C3g, whereas the major EBV surface glycoprotein (gp350/220) binds to the amino-terminal SCR domains I and II (Carel et al. 1990). It is possible by analogy with EBV that measles virus binds to SCR I and SCR II of CD46, but the regions of interaction between H and CD46 remain to be determined. Studies with mutant proteins will be required to map the binding domains for measles virus.

OTHER RECEPTORS FOR MEASLES VIRUS MAY BE INVOLVED IN PENETRATION

CD46 has been conclusively shown to function as a cellular receptor for measles virus (Dörig et al. 1993; Naniche et al. 1993b). Whether it is the sole receptor remains to be explored further. Alternative receptors and/or cofactors are known for other viruses (for review, see Haywood 1994). Semliki forest virus, which utilizes MHC class I as a receptor, also infects MHC-I-negative cells (Marsh and Helenius 1989). HIV-1 can also infect CD4$^-$ cells using galactosyl ceramide as a low-affinity receptor, or via complement-binding proteins and antibodies specific for the retrovirus (Bhat et al. 1991; Dierich et al. 1993; Fantini et al. 1993). In addition to alternative receptors, there are a number of indications that several viruses with pH-independent fusion at the plasma membrane require at least one further cellular component for their productive entry into the host cell. Murine cells expressing human CD4, the receptor for HIV-1, are not susceptible to infection by HIV-1 (Maddon et al. 1986). The virus binds to the host cell, but the nucleocapsid is not transported into the cytoplasm (Signoret et al. 1993). Although it remains a controversial issue, CD26 has recently been suggested as cofactor to CD4/HIV binding, which facilitates fusion of the viral membrane with the plasma membrane of the host cell (Callebaut et al. 1993). Studies with two different strains of mouse hepatitis virus revealed that several cellular factors are required for cell entry (Asanaka and Lai 1993; Yokomori et al. 1993). In the case of the ecotropic murine retrovirus, it is assumed that a second, limiting cellular factor is required for infection (Wang et al. 1991). Measles virus also attaches and fuses to the plasma membrane of its host cell; it seems plausible that an additional receptor or factor may interact with the F protein and facilitate fusion and penetration of the virus into the host cell. No firm evidence for this process exists at this time.

Another recent candidate for a specific receptor for measles virus is the cytoskeletal protein moesin, which is a member of the erythrocyte band 4.1 protein family along with ezrin and radixin. Moesin is associated with intracellular actin, but a small portion of this protein is exposed on the cell surface. Dunster et al. (1994) screened monoclonal antibodies raised against cell-surface proteins and discovered one antibody (mAB119) that inhibited measles virus infections and recognized a 75-kD cellular protein. Microsequencing of the amino terminus of this protein revealed that it was moesin. The monoclonal antibody mAB119, as well as a standard one directed against moesin (mAb38/87), inhibited the binding of measles virus to human monocytes; a control antibody had no effect. Therefore, moesin could function as an additional receptor or a cofactor for measles infection. Interestingly, Lankes et al. (1988) demonstrated that the epitope recognized by mAb38/87 is not expressed on the surface of the Jurkat human T-leukemia cell line, cells which are normally highly susceptible to measles virus infection. However, moesin is widely distributed throughout endothelial, epithelial, skeletal muscle, and smooth muscle cells—a required characteristic for a measles virus receptor. It remains to be seen what the exact role of this protein is in relation to virus attachment and penetration.

PERSPECTIVES AND DIRECTIONS FOR FUTURE RESEARCH

The identification of CD46 as a cellular receptor for measles virus helps explain the primate specificity and wide tissue range exhibited during viral infections. However, many questions regarding virus/host interaction and the mechanism of viral entry remain to be explored. For example, the exact peptide domains on CD46 that interact with the measles virus hemagglutinin protein remain to be elucidated. Analysis of mutant proteins and the production of monoclonal antibodies directed against specific regions of CD46 should facilitate the identification of the virus-binding domain. Of similar interest are the sites of interaction on the measles virus hemagglutinin (H) protein. Future research with other members of the morbillivirus subfamily, including canine distemper virus, rinderpest virus, phocine distemper virus, and PPRV (pestivirus des petits ruminants), should identify specific receptors for these viruses that explain their host range. Attachment of a virus to its specific host-cell receptor is simply the first step in the process of infection. The role of other cellular proteins involved in membrane fusion and penetration of the host cell could prove equally intriguing. Another challenging study concerns the interaction of measles virus with cells of the central nervous system and its implication in neurological disease following intracerebral inoculation of the virus. The differences between neurotropic strains and systemic wild-type measles virus await definition. Finally, transgenic mice expressing human CD46 may provide a deeper understanding of the immunology and pathogenesis of measles virus infections. These mice could serve as the first small animal model for testing measles virus vaccines and antiviral drugs.

REFERENCES

Aaby, P., B. Samb, F. Simondon, K. Knudson, A.M.C. Seck, S. Bennett, and H. Whittle. 1993. Divergent mortality for male and female recipients of low-titer and high titer measles vaccines in rural Senegal. *Am. J. Epidemiol.* **138:** 746.

Abbas, A.K., A.H. Lichtman, and J.S. Pober. 1991. The complement system. In *Cellular and molecular immunology*, p. 259. W.B. Saunders, Philadelphia.

Adams, E.M., M.C. Brown, M. Nunge, M. Krych, and J.P. Atkinson. 1991. Contribution of the repeating domains of membrane cofactor protein (MCP; CD46) of the complement system to ligand binding and cofactor activity. *J. Immunol.* **147:** 3005.

Ahearn, J.M. and D.T. Fearon. 1989. Structure and function of the complement receptors, CR1 (CD35) and CR2 (CD21). *Adv. Immunol.* **46:** 183.

Albrecht, P., D. Lorenz, M.J. Klutch, J.H. Vickers, and F.A. Ennis. 1980. Fatal measles infection in marmosets: Pathogenesis and prophylaxis. *Infect. Immun.* **27:** 969.

Alkhatib, G. and D.J. Briedis. 1986. The predicted primary structure of measles virus hemagglutinin. *Virology* **150:** 479.

Asanaka, M. and M.M.C. Lai. 1993. Cell fusion studies identified multiple cellular factors involved in mouse hepatitis virus entry. *Virology* **197:** 732.

Barclay, A.N., M.L. Birkeland, M.H. Brown, A.D. Beyers, S.J. Davis, C. Somoza, and A. Williams. 1993. *The leukocyte antigen factsbook.* Academic Press, New York, p. 206.

Bhat, S., S.L. Spitalnik, F. Gonzalez-Scarano, and D.H. Silberberg. 1991. Galactosyl ceramide or a derivative is an essential component of the neural receptor for human immunodeficiency virus type I envelope glycoprotein gp120. *Proc. Natl. Acad. Sci.* **88:** 7131.

Billeter, M.A. and R. Cattaneo. 1991. Molecular biology of defective measles virus persisting in the human central nervous system. In *The paramyxoviruses* (ed. D.W. Kingsbury), p. 323. Plenum Press, New York.

Calain, P. and L. Roux. 1988. Generation of measles virus defective interfering particles and their presence in a preparation of attenuated live-virus vaccine. *J. Viol.* **62:** 2589.

Callebaut, C., B. Krust, E. Jacotot, and A.G. Hovanessian. 1993. T cell activation antigen, CD26, as a cofactor for entry of HIV in CD4+ cells. *Science* **262:** 2045.

Carel, J.-C., B.L. Myones, B. Frazier, and V.M. Holers. 1990. Structural requirements for C3d,g/Epstein-Barr virus receptor (CR2/CD21) ligand binding, internalization, and viral infection. *J. Biol. Chem.* **265:** 12293.

Carrigan, D.R. 1986. Round cell variant of measles virus: Neurovirulence and pathogenesis of acute encephalitis in newborn hamsters. *Virology* **148:** 349.

Cervoni, F., P. Fenichel, C. Akhoundi, B.-L. Hsi, and B. Rossi. 1993. Characterization of a cDNA clone coding for human testis membrane cofactor protein (MCP, CD46). *Mol. Reprod. Dev.* **34:** 107.

Cho, S.-W., T.J. Oglesby, B.-L. Hsi, E.M. Adams, and J.P. Atkinson. 1991. Characterization of three monoclonal antibodies to membrane co-factor protein (MCP) of the complement system and quantification of MCP by radioassay. *Clin. Exp. Immunol.* **83:** 257.

Dierich, M.P., C.F. Ebenbichler, P. Marschang, G. Füst, N.M. Thielens, and G.J. Arlaud. 1993. HIV and human complement: Mechanisms of interaction and biological implication. *Immunol. Today* **14:** 435.

Dore-Duffy, P. and C. Howe. 1978. N-acetylneuraminic acid (NANA) in measles virus. *Proc. Soc. Exp. Biol. Med.* **157:** 622.

Dörig, R.E., A. Marcil, A. Chopra, and C.D. Richardson. 1993. The human CD46 molecule is a receptor for measles virus (Edmonston strain). *Cell* **75:** 295.

Dunster, L.M., J. Schneider-Schaulies, S. Löffler, W. Lankes, R. Schwartz-Albiez, F. Lottspeich, and V. ter Meulen. 1994. Moesin: A cell membrane protein linked with susceptibility to measles virus infection. *Virology* **198:** 265.

Esolen, L.M., B.J. Ward, T.R. Moench, and D.E. Griffin. 1993. Infection of monocytes during measles. *J. Infect. Dis.* **168:** 47.

Fantini, J., D.G. Cook, N. Nathanson, S.L. Spitalnik, F. Gonzalez-Scarano. 1993. Infection of colonic epithelial cell lines by type I human immunodeficiency virus is associated with cell surface expression of galactosylceramide, a potential alternative gp120 receptor. *Proc. Natl. Acad. Sci.* **90:** 2700.

Fenger, T.W. and C. Howe. 1979. Isolation and characterization of erythrocyte receptors for measles virus. *Proc. Soc. Exp. Biol. Med.* **162:** 299.

Fraser, K.B. and S.J. Martin. 1978. *Measles virus and its biology.* Academic Press, London.

Garenne, M., O. Leroy, J.P. Bean, and I. Sene. 1991. Child mortality after high-titre measles vaccines: Prospective study in Senegal. *Lancet* **338:** 903.

Gerlier, D., M.-C. Trescol-Biémont, G. Varior-Krishnan, D. Naniche, I. Fugier-Vivier, and C. Rabourdin-Combe. 1994. Efficient major histocompatibility complex class II-restricted presentation of measles virus relies on hemagglutinin-mediated targeting to its cellular receptor human CD46 expressed by murine B cells. *J. Exp. Med.* **179:** 353.

Gordon, D.L., T.A. Sadlon, S.L. Wesselingh, S.M. Russell, R.W. Johnstone, and D.F.J. Purcell. 1992. Human astrocytes express membrane cofactor protein (CD46), a regulator of complement activation. *J. Neuroimmunol.* **36:** 199.

Griffin, D.E. and B.J. Ward. 1993. Differential CD4 T cell activation in measles. *J. In-*

fect. Dis. **168:** 275.

Harrowe, G., M. Mitsuhashi, and D.G. Payan. 1990. Measles virus—Substance P receptor interactions. *J. Clin. Invest.* **85:** 1324.

Harrowe, G., J. Sudduth-Klinger, and D.G. Payan. 1992. Measles virus—Substance P receptor interactions: Jurkat lymphocytes transfected with substance P receptor cDNA enhance measles virus fusion and replication. *Cell. Mol. Neurobiol.* **12:** 397.

Haywood, A.M. 1994. Virus receptors: Binding, adhesion strengthening, and changes in viral structure. *J. Virol.* **68:** 1.

Hilleman, M.R. 1994. Vaccinology, immunology, and comparative pathogenesis of measles in the quest for a preventative against AIDS. *AIDS Res. Hum. Retroviruses* **10:** 3.

Holmes, C.H., K.L. Simpson, H. Okada, N. Okada, S.D. Wainwright, D.F.J. Purcell, and J.M. Houlihan. 1992. Complement regulatory proteins at the feto-maternal interface during human placental development: Distribution of CD59 by comparison with membrane cofactor protein (CD46) and decay accelerating factor (CD55). *Eur. J. Immunol.* **22:** 1579.

Holt, E.A., L.H. Moulton, G.K. Siberry, and N.A. Halsey. 1993. Differential mortality by measles vaccine: Titer and sex. *J. Inf. Dis.* **168:** 1087.

Hourcade, D., V.M. Holers, and J.P. Atkinson. 1989. The regulators of complement activation (RCA) gene clusters. *Adv. Immunol.* **45:** 381.

Howe, C. and L.T. Lee. 1972. Virus-erythrocyte interactions. *Adv. Virus Res.* **17:** 1.

Johnson, P.M. 1993. Immunobiology of the human placental trophoblast. *Exp. Clin. Immunogenet.* **10:** 118.

Kingsbury, D.W. 1991. *The paramyxoviruses.* Plenum Press, New York.

Krah, D.L. and P.W. Choppin. 1988. Mice immunized with measles virus develop antibodies to a cell surface receptor for binding virus. *J. Virol.* **62:** 1565.

Lankes, W., A. Griesmacher, J. Grünwald, R. Schwartz-Albiez, and R. Keller. 1988. A heparin-binding protein involved in inhibition of smooth-muscle cell proliferation. *Biochem. J.* **251:** 831.

Li, B., C. Sallee, M. Dehoff, S. Foley, H. Molina, and V.M. Holers. 1993. Mouse Crry/p65. Characterization of monoclonal antibodies and the tissue distribution of a functional homologue of human MCP and DAF. *J. Immunol.* **151:** 4295.

Liebert, U.G. and V. ter Meulen. 1987. Virological aspects of measles virus-induced encephalomyelitis in Lewis and BN rats. *J. Gen. Virol.* **68:** 1715.

Liszewski, M.K. and J.P. Atkinson. 1992. Membrane cofactor protein. *Curr. Top. Microbiol. Immunol.* **178:** 45.

Liszewski, M.K., T.W. Post, and J.P. Atkinson. 1991. Membrane cofactor protein (MCP or CD46): Newest member of the regulators of complement activation gene cluster. *Annu. Rev. Immunol.* **9:** 431.

Maddon, P.J., A.G. Dalgleish, J.S. McDougal, P.R. Clapham, R.A. Weiss, and R. Axel. 1986. The T4 gene encodes the AIDS virus receptor and is expressed in the immune system and the brain. *Cell* **47:** 333.

Manchester, M., M.K. Liszewski, J.P. Atkinson, and M.B.A. Oldstone. 1994. Multiple isoforms of CD46 (membrane cofactor protein) serve as receptors for measles virus. *Proc. Natl. Acad. Sci.* **91:** 2161.

Markwell, M.A.K. 1991. New frontiers opened by the exploration of host cell receptors. In *The paramyxoviruses.* (ed. D.W. Kingsbury), p. 407. Plenum Press, New York.

Markwell, M.A.K., L. Svennerholm, and J.C. Paulson. 1981. Specific gangliosides function as host cell receptors for Sendai virus. *Proc. Natl. Acad. Sci.* **78:** 5406.

Marsh, M. and A. Helenius. 1989. Virus entry into animal cells. *Adv. Virus Res.* **36:** 107.

Matumoto, M. 1966. Multiplication of measles virus in cell cultures. *Bacteriol. Rev.* **30:** 152.

Naniche, D., T.F. Wild, C. Rabourdin-Combe, and D. Gerlier. 1992. A monoclonal antibody recognizes a human cell surface glycoprotein involved in measles virus binding. *J. Gen. Virol.* **73:** 2617.

―――. 1993a. Measles virus haemagglutinin induces down-regulation of gp57/67, a molecule involved in virus binding. *J. Gen. Virol.* **74:** 1073.

Naniche, D., G. Varior-Krishnan, F. Cervoni, T.F. Wild, B. Rossi, C. Rabourdin-Combe, and D. Gerlier. 1993b. Human membrane cofactor protein (CD46) acts as a cellular receptor for measles virus. *J. Virol.* **67:** 6025.

Nickells, M.W. and J.P. Atkinson. 1990. Characterization of CR1- and membrane cofactor protein-like proteins of two primates. *J. Immunol.* **144:** 4262.

Norrby, E. 1962. Hemagglutination by measles virus. *Arch. Gesamte Virusforsch.* **12:** 164.

Norrby, E. and M.N. Oxman. 1990. Measles virus. In *Virology*, 2nd edition (ed. B.N. Fields et al.), p. 1013. Raven Press, New York.

Paul, M.S., M. Aegerter, K. Cepek, M.D. Miller, and J.H. Weis. 1990. The murine complement receptor gene family. III. The genomic and transcriptional complexity of the Crry and Crry-ps genes. *J. Immunol.* **144:** 1988.

Periés, J.R. and C. Chany. 1960. Activité hémagglutinante et hémolytique du virus morbilleux. *C.R. Acad. Sci.* **251:** 820.

―――. 1962. Mécanisme de l'action hémagglutinante des cultures de virus morbilleux. *C.R. Acad. Sci.* **252:** 2956.

Post, T.W., M.K. Liszewski, E.M. Adams, I. Tedja, E.A. Miller, and J.P. Atkinson. 1991. Membrane cofactor protein of the complement system: Alternative splicing of serine/threonine/proline-rich exons and cytoplasmic tails produce multiple isoforms that correlate with protein phenotype. *J. Exp. Med.* **174:** 93.

Purcell, D.F.J., S.M. Russell, N.J. Deacon, M.A. Brown, D.J. Hooker, and I.F.C. McKenzie. 1991. Alternatively spliced RNAs encode several isoforms of CD46 (MCP), a regulator of complement activation. *Immunogenetics* **33:** 335.

Randall, R.E. and W.C. Russell. 1991. Paramyxovirus persistence. Consequences for host and virus. In *The paramyxoviruses* (ed. D.W. Kingsbury), p. 323. Plenum Press, New York.

Richardson, C.D., D. Hull, P. Greer, K. Hasel, A. Berkovich, G. Englund, W. Bellini, B. Rima, and R. Lazzarini. 1986. The nucleotide sequence of the mRNA encoding the fusion protein of measles virus (Edmonston strain): A comparison of fusion proteins from several different paramyxoviruses. *Virology* **155:** 508.

Rosanoff, E.I. 1961. Hemagglutination and hemadsorption of measles virus. *Proc. Soc. Exp. Biol. Med.* **106:** 563.

Rota, P.A., A.E. Bloom, J.A. Vanchiere, and W.J. Bellini. 1994a. Evolution of the nucleoprotein and matrix genes of wild-type strains of measles virus isolated from recent epidemics. *Virology* **198:** 724.

Rota, J.S., K.B. Hummel, P.A. Rota, and W.J. Bellini. 1992. Genetic variability of the glycoprotein genes of current wild-type measles isolates. *Virology* **188:** 135.

Rota, J.S., Z.-D. Wang, P.A. Rota, and W.J. Bellini. 1994b. Comparison of sequences of the H, F, and N coding genes of measles virus vaccine strains. *Virus Res.* **31:** 317.

Schroeder, C. 1986. Substance P, a neuropeptide, inhibits measles virus replication in cell culture. *Acta Virol.* **30:** 432.

Schumacher, H.P., P. Albrecht, and N.M. Tauraso. 1972. Markers for measles virus. Tissue culture properties. *Arch. Gesamte Virusforsch.* **36:** 296.

Seya, T., L.L. Ballard, N.S. Bora, V. Kumar, W. Cui, and J.P. Atkinson. 1988. Distribution of membrane cofactor protein of complement on human peripheral blood cells. An altered form is found on granulocytes. *Eur. J. Immunol.* **18:** 1289.

Signoret, N., P. Poignard, D. Blanc, and Q.J. Sattentau. 1993. Human and simian immunodeficiency viruses: Virus-receptor interactions. *Trends Microbiol.* **1:** 328.

Tanner, J., J. Weis, D. Fearon, Y. Whang, and E. Kieff. 1987. Epstein-Barr virus gp350/220 binding to the B lymphocyte C3d receptor mediates adsorption, capping, and endocytosis. *Cell* **50:** 203.

Tischer, I. 1967. Erhöhte Empfindlichkeit von neuraminidasebehandelten Affenerythrocyten für den Nachweis der Haemagglutinationsaktivität von Masernviren und einigen Adenoviren. *Zentralbl. Bakteriol. 1 Abt Orig. A Med. Microbiol. Infektionskr. Parasitol.* **204:** 466.

Valdimarsson, H., G. Agnarsdottir, and P.J. Lachmann. 1975. Measles virus receptor on human T lymphocytes. *Nature* **255:** 554.

Wang, H., R. Paul, R.E. Burgeson, D.R. Keene, and D. Kabat. 1991. Plasma membrane receptors for ecotropic murine retroviruses require a limiting accessory factor. *J. Virol.* **65:** 6468.

Weis, W., J.H. Brown, S. Cusack, J.C. Paulson, J.J. Skehel, and D.C. Wiley. 1988. Structure of the influenza virus haemagglutinin complexed with its receptor sialic acid. *Nature* **333:** 426.

Weiss, R. 1992. Measles battle loses potent weapon. *Science* **258:** 546.

Wild, T.F., E. Malvoisin, and R. Buckland. 1991. Measles virus: Both the haemagglutinin and fusion glycoproteins are required for fusion. *J. Gen. Virol.* **72:** 439.

Yang, C., J.L. Jones, and S.R. Barnum. 1993. Expression of decay-accelerating factor (CD55), membrane cofactor protein (CD46) and CD59 in the human astroglioma cell line, D54-MG, and primary rat astrocytes. *J. Neuroimmunol.* **47:** 123.

Yokomori, K., M. Asanaka, S.A. Stohlman, and M.M.C. Lai. 1993. A spike protein-dependent cellular factor other than the viral receptor is required for mouse hepatitis virus entry. *Virology* **196:** 45.

11

Receptor Binding and Membrane Fusion by Influenza Hemagglutinin

John J. Skehel, David Steinhauer,
and Steve A. Wharton
Division of Virology
National Institute for Medical Research
London, NW7 1AA, United Kingdom

Per A. Bullough, Fred M. Hughson,
Stan J. Watowich, and Don C. Wiley
Department of Biochemistry and Molecular Biology
Harvard University
Cambridge, Massachusetts 02138

The influenza component which is involved in receptor recognition and membrane fusion to effect transfer of the RNA genome-transcriptase complex into the cell is the hemagglutinin membrane glycoprotein. The hemagglutinin binds viruses to sialic acid residues on cell-surface glycoconjugates and, following endocytosis of the bound virus, mediates fusion between virus and endosomal membranes. It is a 220-kD trimer of identical subunits, each containing two glycopolypeptides, HA_1 and HA_2 (Fig. 1). The smaller HA_2 chain, from which the carboxy-terminal membrane anchor is removed by bromelain digestion to produce soluble bromelain-released hemagglutinin (BHA) for crystallization, is the major component of a mainly α-helical stem that forms the center of the 140-Å-long molecule. HA_1 also contributes to the stem structure but primarily forms a membrane-distal globular domain containing the receptor-binding site surrounded by variable, antigenically important, surface residues (Wiley and Skehel 1987).

RECEPTOR BINDING

Evidence for the location in the hemagglutinin of the receptor-binding site comes primarily from crystallographic studies of hemagglutinin-receptor analog complexes (Weis et al. 1988; Sauter et al. 1992) which indicate that sialic acid is bound in a shallow pocket at the membrane-distal tip of the molecule. The pocket is defined by the presence of a

Cellular Receptors for Animal Viruses
© 1994 Cold Spring Harbor Laboratory Press 0-87969-429-7/94 $5 + .00

number of conserved amino acid residues: $Tyr-98_1$, $Trp-153_1$, $His-183_1$, and $Leu-194_1$ (residues in HA_1 and HA_2 are numbered with the appropriate subscript). Interactions between these residues and with the substituents of sialic acid are shown in Figure 2. β-Anomers of sialyl glycosides interact very weakly with HA, suggesting the importance for binding of the hydrogen bonds with $Ser-136_1$ OH and main-chain 137_1 NH formed by the 2-carboxylate in the axial position. The equatorial hydroxyl substituent at the carbon-4 position points toward solution and the N-acetyl at carbon 5 is located over the indole ring of conserved Trp-153_1. The hydroxyl substituents at carbon 8 and carbon 9 are in positions to form hydrogen bonds with conserved $Tyr-98_1$ OH and the conserved charged residue, $Glu-190_1$. Dissociation constants for binding of sialic acid derivatives have been determined using nuclear magnetic resonance spectroscopy by observing perturbations of sialic acid resonances in the presence of HA, in particular, an upfield chemical shift of the N-acetyl methyl resonance presumably due to the proximity of the methyl group to $Trp-153_1$. These studies indicated that X-31 HA binds to the α-methyl glycoside of sialic acid with a dissociation constant of 2.8 mM (Sauter et al. 1989).

Crystallographic analysis at 2.1 Å resolution of complexes between a number of high-affinity receptor analogs and HA (S.J. Watowich et al., in prep.) indicates that the sialic-acid-binding site is located between a number of hydrophilic pockets to form a groove across the top of the molecule and that, in addition, the front of the site extends into a hydrophobic channel toward $Arg-224_1$. The hydrophilic groove extends toward the oligosaccharide side chain attached to $Asn-165_1$ of the neighboring subunit and side-chain atoms of $Thr-187_1$, $Gln-189_1$, $Ser-219_1$, and $Trp-222_1$. The floor of the groove in this region is formed by side-chain atoms of $Ser-186_1$ and $Ser-227_1$, and backbone atoms of $Gly-218_1$, $Arg-220_1$, $Ser-227_1$, and $Ser-228_1$. In the opposite direction, the right side of the groove comprises a broad open-ended pocket and two smaller hydrophilic pockets formed by side-chain atoms of $Thr-131_1$, $Trp-153_1$, and $Thr-155_1$, and backbone atoms of $Gln-132_1$, $Asn-133_1$, $Gly-134_1$, $Trp-153_1$, $Leu-154_1$, $Thr-155_1$, and $Leu-194_1$. Studies of the significance of these extensions for binding natural receptors and for the design of receptor analogs are in progress.

MEMBRANE FUSION

The membrane fusion potential of HA is activated in two distinct processes that occur at different stages of virus infection. First, the primary translation product of mRNA for HA is a precursor, HA_0, from which

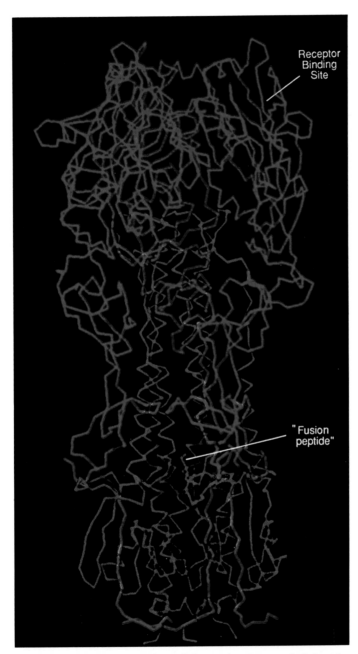

Figure 1 α-Carbon tracing of the native hemagglutinin trimer showing the regions of the molecule implicated in receptor binding and membrane fusion. The HA$_1$ polypeptide chains are colored blue, HA$_2$ chains are red. The virus membrane anchor in complete HA would be at the bottom of the figure.

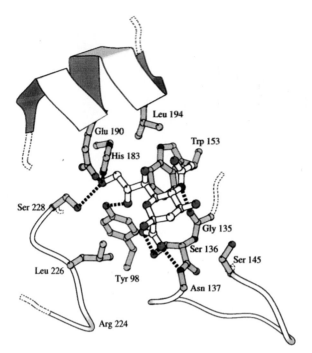

Figure 2 (*See facing page for legend.*)

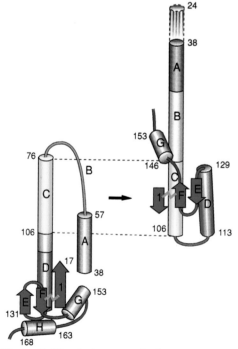

Figure 3 (*See facing page for legend.*)

both HA_1 and HA_2 are derived by a proteolytic cleavage (Klenk et al. 1975; Lazarowitz and Choppin 1975) that generates the carboxyl terminus of HA_1 and the amino terminus of HA_2 (Skehel and Waterfield 1975). Trimers of HA_0 expressed at the surface of cells late in infection, or on virus particles, can bind to receptors but are unable to mediate membrane fusion unless cleaved by extracellular proteases. Second, at the beginning of virus infection following receptor binding, virus is taken into endosomes and, at the low pH of endosomes, fusion activity is induced (White et al. 1983). Incubation of cells with bases such as amino adamantane which elevate endosomal pH prevent HA-mediated fusion and block infection (Miller and Lenard 1981).

The region of HA implicated in membrane fusion is the amino terminus of HA_2, which is known as the "fusion peptide." At the pH of fusion, this conserved, hydrophobic region is extruded from its buried location in the native trimer (Fig. 1) in a conformational change that involves extensive reorganization of HA structure. Protein chemistry, mutation, and site-specific modification studies (Skehel et al. 1982; Daniels et al. 1985; Godley et al. 1992) have given indications of the nature of this reorganization and provided evidence that it is required for membrane fusion. Recent crystallographic analyses of a fragment of HA in the fusion pH conformation address directly the details and the extent of the changes (Bullough et al. 1994 and in prep.).

Incubation of membrane-anchorless BHA, at the pH of fusion, causes its aggregation into protein micelles through the association of extruded fusion peptides (Ruigrok et al. 1988). The micelles can be solubilized by digestion with trypsin to remove HA_1 residues 28_1–328_1 (Skehel et al. 1982) and then with thermolysin to remove the amino-terminal 38 residues of HA_2, which includes the uncharged residues of the fusion peptide, residues 1_2–10_2 (Ruigrok et al. 1988). Figure 3 compares diagrammatically the structure of a subunit of this trimeric thermolytic

Figure 2 Diagram of the receptor-binding site of one HA subunit containing sialic acid to indicate the conserved residues which form the site and hydrogen bonds between HA and sialic acid.

Figure 3 Structural difference between equivalent regions of subunits of native HA (*left*) and HA in the fusion pH conformation (*right*). The fusion pH structure was obtained by analyses of a fragment prepared by thermolytic digestion of HA at the pH of fusion. The equivalent native structure is a partial diagram of the complete native structure. The extension of the fusion pH helix from residue 38_2 to 24_2 is based on electron micrographs of less extensively digested HA fragments.

fragment with the structure of the equivalent region of native HA.

The major feature of the fragment's structure is a trimeric α-helical coiled coil, approximately 100 Å long, extending from its amino terminus, residue 38_2, to residue 106_2. The helices are formed by displacement of the short α helix A of the native helical hairpin to the top of the new α helix and by the refolding into an α helix of the extended chain, B, as an extension of helix C. In each subunit, this ABC helix is followed by a short loop formed by refolding of residues 106_2–113_2, which reverses the direction of the chain, and by a shorter α helix, D, residues 113_2–129_2, which packs antiparallel against the long α helix of the same subunit and that of another subunit. The β hairpin E and F, residues 131_2–140_2, together with the additional antiparallel strand, 1, contributed by the disulfide-linked peptide of HA_1, residues 11_1–16_1, forms a small β sheet packed against helix D. Residues 146_2–153_2 form a short α helix that packs against the coiled coil. Residues beyond 152_2 of one subunit and 162_2 of the other two subunits of the trimer appear to be disordered. Only 30 residues corresponding to the top half of the long α helix of native HA, helix C, which form a coiled coil in both structures, have the same structure in both native HA and fusion pH conformations.

These structural data suggest that at the pH of fusion the fusion peptide may be delivered over 100 Å toward the target membrane to form a bridge between viral and endosomal membranes. They do not rule out the possibility that the molecule inverts to place the fusion peptide in the viral membrane, since the consequences for the orientation of the molecule of the reversal in direction that results from the 180° turn following helix C are uncertain; no data are available on the location of residues from 160_2 to the viral membrane at 185_2, a segment of 25 residues that could extend about 100 Å. Does the chain direction reverse again? Are HAs in both orientations involved in membrane fusion?

ACKNOWLEDGMENTS

We acknowledge the support of Rose Gonsalves, David Stevens, and Alan Douglas. This work was supported by the Medical Research Council and by National Institutes of Health grant AI-13654. D.C.W. is an investigator of the Howard Hughes Medical Institute.

REFERENCES

Bullough, P.A., F.M. Hughson, A.C. Treharne, R.W.H. Ruigrok, J.J. Skehel, and D.C. Wiley. 1994. Crystals of a fragment of influenza haemagglutinin in the low pH induced conformation. *J. Mol. Biol.* **236:** 1262.

Daniels, R.S., J.C. Downie, A.J. Hay, M. Knossow, J.J. Skehel, M.L. Wang, and D.C. Wiley. 1985. Fusion mutants of the influenza virus hemagglutinin glycoprotein. *Cell* **40:** 431.

Godley, L., J. Pfeifer, D. Steinhauer, B. Ely, G. Shaw, R. Kaufmann, E. Suchanek, C. Pabo, J.J. Skehel, D.C. Wiley, and S. Wharton. 1992. Introduction of intersubunit disulfide bonds in the membrane-distal region of the influenza hemagglutinin abolishes membrane fusion activity. *Cell* **68:** 635.

Klenk, H.-D., R. Rott, M. Orlich, and J. Blodorn. 1975. Activation of influenza A viruses by trypsin treatment. *Virology* **68:** 426.

Lazarowitz, S.G. and P.W. Choppin. 1975. Enhancement of the infectivity of influenza A and B viruses by proteolytic cleavage of the hemagglutinin polypeptide. *Virology* **68:** 440.

Miller, K.M. and J. Lenard. 1981. Antihistaminics, local anesthetics, and other amines as antiviral agents. *Proc. Natl. Acad. Sci.* **78:** 3605.

Ruigrok, R.W.H., A. Aitken, L.J. Calder, S.R. Martin, J.J. Skehel, S.A. Wharton, W. Weis, and D.C. Wiley. 1988. Studies on the structure of the influenza virus haemagglutinin at the pH of membrane fusion. *J. Gen. Virol.* **69:** 2785.

Sauter, N.K., M.D. Bednarski, B.A. Wurzburg, J.E. Hanson, G.M. Whitesides, J.J. Skehel, and D.C. Wiley. 1989. Hemagglutinins from two influenza virus variants bind to sialic acid derivatives with millimolar dissociation constants: A 500-MHz proton nuclear magnetic resonance study. *Biochemistry* **28:** 8388.

Sauter, N.K., J.E. Hanson, G.D. Glick, J.H. Brown, R.L. Crowther, S.-J. Park, J.J. Skehel, and D.C. Wiley. 1992. Binding of influenza virus hemagglutinin to analogs of its cell-surface receptor, sialic acid: Analysis by proton nuclear magnetic resonance spectroscopy and X-ray crystallography. *Biochemistry* **31:** 9609.

Skehel, J.J. and M.D. Waterfield. 1975. Studies on the primary structure of the influenza virus hemagglutinin. *Proc. Natl. Acad. Sci.* **72:** 93.

Skehel, J.J., P.M. Bayley, E.B. Brown, S.R. Martin, M.D. Waterfield, J.M. White, I.A. Wilson, and D.C. Wiley. 1982. Changes in the conformation of influenza virus hemagglutinin at the pH optimum of virus-mediated membrane fusion. *Proc. Natl. Acad. Sci.* **79:** 968.

Weis, W., J.H. Brown, S. Cusack, J.C. Paulson, J.J. Skehel, and D.C. Wiley. 1988. Structure of the influenza virus haemagglutinin complexed with its receptor, sialic acid. *Nature* **333:** 426.

White, J., M. Kielian, and A. Helenius. 1983. Membrane fusion proteins of enveloped animal viruses. *Q. Rev. Biophys.* **16:** 151.

Wiley, D.C. and J.J. Skehel. 1987. The structure and function of the hemagglutinin membrane glycoprotein of influenza virus. *Annu. Rev. Biochem.* **56:** 365.

12

Interaction of Rhinovirus with Its Receptor, ICAM-1

Jeffrey M. Greve
Miles Biotechnology
West Haven, Connecticut 06516

Michael G. Rossmann
Department of Biological Sciences
Purdue University
West Lafayette, Indiana 47907

The rhinovirus is the single major infectious agent causing acute upper respiratory infections in humans. The rhinovirus has also emerged, following the determination of its atomic structure and identification of its major receptor, as a useful virus with which to study the molecular basis of virus/receptor interaction and the mechanism of virus entry into cells. In this chapter, we review the aspects of the structure and function of both rhinoviruses and the major receptor relevant to virus entry into host cells. We then describe recent studies directed toward defining the molecular basis of the interaction of rhinoviruses with this receptor and discuss how conformational changes in the virion may be involved in virus entry and uncoating.

Rhinoviruses belong to the family Picornaviridae and comprise a group of approximately 100 serologically distinct viruses. Of these viruses, 90% utilize a single common cell-surface receptor (Abraham et al. 1984; Uncapher et al. 1991), the major rhinovirus receptor, which has been identified as ICAM-1, or *i*nter*c*ellular *a*dhesion *m*olecule-1 (Greve et al. 1989; Staunton et al. 1989). The remaining 10% of the serotypes bind to a second receptor class, designated the minor receptor. The minor rhinovirus receptor appears to be a protein with an apparent molecular weight of 100 kD whose identity has not yet been determined (Mischak et al. 1988; Hofer et al. 1992). One rhinovirus serotype, HRV87, apparently binds to a third receptor (Uncapher et al. 1991). In addition to rhinoviruses, some coxsackie A viruses also utilize ICAM-1 as a receptor (Lonberg-Holm et al. 1976a). The ability of the rhinovirus family to maintain selectivity for the major receptor ICAM-1 in the face of the high degree of capsid protein amino acid sequence diversity underscores the degree to which the virus has adapted to its human host. Elucidation of the manner in which rhinovirus interacts with its receptor will lead to a greater understanding of the initial steps of virus infection, of the adaptive nature of its relationship with its human host, and possibly of the natural function of the receptor, ICAM-1.

STRUCTURE OF THE VIRUS

The three-dimensional structure of rhinovirus was determined by X-ray crystallographic studies of HRV-14 (Rossmann et al. 1985). The rhinovirus capsid is composed of an icosahedral protein shell surrounding a core containing a single (+) sense strand of RNA. The protein shell is composed of four subunits, VP1–4. VP1, VP2, and VP3 are the major surface proteins, and VP4 is internal in the mature infectious virion (Fig. 1). The subunit structures of VP1, VP2, and VP3 exhibit a similar folding topology, described as an eight-stranded antiparallel β-barrel or a "jelly-roll." The basic arrangement of the subunits and the basic fold of the capsid proteins themselves are conserved among the other picornaviruses that have been examined to date, such as poliovirus (Hogle 1985), Mengo virus (Luo et al. 1987), and foot-and-mouth disease virus (FMDV) (Acharya et al. 1989). External protrusions formed by loops inserted between the β strands form the major antigenic sites. These epitopes have been mapped by selecting and sequencing virus mutants which have escaped from neutralization by monoclonal antibodies (Sherry and Rueckert 1985; Sherry et al. 1986) and more recently by cryoelectron microscopic image reconstruction of a virus/Fab complex (Smith et al. 1993).

A surface depression or "canyon" encircles each fivefold vertex; portions of this canyon are represented on each of the 60 identical faces of the virion. The dimensions of this canyon (~20 Å deep and 15 Å wide) are such that an antibody-combining site is incapable of penetrating it (Fig. 2). The inaccessibility of the canyon to antibody thus makes the amino acid residues lining the canyon resistant to the continual selective pressure imposed on the virus by the host immune system to alter these residues. These characteristics led to the hypothesis that this canyon is the receptor-binding site on the virion (Rossmann et al. 1985; Rossmann 1989).

A number of lines of evidence have emerged to support this model. First, a comparison of the variability of surface-exposed residues between a number of picornaviruses indicated that amino acid residues lining the canyon are significantly more conserved than other surface-exposed residues (Rossmann and Palmenberg 1988). Second, site-

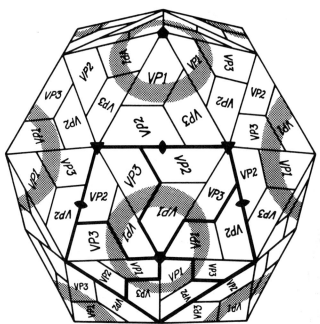

Figure 1 Diagrammatic representation of the structure of the rhinovirus capsid. The icosahedral capsid is composed of 60 identical protomeric units. The assembly protomer, composed of VP1, VP2, VP3 (VP4 is internal and not shown here), and the pentamer surrounding the fivefold axis of symmetry is shown in thick outline. The stippled circle indicates the canyon which encircles the fivefold axis of symmetry. (Reprinted, with permission, from Rossmann et al. 1985 copyright by Macmillan Magazines.)

directed mutagenesis of HRV-14 has indicated that modification of several amino acid residues located in the base of the canyon has an impact on virus/receptor affinity (Colonno et al. 1988). Specifically, mutants with substitutions at residues 1273,[1] 1223, 1103, and 1220 exhibited an alteration in virus/receptor affinity. Third, WIN capsid-binding antiviral compounds block the binding of some of the major receptor rhinoviruses, including HRV-14 (Pevear et al. 1989). These compounds bind to many picornaviruses in a hydrophobic pocket located under the canyon floor and, in most cases, block virus from uncoating once inside the cell (Smith et al. 1986; Badger et al. 1988; Kim et al. 1993). Upon binding to HRV-14, a conformational change occurs in which several amino acid residues are displaced by as much as 4 Å. These findings suggest that the conformational change in the shape of the canyon can pre-

[1]The numbering system for picornavirus capsid protein amino acid residues indicates the capsid protein number x 1000 + amino acid residue number (i.e., residue 273 of VP1 is designated 1273).

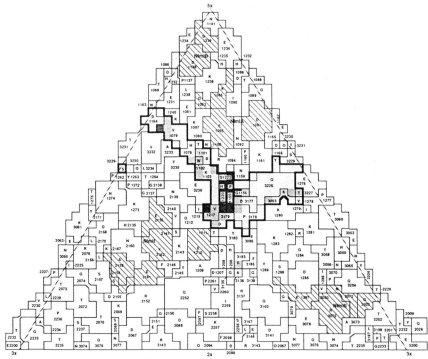

Figure 2 A "roadmap" of the surface of one triangular face of the virion. Note that this protomer is different from the assembly protomer shown in Fig. 1 in that it is composed of VP1 and VP2 from the assembly protomer and VP3 from the protomer to the right. Residues are shaded progressively darker to represent their depth below the rim of the canyon. (Reprinted, with permission, from Rossmann and Palmenberg 1988.)

vent ICAM-1 binding. In poliovirus, a related picornavirus, another region of the capsid has been implicated in determination of host range, a phenotype which is likely to be related to receptor specificity (Martin et al. 1988; Yeates et al. 1991). In this study, the determinant for adapting the host range of poliovirus from human to mouse was assigned to the BC loop in VP1, which is on the viral surface close to the fivefold axis of symmetry and outside the poliovirus canyon.

Although the observations for rhinovirus are consistent with the canyon's being the receptor-binding site, they do not provide conclusive proof, nor do they identify a complete footprint of the receptor on the virus surface. The concave structure of the canyon covers a large amount of surface area, encompassing approximately 100 Å^2 and 17 amino acid residues contributed by three different capsid proteins, which can potentially interact with a correspondingly convex surface area available on the receptor.

In principle, sequence comparisons between different rhinovirus serotypes and with other picornaviruses should be helpful in identifying highly conserved residues that would be potential receptor contact residues. The sequences of two rhinovirus serotypes of the major receptor class (HRV-14, HRV-89) and three serotypes of the minor receptor class (HRV-1A, HRV-1B, and HRV-2) have been reported to date (Stanway et al. 1984; Skern et al. 1985; Duechler et al. 1987; Hughes et al. 1988). Although surface-exposed residues lining the canyon are more conserved among picornaviruses than other surface-exposed residues, the degree of conservation of canyon residues between two major receptor viruses, HRV-14 and HRV-89, is less than the degree of conservation between a major and a minor rhinovirus (i.e., HRV-14 and HRV-1A or HRV-89 and HRV-1A) (Rossmann and Palmenberg 1988). In fact, the degree of conservation between the major receptor rhinoviruses HRV-14 and HRV-89 is approximately the same as that between HRV-14 and poliovirus, which belongs to a different genus of the picornavirus family and utilizes a different receptor. Thus, the high degree of sequence diversity in the rhinovirus family and an apparent lack of a linkage between receptor specificity and phylogenetic relatedness has, at this point, made this kind of sequence analysis less than informative. A structural comparison between HRV-14 (major receptor) and HRV-1A (minor receptor) indicates significant differences between these two viruses in the shape of the base of the canyon and, most importantly, the charge distribution (Kim et al. 1989). Clearly, the basis of recognition between virus and receptor is complex, and elucidation of their contacts will require more direct approaches.

STRUCTURE OF THE RECEPTOR

The major rhinovirus receptor was identified by amino acid sequence identity between a protein isolated from HeLa cells with virus-binding activity and ICAM-1 (Greve et al. 1989). ICAM-1 is an integral membrane protein with a 453-amino-acid extracellular region, a 24-amino-acid membrane-spanning domain, and a short 28-amino-acid carboxy-terminal cytoplasmic domain (Simmons et al. 1988; Staunton et al. 1988) (Fig. 3A). The sequence of the extracellular portion can be divided into five domains having low homology with immunoglobulin-type domains, and the intron-exon organization of the genomic sequence has indicated that the individual immunoglobulin-like domains are encoded by separate exons (Voraberger et al. 1991). ICAM-1 is heavily glycosylated, containing seven to eight N-linked oligosaccharide chains (Greve et al.

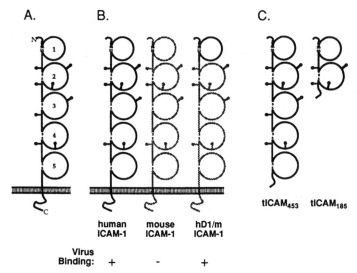

Figure 3 Domain organization of ICAM-1. (*A*) The structure of human ICAM-1, with immunoglobulin-like domains indicated as circles, numbered from the amino to the carboxyl terminus. N-linked oligosaccharides are indicated as lollipop-like structures. (*B*) Localization of the virus binding within domain 1. Human ICAM-1 is in dark line, mouse ICAM-1 is in gray line. The virus-binding properties of the receptors are indicated below. (*C*) Soluble truncated forms of ICAM-1. tICAM$_{453}$ and tICAM$_{185}$ indicate the five-domain and two-domain forms of ICAM-1, respectively.

1989), although the fifth domain and, notably, the first amino-terminal domain are deficient in glycosylation sites; the oligosaccharides play no role in rhinovirus binding (McClelland et al. 1991). The physiological function of ICAM-1 is to serve as the counterreceptor of the leukocyte adhesion molecules LFA-1 and Mac-1, both of whom are members of the integrin family of receptors (Springer 1990). The cytokine-inducible expression of ICAM-1 on vascular endothelial cells is one of the major steps leading to the extravasation of leukocytes at sites of inflammation. ICAM-1 can also be expressed by epithelial cells, fibroblasts, and some leukocytes (Dustin et al. 1986; Pober et al. 1986).

The location of the virus-binding portion of the receptor has been determined by several approaches. First, capitalizing on the fact that mouse ICAM-1 is not capable of binding rhinovirus, interspecies (mouse-human) chimeric ICAM-1 receptors have been created and the virus-binding site has been mapped by determining their ability to bind rhinovirus (Staunton et al. 1990; McClelland et al. 1991). The smallest portion of human ICAM-1 that can positively support rhinovirus binding to cells in such chimeric receptors is the amino-terminal 88 amino acids (McClelland et al. 1991) (Fig. 3B). A second approach has been to produce soluble truncated ICAM-1 molecules and to study their virus-binding and virus-neutralizing properties in solution. The smallest active fragment of ICAM-1 that has been produced is a 185-amino acid species comprising the two amino-terminal domains (Greve et al. 1991). The ability of this fragment to bind to rhinovirus, as determined by its ability to competitively inhibit the binding of rhinovirus to ICAM-1, was essentially the same as that of the entire five-domain extracellular portion (Fig. 3C). A third approach has been to subject the ICAM-1 molecule to site-directed mutagenesis (Staunton et al. 1990) or to perform systematic mouse-human exchanges throughout the first domain (McClelland et al. 1991; Register et al. 1991) to identify regions critical to virus binding. The results from these three studies are summarized in Figure 4A. Positions in which a major reduction of virus binding (>90%) was observed were found in seven regions or clusters: residues 1–2 (the amino terminus), residues 26–29 (in the BC loop), residues 40–43 (in strand bD), residues 46–48 (in the DE loop), residue 67 (in strand βF), residues 70–72 (in the FG loop), and residues 75–77 (in strand βG).

Immunoglobulin-like domains consist of seven β strands (βA–βG), arranged into two β sheets that form a β sandwich (Fig. 4B). The sequence of the first domain of ICAM-1 (D1) has two unusual features for an immunoglobulin-like domain. First, it is relatively short, being 88 residues instead of the more typical size of approximately 100 residues. Second, instead of the typical two cysteine residues, located in the βB strand and the βF strands, there are four cysteines. The βB and the βF cysteines usually participate in an intrachain disulfide bond across the β sandwich in most members of the immunoglobulin supergene family. However, the two additional cysteine residues in ICAM-1 D1 have an i+4 spacing relative to C21 and C65, which in a β strand would place them in proper register for forming a second disulfide bond between the βB and βF strands. Interestingly, these sequence features are conserved in domains present in a small family of cell-surface receptors that are related by sequence homology and by their ability to serve as ligands for various members of the heterodimeric integrin receptor family. ICAM-1, ICAM-2, and ICAM-3 all serve as counterreceptors for the integrin receptor LFA-1 (Springer 1990); and VCAM-1 and its alternatively spliced variant, VCAM-AS1, serve as counterreceptors to the integrin VLA-4 (Cybulsky et al. 1991; Hession et al. 1991). The amino acid sequences of ICAM-2 D1, ICAM-3 D1, VCAM-1 D1, and VCAM-1 DAS are all closely related to ICAM-1 D1, and all possess the novel four-cysteine sequence motif. Since these domains all have been either impli-

A.

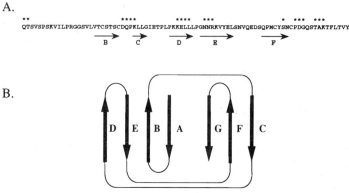

B.

Figure 4 ICAM-1 domain 1. (*A*) The sequence of ICAM-1 D1 with asterisks indicating those amino acid residues which are involved in virus binding by site-
directed mutagenesis. The criterion for involvement is a reduction of ~90% or
more in virus binding to ICAM-1 mutants in the absence of evidence for gross
structural defects (Staunton et al. 1990; McClelland et al. 1991; Register et al.
1991). Positions identified by Staunton et al. (1990) are: 1–2, 26–29, and 46–48;
positions identified by McClelland et al. (1991) are: 40–43, 70–72, and 75–77;
positions identified by Register et al. (1991) are: 26–30, 67, and 70. Predicted β
strands are indicated by arrows underneath. (*B*) Diagram of the secondary structure and connectivity of an immunoglobulin-like domain motif. The heavy arrows indicate β strands.

cated or directly shown to contain the binding sites for their integrin
counterreceptors, it is possible that ICAM-1 D1 represents a prototype
for an integrin-binding domain. The recently determined three-dimensional structure of another integrin-binding domain, the fibronectin type
III domain, has indicated that it also possesses an immunoglobulin-type
fold. The tripeptide sequence RGD, which contains the critical site for
recognition by many integrin receptors, is exposed on the loop between
the βF and the βG strands (Leahy et al. 1992; Main et al. 1992). Interestingly, a number of the mutations that reduce rhinovirus binding to
ICAM-1 cluster in a homologous region of ICAM-1 D1 (Fig. 4A).

STRUCTURE OF RHINOVIRUS/RECEPTOR COMPLEXES

To directly study the structural basis of rhinovirus/ICAM-1 interaction,
we have begun to determine the structure of both the receptor and the
virus/receptor complex. Two species of ICAM-1 have been produced in
large amounts in mammalian cells, one comprising the entire five-
domain extracellular portion, designated $tICAM_{453}$, and a smaller one
containing the virus-binding site, comprising the two amino-terminal
domains (D1D2), designated $tICAM_{185}$ (Fig. 3C). The five-domain form

appears to be an extended molecule, as determined by electron microscopic (Staunton et al. 1990; N.H. Olson et al., unpubl.) and hydrodynamic properties (Staunton et al. 1990; Greve et al. 1991). Electron micrographs of rotary shadowed five-domain soluble ICAM-1 indicates a length of 187 Å, with a slight bend in the molecule 69 Å from one of the ends (Staunton et al. 1990). The length is consistent with that of five end-to-end immunoglobulin-like domains approximately 3.7 nM in the long axis. The hydrodynamic properties of D1D2 also indicate an asymmetric structure (Greve et al. 1991). D1D2 has recently been crystallized (Kolatkar et al. 1992), and structure determination is in progress.

Efforts have also been directed toward determination of the structure of the virus/receptor complex (Olson et al. 1993). To accomplish this, however, several conditions need to be met. First, stable virus/receptor complexes need to be obtained. Second, these complexes must be stoichiometric; in principle, if the canyon serves as a receptor-binding site, each virion should be capable of binding 60 molecules of receptor, since the canyon is present on each of the 60 icosahedral faces of the virion.

Initial studies on the interaction of soluble ICAM-1 with rhinovirus in vitro have indicated that the stability of the complexes was highly dependent on the serotype of rhinovirus. In the experiment shown in Figure 5, two serotypes, HRV-14 and HRV-16, were incubated with an excess of $tICAM_{453}$ and then sedimented through a sucrose gradient to separate virus-bound from free ICAM-1. Two peaks were observed, depending on the serotype. Both serotypes formed a peak at 135S, sedimenting more slowly than the peak for uncomplexed virus at 149S. This 135S peak contained all four viral capsid proteins and $tICAM_{453}$. However, whereas HRV-16 formed a single peak at 135S, HRV-14 formed a second peak at 80S, which appeared to increase in size with incubation time. The 80S peak contained an "uncoated" virion, lacking RNA and VP4, and did not contain $tICAM_{453}$ (Greve et al. 1991; Hoover-Litty and Greve 1993). Thus, soluble receptor is uncoating rhinovirus, mimicking a process which must take place in vivo for successful infection to occur. Although the physiological relevance of this receptor-mediated uncoating is presently unclear, empty capsids are in fact natural products of infection in vivo (Lonberg-Holm and Konort 1972; Abraham and Colonno 1988), and these results demonstrate that receptor can destabilize the virion and may play an active role in the uncoating of virus. These data demonstrate in a dramatic fashion that conformation changes in the virion take place upon binding receptor, but they also indicate that these conformational changes must differ quite significantly in magnitude among serotypes.

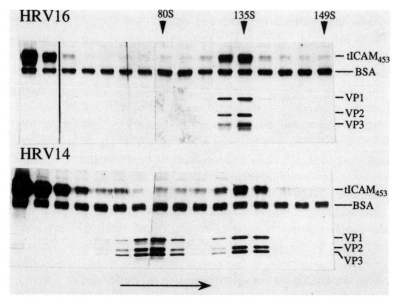

Figure 5 Soluble ICAM-1 can form saturated virus/receptor complexes and can induce viral uncoating. 50 μg of HRV-16 or HRV-14 was incubated with a 480-fold molar excess of tICAM$_{453}$ over virions for 2 hr at 34°C before centrifugation through sucrose gradients. Aliquots were analyzed by SDS-PAGE and silver stained. Positions of 80S empty capsids, the 135S virus/receptor complex, and the 149S native virus are indicated, and the horizontal arrow on the bottom indicates the direction of sedimentation. (Reprinted, with permission, from Hoover-Litty and Greve 1993.)

HRV-16 was thus chosen for further analysis, since it formed the most stable virus/receptor complexes. With the D1D2 form of soluble ICAM-1, tICAM$_{185}$, HRV-16 formed a peak with an intermediate sedimentation coefficient of 140S, suggesting that the slower sedimentation of the complex was due to the hydrodynamic properties of the virus/receptor complex. The rhinovirus/D1D2 complex proved to be close to a stoichiometric complex between virus and receptor, with approximately 60 mole of ICAM-1 per mole of HRV-16, as determined by amino acid analysis (Hoover-Litty and Greve 1993). HRV-16/D1D2 complexes were then subjected to cryoelectron microscopy and three-dimensional image reconstruction procedures to produce the electron density map shown in Figure 6. This reconstruction, although of relatively low (~25 Å) resolution, has provided a great deal of information that confirms and extends our knowledge about rhinovirus/receptor interaction. Comparison of the reconstruction of the complex and the un-complexed image of HRV-14, computed to a comparable resolution from X-ray data, clearly shows the projection of 60 ICAM-1 molecules from

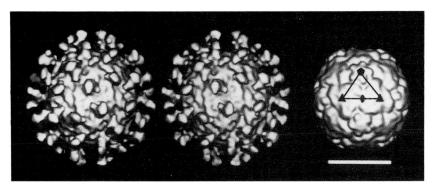

Figure 6 Cryoelectron microscopy of the HRV-16/D1D2 complex. (*Left, middle*) Stereoview of the reconstruction of the HRV-16/D1D2 complex, viewed along an icosahedral twofold axis. Sixty D1D2 molecules are bound to symmetry-equivalent positions at the 12 canyon regions on the virion. (*Right*) Shaded-surface view of HRV-14, computed from the known atomic structure truncated to 20 Å resolution. The triangular outline of one icosahedral asymmetric unit is indicated. Bar, 200 Å. (Adapted, with permission, from Olson et al. 1993.)

the virion surface. The D1D2 ICAM-1 fragment projects approximately 55 Å from the virion surface, showing that each icosahedral face is capable of binding a receptor molecule. A slight bend is apparent in the portion of ICAM-1 projecting from the virion, allowing the symmetry relationships of the bound molecules to be discerned and indicating that the ICAM-1 molecules are bound in a specific orientation consistent with the internal symmetry of the virus. Even though the reconstructed complex is with HRV-16 and not HRV-14, the orientation of the ICAM-1 molecules relative to landmarks seen in HRV-14, such as the fivefold and threefold axes of symmetry, clearly indicates that the receptor is bound in the center of the triangle formed by the fivefold and the two adjacent threefold axes, thus being in the canyon.

To specifically visualize ICAM-1, a difference map was constructed by subtracting the calculated HRV-14 structure from the D1D2/HRV-16 complex reconstruction (Fig. 7A). The length of the receptor fragment in this difference map is approximately 75 Å, consistent with that predicted by two end-to-end immunoglobulin-like domains and indicating that approximately 15–20 Å is buried below the surface of the virion. The ICAM-1 density fits well within the space created by the virus canyon (Fig. 7B). The only exception was the BC loop of VP1, which overlapped by about 3 Å the density assigned to ICAM-1. However, the BC loop is highly variable in structure between HRV-14 and HRV-1A (Kim et al. 1989), and it has now been shown (W.M. Lee and R.R. Rueckert,

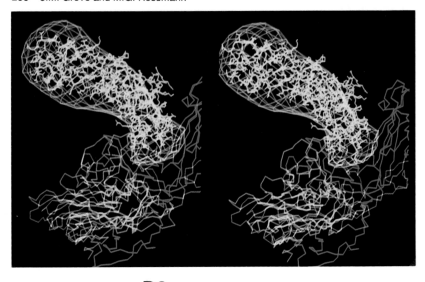

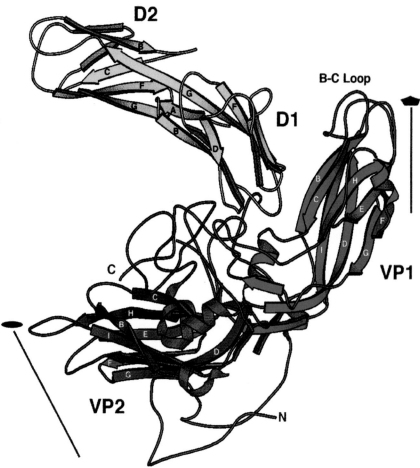

Figure 7 (See facing page for legend.)

unpubl.) that the structure of this region in HRV-16 has a deletion relative to HRV-14.

The electron microscopic and X-ray crystallographic studies have shown the interaction of rhinovirus with its receptor, ICAM-1, at the molecular level. The biochemical studies suggest that this interaction is dynamic and that major conformational changes in the virion occur upon receptor binding. The molecular details of the binding, and the conformational changes and postbinding events, can be examined. Higher resolution structures will clearly be necessary to elucidate these interactions.

VIRUS ENTRY AND POSTBINDING EVENTS

Virus entry into the host cell involves four separable physical events: (1) virus/receptor binding, (2) movement of the virus to the appropriate cellular compartment, (3) uncoating of the viral genome, and (4) delivery of the genome through the limiting membrane. Little is known about the latter three steps of the pathway for rhinovirus. However, examination of the behavior of rhinovirus in vitro and some in vivo observations provide some insight into the process.

The entry pathways of some enveloped viruses, particularly influenza virus, are well characterized (Marsh and Helenius 1989). Influenza virus binds to sialic acid-containing receptors on the host cell surface and then enters the endosomal compartment by receptor-mediated endocytosis. In endosomes, the increasingly acidic environment induces conformational changes in the viral coat protein HA that expose a hydrophobic "fusion" peptide at the amino terminus of HA2, conferring upon the virus a fusion-competent state and promoting the fusion of the viral envelope with the endosomal membrane. Although such a detailed characterization of the cellular and molecular events in the entry pathway of picornaviruses has not yet been performed, influenza provides a useful paradigm for considering the mechanism of rhinovirus entry.

Figure 7 Stereo diagram showing the fit of the CD4 structure into the difference density between the HRV-16/D1D2 reconstruction (Fig. 5A) and the X-ray map of HRV-14 (Fig. 5B). (*Top*) The difference electron density is shown in scarlet hatching and the HRV-14 backbone is shown in blue (VP1), green (VP2), and red (VP3). The structure of domains 1 and 2 of CD4 (Ryu et al. 1990; Wang et al. 1990) is superimposed onto the density of ICAM-1; the strands $\beta C'$ and $\beta C''$ of domain 1 of CD4 (which would not be present in ICAM-1) lie outside the difference density. (*Bottom*) Diagrammatic drawing of the predicted structure of ICAM-1 D1D2 fitted into the rhinovirus canyon, based on the electron density in top figure. The predicted structure of ICAM-1 D1 (Giranda et al. 1990) was superimposed on the backbone of CD4 D1D2. (Reprinted, with permission, from Olson et al. 1993.)

An intracellular low-pH step is likely to be an important step in rhinovirus entry. Studies with poliovirus (Madshus et al. 1984a), FMDV (Carrillo et al. 1984, 1985), and a minor receptor rhinovirus (Madshus et al. 1984b; Neubauer et al. 1987) have indicated that infection by these picornaviruses is inhibited by drugs that prevent the acidification of endosomes, suggesting that they have an obligatory low-pH step, and enter the host cell through the endosomal pathway. Similarly, an early step in the infection of HeLa cells by the major receptor rhinoviruses HRV-14 and HRV-16 is sensitive to the drugs chloroquine and monensin, which prevent the acidification of endosomes (J.M. Greve, unpubl.). In vitro, mildly acidic pH can induce conformational changes and even complete uncoating of rhinovirus (Hoover-Litty and Greve 1993). pH 5.0 (a pH likely to be encountered in the endosome) induces formation of the 135S VP4 (–) RNA (+) form with HRV-14, whereas with HRV-16 the same treatment induces formation of 80S VP4 (–) RNA (–) empty capsids (Fig. 8B). These results, combined with the in vivo observations, suggest that low-pH-induced conformational changes are a critical step in rhinovirus entry. However, the fact that low pH cannot induce the appropriate in vitro conformational changes in all rhinovirus serotypes indicates that it is unlikely that low pH alone is responsible for the uncoating.

Receptor-mediated destabilization of the virion is also potentially involved in the uncoating and entry of rhinovirus into the cell. The observation that soluble ICAM-1 can catalyze the uncoating of rhinovirus is consistent with such a role for the receptor. However, similar to the situation with low pH, soluble receptor-mediated destabilization does not occur efficiently in all serotypes. For example, although HRV-14 is rapidly uncoated to the 80S VP4 (–) RNA (–) empty capsid, HRV-16 forms a stable virus/receptor complex (Hoover-Litty and Greve 1993) (Fig. 8A). Since the in vivo drug experiments suggest an obligatory intracellular low-pH step, productive uncoating in vivo presumably requires an orchestration of both receptor-mediated and low-pH-mediated conformational changes in the rhinovirus virion, perhaps even in concert with other cellular factors. These observations on the factors that destabilize rhinovirus in vitro will serve to illustrate the steps which are likely to be important in virus entry. Different rhinovirus serotypes exhibit different phenotypes with regard to their destabilization by low soluble receptor and low pH in vitro (Hoover-Litty and Greve 1993), and it is therefore likely that different serotypes have evolved different efficiencies for various steps of the entry process in vivo. Rhinovirus must tread a delicate balance between having an affinity for the receptor that is high enough to bind efficiently at the surface of the host cell while still allowing the uncoating and release of the viral genome into the cytoplasm.

A.

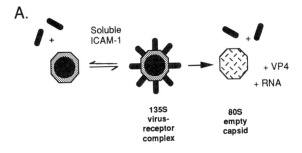

B.

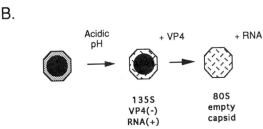

Figure 8 In vitro conformational transitions in rhinovirus. (*A*) Soluble-receptor-mediated transitions. Soluble ICAM-1 form saturated virus/receptor complexes with rhinovirus that can spontaneously uncoat; HRV-16 is apparently blocked at the virus/receptor complex step. (*B*) Low-pH-mediated transitions. Incubation of HRV-14 at pH 5.0 results in the formation of a 135S VP4(–) RNA(+) species; incubation of HRV-16 under the same conditions results in the formation of a 80S VP4(–) RNA(–) empty capsid.

To translocate the RNA genome into the cytoplasm, it is likely that rhinovirus must have an intimate, hydrophobic interaction with the limiting membrane. It has been reported that subviral particles of rhinovirus induced by low pH have hydrophobic properties allowing interaction with liposomes (Korant et al. 1972; Lonberg-Holm et al. 1976b). In poliovirus, it has been reported that the amino terminus of poliovirus VP1, which is exposed as a result of a cell-induced conformational change in the virion, acts as a hydrophobic peptide capable of interaction with lipid membranes (Fricks and Hogle 1990). This poliovirus VP1 sequence has the potential to form an amphipathic α helix, which in principle could function in a manner similar to the role the influenza HA fusion peptide plays in promoting membrane fusion. The homologous sequence in HRV-14 also has the potential to form an amphipathic α helix. Although a role for such a fusion sequence in membrane penetration is attractive, the existence of a fusion-competent form of rhinovirus has not yet been directly demonstrated.

The manner in which these conformational transitions are orchestrated during the entry of rhinovirus into its host cell will require greater knowledge of the cell biology of the entry pathway as well as biochemical reconstitution of the various steps of the pathway in vitro. Combining this information with structural information on the virus and the receptor will allow us to understand these processes at the molecular level.

ACKNOWLEDGMENTS

We particularly thank Prasanna Kolatkar, Norman Olson, Holland Cheng, Tim Baker (Purdue), Art Robbins, and Helana Hoover-Litty (Miles) for their active participation in the studies described here. The work in M.G.R.'s laboratory was supported by a grant from the National Institutes of Health, the Sterling Winthrop Company, a Lucille P. Markey Award, and a Jane Coffin Childs postdoctoral fellowship to Prasanna Kolatkar.

REFERENCES

Abraham, G. and R.J. Colonno. 1984. Many rhinovirus serotypes bind to the same cellular receptor. *J. Virol.* **51:** 340.

————. 1988. Characterization of human rhinoviruses displaced by an anti-receptor monoclonal antibody. *J. Virol.* **62:** 2300.

Acharya, R., E. Fry, D. Stuart, G. Fox, D. Rowlands, and F. Brown. 1989. The three-dimensional structure of foot-and-mouth disease virus at 2.9 Å resolution. *Nature* **337:** 709.

Badger, J., I. Minor, M. Kremer, M.A. Oliveira, T.J. Smith, J.P. Griffith, D.M.A. Guerin, S. Krishnaswamy, M. Luo., M.G. Rossmann, M.A. McKinlay, G.D. Diana, F.J. Dutko, M. Fancher, R.R. Rueckert, and B.A. Heinz. 1988. Structural analysis of a series of antiviral agents complexed with human rhinovirus 14. *Proc. Natl. Acad. Sci.* **85:** 3304.

Carrillo, E.C., C. Giachetti, and R.H. Campos. 1984. Effect of lysosomotropic agents on the foot-and-mouth disease virus. *Virology* **135:** 542.

————. 1985. Early steps in FMDV replication: Further analysis on the effects of chloroquine. *Virology* **147:** 118.

Colonno, R.J., J.H. Condra, S. Mizutani, P.L. Callahan, M.-E. Davies, and M.A. Murcko. 1988. Evidence for the direct involvement of the rhinovirus canyon in receptor binding. *Proc. Natl. Acad. Sci.* **85:** 5449.

Cybulsky, M.I., J.W.U. Fries, A.J. Williams, P. Sultan, V.M. Davis, M.A. Gimbrone, and T. Collins. 1991. Alternative splicing of human VCAM-1 in activated vascular endothelium. *Am. J. Pathol.* **138:** 815.

Duechler, M., T. Skern, W. Sommergruber, C. Neubauer, P. Gruendler, I. Fogy, D. Blaas, and E. Kuechler. 1987. Evolutionary relationships within the human rhinovirus genus: Comparison of serotypes 89, 2, and 14. *Proc. Natl. Acad. Sci.* **84:** 2605.

Dustin, M.L., R. Rothlein, A.K. Bhan, C.A. Dinarello, and T.A. Springer. 1986. Induction by IL1 and interferon-γ: Tissue distribution, biochemistry, and function of a natural adherence molecule (ICAM-1). *J. Immunol.* **137:** 245.

Fricks, C.E. and J.M. Hogle. 1990. Cell-induced conformational change in poliovirus: Externalization of the amino terminus of VP1 is responsible for liposome binding. *J. Virol.* **64:** 1934.

Giranda, V.L., M.S. Chapman, and M.G. Rossmann. 1990. Modeling of the human intercellular adhesion molecule-1, the human major group receptor. *Proteins* **7:** 227.

Greve, J.M., C.P. Forte, C.W. Marlor, A.M. Meyer, H. Hoover-Litty, D. Wunderlich, and A. McClelland. 1991. Mechanisms of receptor-mediated rhinovirus neutralization defined by two soluble forms of ICAM-1. *J. Virol.* **65:** 6015.

Greve, J.M., G. Davis, A.M. Meyer, C.P. Forte, S.C. Yost, C.W. Marlor, M.E. Kamarck, and A. McClelland. 1989. The major human rhinovirus receptor is ICAM-1. *Cell* **56:** 839.

Hession, C., R. Tizard, C. Vassalo, S.B. Schiffer, D. Goff, P. Moy, G. Chi-Rosso, S. Luhowskyj, R. Lobb, and L. Osborn. 1991. Cloning of an alternative form of vascular adhesion molecule-1 (VCAM1). *J. Biol. Chem.* **266:** 6682.

Hofer, F., B. Berger, M. Gruenberger, H. Machat, R. Dernick, U. Tessmer, E. Kuechler, and D. Blaas. 1992. Shedding of a rhinovirus minor group binding protein: Evidence for a Ca^{++}-dependent process. *J. Gen. Virol.* **73:** 627.

Hogle, J.M., M. Chow, and D.J. Filman. 1985. Three-dimensional structure of poliovirus at 2.9 Å resolution. *Science* **229:** 1358.

Hoover-Litty, H. and J.M. Greve. 1993. Formation of rhinovirus-soluble ICAM-1 complexes and conformational changes in the virion. *J. Virol.* **67:** 390.

Hughes, P.J., C. North, C.H. Jellis, P.D. Minor, and G. Stanway. 1988. The nucleotide sequence of human rhinovirus 1B: Molecular relationships within the rhinovirus genus. *J. Gen. Virol.* **69:** 49.

Kim, S., T.J. Smith, M.M. Chapman, M.G. Rossmann, D.C. Pevear, F.J. Dutko, P.J. Felock, G.D. Diana, and M.A. McKinlay. 1989. Crystal structure of human rhinovirus serotype 1A (HRV1A). *J. Mol. Biol.* **210:** 91.

Kim, K.H., P. Willingmann, Z.-X. Gong, M.J. Kremer, M.S. Chapman, I. Minor, M.A. Oliveira, M.G. Rossmann, K. Andries, G.D. Diana, F.J. Dutko, M.A. McKinlay, and D.C. Pevear. 1993. A comparison of the anti-rhinoviral drug binding pocket in HRV14 and HRV1A. *J. Mol. Biol.* **230:** 206.

Kolatkar, P.R., M.A. Oliveira, M.G. Rossmann, A.H. Robbins, S.K. Katti, H. Hoover-Litty, C. Forte, J.M. Greve, A. McClelland, and N.H. Olson. 1992. Preliminary X-ray crystallographic analysis of intercellular adhesion molecule-1. *J. Mol. Biol.* **225:** 1127.

Korant, B.D., K. Lonberg-Holm, J. Noble, and J.T. Stasny. 1972. Naturally occurring and artifically produced components of three rhinoviruses. *Virology* **48:** 71.

Leahy, D.J., W.A. Hendrickson, I. Aukhil, and H.P. Erickson. 1992. Structure of a fibronectin type III domain from tenascin phased by MAD analysis of the selenomethionyl protein. *Science* **258:** 987.

Lonberg-Holm, K. and B.D. Korant. 1972. Early interactions of rhinoviruses with host cells. *J. Virol.* **9:** 29.

Lonberg-Holm, K., R.J. Crowell, and L. Philipson. 1976a. Unrelated animal viruses share receptors. *Nature* **259:** 679.

Lonberg-Holm, K., L.B. Gosser, and J. Shimshick. 1976b. Interaction of liposomes with subviral particles of poliovirus type 2 and rhinovirus type 2. *J. Virol.* **19:** 746.

Luo, M, G. Vriend, G. Kamer, I. Minor, E. Arnold, M.G. Rossmann, U. Boege, D.G. Scraba, G.M. Duke, and A.C. Palmenbeg. 1987. The atomic structure of Mengo virus at 3.0 Å resolution. *Science* **235:** 182.

Madshus, I.H., S. Olsnes, and K. Sandvig. 1984a. Requirements for entry of poliovirus

RNA into cells at low pH. *EMBO J.* **3:** 1945.

―――. 1984b. Different pH requirements for entry of the two picornaviruses, human rhinovirus 2 and murine encephalomyocarditis virus. *Virology* **139:** 346.

Main, A.L., T.S. Harvey, M. Baron, J. Boyd, and I.D. Campbell. 1992. The three-dimensional structure of the tenth type III module of fibronectin: An insight into RDG-mediated interactions. *Cell* **71:** 671.

Marsh, M. and A. Helenius. 1989. Virus entry into animal cells. *Adv. Virus Res.* **36:** 107.

Martin, A., C. Wyshowski, T. Couderc, R. Crainic, J. Hogle, and M. Girard. 1988. Engineering a poliovirus type 2 antigenic site on a type 1 capsid results in a chimeric virus which is neurovirulent for mice. *EMBO J.* **7:** 2839.

McClelland, A, J. deBear, S. Connonly Yost, A.M. Meyer, C.W. Marlor, and J.M. Greve. 1991. Identification of monoclonal antibody epitopes and critical residues for rhinovirus binding in domain 1 of ICAM-1. *Proc. Natl. Acad. Sci.* **88:** 7993.

Mischak, H., C. Neubauer, B. Berger, E. Kuechler, and D. Blaas. 1988. Detection of the human rhinovirus minor group receptor on renaturing western blots. *J. Gen. Virol.* **69:** 2653.

Neubauer, C., L. Frasel, E. Kuechler, and D. Blass. 1987. Mechanism of entry of human rhinovirus 2 into Hela cells. *Virology* **158:** 255.

Olson, N.H., P.R. Kolatkar, M.A. Oliveira, R.H. Cheng, J.M. Greve, A. McClelland, T.S. Baker, and M.G. Rossmann. 1993. Structure of a human rhinovirus complexed with its receptor molecule. *Proc. Natl. Acad. Sci.,* **90:** 507.

Pevear, D.C., M.J. Fancher, P.J. Felock, M.G. Rossmann, M.S. Miller, G. Diana, A.M. Treasurywala, M.A. McKinaly, and F.J. Dutko. 1989. Conformational change in the floor of the human rhinovirus canyon blocks absorption to HeLa cell receptors. *J. Virol.* **63:** 2002.

Pober, J.S., M.A. Gimbrone, L.A. LaPierre, D.L. Mendrick, W. Fiers, R. Rothlein, and T.A. Springer. 1986. Overlapping patterns of activation of human endothelial cells by interleukin 1, tumor necrosis factor, and immune interferon. *J. Immunol.* **137:** 1893.

Register, R.B., C.R. Uncapher, A.M. Naylor, D.W. Lineberger, and R.J. Colonno. 1991. Human-murine chimera of ICAM-1 identify amino acid residues critical for rhinovirus and antibody binding. *J. Virol.* **65:** 6589.

Rossmann, M.G. 1989. The canyon hypothesis. Hiding the host cell receptor attachment site on a viral surface from immune surveillance. *J. Biol. Chem.* **264:** 14587.

Rossmann, M.G. and A.C. Palmenberg. 1988. Conservation of the putative receptor attachment site in picornaviruses. *Virology* **164:** 373.

Rossmann, M.G., E. Arnold, J.W. Erickson, E.A. Frankenberger, J.P. Griffith, H.J. Hecht, J.E. Johnson, G. Kamer, M. Luo, A.G.. Mosser, R.R. Rueckert, B. Sherry, and G. Vriend. 1985. Structure of a common cold virus and functional relationship to other picornaviruses. *Nature* **317:** 145.

Ryu, S., P.D. Kwong, A. Truneh, T.G. Porter, J. Arthos, M. Rosenberg, X. Dai, N. Xuong, R. Axel, R.W. Sweet, and W.A. Hendrickson. 1990. Crystal structure of an HIV-binding recombinant fragment of human CD4. *Nature* **348:** 419.

Sherry, B. and R. Rueckert. 1985. Evidence for at least two dominant neutralization antigens on human rhinovirus 14. *J. Virol.* **53:** 137.

Sherry, B., A.G. Mosser, R.J., Colonno, and R.R. Rueckert. 1986. Use of monoclonal antibodies to identify four neutralization immunogens on a common cold picornavirus, human rhinovirus 14. *J. Virol.* **57:** 246.

Simmons, D., M.W. Makgoba, and B. Seed. 1988. ICAM, an adhesion ligand of LFA-1, is homologous to the neural cell adhesion molecule NCAM. *Nature* **331:** 624.

Skern, T., W. Sommergruber, D. Blaas, P. Gruendler, F. Fraundorfer, C. Pieler, I. Fogy, and E. Kuechler. 1985. Human rhinovirus 2: Complete nucleotide sequence and proteolytic processing signals in the capsid protein region. *Nucleic Acids Res.* **6:** 2111.

Smith, T. J., M.J. Kremer, M. Luo, G. Vriend, E. Arnold, G. Kamer, M.G. Rossmann, M.A. McKinlay, G.D. Diana, and M.J. Otto. 1986. The site of attachment in human rhinovirus 14 for antiviral agents that inhibit uncoating. *Science* **233:** 1286.

Smith, T.J., N.H. Olson, R.H. Cheng, H. Liu, E.S. Chase, W.M. Lee, D.M. Leippe, A.G. Mosser, R.R. Rueckert, and T.S. Baker. 1993. Structure of human rhinovirus complexed with Fab fragments from a neutralizing antibody. *J. Virol.* **67:** 1148.

Springer, T.A. 1990. Adhesion receptors of the immune system. *Nature* **346:** 425.

Stanway, G., P.J. Hughes, R.C. Mountford, P.D. Minor, and J.W. Almond. 1984. The complete nucleotide sequence of a common cold virus: Human rhinovirus 14. *Nucleic Acids Res.* **12:** 7859.

Staunton, D.E., M.L. Dustin, H.P. Erickson, and T.A. Springer. 1990. The arrangement of immunoglobulin-like domains of ICAM-1 and the binding sites for LFA-1 and rhinovirus. *Cell* **61:** 243.

Staunton, D.E., S.D. Marlin, C. Stratowa, M.L. Dustin, and T.A. Springer. 1988. Primary structure of intercellular adhesion molecule 1 (ICAM-1) demonstrates interaction between the immunoglobulin and integrin supergene families. *Cell* **52:** 925.

Staunton, D.E., V.J. Merluzzi, R. Rothlein, R. Barton, S.D. Marlin, and T.A. Springer. 1989. A cell adhesion molecule, ICAM-1, is the major surface receptor for rhinoviruses. *Cell* **56:** 849.

Uncapher, C.R., C.M. DeWitt, and R.J. Colonno. 1991. The major and minor group receptor families contain all but one rhinovirus serotype. *Virology* **180:** 814.

Voraberger, G., R. Shafer, and C. Stratowa. 1991. Cloning of the human gene for intercellular adhesion molecule-1 and analysis of its 5′-regulatory region. *J. Immunol.* **147:** 2777.

Wang, J., Y. Yan, T.P.J. Garrett, J. Liu, D.W. Rodgers, R.L. Garlick, G.E. Tarr, Y. Husain, E.L. Rheinherz, and S.C. Harrison. 1990. Atomic structure of a fragment of human CD4 containing two immunoglobulin-like domains. *Nature* **348:** 411.

Yeates, T.O., D.H. Jacobson, A. Martin, C. Wychowski, M. Girard, D.J. Filman, and J.M. Hogle. 1991. Three-dimensional structure of a mouse-adapted type 2/type 1 poliovirus chimera. *EMBO J.* **10:** 2331.

13

The Endocytic Pathway and Virus Entry

Mark Marsh and Annegret Pelchen-Matthews
MRC Laboratory for Molecular Cell Biology
and Department of Biology
University College London
London WC1E 6BT, United Kingdom

Endocytosis is an essential component of the strategies employed by many animal viruses to enter their host cells. For Semliki forest virus (SFV) or influenza virus, for example, the acidic environment in endocytic organelles triggers conformational changes in the envelope glycoproteins that initiate the membrane fusion events leading to penetration. As fusion is absolutely dependent on exposure to acid pH, and can only occur within endocytic organelles, endocytosis is a prerequisite for the productive entry of these viruses (Marsh and Helenius 1989).

Weak bases, carboxylic ionophores, or specific inhibitors of vacuolar proton ATPases, which neutralize acidic endocytic organelles, inhibit the entry of pH-dependent viruses and can distinguish enveloped and non-enveloped viruses that require exposure to acid pH from those that do not (see, e.g., McClure et al. 1988, 1990). As the entry of this latter group is pH-independent, it is frequently assumed that their entry is also independent of endocytosis and occurs by penetration of the plasma membrane (see, e.g., Stein et al. 1987). However, the evidence that penetration at the cell surface can lead to productive infection is scant and often equivocal. In this chapter, we discuss the notion that endocytosis may facilitate the productive entry of both pH-dependent and pH-independent viruses. Furthermore, we discuss the evidence that endocytosis may play additional roles in viral infection and pathology.

ENDOCYTOSIS AND ENDOCYTIC PATHWAYS

Phagocytic and Constitutive Endocytosis

Endocytosis describes the uptake of solutes, small particles, and fluid into membrane-bound intracellular vesicles. Different forms of endocytosis, mediated by distinct biochemical mechanisms, operate in animal cells. The most spectacular of these is the phagocytic uptake of large (>200 nm diameter) particulate ligands, such as yeast or bacteria.

Phagocytosis is often a property of professional phagocytes, such as macrophages, and is induced by opsonized particles binding to specific receptors on the surface of the phagocytic cell, the subsequent actin-dependent envelopment of the particle, and the formation of the phagocytic vesicle (for review, see Watts and Marsh 1992).

In contrast to the ligand-induced formation of phagocytic vesicles, virtually all nucleated cells continually internalize fluid from their environment in smaller pinocytic vesicles (Watts and Marsh 1992). This process occurs without the involvement of inductive signals, primarily through clathrin-coated pits that invaginate from the plasma membrane to form coated vesicles. These vesicles, which have an average internal diameter of 100 nm, also take up membrane and macromolecular or small particulate (<150 nm diameter) ligands bound to the cell surface. In baby hamster kidney (BHK) cells, coated pits occupy about 2% of the plasma membrane area and form approximately 1200 coated vesicles per minute (Marsh and Helenius 1980). In smaller lymphocytic cells, coated pits also account for about 2% of the cell surface area and form approximately 100 vesicles per minute (Pelchen-Matthews et al. 1991). With this number of vesicles, both BHK and lymphoid cells can internalize the equivalent of 50–100% of the cell surface per hour, and a similar area of membrane must recycle during this time to maintain the dimensions of the cell. Thus, the plasma membrane is highly dynamic and continually undergoes endocytosis and recycling.

Besides this nonspecific or bulk flow internalization of fluid and membrane, clathrin-coated pits have the capacity to bind specific plasma membrane components and receptors. These receptors concentrate in coated pits and, because the pits continuously invaginate to form coated vesicles, internalize at rates severalfold higher than molecules internalized by bulk flow (Goldstein et al. 1985). The list of cell-surface receptors known to interact with coated pits, and to be capable of receptor-mediated endocytosis, is now extensive and includes receptors for nutrients or nutrient carriers (e.g., low density lipoprotein [LDL], transferrin [Tf], and cobalamin), growth factors (e.g., epidermal growth factor [EGF], platelet-derived growth factor [PDGF]), immunoglobulins (Ig), mannose 6-phosphate (M6P)-containing lysosomal hydrolases, and protease inhibitors (e.g., α_2-macroglobulin). Thus, the coated vesicle pathway is responsible for fluid-phase endocytosis, receptor-mediated endocytosis, and bulk membrane turnover (Watts and Marsh 1992).

Other routes of endocytosis may exist. In some cells, growth factors induce large noncoated macropinocytic vesicles (van Deurs et al. 1989; Watts and Marsh 1992). Furthermore, clathrin-independent routes may contribute to constitutive endocytosis in various cells (see Watts and

Marsh 1992). Significantly, these noncoated vesicles appear capable of delivering endocytic tracers to endosomes and lysosomes. However, the extent of their activity and the underlying biochemical mechanisms are unclear. Finally, recent observations have led to the suggestion that caveolae might also be endocytic (Anderson 1993). These structures have been implicated in transcytosis in endothelial cells, but there is currently little evidence that they are involved in the delivery of endocytic markers to the endosomal and lysosomal compartments of the endocytic pathway or that they play a role in virus entry.

Coated Pits and Endocytosis Signals

The mechanisms involved in endocytic coated-pit formation and the interactions of specific receptors with components of the clathrin coat have been analyzed in detail. The coat itself consists of the structural protein complex, clathrin, which forms a well-characterized polyhedral lattice on the cytoplasmic aspect of the plasma membrane (Schmid 1992). Associated with the clathrin lattice are multiple copies of another protein complex, the adapters (Robinson 1992), which can interact specifically with endocytosis signals displayed on the cytoplasmic tails of certain cell-surface molecules, thus mediating their recruitment into coated pits. One such endocytosis signal has recently been identified as a short stretch of 4–6 amino acids with flanking aromatic or large hydrophobic residues, frequently including at least one tyrosine (e.g., FDNPVY in the LDLR and YXRF in the Tf-R), and predicted to form tight β turns (Vaux 1992; Trowbridge et al. 1993). However, plasma membrane proteins that lack these motifs, such as the T-cell glycoprotein CD4, are capable of efficient endocytosis and appear to use alternative signals (Pelchen-Matthews et al. 1993). The number and precise nature of these alternative signals are at present unknown. However, one candidate, a pair of leucine residues frequently separated by 3–4 amino acids from a charged amino acid or phosphoserine residue, has been identified (Letourneur and Klausner 1992; Dietrich et al. 1994). Although the majority of endocytosis signals have been identified in type I and II integral membrane proteins, coated-pit localization signals are present in some multispanning integral membrane proteins (Piper et al. 1993).

Endocytosis signals are required for the rapid and efficient uptake of receptors and their ligands into coated pits, but they are not essential for endocytosis. Membrane proteins that lack endocytosis signals, or receptors from which an endocytosis signal has been deleted, are not excluded from coated pits but are equally distributed over both coated and noncoated domains of the plasma membrane and are internalized with bulk flow kinetics (Jing et al. 1990; Miettinen et al. 1990; Pelchen-Matthews et al. 1991). A third class of plasma membrane proteins, which includes CD8 and the B lymphocyte B1 form of the murine FcRII, does not undergo significant endocytosis (Miettinen et al. 1990; P.A. Reid and M. Marsh, unpubl.). These proteins are excluded from coated pits through mechanisms that remain to be established. However, in some cases, association with components of the cytoskeleton appears to prevent these proteins from entering the endocytic pathway (Hammerton 1991; Miettinen et al. 1992). Glycophosphatidylinositol (GPI)-linked cell-surface glycopro-teins, which do not span the lipid bilayer and therefore do not contain endocytosis signals, appear to be excluded from coated pits (Bretscher et al. 1980). Nevertheless, a number of these proteins do internalize (van den Bosch et al. 1988; Keller et al. 1992), although the rates of uptake can be slow (Bamezai et al. 1989). The proposed association of GPI-linked molecules with lipid-rich microdomains or with other integral membrane proteins (Robinson 1991; Brown and Rose 1992) may account for these slow internalization rates.

Whereas many cell-surface proteins constitutively interact with coated pits, others undergo regulated endocytosis. For example, many growth factor receptors (e.g., those for EGF, PDGF, or insulin) must bind their specific ligand to undergo endocytosis (Carpenter and Cohen 1976). Ligand binding can induce dimerization of these receptors, which may in turn facilitate the display of endocytosis signals (Cochet et al. 1988). Multivalent cross-linking of other cell-surface glycoproteins can modulate their interactions with the endocytic pathway (see, e.g., Ukkonen et al. 1986) and may also induce their internalization (see Schmid 1992). Examples of other mechanisms for the regulation of endocytic trafficking are also emerging. For example, CD4 is excluded from coated pits by association with the T-lymphocyte-specific protein tyrosine kinase p56[lck] and is only constitutively endocytosed in p56[lck]-negative cells (e.g., cells of the macrophage lineage or transfected nonlymphoid cells). Since the interaction of CD4 and p56[lck] is noncovalent, agents that cause the dissociation of the complex can induce CD4 internalization (Pelchen-Matthews et al. 1992, 1993).

The interaction of proteins with endocytic pathways is complex. Plasma membrane components can be internalized efficiently through signals that are constitutively active or that can be switched on by, for example, dimerization or phosphorylation. Some components are internalized by bulk flow mechanisms, whereas others are retained at the cell surface. Moreover, the endocytic properties of cell-surface components in each of these categories can be modulated by physiological and experimental stimuli or by the binding of extracellular ligands. The factors that

regulate the interactions of membrane components with endocytic pathways are not fully understood, and we cannot predict how they might be
modified by the binding of multivalent ligands such as viruses.

Endosomes and Other Endocytic Organelles

After pinching off from the plasma membrane, coated vesicles are rapidly uncoated through the action of uncoating enzymes (Schmid 1992).
The uncoated vesicles then fuse with early endosomes in the cell
periphery (Fig. 1). Endosomes have a complex morphology, consisting
of highly plastic networks of interconnected vacuolar and tubular structures. The main function of the early endosome appears to be the sorting
of internalized proteins for recycling to the cell surface, transport to late
endosomes and lysosomes, or, in appropriate cell types, transcytosis or
delivery to synaptic vesicles. Currently, the intricacies of the endosome
compartment are still being uncovered, and it is apparent that some of the
sorting functions may occur within specialized subcomponents of the
endosome system. Thus, the tubular extensions are believed to be involved in recycling of membrane and receptors, whereas proteins
destined for degradation are sequestered onto the internal vesicles of
multivesicular bodies and are transported to the more juxtanuclear late
endosome, or prelysosomal compartment, before reaching the lysosomes
where they are degraded (see Trowbridge et al. 1993).

Late endosomes become labeled with endocytic tracers after the early
endosomes and can be distinguished from early endosomes both biochemically (e.g., they contain significant amounts of the cation-inde-
pendent M6P-receptor and, on the cytoplasmic aspect, label for the small
GTP-binding protein Rab7) and by cell fractionation (Griffiths and
Gruenberg 1991). They are also morphologically complex, consisting of
both vesicular and tubular components, with the vesicular elements frequently containing considerable amounts of membrane that appears as
myelin-like profiles in electron micrographs. Late endosomes are frequently located in the perinuclear region of the cell and appear to be the
last station on the endocytic pathway before the hydrolytic lysosome
compartment. As with transport from the cell surface to early endosomes,
transport between early and late endosomes is believed to occur through
vesicular intermediates. These carriers appear as large (>200 nm
diameter) vesicles termed multivesicular bodies or endosomal carrier
vesicles (Griffiths and Gruenberg 1991; Trowbridge et al. 1993), and
their relocation is dependent on interactions with microtubules.

Acidification of intracellular organelles including endosomes and
lysosomes occurs through membrane-bound vacuolar H^+-ATPases. The

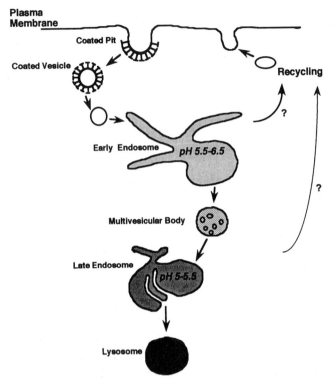

Figure 1 The constitutive endocytic pathway. Coated pits invaginate from the cell surface and pinch off to form coated vesicles, which are uncoated before fusing with early endosomes located primarily in the cell periphery. Multi-vesicular bodies may function as endosomal carrier vesicles on the route to the late endosomes (prelysosomal compartment) and lysosomes, both of which are found in a more juxtanuclear location. Recycling is believed to occur primarily from the early endosomes, although the exact structures and pathways involved have not yet been clearly identified.

pH in the lumen of early endosomes is about 6, and in lysosomes and late endosomes ranges from 4.8 to 5.5 (Mellman et al. 1986). The sorting events that occur in endosomes are, at least in part, dependent on this acidification. Thus, LDL dissociates from the LDLR at mildly acid pH and is sorted to lysosomes, whereas the LDLR recycles to the plasma membrane. Similarly, ferric iron dissociates from diferric transferrin at endosomal pH. The iron remains in the cell, but the TfR and apotransferrin recycle to the cell surface. Weak bases (e.g., NH_4Cl, chloroquine), carboxylic ionophores (e.g., monensin), and specific inhibitors of vacuolar H^+-ATPases, such as Bafilomycin A, neutralize the acidic environment of endocytic organelles. As a consequence, these reagents can modulate the sorting properties of endocytic organelles by inhibiting the dissociation of low-pH-sensitive receptor/ligand complexes and influencing the trafficking of certain receptors (Mellman et al. 1986). However, with the exceptions of primaquine (Hiebsch et al. 1991) and Bafilomycin A (Clague et al. 1994), none of these agents has been shown to have major effects on vesicular transport through the endocytic pathway.

Other compartments of the vacuolar apparatus, including secretory vesicles and the *trans* Golgi network (TGN), are also believed to be acidified by vacuolar H^+-ATPases and to be functionally compromised by weak bases, etc. (Mellman et al. 1986). Entry of endocytic tracers into these organelles is inefficient, and there is no evidence that they play a role in virus entry.

VIRUS ENTRY: FUSION, PENETRATION, AND UNCOATING

In general, the mechanisms of membrane penetration and entry are best understood for enveloped viruses (Marsh and Helenius 1989), and much of the following discussion leans heavily on studies of these viruses. Nevertheless, the role of endocytosis in productive virus entry is equally relevant to nonenveloped viruses.

pH-dependent Viruses

The role of endocytosis in virus entry has been controversial. Studies which indicated that a number of enveloped and nonenveloped viruses could associate with endocytic organelles were contradicted by morphological observations of virions seemingly entering cells by direct fusion with the plasma membrane. Experiments with SFV in the early 1980s indicated that, following binding to cell-surface receptors, virions undergo receptor-mediated endocytosis through coated pits and vesicles and are delivered intact into endosomes (Helenius et al. 1980; Marsh and Helenius 1980; Marsh et al. 1983). However, the key observations which indicated that these endocytic events could lead to productive infection were (1) that the weak bases and carboxylic ionophores that neutralize acidic organelles inhibit SFV infection (Helenius et al. 1980, 1982) and (2) that virions could be induced to fuse with plasma membranes of liposomes by brief exposure to acidic media (Helenius et al. 1980; White and Helenius 1980). The observation that the neutralization of endocytic organelles by weak bases and carboxylic ionophores could be used to inhibit SFV infection was quickly exploited to examine the pH-dependence for entry of other viruses. These experiments indicated that acid-dependent entry was not restricted to α viruses and occurred for a number of enveloped and nonenveloped viruses (Table 1), including influ-

Table 1 pH-Dependence of virus entry

Virus group	Virus
Acid-dependent viruses	
alpha	SFV, Sindbis
orthomyxo	influenza A, B, C
flavi	West Nile virus
rhabdo	VSV, rabies
bunya	La Crosse virus
retro	MMTV
irido	African swine fever
picorna	rhino, FMDV
adeno	adenovirus type 2
reo	reovirus type 3
parvo	canine parvovirus
astro	human type 1[a]
herpes	human herpes 6[b]
Possibly acid-dependent viruses	
corona	MHV-3
baculo	nuclear polyhedrosis virus
retro	ecoMLV[c]
pox	vaccinia
arenavirus	Junin virus
Acid-independent viruses	
paramyxo	Sendai, Newcastle disease virus
retro (avian)	Rous sarcoma virus
retro (primate)	Mason-Pfizer monkey virus, HTLV-1
retro (lenti)	HIV-1, HIV-2, SIV
herpes	herpes simplex virus 1
papova	SV40, polyomavirus
rota	porcine rotavirus
hepadna	duck hepatitis B
picorna	hepatitis A, murine encephalomyocarditis virus
baculo	lepidopteran nuclear polyhedrosis virus (polyhedron-derived virus)[d]

Unless indicated, references can be found in Marsh and Helenius (1989) or Marsh and Pelchen-Matthews (1993).

[a]Donnelli et al. (1992).

[b]Cirone et al. (1992).

[c]Ecotropic murine leukemia virus exhibits pH-dependent entry in some cell lines but not others (McClure et al. 1990).

[d]Horton and Burand (1993).

enza, vesicular stomatitis virus (VSV), and adenovirus. Subsequent experiments showed that entry involves receptor-mediated internalization, delivery to endosomes, and acid-induced conformational changes in the envelope glycoproteins or capsid structures that trigger membrane fusion or penetration reactions (see Marsh and Helenius 1989).

The conformational changes induced by exposure to low pH have been most thoroughly characterized for the envelope proteins of influenza (see, e.g., Stegmann et al. 1990; Carr and Kim 1993) and SFV (Kielian and Helenius 1985; Wahlberg et al. 1992). However, the precise molecular mechanisms that trigger the lipid reorganization in the two opposing membrane systems that result in membrane fusion are not established. In addition to the role in penetration, recent experiments with influenza A viruses indicate that exposure to low pH also opens a proton channel in the viral membrane. This channel, formed by the viral M2 protein, allows acidification of the viral core and facilitates the uncoating of the viral ribonucleoprotein complexes after fusion (Martin and Helenius 1991; Pinto et al. 1992). Whether similar mechanisms are involved in the uncoating of other viral capsid structures is unclear.

The molecular events involved in penetration and uncoating of pH-dependent nonenveloped viruses are less well understood. However, studies with adenovirus and with pH-dependent picornaviruses indicate that changes in the structure of the capsid induced at pH values equivalent to those found in endosomes affect the integrity and hydrophobic properties of the virions (Fricks and Hogle 1990; Varga et al. 1991; Greber et al. 1993).

As the various endocytic mechanisms discussed above provide an efficient mechanism to deliver virions into an acid environment, the entry of pH-dependent viruses is also endocytosis-dependent. This coupled dependence on both endocytosis and exposure to acid pH has important consequences for the virions. In tissue culture and in vivo, with the exception of the gastrointestinal tract, the principal acidic locations are within endocytic organelles. Since the acidic pH in these organelles is maintained by vacuolar H^+-ATPases, acidic organelles are only found in viable cells. Furthermore, as the conformational changes involved in the fusion or penetration reactions of a number of viruses are either irreversible or exhibit only limited reversibility, premature activation of the fusion/penetration reactions leads to inactivation of the virus. Thus, the low pH and endocytosis dependence ensures that the penetration reactions are only activated after encounter with a cell. In addition, as endocytosis is a constitutive property of nucleated cells, acid-induced penetration enhances the chance that a virus will enter a cell in which it can replicate.

pH-independent Viruses

The weak bases and carboxylic ionophores not only identified pH-dependent viruses, but also indicated that a number of other enveloped and nonenveloped viruses do not require exposure to acid pH for entry (Table 1). Thus, for paramyxoviruses such as Sendai, or for the human immunodeficiency viruses (HIV-1 and -2), entry is not affected by weak bases or carboxylic ionophores (White et al. 1983; Stein et al. 1987; McClure et al. 1988) and the virions are not inactivated by treatment with acidic media (McClure et al. 1988). Furthermore, cells infected with pH-independent enveloped viruses can form syncytia (fusion from within) in neutral or mildly alkaline media (McClure et al. 1988).

Although the fusion and penetration reactions of these viruses are not dependent on exposure to low pH, there is evidence that they may be subject to alternative controls. The clearest example for this is with HIV-1, where it is apparent that HIV-1[VSV] pseudotypes (VSV nucleocapsids in an envelope containing the HIV-1 envelope glycoprotein), which can infect human CD4$^+$ cells, can bind to murine cells expressing human CD4$^+$ but do not fuse with or infect these cells (Maddon et al. 1986). The endocytic properties of human CD4 expressed in human and murine cells are comparable (Pelchen-Matthews et al. 1989, 1992), and it has been concluded that the murine cells must lack a critical component required for HIV-1 fusion. A similar explanation might also account for some of the observed tropisms exhibited by specific HIV strains for various CD4$^+$ cells (see, e.g., Cann et al. 1992). Although experiments with the pH-independent ecotropic murine leukemia virus and with HIV-1 have led to the suggestion that a protease might function as a fusion trigger (Andersen 1983; Moore and Nara 1992) and receptor binding appears to initiate poliovirus penetration (Hogle 1993), the mechanisms involved in activating the fusion or penetration of pH-independent viruses are obscure. Whether fusion/penetration must be activated for all pH-independent viruses is unclear. Sendai virus, for instance, can fuse with liposomes across a range of pH values without a requirement for proteins in the liposome membrane (White et al. 1983).

The facts that some viruses do not require low pH to activate fusion/penetration and that pH-independent enveloped viruses can induce syncytium formation, along with the observation of fusion figures at the cell surface (see below), have led to the assumption that pH-independent viruses can productively infect cells by direct penetration through the plasma membrane. However, the lack of detailed knowledge of the mechanisms responsible for activating the fusion/penetration of these viruses has prevented clear identification of the site(s) relevant for productive infection. Furthermore, although syncytium formation and cell-surface fusion figures indicate that the triggers that activate the penetration of at least some pH-independent viruses can be present at the cell surface, the known cycling properties of the plasma membrane may allow these factors to be present in endocytic vesicles and to be capable of redistribution.

VIRUS ENDOCYTOSIS

Morphological Observations

Virus Uptake Pathways

Electron microscopic observations in different virus and cell systems have demonstrated the internalization of pH-dependent viruses in endocytic vesicles. Frequently, uptake is observed in clathrin-coated vesicles (see, e.g., Helenius et al. 1980; Matlin et al. 1981). SFV, which has a virion diameter (75 nm) less than that of the average endocytic coated vesicle and can be bound to cells in large numbers, has been used to quantitate coated vesicle formation (see above) and is internalized with kinetics similar to those of physiological ligands taken up by receptor-mediated endocytosis (Marsh and Helenius 1980). Significantly, pH-independent viruses including Sendai, RSV, and HIV-1 are also internalized in coated vesicles (see, e.g., Dales 1973; Grewe et al. 1990), although quantitative data on these endocytic events are not available.

The role of noncoated vesicles in viral endocytosis is less well documented. Influenza virions, for example, are frequently observed in apparently noncoated plasma membrane invaginations and in noncoated vesicles (see, e.g., Patterson et al. 1979; Matlin et al. 1981). Although oblique sections through invaginations of the plasma membrane can appear as vesicles, non-clathrin-mediated constitutive endocytic mechanisms have been reported in various cell types (van Deurs et al. 1989) and may provide a portal for virus uptake. Viruses that use sialic acid as a receptor (e.g., influenza virus) can bind to a variety of cell-surface glycolipids and glycoproteins and may be able to utilize different endocytic routes. Furthermore, virions with multiple receptor-binding sites may be able to induce invagination through receptor-ligand "zippering" effects similar to those described for phagocytosis. However, it is not clear that virus-containing noncoated invaginations do form endocytic vesicles, nor has it been demonstrated that the noncoated vesicle profiles do not derive from uncoated clathrin-coated vesicles.

A number of studies describe the uptake of virions into larger phagocyte-like or macropinocytic vesicles (Pauza and Price 1988; Bourinbaiar and Phillips 1991). Although virions may induce the formation of macropinocytic vesicles, it is often difficult, without appropriate controls, to distinguish these structures from endosomes that have received virions from endocytic coated or noncoated vesicles.

Penetration

Following uptake from the cell surface, both clathrin-coated and noncoated vesicles fuse with, and deliver their membrane and contents to, early endosomes. Both pH-dependent and pH-independent viruses are delivered to these structures and can subsequently be seen in late endosomes and lysosomes (see, e.g., Helenius et al. 1980; Matlin et al. 1981).

Although virions are frequently observed in endocytic vesicles and these sites have been identified biochemically as a location for fusion (Marsh et al. 1983), profiles of virions undergoing fusion or penetration are often difficult to see. The fusion reactions of pH-dependent enveloped viruses occur very rapidly. With SFV and influenza, for example, the fusion reactions can be completed within a few seconds of the virions' being exposed to an appropriate low-pH environment (White and Helenius 1980; Stegmann et al. 1990). Furthermore, once the viruses have undergone fusion, the morphological integrity of the capsid is often rapidly lost. The rapid fusion kinetics, the asynchronous delivery of virions to acidic compartments, and the fact that only about 50% of the best virus preparations undergo fusion with cellular membranes results in limited numbers of fusion events at a given time. The fraction of virions that fail to fuse and remain intact within endocytic vesicles, or are delivered to lysosomes, can give the impression that endocytosis is a means of disposing of viruses rather than an infectious route into the cell. Nevertheless, images of virions undergoing fusion with endosomal membranes have been observed, both for pH-dependent and pH-independent viruses (see, e.g., Helenius 1984; Pauza and Price 1988; Grewe et al. 1990). For the pH-dependent viruses, the frequency with which these structures are observed can be increased by loading virions into endocytic vesicles in the presence of a weak base and viewing the synchronized fusion of virions at short times after the re-acidification of endocytic organelles following the removal of the weak base (Helenius 1984).

Penetration figures can also be observed at the cell surface. With pH-dependent enveloped viruses, for example, incubation of cells with bound virus in mildly acidic medium can induce fusion at the cell surface (White et al. 1980; Matlin et al. 1981). Similar figures can be observed for pH-independent viruses (Grewe et al. 1990). However, as morphological experiments must be done with relatively high titers of virus where the pfu-to-particle ratio of the preparation is often low, it is impossible to determine whether particular fusion/penetration events give rise to productive infections, regardless of whether these events are observed at the cell surface or within endocytic vesicles. It is only when microscopy studies are coupled with biochemical and cell biological analysis of virus entry that morphological observations can be related to infectious entry.

Endocytosis of Virus Receptors

The identification of the cell-surface receptors responsible for virus binding and entry has long been a focus for research, and the literature is replete with candidate virus receptors. However, the demonstration that a particular component can mediate the productive infection of a given virus is frequently lacking. The recent advances in cloning and expression technologies have enabled putative receptors to be expressed in receptor-negative cell lines and have allowed direct analysis of their functional activity (Maddon et al. 1986; Mendelsohn et al. 1989; Staunton et al. 1989; Dveksler et al. 1991). Although the number of viruses for which functional receptors have been identified is small, the current list (Table 2) indicates that a range of different cell-surface proteins, from multiple membrane-spanning channels or transporters to single-spanning type I and II integral membrane proteins can be used as virus receptors. The strategies employed to express these receptors have also been used to analyze the properties of mutant receptors and to try to determine whether or not specific signals influence the activity of the molecule as a virus receptor.

As discussed above, the interaction of cell-surface proteins with endocytic pathways is complex. Endocytosis signals are multiple and not yet fully characterized. Many signals are only essential for rapid internalization, and tailless mutants of endocytic receptors or GPI-linked membrane proteins can be internalized to some extent. In some cases, data on well-characterized virus receptors are available from endocytosis experiments using antibodies or physiological ligands. However, there is, for the most part, very little information on how these receptors behave following their binding and cross-linking by multivalent viruses. From the data that are available, there is some indication that virus binding may alter the constitutive trafficking properties of the receptor molecules. For example, MHC class I antigens are believed to function as the primary receptors for SFV on murine cells. These molecules normally exhibit slow rates of constitutive internalization (Reid and Watts 1990) but mediate the rapid and efficient endocytosis of SFV (Marsh and Helenius 1980). Similarly, the influenza HA molecule is used as a model nonendocytic cell-surface antigen and appears to be excluded from coated pits on CV1 cells (Lazarovits and Roth 1988), yet this protein can clearly function as an endocytic receptor for the pH-dependent VSV (Fuller et al. 1985). Thus, the constitutive endocytic properties of cell-surface antigens do not necessarily tell us how these molecules will behave after binding a virus.

It is clear that pH-dependent viruses must bind to receptors capable of mediating their endocytosis. In the cases where receptors for pH-depen-

Table 2 Virus-binding cell-surface components and receptors

Virus group	Virus	Binding component
Enveloped viruses		
paramyxo	Sendai	sialic acid (glycoprotein/glycolipid)
	measles	membrane cofactor protein (CD46)[a,b]
orthomyxo	influenza A, B and C	sialic acid (glycoprotein/glycolipid)
toga	Semliki forest virus	class I MHC
	Sindbis virus	catecholinergic receptor; high-affinity laminin receptor[c]
	lactate dehydrogenase virus	class II MHC
	West Nile virus	Fc receptor (via bound IgG)
rhabdo	rabies virus	acetylcholine receptor
	vesicular stomatitis virus	phosphatidyl serine and other negatively charged lipids
retro	ecotropic murine leukemia virus (EcoMLV)	cationic amino acid transporter[a]
	radiation leukemia virus	CD4/T-cell receptor complex
	gibbon ape leukemia virus, and feline leukemia virus (subgroup B)	multi-spanning membrane protein (phosphate transporter?)[a]
	human T-cell leukemia virus 1	40-75-kD glycoprotein
	bovine leukemia virus	80-kD protein[a,d]
	Rous sarcoma virus (subgroup A)	low-density lipoprotein receptor-like protein[a,e]
lentiviruses	human immunodeficiency virus-1 and -2	CD4[a]
	human immunodeficiency virus-1	galactosyl ceramide
	visna virus	50-kD glycoprotein; MHC class II
herpes	Epstein-Barr virus	CR2[CD21][a]
	human cytomegalovirus	30, 32-kD glycoprotein, 92-kD protein
		heparan sulfate proteoglycan
	herpes simplex virus	heparan sulfate proteoglycan (syndecan?)[f]

pox	varicella-zoster virus	mannose-6-phosphate receptor
	vaccinia	epidermal growth factor receptor
corona	mouse hepatitis virus	carcinoembryonic antigen (Ig family)[a]
	transmissible gastroenteritis virus (TGEV) and human coronavirus 229E	aminopeptidase N[a]
	human coronavirus OC43, bovine coronavirus	N-acetyl-9-O-acetylneuraminic acid[g]
irido	African swine fever virus	12, 17-kD protein
Nonenveloped viruses		
picorna	coxsackie B	49-kD glycoprotein
	rhinovirus (major group)	intracellular adhesion molecule (ICAM)-1[a]
	rhinovirus (minor group)	85-kD glycoprotein
	poliovirus	poliovirus receptor (VPR)[a]
	encephalomyocarditis virus	glycophorin A
	Theiler's murine encephalomyelitis virus	34-kD glycoprotein
	foot and mouth disease virus	integrin-type receptor
	echovirus 1	integrin VLA-2 ($\alpha_2\beta_1$)[h]
reo	reovirus type 3	67-kD glycoprotein, 54-kD protein
	reovirus type 1	54-kD protein
	reovirus type 1 and 3	sialic acid
papova	polyomavirus	24, 30–40, 50, 95-kD glycoproteins
adeno	adenovirus type 2	78, 42, 34-kD glycoproteins, second receptor $\alpha_v\beta_3$ and $\alpha_v\beta_2$ vitronectin receptors[i]
rota	rhesus rotavirus (group A)	300/330-kD enterocyte glycoprotein

Unless indicated otherwise, references can be found in Marsh and Helenius (1989) or Marsh and Pelchen-Matthews (1993). [a]Indicates cell-surface proteins that have been demonstrated to function as virus receptors by expression in receptor-negative cells or animals; [b]Dörig et al. (1993); [c]Naniche et al. (1993); [c]Wang et al. (1992); [d]Ban et al. (1993); [e]Bates et al. (1993); [f]Bernfield et al. (1992); [g]Vlasak et al. (1988); [h]Bergelson et al. (1992); [i]Wickham et al. (1993).

dent viruses have been clearly identified (e.g., major group rhinoviruses and two coronaviruses), these receptors do not contain known endocytosis signals, nor have they been demonstrated to undergo rapid endocytosis, although aminopeptidase has been shown to internalize and recycle when cross-linked with two layers of antibodies (Louvard 1980). In a number of cases, virus receptors have been identified for which constitutive endocytic activity has been clearly demonstrated. For vaccinia, there is evidence that entry may be pH-dependent, and since the virus binds to the EGFR in a manner similar to native EGF, it must presumably induce internalization of the receptor. The flavivirus West Nile is clearly pH-dependent and, during antibody-enhanced infection, can utilize a receptor with both constitutive endocytic and phagocytic activity. For varicella-zoster virus, which is believed to bind to an M6P receptor, and HIV-1 and -2, which bind CD4, entry is pH-independent, although not necessarily endocytosis-independent. Similarly, Epstein-Barr virus is reported to be pH-independent for entry through the CD21/complement receptor 2. This molecule can mediate phagocytosis and requires an intact cytoplasmic domain to function as a virus receptor (Carel et al. 1990).

The endocytic activity of other virus receptors is less well characterized. Several retroviruses (ecotropic murine leukemia virus, gibbon-ape leukemia virus, and subgroup B feline leukemia virus) have recently been found to bind to multispanning membrane proteins (a cationic amino acid transporter and a putative phosphate transporter). These viruses are all pH-independent for entry (McClure et al. 1990) and multispanning membrane proteins similar to these receptors are often considered as undergoing minimal endocytosis. Nevertheless, the multispanning glucose transporter GLUT 4 does clearly internalize through coated pits (Piper et al. 1993), and the β-adrenergic receptor can be induced to internalize (Collins et al. 1992).

In a few cases, viruses have been suggested to use lipids as receptors. For example, VSV is claimed to bind to negatively charged phospholipids and HIV-1 may use galactosyl ceramide as an alternative receptor to CD4. These molecules clearly have no inherent endocytosis signal, but nevertheless, they do undergo bulk flow endocytosis. The uptake of certain gangliosides through endocytic coated pits and coated vesicles has been demonstrated previously (Sandvig et al. 1989). In the case of VSV at least, entry is pH-dependent and therefore dependent on endocytosis. Thus, there is no clear indication that pH-dependent viruses utilize specialized endocytic receptors. Furthermore, some pH-independent viruses exploit receptors with demonstrated endocytic properties.

CELL-SURFACE VERSUS ENDOSOMAL PENETRATION

It is frequently assumed that pH-independent viruses do not require endocytosis for productive infection. However, in most cases where cell-surface fusion/penetration is observed, the endocytic pathway is also active and cannot be excluded as the route of productive infection.

Endocytosis is constitutively active in most cells, and currently, there are few ways of inhibiting the process. As with other membrane transport events, endocytosis is blocked when cells are kept at 4°C or depleted of ATP. At 37°C, phagocytosis, macropinocytosis, and some non-clathrin-mediated constitutive endocytic activity can be inhibited by cytochalasins. However, coated vesicle formation is only inhibited when cells are incubated in hypertonic or mildly acidic media or depleted of potassium ions (see van Deurs et al. 1989). These treatments, although effective in some cells, can cause significant loss of viability (A. Pelchen-Matthews and M. Marsh, unpubl.) or may induce alternative endocytic mechanisms that are independent of clathrin (P. Courtoy, pers. comm.). Thus, in most studies of the entry of pH-independent viruses, the endocytic pathway is active and it is difficult to devise effective experimental strategies to inhibit this endocytic activity.

For the few pH-independent viruses for which some information exists, it is apparent that fusion or penetration can occur across a range of mildly acidic and alkaline pH values (see White et al. 1983; Sinangil et al. 1988), and the viruses show little or no enhanced penetration activity at neutral pH. Thus, at least as far as pH is concerned, virus fusion or penetration should be equally efficient in endosomes and at the cell surface and, although weak bases, carboxylic ionophores, etc. neutralize acidic organelles and block the fusion/penetration of pH-dependent viruses, they would not block the fusion/penetration of pH-independent viruses. Furthermore, they do not affect the formation of endocytic vesicles nor the internalization of most endocytic receptors. Thus, resistance to these reagents does not indicate that penetration occurs at the cell surface.

With pH-dependent enveloped viruses, the site of fusion can be controlled experimentally. Under normal circumstances, fusion occurs in acidic intracellular vesicles, primarily endosomes, following endocytosis from the cell surface. This fusion can be blocked by reagents that neutralize acidic organelles. Fusion can be induced at the plasma membrane by briefly treating cells with bound virus with mildly acidic medium (White et al. 1980). Fusion is very rapid, and the cells can be returned to normal medium after 1 minute without the low-pH treatment having a significant effect on their viability. One can then ask whether virus fused at the cell surface is able to infect the cell. When this experi-

ment is done with SFV in BHK cells, fusion at the cell surface does lead
to productive infection (White et al. 1980; Helenius et al. 1982). However, when the same experiment is performed on Chinese hamster ovary
(CHO) cells, which can be infected through the normal endocytic route,
fusion at the cell surface does not lead to productive infection (Marsh
and Pelchen-Matthews 1992 and unpubl.). Similar results have been obtained with an avian influenza virus (fowl plague virus) or with VSV
fused to Madin Darby canine kidney cells, and with a flavivirus (West
Nile) fused to the surface of the murine macrophage-like cell line
P338D1 (Matlin et al. 1981, 1982; Gollins and Porterfield 1986).

Together, these results indicate that in certain normally permissive
cells, viruses fused at the plasma membrane do not infect the cell.
Presumably, the viral genome does not reach the appropriate replicative
machinery, although the reason for this failure is unclear. One possible
explanation is that the cortical cytoskeleton may present an additional
barrier to infection. Thin-section electron micrographs of, for example,
leukocytes indicate that the cytoplasmic aspect of the plasma membrane
is underlaid by a prominent cortical cytoskeleton (see, e.g., Alberts et al.
1989). This structure is present to a greater or lesser extent in most cells
and can be seen to exclude ribosomes and other cytoplasmic organelles
from the area immediately adjacent to the plasma membrane. Thus,
viruses may encounter more than just the barrier imposed by the limiting
membrane of the cell, and they may use endocytic vesicles, which clearly
have a capacity to cross the cortical layer, to overcome this additional
barrier. Electron micrographs suggest that BHK cells, in which virus fusion at the cell surface is permissive for infection, may be a cell line in
which the cortical cytoskeleton is less well developed and may present a
less effective barrier to virions fused at the cell surface.

In addition to the possible barrier imposed by the cortical cytoskeleton, there are further reasons for believing that the endocytic pathway may play a role in facilitating virus entry. It is clear that different
virus groups make different demands on the cell in terms of the sites and
components that they use to replicate. SFV, for example, uses the 60S
ribosomal RNA to bind the capsid protein and uncoat the viral
nucleocapsid (Singh and Helenius 1992). For influenza viruses, the incoming ribonucleoproteins must be transported into the nucleus. For the
HIVs, the incoming RNA must be reverse-transcribed and the viral DNA
and integrase must be imported into the nucleus. Because HIVs can infect nondividing cells, they must have a capacity to enter the nucleus
without disruption of the nuclear membrane. In general, cells are highly
ordered structures in which the distribution of organelles and molecules
is regulated by their interaction with various elements of the cyto-

skeleton. The endocytic organelles tend to be found in specific locations, with early endosomes primarily distributed in the periphery of the cell and late endosomes and lysosomes found in the perinuclear region. Furthermore, these organelles are shuttled from one site to another by association with motor proteins that interact with components of the cytoskeleton. Thus, the endocytic pathway may provide a route for shuttling viruses or viral components to appropriate cellular locations. SFV, for example, can fuse out of endosomes into a region of the cytoplasm where ribosomes are present and are able to mediate uncoating. Similarly, the movement of influenza or HIVs through the endocytic pathway to the perinuclear region may facilitate delivery of the viral genome to the nucleus. In a more extreme example, the infection of neurons by poliovirus, penetration through the plasma membrane at the neuromuscular junction would put the virions into a location that cannot support protein synthesis, whereas uptake into endocytic vesicles and retrograde transport to the cell body would deliver the virions to sites that can support replication. In fact, neurotropic strains of Sindbis virus show a decreased pH threshold for fusion, which might be an advantage to viruses that need to delay fusion until entering late stages of the endocytic pathway in the cell body (Boggs et al. 1989).

Given the different types of cell-surface molecules used as virus receptors and the differences in the viral fusion and uncoating reactions, comparisons between the efficiencies of entry of pH-dependent and pH-independent viruses are not usually informative. However, in a recent experiment, viruses containing an RSV core, but the envelope glycoproteins of either the pH-independent RSV or the pH-dependent influenza virus, were generated. When the infectivity of these virus preparations was compared, the viruses exhibited similar titers on avian cells, suggesting that both use the same entry pathway. As the HA-coated viruses must use the endocytic pathway, this would imply that the pH-independent RSV-coated particles which productively infect the cell would also use the endocytic pathway (Dong et al. 1992).

HIV ENTRY AND ADDITIONAL ROLES FOR ENDOCYTOSIS
IN VIRAL PATHOGENESIS

Although the role of endocytosis in the productive entry of the HIVs and other pH-independent viruses remains controversial (see, e.g., Maddon et al. 1988; Pauza and Price 1988; Orloff et al. 1991), it is apparent that endocytosis can play a significant role in other aspects of the infection cycle of these viruses. With HIV it is apparent that virus may be transmitted between individuals as both cell-borne and free virions. Although physical trauma may provide direct access across the rectal or vaginal epithelium, or infected cells may have the facility to migrate through the epithelia, it is apparent that M cells can provide a transcytotic route. These specialized epithelial cells overlie lymphoid follicles and provide a continual source of antigens to the antigen-presenting cells (APCs) and lymphocytes that lie beneath. M cells have been demonstrated to transport a number of viral and bacterial pathogens across the gut epithelia in a process that involves the endocytosis of particles from the lumen, transcytosis, and release of the intact particle into the follicle. Significantly, in humans the highest density of M cells is found in the rectal epithelium, and M cells from rabbits and mice have been demonstrated to internalize and transcytose intact HIV-1 particles by a CD4-independent mechanism (Amerongen et al. 1991). Furthermore, it has been demonstrated in tissue-culture systems that HIV-infected cells can deliver infectious virions to epithelial cells in a polarized manner (Bourinbaiar and Phillips 1991). Although it is unclear whether infection of enterocytes occurs in vivo, it seems likely that infected lymphoid cells or macrophages might mediate similar delivery to M cells.

The M-cell-mediated transport of HIV through the epithelium directly delivers the viruses to an environment containing a range of potential target cells, including CD4$^+$ T cells, macrophages, and monocytes. The fact that the virions involved in HIV transmission exhibit macrophage tropisms suggests that follicular monocytic and dendritic cells may be the primary targets for infection by these incoming viruses. Furthermore, the demonstration that monocytic cell lines efficiently endocytose CD4 (Pelchen-Matthews et al. 1991) also suggests that this subpopulation of follicular cells may efficiently sequester incoming virus. Dendritic cells in particular appear to be able to sequester virus that can subsequently be released to infect T cells, although it has not been demonstrated that this sequestration involves endocytosis (Cameron et al. 1992).

The endocytosis and recycling pathways thus may play significant roles in the initial infection of a host by HIV and may also influence the systemic dissemination of these viruses to sites of transmission to CD4$^+$ lymphoid cells in the lymph nodes and thymus (Aldovandi et al. 1993; Bonyhadi et al. 1993; Embretson et al. 1993; Pantaleo et al. 1993).

CONCLUSIONS

The most effective way of preventing virus infection and disease is to prevent the initial entry of virions into their target cells. The analysis of viral receptors and penetration mechanisms have begun to identify means through which this aim might be rationally achieved. One of the major gaps in our understanding of virus entry is the knowledge of the cellular pathways utilized by the pH-independent viruses; we have argued that, although essential for pH-dependent viruses, endocytosis may also facilitate the entry of pH-independent viruses. As yet, we know little of the factors that activate the fusion or penetration reactions of pH-independent viruses, and it is conceivable that these may be components that are associated with endocytic organelles. Thus, if we are to devise strategies to effectively combat viruses such as HIV, it will be essential to understand the mechanisms involved in productive infection. If these reactions are occurring inside the cell rather than at the cell surface, a different set of problems will have to be addressed.

As with many other aspects of their replication, the pH-dependent viruses have left nothing to chance and have evolved a mechanism that exploits the properties of endocytic organelles to maximize their productive entry into cells. We cannot rule out the possibility that pH-independent viruses have similar requirements and have evolved similar, although not identical, entry strategies.

ACKNOWLEDGMENTS

The authors are supported by a grant from the Medical Research Council AIDS Directed Programme. We thank Debbie Wheeler and Dan Cutler for helpful criticism and discussion.

REFERENCES

Alberts, B., D. Bray, J. Lewis, M. Raff, K. Roberts, and J.D. Watson. 1989. *Molecular biology of the cell*, p. 629. Garland Publishing, London.

Aldrovandi, G.M., G. Feuer, L. Gao, B. Jamieson, M. Kristeva, I.S.Y. Chen, and J.A. Zack. 1993. The SCID-hu mouse as a model for HIV-1 infection. *Nature* **363**: 732.

Amerongen, H.M., R. Weltzin, C.M. Farnet, P. Michetti, W.A. Haseltine, and M.R. Neutra. 1991. Transepithelial transport of HIV-1 by intestinal M cells: A mechanism for transmission of AIDS. *J. Acquired Immune Defic. Syndr.* **4**: 760.

Andersen, K.B. 1983. Leupeptin inhibits retrovirus infection in mouse fibroblasts. *J. Virol.* **48**: 765.

Anderson, R.G.W. 1993. Potocytosis of small molecules and ions by caveolae. *Trends Cell Biol.* **3**: 69.

Bamezai, A., V. Goldmacher, H. Reiser, and K.I. Rock. 1989. Internalization of phosphatidylinositol-anchored lymphocyte proteins: I. Documentation and potential significance for T cell stimulation. *J. Immunol.* **143**: 3107.

Ban, J., D. Portetelle, C. Altaner, B. Horion, D. Milan, V. Krchnak, A. Burny, and R. Kettmann. 1993. Isolation and characterisation of a 2.3 kilobase-pair cDNA fragment encoding the binding domain of the bovine leukaemia virus cell receptor. *J. Virol.* **67**: 1050.

Bates, P., J.A.T. Young, and H.E. Varmus. 1993. A receptor for subgroup A Rous sarcoma virus is related to the low density lipoprotein receptor. *Cell* **74:** 1043.

Bergelson, J.M., M.P. Shepley, B.M. Chan, M.E. Hemler, and R.W. Finberg. 1992. Identification of the integrin VLA-2 as a receptor for echovirus 1. *Science* **255:** 1718.

Bernfield, M., R. Kokenyesi, M. Kato, M.T. Hinkes, J. Spring, R.L. Gallo, and E.J. Lose. 1992. Biology of the syndecans: A family of transmembrane heparan sulphate proteoglycans. *Annu. Rev. Cell Biol.* **8:** 365.

Boggs, W.M., C.S. Hahn, E.G. Strauss, J.H. Strauss, and D.E. Griffin. 1989. Low pH-dependent Sindbis virus-induced fusion of BHK cells: Differences between strains correlate with amino acid changes in the E1 glycoprotein. *Virology* **169:** 485.

Bonyhadi, M.L., L. Rabin, S. Salimi, D.A. Brown, J. Kosek, J.M. McCune, and H. Kaneshima. 1993. HIV induces thymus depletion in vivo. *Nature* **363:** 728.

Bourinbaiar, A. S. and D.M. Phillips. 1991. Transmission of human immunodeficiency virus from monocytes to epithelia. *J. Acquired Immune Defic. Syndr.* **4:** 56.

Bretscher, M.S., J.N. Thomson, and B.M.F. Pearse. 1980. Coated pits act as molecular filters. *Proc. Natl. Acad. Sci.* **77:** 4156.

Brown, D.A. and J.K. Rose. 1992. Sorting of GPI-anchored proteins to glycolipid-enriched membrane subdomains during transport to the apical cell-surface. *Cell* **68:** 533.

Cameron, P.U., P.S. Freudenthal, J.M. Barker, S. Gezelter, K. Inaba, and R.M. Steinman. 1992. Dendritic cells exposed to human immunodeficiency virus type-1 transmit a vigorous cytopathic infection to CD4[+] T cells. *Science* **257:** 383.

Cann, A.J., M.J. Churcher, M. Boyd, W. O'Brien, J.Q. Zhao, J. Zack, and I.S. Chen. 1992. The region of the envelope gene of human immunodeficiency virus type 1 responsible for determination of cell tropism. *J. Virol.* **66:** 305.

Carel, J.C., B.L. Myones, B. Frazier, and V.M. Holers. 1990. Structural requirements for C3d,g/Epstein-Barr virus receptor (CR2/CD21) ligand binding internalisation and viral infection. *J. Biol. Chem.* **265:** 12293.

Carpenter, G. and S. Cohen. 1976. ^{125}I-labeled human epidermal growth factor. Binding internalization and degradation in human fibroblasts. *J. Cell Biol.* **71:** 159.

Carr, C.M. and P.S. Kim. 1993. A spring-loaded mechanism for the conformational change of influenza hemagglutinin. *Cell* **73:** 823.

Cirone, M., C. Zompetta, A. Angeloni, D.V. Ablashi, S.Z. Salahuddin, A. Pavan, M.R. Torrisi, L. Frati, and A. Faggioni. 1992. Infection by human herpesvirus 6 (HHV-6) of human lymphoid T cells occurs through an endocytic pathway. *AIDS Res. Hum. Retroviruses* **8:** 2031.

Clague, M.J., S. Urbe, F. Aniento, and J. Gruenberg. 1994. Vacuolar ATPase activity is required for endosomal carrier vesicle formation. *J. Biol. Chem.* **269:** 21.

Cochet, C., O. Kashles, E.M. Chambaz, I. Borrello, C.R. King, and J. Schlessinger. 1988. Demonstration of epidermal growth factor-induced receptor dimerization in living cells using a chemical covalent cross-linking agent. *J. Biol. Chem.* **263:** 3290.

Collins, S., M.G. Caron, and R.J. Lefkowitz. 1992. From ligand binding to gene expression: New insights into the regulation of G-protein-coupled receptors. *Trends Biochem. Sci.* **17:** 37.

Dales, S. 1973. Early events in cell-animal virus interactions. *Bacteriol. Rev.* **37:** 103.

Dietrich, J., X. Hou, A.-M. Wegener, and C. Geisler. 1994. CD3g contains a phosphoserine-dependent di-leucine motif involved in down-regulation of the T cell receptor. *EMBO J.* **13:** 2156.

Donelli, G., F. Superti, A. Tinari, and M.L. Marziano. 1992. Mechanism of astrovirus entry into Graham 293 cells. *J. Med. Virol.* **38:** 271.

Dong, J., M.G. Roth, and E. Hunter. 1992. A chimeric avian retrovirus containing the influenza virus hemagglutinin has an expanded host range. *J. Virol.* **66:** 7374.

Dörig, R.E., A. Marcil, A. Chopra, and C.D. Richardson. 1993. The human CD46 molecule is a receptor for measles virus (Edmonston strain). *Cell* **75:** 295.

Dveksler, G.S., M.N. Pensiero, C.B. Cardellichio, R.K. Williams, G.S. Jiang, K.V. Holmes, and C.W. Dieffenbach. 1991. Cloning of the mouse hepatitis virus (MHV) receptor: Expression in human and hamster cell lines confers susceptibility to MHV. *J. Virol.* **65:** 6881.

Embretson, J., M. Zupancic, J.L. Ribas, A. Burke, P. Racz, K. Tenner-Racz, and A.T. Haase. 1993. Massive covert infection of helper T lymphocytes and macrophages by HIV during the incubation period of AIDS. *Nature* **362:** 359.

Fricks, M.L. and J.M. Hogle. 1990. Cell-induced conformational change in poliovirus: Externalization of the amino terminal of VP1 is responsible for liposome binding. *J. Virol.* **64:** 1934.

Fuller, S., C.-H. von Bonsdorff, and K. Simons. 1985. Cell-surface hemagglutinin can mediate infection by other animal viruses. *EMBO J.* **4:** 2475.

Goldstein, J.L., M.S. Brown, R.G.W. Anderson, and D.W. Russell. 1985. Receptor mediated endocytosis: Concepts emerging from the LDL receptor system. *Annu. Rev. Cell Biol.* **1:** 1.

Gollins, S.W. and J.S. Porterfield. 1986. The uncoating and infectivity of the flavivirus West Nile on interaction with cells: Effects of pH and ammonium chloride. *J. Gen. Virol.* **67:** 1941.

Greber, U.F., M. Willetts, P. Webster, and A. Helenius. 1993. Stepwise dismantling of adenovirus 2 during entry into cells. *Cell* **75:** 477.

Grewe, C., A. Beck, and H.R. Gelderblom. 1990. HIV: Early virus-cell interactions. *J. AIDS.* **3:** 965.

Griffiths, G. and J. Gruenberg. 1991. The arguments for pre-existing early and late endosomes. *Trends Cell Biol.* **1:** 5.

Hammerton, R.W., K.A. Krzeminski, R.W. Mays, R.A. Ryan, D.A. Wollner, and W.J. Nelson. 1991. Mechanisms for regulating cell-surface distribution of Na^+, K^+-ATPase in polarized epithelial cells. *Science* **254:** 847.

Helenius, A. 1984. Semliki Forest virus penetration from endosomes: A morphological study. *Biol. Cell.* **51:** 181.

Helenius, A., M. Marsh, and J. White. 1982. Effect of lysosomotropic weak bases on Semliki Forest virus penetration into host cells. *J. Gen. Virol.* **58:** 47.

Helenius, A., J. Kartenbeck, K. Simons, and E. Fries. 1980. On the entry of Semliki Forest virus into BHK-21 cells. *J. Cell Biol.* **84:** 404.

Hiebsch, R.R., T.J. Raub, and B.W. Wattenberg. 1991. Primaquine blocks transport by inhibiting the formation of functional transport vesicles. Studies in a cell-free assay of protein transport through the Golgi apparatus. *J. Biol. Chem.* **266:** 20323.

Hogle, J. 1993 The viral canyon. *Curr. Biol.* **3:** 278.

Horton, H.M. and J.P. Burand. 1993. Saturable attachment sites for polyhedron-derived baculovirus on insect cells and evidence for entry via direct membrane fusion. *J. Virol.* **67:** 1860.

Jing, S., T. Spencer, K. Miller, C. Hopkins, and I.S. Trowbridge. 1990. Role of the human transferrin receptor cytoplasmic domain in endocytosis: Localization of a specific signal sequence for internalization. *J. Cell Biol.* **110:** 283.

Keller, G.-A., M.W. Siegel, and I.W. Caras. 1992. Endocytosis of glycosphingolipid-anchored and transmembrane forms of CD4 by different endocytic pathways. *EMBO J.* **11:** 863.

Kielian, M. and A. Helenius. 1985. pH-induced alterations in the fusogenic spike protein of Semliki Forest virus. *J. Cell Biol.* **101:** 2284.

Lazarovits, J. and M. Roth. 1988. A single amino acid change in the cytoplasmic domain allows the influenza virus hemagglutinin to be endocytosed through coated pits. *Cell* **53:** 743.

Letourneur, F. and R.D. Klausner. 1992. A novel di-leucine motif and a tyrosine-based motif independently mediate lysosomal targetting and endocytosis of CD3 chains. *Cell* **69:** 1143.

Louvard, D. 1980. Apical membrane aminopeptidase appears at site of cell-cell contact in cultured kidney epithelial cells. *Proc. Natl. Acad. Sci.* **77:** 4132.

Maddon, P. J., A.G. Dalgleish, J.S. McDougal, P.R. Clapham, R.A. Weiss, and R. Axel. 1986. The T4 gene encodes the AIDS virus receptor and is expressed in the immune system and the brain. *Cell* **47:** 333.

Maddon, P.J., J.S. McDougal, P.R. Clapham, A.G. Dalgleish, S. Jamal, R.A. Weiss, and R. Axel. 1988. HIV infection does not require endocytosis of its receptor, CD4. *Cell* **54:** 865.

Marsh, M. and A. Helenius. 1980. Adsorptive endocytosis of Semliki Forest virus. *J. Mol. Biol.* **142:** 439.

―――. 1989. Virus entry into animal cells. *Adv. in Virus Res.* **36:** 107.

Marsh, M. and A. Pelchen-Matthews. 1992. On the role of endocytosis in the entry of animal viruses. *NATO ASI Ser. H Cell Biol.* **62:** 399.

―――. 1993 Animal virus entry into cells. *Rev. Med. Virol.* **3:** 173.

Marsh, M., E. Bolzau, and A. Helenius. 1983. Semliki Forest virus penetration occurs from acid prelysosomal vacuoles. *Cell* **32:** 931.

Martin, K. and A. Helenius. 1991. Transport of incoming influenza virus nucleocapsids into the nucleus. *J. Virol.* **65:** 232.

Matlin, K. S., H. Reggio, A. Helenius, and K. Simons. 1981. Infectious entry pathway of influenza virus in a canine kidney cell line. *J. Cell Biol.* **91:** 601.

―――. 1982. Pathway of vesicular stomatitis virus entry leading to infection. *J. Mol. Biol.* **156:** 609.

McClure, M.O., M. Marsh, and R.A. Weiss. 1988. Human immunodeficiency virus infection of CD4-bearing cells occurs by a pH-independent mechanism. *EMBO J.* **7:** 513.

McClure, M.O., M.A. Sommerfelt, M. Marsh, and R.A. Weiss. 1990. The pH independence of mammalian retrovirus infection. *J. Gen. Virol.* **71:** 767.

Mellman, I., R. Fuchs, and A. Helenius. 1986. Acidification of the endocytic and exocytic pathways. *Annu. Rev. Biochem.* **55:** 663.

Mendelsohn, C.L., E. Wimmer, and V.R. Racaniello. 1989. Cellular receptor for poliovirus: Molecular cloning, nucleotide sequence and expression of a new member of the immunoglobulin superfamily. *Cell* **56:** 855.

Miettinen, H.M., J.K. Rose, and I. Mellman. 1990. Fc receptor isoforms exhibit distinct abilities for coated pit localization as a result of cytoplasmic domain heterogeneity. *Cell* **58:** 317.

Miettinen, H.M., K. Matter, W. Hunziker, J.K. Rose, and I. Mellman. 1992. Fc receptor endocytosis is controlled by a cytoplasmic domain determinant that actively prevents coated pit localization. *J. Cell Biol.* **116:** 875.

Moore, J.P. and P.L. Nara. 1992. The role of the V3 loop of gp120 in HIV infection. *AIDS.* **6:** S21.

Naniche, D., G. Varior-Krishnan, F. Cervoni, T.F. Wild, B. Rossi, C. Rabourdin-Combe, and D. Gerlier. 1993. Human membrane cofactor protein (CD46) acts as a cellular receptor for measles virus. *J. Virol.* **67:** 6025.

Orloff, G.M., S.L. Orloff, M.S. Kennedy, P.J. Maddon, and J.S. McDougal. 1991. Penetration of CD4 T cells by HIV-1. The CD4 receptor does not internalize with HIV, and CD4-related signal transduction events are not required for entry. *J. Immunol.* **146:** 2578.

Pantaleo, G., C. Graziosi, J.F. Demarest, L. Butini, M. Montroni, C.H. Fox, J.M. Orenstein, D.P. Kotler, and A.S. Fauci. 1993. HIV infection is active and progressive in lymphoid tissue during the clinically latent stage of disease. *Nature* **362:** 355.

Patterson, S., J.S. Oxford, and R.R. Doourmashkin. 1979. Studies on the mechanism of influenza virus entry into cells. *J. Gen. Virol.* **43:** 223.

Pauza, C.D. and T.M. Price. 1988. Human immunodeficiency virus infection of T cells and monocytes proceeds via receptor-mediated endocytosis. *J. Cell Biol.* **107:** 959.

Pelchen-Matthews, A., J.E. Armes, and M. Marsh. 1989. Internalization and recycling of CD4 transfected into HeLa and NIH-3T3 cells. *EMBO J.* **8:** 3641.

Pelchen-Matthews, A., I.J. Parsons, and M. Marsh. 1993. Phorbol ester-induced down-regulation of CD4 is a multi-step process involving dissociation from p56^{lck}, increased association with clathrin-coated pits and altered endosomal sorting. *J. Exp. Med.* **178:** 1209.

Pelchen-Matthews, A., I. Boulet, D. Littman, R. Fagard, and M. Marsh. 1992. The protein tyrosine kinase p56^{lck} inhibits CD4 endocytosis by preventing entry of CD4 into coated pits. *J. Cell Biol.* **117:** 279.

Pelchen-Matthews, A., J.E. Armes, G. Griffiths, and M. Marsh. 1991. Differential endocytosis of CD4 in lymphocytic and non-lymphocytic cells. *J. Exp. Med.* **173:** 575.

Pinto, L.H., L.J. Holsinger, and R.A. Lamb. 1992. Influenza virus M$_2$ protein has ion channel activity. *Cell* **69:** 517.

Piper, R.C., C. Tai, P. Kulesza, S. Pang, D. Warnock, J. Baenziger, J.W. Slot, H.J. Geuze, C. Puri, and D.E. James. 1993. GLUT-4 NH$_2$ terminus contains a phenylalanine-based targetting motif that regulates intracellular sequestration. *J. Cell Biol.* **121:** 1221.

Reid, P.A. and C. Watts. 1990. Cycling of cell-surface MHC glycoproteins through primaquine-sensitive intracellular compartments. *Nature* **346:** 655.

Robinson, M. 1992. Adaptins. *Trends Cell Biol.* **2:** 293.

Robinson, P.J. 1991. Phosphatidyl inositol membrane anchors and T-cell activation. *Immunol. Today* **12:** 35.

Sandvig, K., S. Olsnes, J.E. Brown, O.W. Peterson, and B. van Deurs. 1989. Endocytosis from coated pits of Shiga toxin: A glycolipid-binding protein from *Shigella dysenteriae*. *J. Cell Biol.* **108:** 1331.

Schmid, S.L. 1992. The mechanism of receptor-mediated endocytosis: More questions than answers. *BioEssays* **14:** 589.

Sinangil, F., A. Loyter, and D.J. Volsky. 1988. Quantitative measurement of fusion between human immunodeficiency virus and cultured cells using membrane fluorescence dequenching. *FEBS Letters* **239:** 88.

Singh, I. and A. Helenius. 1992. Role of ribosomes in Semliki Forest virus nucleocapsid uncoating. *J. Virol.* **66:** 7049.

Staunton, D.E., V.J. Merluzzi, R. Rothlein, R. Barton, S.D. Marlin, and T.A. Springer. 1989. A cell adhesion molecule, ICAM-1, is the major surface receptor for rhinovirus. *Cell* **56:** 849.

Stegmann, T., J.M. White, and A. Helenius. 1990. Intermediates in influenza induced membrane fusion. *EMBO J.* **9:** 4231.

Stein, B.S., S.D. Gowda, J.D. Lifson, R.C. Penhallow, K.G. Bensch, and E.G. Engleman. 1987. pH-independent HIV entry into CD4-positive cells via virus envelope fusion to the plasma membrane. *Cell* **49:** 659.

Trowbridge, I.S., J.F. Collawn, and C.R. Hopkins. 1993. Signal-dependent membrane protein trafficking in the endocytic pathway. *Annu. Rev. Cell Biol.* **9:** 129.

Ukkonen, P., V. Lewis, M. Marsh, A. Helenius, and I. Mellman. 1986. Transport of macrophage Fc receptors and Fc receptor-bound ligands to lysosomes. *J. Exp. Med.* **163:** 952.

van den Bosch, R., A.P.M. du Maine, H.J. Geuze, A. van der Ende, and G.J. Strous. 1988. Recycling of 5′-nucleotidase in a rat hepatoma cell line. *EMBO J.* **7:** 3345.

van Deurs, B., O.W. Petersen, S. Olsnes, and K. Sandvig. 1989. The ways of endocytosis. *Int. Rev. Cytol.* **117:** 131.

Varga, M.J., C. Weibull, and E. Everitt. 1991. Infectious entry pathway of adenovirus type 2. *J. Virol.* **65:** 6061.

Vaux, D. 1992. The structure of an endocytosis signal. *Trends Cell Biol.* **2:** 189.

Wahlberg, J.M., R. Bron, J. Wischut, and H. Garoff. 1992. Membrane fusion of Semliki Forest virus involves homotrimers of the fusion protein. *J. Virol.* **66:** 7309.

Wang, K.S., R.J. Kuhn, E.G. Strauss, and J.H. Strauss. 1992. High-affinity laminin receptor is a receptor for Sindbis virus in mammalian cells. *J. Virol.* **66:** 4992.

Watts, C. and M. Marsh. 1992. Endocytosis: What goes in and how? *J. Cell Sci.* **103:** 1.

White, J.M. and A. Helenius. 1980. pH dependent fusion between the Semliki Forest virus membrane and liposomes. *Proc. Natl. Acad. Sci.* **77:** 3273.

White, J.M., J. Kartenbeck, and A. Helenius. 1980. Fusion of Semliki Forest virus with the plasma membrane can be induced by low pH. *J. Cell Biol.* **87:** 264.

White, J., M. Kielian, and A. Helenius. 1983. Membrane fusion proteins of enveloped viruses. *Q. Rev. Biophys.* **16:** 151.

Wickham, T.J., P. Mathias, D.A. Cheresh, and G.R. Nemerow. 1993. Integrins $\alpha_v\beta_3$ and $\alpha_v\beta_5$ promote adenovirus internalization but not virus attachment. *Cell* **73:** 309.

Vlasak, R., W. Luytjes, W. Spaan, and P. Palese. 1988. Human and bovine coronaviruses recognize sialic acid-containing receptors similar to those of influenza C viruses. *Proc. Natl. Acad. Sci.* **85:** 4526.

14

Activation Cleavage of Viral Spike Proteins by Host Proteases

Hans-Dieter Klenk and Wolfgang Garten
Institut für Virologie
Philipps-Universität Marburg
35037 Marburg, Germany

Endoproteolytic cleavage, usually at arginine residues, is a common posttranslational modification of membrane and secretory proteins on the exocytotic transport route. Such proteins include precursors of peptide hormones, neuropeptides, growth factors, coagulation factors, serum albumin, cell-surface receptors, and adhesion molecules. All of these proteins play important roles in a large variety of different biological processes, and these functions depend on proteolytic cleavage of the proteins (for review, see Barr 1991). The same type of processing has also been observed with many viral membrane proteins (Fig. 1) and, in some instances, proved to be a crucial factor in determining organ and host tropism, spread of infection, and pathogenicity of these viruses.

VIRUSES WITH SPIKE PROTEINS UNDERGOING POSTTRANSLATIONAL PROTEOLYTIC CLEAVAGE

Paramyxoviridae

The concept that proteolytic activation of a viral glycoprotein is an important factor in virus replication was first established with the fusion (F) protein of Sendai virus (Homma and Ohuchi 1973; Scheid and Choppin 1974). Cleavage of this protein results in the exposition of a highly conserved hydrophobic sequence at the amino terminus of the F1 fragment (Fig. 1) (Gething et al. 1978; Scheid et al. 1978) which induces fusion of the viral envelope with the plasma membrane of the target cell, thereby allowing entry of the viral genome into the cytoplasm. Cleavage of F is therefore necessary for virus infectivity. Evidence from various biochemical and biophysical data indicates that the membrane fusion characteristic of paramyxoviruses is driven by a hydrophobic interaction of the F1 amino terminus with the lipid bilayer of the target membrane (for references, see Nagai et al. 1989).

Preceding the fusion-inducing hydrophobic sequence there is a

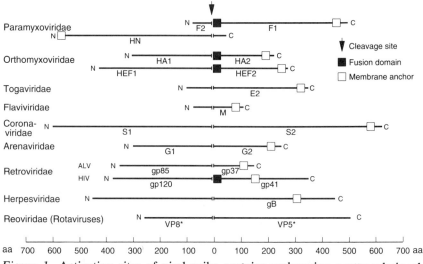

Figure 1 Activation sites of viral spike proteins undergoing posttranslational proteolytic cleavage.

teolytic cleavage signal. With Sendai virus and the apathogenic New-castle disease virus (NDV) strains, it consists of a single basic residue, occasionally with another isolated arginine or lysine residue in position −4 (Table 1). The F proteins of all other paramyxoviruses have a multi-basic cleavage site with as many as six arginine and lysine residues in a row (Table 2). Precursor proteins with multibasic cleavage sites are efficiently cleaved in many cells of various origin, whereas precursors containing a single basic residue at the cleavage site can be cleaved only in a few types of cells, such as the allantoic cells of the chick embryo. Since cleavage of F is not necessary for virus maturation, in the latter case many host cells produce particles with uncleaved F_0 that can be activated in vitro with trypsin or other suitable proteases (for review, see Rott and Klenk 1988; Nagai et al. 1989). If the F_0 protein has a multibasic activation site, cleavage occurs in the *trans* Golgi membranes, or in a cell compartment occupied by the proteins quite soon after their transit through the *trans* Golgi membranes (Nagai et al. 1976b; Morrison et al. 1985; Yoshida et al. 1986). In contrast, the available evidence indicates that F proteins with a single arginine at the cleavage site are activated after arrival at the cell surface (Gotoh et al. 1990). Studies on cleavage site variants of the F protein of Simian virus 5 (SV5) obtained by site-directed mutagenesis indicated that the number of basic residues is critical for high cleavability (Paterson et al. 1989), and comparison of all data available to date shows that the consensus sequence R-X-K/R-R is required (Table 2). The differential sensitivity of the F_0 precursor to

Table 1 Monobasic cleavage sites of viral glycoproteins with restricted cleavability

Virus	Glycoprotein	Cleavage site	Reference
Orthomyxoviridae			
A/WSN/33 (H1)	HA	PSIQYR GL	Hiti et al. (1981)
A/Japan/305/57 (H2)	HA	PQIESR GL	Gething et al. (1980)
A/Memphis/102/72 (H3)	HA	PEKQTR GL	Sleigh et al. (1979)
A/seal/Mass/133/82 (H4)	HA	PEKATR GL	Donis et al. (1989)
A/seal/Mass/1/80 (H7)	HA	ENPKTR GL	Naeve and Webster (1983)
A/chick/Germany/49 (H10)	HA	EVVQGR GL	Feldmann et al. (1988)
A/gull/Maryland/704/77 (H13)	HA	PAISNR GL	Chambers et al. (1989)
A/mallard/Gurjev/263/82 (H14)	HA	PGKQAK GL	Kawaoka et al. (1990)
B/Lee/40	HA	KLLKER GF	Krystal et al. (1982)
C/JHB/1/66	HEF	TKPKSR IF	Pfeifer and Compans (1984)
Paramyxoviridae			
Sendai Virus	F	GAPQSR FF	Hidaka et al. (1984)
NDV La Sota	F	GGRQSR LI	Pritzer et al. (1990)
NDV Ulster	F	GGKQSR LI	Toyoda et al. (1987)

proteolytic cleavage is of primary importance for the virulence of NDV, as discussed below.

Paramyxoviridae have a second glycoprotein spike that contains both hemagglutinin (H) and neuraminidase (N) activities with the members of the paramyxovirus genus (Scheid et al. 1972). The HN glycoprotein has a single hydrophobic domain that serves as signal sequence as well as membrane anchor (Fig. 1). Proteolytic processing of this glycoprotein has been observed with some avirulent NDV strains (Nagai et al. 1976a; 1980; Nagai and Klenk 1977). Resulting from a shifted stop codon (Nagai et al. 1989), there is a larger precursor HN_0 with these viruses that is converted into biologically active HN by removal of a small carboxy-terminal glycopeptide (Garten et al. 1980; Schuy et al. 1984). This cleavage is accomplished not only by arginine-specific enzymes, but also by various other proteases of different specificities (Nagai and Klenk 1977). However, the cleavage activation site has not been identified on the amino acid sequence.

Orthomyxoviridae

The hemagglutinin of influenza A and B viruses is composed of the subunits HA1 and HA2 that are derived by proteolytic cleavage from the

Table 2 The consensus sequence R-X-K/R-R at the multibasic cleavage sites of viral glycoproteins with high cleavability

Virus	Glycoprotein	Cleavage site	Reference
Orthomyxoviridae			
A/FPV/Rostock/34 (H7)	HA	KKREKR GL	Porter et al. (1979)
A/FPV/Rostock/34 (H7)	HA	KKRKKR GL	Garten et al. (1985)
A/FPV/Dutch/27 (H7)	HA	KKRRKR GL	Munk et al. (1992)
A/Tern/SA/61 (H5)	HA	TRRQKR GL	Kawaoka et al. (1987)
Paramyxoviridae			
NDV (Miyadera)	F	GRRQRR FI	Toyoda et al. (1987)
parainfluenza virus	F	DPRTKR FF	Spriggs et al. (1986)
parainfluenza virus	F	KTRQKR FA	Hu et al. (1990)
mumps virus	F	SRRHKR FA	Waxham et al. (1987)
measles virus	F	SRRHKR FA	Richardson et al. (1986)
simian virus 5	F	TRRRRR FA	Paterson et al. (1984)
canine distemper virus	F	GRRQRR FA	Barrett et al. (1987)
rinderpest virus	F	SRRHKR FA	Tsukiyama et al. (1988)
respiratory-syncytial virus	F	KKRKRR FL	Collins et al. (1984)
rhinotracheitis virus	F	SPRRRR FV	Yu et al. (1991)
Flaviviridae			
yellow fever virus	M	SGRSRR SV	Rice et al. (1985)
west Nile virus	M	SRRSRR SL	Castle et al. (1985)
Kunjin virus	M	SRRSRR SL	Coia et al. (1988)
Japan B encephalitis virus	M	SKRSRR SV	Sumiyoshi et al. (1986)
Togaviridae			
Sindbis virus	E2	SGRSKR SV	Rice and Strauss (1981)
Semliki forest virus	E2	GTRHRR TV	Jain et al. (1991)
Coronaviridae			
infectious bronchitis virus	E2	TRRFRR SI	Cavanagh et al. (1986)
mouse hepatitis virus JHM	E2	SRRARR SV	Schmidt et al. (1987)
Toroviridae			
Berne-virus	P	TRRRRR AV	Snijder et al. (1990)
Retroviridae			
HIV-1	env	VQREKR AV	McCune et al. (1988)
Rous sarcoma virus	env	GIRRKR SV	Schwartz et al. (1983)
feline leukemia virus	env	AARFRR EP	Wünsch et al. (1983)
Friend leukemia virus	env	SYRHKR EP	Koch et al. (1983)
visna virus	env	LQRKKR GI	Sonigo et al. (1985)
mouse mammary tumor virus	env	LIRAKR FV	Perez and Hunter (1987)
bovine leukemia virus	env	PTRVRR SP	Perez and Hunter (1987)
Herpesviridae			
human cytomegalovirus	gB	THRTRR ST	Spaete et al. (1988)
pseudorabies virus	gB	ARRARR SP	Robbins et al. (1987)
varicella zoster virus	gB	NTRSRR SV	Keller et al. (1986)
Marek disease virus	gB	LSRLRR DI	Ross et al. (1989)
Epstein-Barr virus	gB	LRRRRR DA	Pellett et al. (1985a)
equine herpes virus	gB	TTRRRR SL	Whalley et al. (1989)

precursor HA (Fig. 1) (Lazarowitz et al. 1971). The hemagglutinin has two different functions in the initiation of infection. It is responsible for the attachment of the virus to neuraminic-acid-containing receptors at the cell surface and is involved in penetration by triggering fusion of the viral envelope with cellular membranes. The first indication that the hemagglutinin possesses a function in addition to adsorption came from the observation that cleavage of the precursor HA, although irrelevant for adsorption, is necessary for infectivity (Klenk et al. 1975; Lazarowitz and Choppin 1975). Subsequently it has been shown that cleavage is necessary for the fusion capacity (Huang et al. 1981). The amino terminus of HA_2 that is created in the cleavage reaction has attracted special attention as the crucial site for this activity. It is hydrophobic, highly conserved among the hemagglutinin subtypes, and shows structural similarity with the amino terminus of another fusion factor, the F1 polypeptide of paramyxoviruses (Gething et al. 1978; Scheid et al. 1978). The fusion capacity of the hemagglutinin is expressed only at low pH (Maeda and Ohnishi 1980; Huang et al. 1981) which has led to the concept that entry of the virus involves receptor-mediated endocytosis (White et al. 1981), and it has been shown that under these conditions the molecule undergoes a conformational change allowing exposure of the hydrophobic amino terminus of HA_2 (Skehel et al. 1982). It is reasonable to assume that the amino terminus of HA_2 is exposed in such a way that it can insert into the target membrane, thereby forming a bridge between the two membranes. However, other models have also been proposed, and despite extensive studies in this field (for review, see White 1992), important details of the fusion mechanism are still not fully understood.

As is the case with paramyxovirus F protein, monobasic (Table 1) and multibasic (Table 2) cleavage sites are found with influenza virus hemagglutinins. These and several other quite well understood structural differences also account for differences in cleavability and are important determinants for virus pathogenicity, as shown below. Whereas monobasic cleavage sites usually consist of an arginine, the H14 hemagglutinin (Kawaoka et al. 1990) and some human H1 isolates (Günther et al. 1993) have a lysine in this position. The lysine site differs from the arginine site in its protease sensitivity, but the biological significance of this difference is not known (Günther et al. 1993). Finally, again like paramyxovirus F proteins, hemagglutinin with a multibasic cleavage site, such as the one of fowl plague virus (FPV), is cleaved on the exocytotic transport route before it reaches the cell surface (Klenk et al. 1974), whereas hemagglutinin with a monobasic cleavage site is activated on virus particles either in the extracellular space or at the stage of virus entry (see below).

The single glycoprotein of influenza C virus HEF, which has the functions of a hemagglutinin, a fusion protein, and a 9-0-acetyl neuraminate esterase, undergoes proteolytic cleavage into the subunits

HEF_1 and HEF_2 (Fig. 1) (Herrler and Klenk 1991). In contrast to hemagglutinating and esterase activities, fusion activity requires cleavage (Kitame et al. 1982; Ohuchi et al. 1982). The cleavage site consists of a single arginine and is susceptible to proteases present in only a limited number of host cells.

Togaviridae

Togaviruses contain two glycoproteins, designated E1 and E2. They are arranged such that three heterodimers form a trimer spike. E2 is derived from a precursor PE2 (Fig. 1) by proteolytic cleavage at a multibasic cleavage motif (Table 2) (Simons and Garoff 1980). Cleavage has been shown to occur in Golgi vesicles (Hakimi and Atkinson 1982) and in the *trans* Golgi network (de Curtis and Simons 1989; Watson and Moehring 1991). The PE2 (E2) subunit of the spike plays a major role in virus assembly. Proteolytic cleavage appears not to be essential for this function (Presley et al. 1991). E1, on the other hand, promotes receptor binding and fusion and is thus the major component responsible for virus entry (for references, see Salminen et al. 1992). Fusion occurs only at low pH, which is thought to be necessary for loosening the heterodimeric interactions of E1 (Wahlberg et al. 1989; Lobigs et al. 1990b). Studies with cleavage-deficient PE2 obtained by site-directed mutagenesis of subgenomic or complete Semliki forest virus cDNA have shown that release of the heterodimeric bonds depends on cleavage of PE2. Processing of PE2 therefore regulates the entry functions of the E1 subunit by controlling the heterodimer stability under acidic conditions (Lobigs and Garoff 1990; Lobigs et al. 1990a; Salminen et al. 1992).

Flaviviridae

Flaviviruses contain two envelope proteins, E and M. The latter has a precursor glycoprotein, prM, from which a glycopeptide is removed by posttranslational cleavage, leaving the unglycosylated M protein in the envelope (Fig. 1). Cleavage occurs at a multibasic cleavage site (Table 2), presumably in the Golgi apparatus. Little is known about the biological function of M and the role of proteolytic cleavage (Schlesinger and Schlesinger 1990).

Coronaviridae

The peplomers or spikes of the coronavirus envelope consist of the glycoprotein S, which is synthesized as a 200-kD protein. With some coronaviruses, such as infectious bronchitis virus (IBV) and mouse hepatitis virus (MHV) (strain JHM) (Table 2), E2 is cleaved at the multibasic motif R-X-R-R into the amino-terminal fragment S1 and the carboxy-terminal fragment S2 (Fig. 1). MHV A59 has the sequence R-A-H-R at the cleavage site (Luytjes et al. 1987). Cleavage occurs in the Golgi apparatus or at the plasma membrane (Frana et al. 1985; Deregt et al. 1987; Luyties et al. 1987). With the coronaviruses transmissible gastro-enteritis virus (TGEV) and feline infectious peritonitis virus (FIPV), the multibasic site R-X-R-R has been replaced by the sequence R-T-R-G (Rasschaert and Laude 1987). Cleavage of these glycoproteins has so far not been observed, although the R-T-R motif with its isolated arginine residues may allow restricted cleavage in some host systems. E2 has receptor-binding function (Boyle et al. 1987; Schultze et al. 1991) and induces cell fusion at neutral pH, suggesting that penetration occurs at the plasma membrane (Collins et al. 1982; Sturman et al. 1985). Cleavage has been found to stimulate fusion activity and infectivity of MHV A59 (Sturman et al. 1985) and bovine coronavirus (BCV) (Storz et al. 1981). Thus, it appears that cleavage is necessary for the full biological activity of the S protein of MHV A59. However, fusion of the S protein of the JHM strain of MHV does not depend on cleavage (Stauber et al. 1993). With other coronaviruses (FIPV and TGEV) a strict correlation between cleavage of S and fusion has not been observed, either.

Arenaviridae

The arenavirus genome codes for one glycoprotein GPC from which the fragments G1 and G2 are derived by posttranslational proteolytic cleavage. Although the amino terminus of G2 created by the cleavage reaction is hydrophobic, it is not known if cleavage is necessary for a fusion function. The proteolytic cleavage site of the GPC protein of lymphocytic choriomeningitis (LCM) virus has been localized to a 9-amino-acid stretch corresponding to positions 263–271 (Buchmeier et al. 1987). This region contains a dibasic sequence, which is R-R in Lassa virus (Clegg and Lloyd 1983) and R-K in Pichinde virus (Harnish et al. 1983). The observation that cleavage occurred in BHK and Vero cells is puzzling, because there is so far no direct evidence that these cells contain proteases recognizing such cleavage sites (see below). One possible explanation is that these glycoproteins were cleaved by plasmin or another serum protease that may cleave at such sites (see below). The glycoprotein of Tacaribe virus has the sequence R-T at the putative cleavage site, but so far there is no clear evidence that cleavage occurs with this virus (Franze-Fernandez et al. 1987).

Retroviridae

With retroviruses, receptor binding and fusion are exerted by the single envelope glycoprotein. A common feature of all retrovirus glycoproteins, which otherwise show large variations in structure, is proteolytic cleavage of a precursor into an amino-terminal fragment and a carboxy-terminal fragment that form the ectodomain and the transmembrane protein in the mature spike, respectively (Fig. 1). The cleavage site is rich in arginine and lysine and usually has the consensus sequence R-X-K/R-R (Table 2). An exception is human immunodeficiency virus type 2 (HIV-2) gp, which has the sequence R-H-T-R at the cleavage site (Freed and Myers 1992). The transmembrane proteins of some retroviruses, such as HIV, have a hydrophobic domain at the amino terminus that has been shown to be responsible for fusion (Kowalski et al. 1987; Freed and Myers 1992), but hydrophobicity of this region is not a general property of all retroviruses, and there are sequences distant from the cleavage site, such as the V3 loop of HIV-1 (Freed and Myers 1992), that may also be involved in fusion. Nevertheless, cleavage appears to be generally necessary for fusion and, thus, for virus infectivity. This could be shown in studies in which the consensus sequence at the cleavage site had been altered by site-directed mutagenesis. Such mutants were no longer susceptible to cleavage activation by endogenous cellular enzymes. However, some of the mutants could have been cleaved by exogenous proteases, such as chymotrypsin and trypsin, and then have regained activity (McCune et al. 1988; Dong et al. 1992). Furthermore, studies with specific protease inhibitors clearly demonstrated that glycoprotein cleavage was necessary for fusion ability and infectivity of HIV-1 (Hallenberger et al. 1992). Although there have been reports that cleavage may be necessary for surface transport of the Env glycoprotein (Guo et al. 1990), evidence is increasing that this is probably not the case (Perez and Hunter 1987; Willey et al. 1991; Hallenberger et al. 1992). Upstream of the cleavage site, the envelope glycoprotein of HIV-1 has a second site consisting of several arginine and lysine residues, but not showing the correct consensus sequence. Cleavage at this position, which has been observed with a minor fraction of the gp160 molecules, does not result in activation (Fenouillet and Gluckman 1992). Several studies using sensitivity to endo H and other glycosidases as markers have addressed the question at which transport stage proteolytic cleavage occurs. Some suggested that it took place relatively early, e.g., in a distal Golgi compartment (Ulmer and Palade 1991). In most cases, however, cleavage has been localized in the *trans* Golgi area (Tsai and Oroszlan 1988; Merkle et al. 1991; Bedgood and Stallcup 1992). That a relatively large proportion of the HIV-1 glycoprotein is often found uncleaved in cells appears to be due to retention in the endoplasmic reticulum as a result of incorrect folding (Willey et al. 1988; Owens and Compans 1989).

Herpesviridae

Among the better-characterized glycoproteins of the herpesvirus envelope is the gB protein that is encoded by a gene conserved with all subgroups. With human cytomegalovirus (HCMV), the primary translation product of this gene is a precursor glycoprotein about 900 amino acids long that is posttranslationally cleaved into an amino-terminal 90–116-kD fragment and a carboxy-terminal 55-kD fragment, usually designated gB (Fig. 1). Both fragments are present in the virion, linked to each other by disulfide bonds (Meyer et al. 1990). Inhibitor studies employing the ionophores A23187 and monensin indicated that cleavage is calcium-dependent and occurs in *trans* Golgi compartments (Spaete et al. 1990). When transport into this compartment was blocked by glycosylation inhibitors, cleavage did not occur (Radsak et al. 1990). The cleavage site of HCMV gB has the sequence R-T-K-R, and site-directed mutagenesis has shown that the motif R-X-K/R-R- is necessary for cleavage (Spaete et al. 1990). The processing of HCMV gB is reminiscent of the processing observed with the gB homolog of varicella zoster virus (VZV), which also displays this consensus sequence (Keller et al. 1986). In contrast, Epstein-Barr virus (EBV) has the sequence V-L-R-R (Cranage et al. 1986), whereas herpes simplex virus (HSV) has no basic acids at all in this position (Pellett et al. 1985b), and proteolytic cleavage of the gB homologs of these viruses has not been observed. HSV gB has been implicated in the attachment of the virus to the cell surface (WuDann and Spear 1989), but evidence for such a function has not been obtained with other viruses. A study employing protease inhibition indicated that cleavage was not necessary for surface transport of gB and for infectivity of HCMV (Brücher et al. 1990). Thus, the biological function of gB and the role of proteolytic cleavage in herpes virus replication remain to be elucidated.

Reoviridae

Rotaviruses have an outer capsid protein, VP4, that is a hemagglutinin. Although a minor component of the virus, VP4 is an important determinant of virulence and growth in cell culture, and it is an important neutralizing antigen. Rotaviruses do not have a lipid envelope, but the available evidence indicates that they utilize the exocytotic transport machinery for maturation. Furthermore, maturation involves proteolytic cleavage of VP4 into the amino-terminal cleavage product VP8* and the carboxy-terminal cleavage product VP5* (Fig. 1), and this cleavage event greatly enhances infectivity in vitro. Cleavage occurs presumably by host-cell proteases at an arginine-containing cleavage site. This site shows considerable amino acid variation, which appears to influence rotavirus virulence in much the same manner as is known to occur with influenza virus and some paramyxoviruses (for review, see Both et al. 1994).

PROTEOLYTIC CLEAVAGE AS A DETERMINANT FOR SPREAD OF INFECTION AND PATHOGENESIS

Cleavage Activation by Host Proteases as Pathogenicity Determinant of Paramyxoviruses

The concept that cleavage activation is an important determinant for virus pathogenicity was first established with NDV, of which a large number of strains widely varying in virulence are available. As has been pointed out above, the F proteins of the virulent and the avirulent NDV strains differ in the structure of the cleavage site. The avirulent strains have two isolated arginines in this position (Table 1), whereas virulent strains have two pairs of basic amino acids separated by a non-basic amino acid (Table 2). These structural differences account for differences in cleavability. The F proteins of the virulent strains are cleaved in almost all host cells analyzed by a ubiquitous protease whose nature is described below. Thus, all host cells produce infectious virus with activated F protein, allowing rapid spread of infection. The F proteins of the avirulent strains, in contrast, are activated by proteases present only in a few host systems. In most cells, infection therefore does not spread beyond the first round of replication (Nagai et al. 1976a). The least virulent strains also have an HN protein that has to be activated from the precursor HN_0. When HN_0 is not cleaved, as is again the case in most cells, the virus is unable even to attach to cell receptors. Moreover, the masking of neuraminidase activity in HN_0 may result in less efficient virus elution from the host cell, which also would interfere with spread of infection (Nagai and Klenk 1977).

The concept of this relatively simple mechanism of pathogenicity was verified by experiments in an intact organism, the chicken embryo (Nagai et al. 1979). After infection of the chorioallantoic membrane, the glycoproteins of the velogenic strains were activated in each germinal layer of this membrane, regardless of the route of infection, whereas the glycoproteins of the lentogenic viruses were cleaved only in the endodermal cells. Accordingly, there were differences between velogenic and lentogenic strains in their spread through the membrane. Multiplication of nonpathogenic viruses was restricted to the cell layer that was inoculated. Spread of newly synthesized virus was inhibited as soon as the virus reached the barrier of nonpermissive cells. On the other hand, the pathogenic virus spread through the whole membrane and gained entrance into the blood vessels, and the embryo died.

The data, taken together, underline the important role of proteolytic activation of the glycoproteins in pathogenicity. Spread of the lentogenic strains of NDV in the organism is inhibited as soon as the virus infects cells which are unable to activate the glycoprotein. The result is a local infection, which usually does not result in the manifestation of an overt disease. On the other hand, cleavability of the F glycoprotein in a wide spectrum of different cells, as is the case with the velogenic strains, permits rapid production of infectious virus in all organs to high amounts. This allows spread of the virus throughout the organism and results in fatal systemic infection.

Proteolytic cleavage of the fusion glycoprotein has also been found to be a primary determinant for organ tropism and pathogenicity of Sendai virus in mice (Tashiro and Homma 1983a,b; Mochizuki et al. 1988; Tashiro et al. 1988a,b, 1990a, 1991). After intranasal inoculation, wild-type Sendai virus undergoes multiple cycles of replication in mouse lungs, owing to the F protein of progeny virus that is activated at the Ser-Arg cleavage site (Table 1) by a tissue-specific endoprotease. When mouse organs other than the lung are infected by wild-type virus, infection terminates after one cycle of replication because an appropriate protease is lacking (Tashiro et al. 1990a, 1991). Wild-type Sendai virus is therefore strictly pneumotropic in mice. On the other hand, a protease activation mutant, F1-R, has been isolated that has an F protein cleavable by ubiquitous host proteases and is thus able to undergo multiple replication cycles in several cell lines and in various mouse organs. F1-R therefore causes systemic infection in mice following intranasal inoculation (Tashiro et al. 1988b, 1989). Comparative sequence analysis of wild-type virus, mutant F1-R, and a number of revertants revealed that the high cleavability of the F protein of F1-R could be attributed to the exchange of serine at position -1 by proline (Tashiro et al. 1988b, 1991; Middleton et al. 1990). This mutant differs therefore from most other highly cleavable glycoproteins by not possessing a multibasic cleavage site. Although polarity of virus budding was also found to be important for pathogenicity in this system (Tashiro et al. 1990 a,b; 1991, 1992a), these studies demonstrate clearly that organ tropism and pathogenicity of Sendai virus in mice are primarily determined by the distribution of appropriate activating proteases in mouse organs and the cleavability of the F protein by these proteases.

Cleavage Activation by Host Proteases as a Pathogenicity Determinant of Influenza Viruses

As has been observed with NDV, proteolytic activation proved also to be a prime determinant for the pathogenicity of influenza viruses. The mammalian and the apathogenic avian influenza virus strains have hemagglutinins that are cleaved only in a restricted number of cell types. These viruses therefore cause local infection. On the other hand, the pathogenic avian strains have hemagglutinins activated in a broad range of different host cells and, thus, cause systemic infection. There are several structural properties of the hemagglutinin that determine the differential cleavability, but the prime determinant appears to be the structure linking the cleavage products HA1 and HA2 in the uncleaved precursor HA. With hemagglutinins of restricted cleavability, the linker consists usually of a single arginine, whereas highly cleavable hemagglutinins have mostly multiple basic residues in this position (Fig. 2). This concept was first derived from comparisons of naturally occurring strains (Bosch et al. 1981; Garten et al. 1981; Klenk and Rott 1988) and was later further corroborated, when acquisition of high cleavability parallelled by an increase in the number of basic residues at the cleavage site was observed in studies on hemagglutinin mutants generated by site-directed mutagenesis (Kawaoka and Webster 1988) or on virus mutants adapted in vitro to new host cells (Li et al. 1990). Although derived from a wild-type virus of mammalian origin, the mutants analyzed in the latter study became pathogenic for chickens. Thus, the change in cleavability made the virus highly virulent for a new host.

To see whether the basic amino acids have to be present in a specific consensus sequence, further studies employing site-directed mutagenesis have been performed. They showed clearly that the motif R-X-K/R-R upstream of the cleavage site is required for high cleavability (Vey et al. 1992). This consensus sequence is found with the hemagglutinins of all H7 and most H5 strains with a multibasic cleavage site. The only exception to these rules is the H5 hemagglutinin of the strain A/chick/Pennsylvania/83, which contains the unusual tetrapeptide K-K-K-R (Kawaoka and Webster 1989). However, it is not yet clear whether such a motif is recognized by the same endoprotease activating all the other highly cleavable H5 and H7 hemagglutinins or whether it is the particular structure of this H5 hemagglutinin that allows cleavage by another widespread protease.

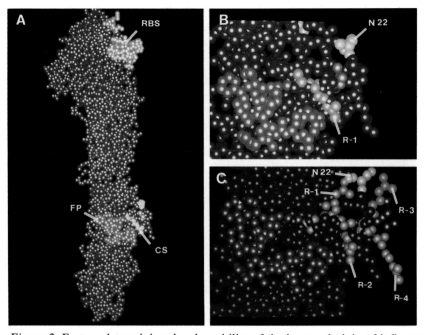

Figure 2 Factors determining the cleavability of the hemagglutinin of influenza A virus. (*A*) Three-dimensional structure of a hemagglutinin (H3) monomer. Receptor-binding site (RBS), fusion peptide (FP), and cleavage site (CS) are shown. (*B*) Monobasic cleavage site. The arginine at position –1 (R-1) of the cleavage site and the glycosylation site at Asn-22 of HA1 (N22) are indicated. (*C*) Multibasic cleavage site. The arginine at position –1 (R-1) and an insertion of 3 additional arginine residues at positions –2 (R-2), –3 (R-3), and –4 (R-4) are shown. Note that arginine –1 has different orientations in the monobasic and the multibasic cleavage site. The structure of the cleaved hemagglutinin was obtained by X-ray crystallography (Wilson et al. 1981). The orientation of the arginine residues that were removed after cleavage was determined by molecular modeling using the H3 coordinates deposited in the Brookhaven Protein Data Bank and a software program kindly provided by Gerrit Vriend, EMBL, Heidelberg.

The relationship between cleavage site, hemagglutinin cleavability, and the virulence of avian influenza A viruses was further assessed when a series of cleavage mutants from a virulent virus was generated by reversed genetics. A transfectant virus containing the wild-type hemagglutinin with R-R-R-K-K-R at the cleavage site, which was readily cleaved by endogenous proteases in chicken embryo fibroblasts, was highly virulent in intramuscularly or intranasally inoculated chickens. In contrast, a mutant containing hemagglutinin with an avirulent-like sequence (R-E-T-R) at the cleavage site, which was not cleaved by the fibroblast protease, was avirulent in chickens (Horimoto and Kawaoka 1994).

Besides the number and sequence of basic residues at the cleavage site, other factors determining cleavability have also been identified. Point mutations at some distance from the cleavage site have been found to increase the spectrum of permissive host cells to a certain degree (Rott et al. 1984; Orlich et al. 1990). Another important determinant is a carbohydrate side chain that is present in the vicinity of the cleavage site and interferes with protease accessibility (Fig. 2). Loss of this carbohydrate resulted in enhanced hemagglutinin cleavability and pathogenicity of the avian influenza virus A/chick/Pennsylvania/83 (H5N2) (Kawaoka et al. 1984; Deshpande et al. 1987). The interaction of this oligosaccharide with the cleavage site has been further corroborated in a study employing plaque variants of the apathogenic strain A/chick/Pennsylvania/1/83 (Ohuchi et al. 1989). Unlike the wild type, the plaque variants contain a hemagglutinin that is cleaved in chick embryo cells and MDCK cells. The variants differ also from the wild type by their pathogenicity for chickens. Nucleotide sequence and oligosaccharide analysis of the hemagglutinin have revealed that, unlike natural isolates with increased pathogenicity (Kawaoka et al. 1984), the variants obtained in vitro have retained an oligosaccharide at Asn-11 that is believed to interfere with the cleavage site of the wild type. However, all variants showed mutations in the hemagglutinin, resulting in an increased number of basic groups at the cleavage site. These observations demonstrate that masking of the cleavage site by an oligosaccharide is overcome by an enhancement of the basic charge at the cleavage site.

The studies described so far were performed on hemagglutinins originating from avian viruses. Even more remarkably, all of the highly cleavable hemagglutinins with multiple basic residues at the cleavage site belong to just 2 of the 14 subtypes known to date, H5 and H7. It was therefore of interest to find out whether high cleavability is a specific trait compatible only with the structural features of these two serotypes, or whether it may also be acquired by other hemagglutinins. It was of particular interest to find out if this is the case with hemagglutinins of human influenza viruses, because of the high pathogenic potential such a virus might have. In a study on the hemagglutinin of the human strain A/Port Chalmers/1/73 (H3N2) it was shown that this hemagglutinin, indeed, can undergo a change in substrate specificity and become sensitive to the ubiquitous proteases (Ohuchi et al. 1991). This has been accomplished by designing hemagglutinin mutants that varied in the number of arginine residues at the cleavage site and in the presence of the oligosaccharide at Asn-22 of HA_1 (Table 3). The results indicated that, in

Table 3 Hemagglutinin variants of influenza virus A/Port Chalmers/1/73 (H3) obtained by site-directed mutagenesis

Hemagglutinin	Oligosaccharide at Asn-22 of HA1	Cleavage site HA1 326 327 328	HA2 329	1	Activation in CV1 cells
Wild type	+	Lys-Gln-Thr------------------------	Arg	Gly	–
Mutant I2+	+	Lys-Gln-Thr-----------**ARG-ARG**-Arg	Arg	Gly	–
Mutant I3+	+	Lys-Gln-Thr------**ARG-ARG-ARG**-Arg	Arg	Gly	–
Mutant I4+	+	Lys-Gln-Thr-**ARG-ARG-ARG-ARG**-Arg	Arg	Gly	+
Mutant S1+	+	Lys-Gln-**ARG**-------------------	Arg	Gly	–
Mutant S2+	+	Lys-**ARG-ARG**-------------------	Arg	Gly	–
Mutant I2–	–	Lys-Gln-Thr-----------**ARG-ARG**-Arg	Arg	Gly	–
Mutant I3–	–	Lys-Gln-Thr------**ARG-ARG-ARG**-Arg	Arg	Gly	+
Mutant S2–	–	Lys-**ARG-ARG**-----------------	Arg	Gly	–
Mutant S3–	–	**ARG-ARG-ARG**-----------------	Arg	Gly	–

Inserted and substituted amino acids are indicated by bold letters. Data from Ohuchi et al. (1991).

the presence of the carbohydrate at Asn-22, an insertion of four additional arginines, i.e., a total sequence of five arginines, is required at the cleavage site to obtain cleavage in CV1 cells. This observation was in good agreement with a report by Gething and coworkers (1989) who, using the same approach, observed cleavage of another human H3 hemagglutinin after insertion of four arginines, whereas one additional arginine had no effect. It also became clear from these data that the number of inserted basic amino acids can be reduced by one, but not by more, residues when the oligosaccharide at Asn-22 is missing. Two conclusions can be drawn from these observations: (1) In agreement with the studies on H7 hemagglutinin described above, the consensus sequence R-X-K/R-R is the minimal requirement for recognition by the ubiquitous proteases. (2) By the insertion of an additional arginine at the cleavage site the masking effect of the oligosaccharide at Asn-22 of HA1 can be abolished, exactly as has been observed with the H5 hemagglutinin (Kawaoka and Webster 1989; Ohuchi et al. 1989). Thus, interplay between this carbohydrate and the cleavage site is a feature common to H5 and H3 hemagglutinins. The study by Ohuchi et al. (1991) showed also that the H3 hemagglutinin can acquire high cleavability only if the basic sequence is introduced by an insertion mechanism. The basic sequence could not be generated at the expense of the carboxy-terminal end of HA1. Since the carboxy-terminal amino acids are not conserved, one can conclude that their number is more important than their individual structures. Thus, it appears that the carboxyl terminus of HA1 has a spacer function which, in addition to the basic residues and the oligosaccharide at Asn-22 of HA1, is another determinant of cleavability.

Cleavage Activation by Bacterial Coinfection

Not only proteases of the eukaryotic host, but also microbial enzymes have been found to be involved in the activation of viral glycoproteins. This concept has been established with influenza virus which, upon coinfection with bacteria, has the potential to cause severe pneumonia in man. First, it was shown that *Staphylococcus aureus* secretes a protease capable of activating the hemagglutinin and of promoting virus replication in the respiratory tract and the development of pneumonia in mice. Interestingly, only proteases of certain *S. aureus* strains were able to activate a given influenza virus strain. Thus, the right virus had to encounter the right bacterium to develop the cooperative effect (Tashiro et al. 1987b,c). Inhibitor studies revealed that the bacterial enzymes were serine proteases, and one of these inhibitors, leupeptin, also showed therapeutic effects in mice (Tashiro et al. 1987a). In another study,

Aerococcus viridans, isolated from a patient with pneumonia, was found to secrete a protease that could activate hemagglutinin directly (Scheiblauer et al. 1992). Proteases from *Serratia marescens* (Akaike et al. 1989) and *Pseudomonas aeruginosa* (Scheiblauer et al. 1992) could not activate hemagglutinin directly, but application of influenza virus together with these enzymes into mice enhanced virus titers and pathogenicity. Generation of trypsin-like activity in bronchoalveolar lavages of these animals was thought to be responsible for hemagglutinin activation. Similar indirect effects were induced by streptokinase and staphylokinase known to generate plasmin by plasminogen activation. These observations taken together suggest three different activation mechanisms resulting from combined viral-bacterial infection. First, bacterial proteases cleave hemagglutinin directly. Second, bacterial proteases activate in the lung a zymogen, such as plasminogen, that in turn is able to activate the hemagglutinin. Finally, during combined viral-bacterial infection, host proteases present in inflammatory lesions are scaled up, thus activating influenza virus again by hemagglutinin cleavage (Scheiblauer et al. 1992).

PROTEASES INVOLVED IN CLEAVAGE

Proteolytic activation of viral glycoproteins involves cleavage at a specific cleavage site, usually the carboxyl terminus of an arginine residue, by the sequential action of an endoprotease and a carboxypeptidase that are both provided by the host. As indicated by studies using the influenza virus hemagglutinin as substrate, the carboxypeptidase appears to be a host component resembling in many respects carboxypeptidase N, which is incorporated into the viral envelope. Studies with specific inhibitors have revealed that, in contrast to the initial endoprotease cleavage, removal of the carboxy-terminal basic residues by the carboxypeptidase is not necessary for glycoprotein activation (Garten and Klenk 1983). It has been known for a long time that the endoproteases, which for their general substrate specificity often have been termed "trypsin-like" enzymes, vary significantly in their individual substrate specificities and their distribution in the organism (Klenk et al. 1975; Garten et al. 1982). However, only recently some of the biologically relevant cleavage enzymes have been identified at the molecular level.

Endoproteinases Cleaving at Single Arginine Sites

According to the information available so far, viral glycoproteins containing a monobasic cleavage site (see Table 1) appear to be activated, in general, by enzymes secreted from epithelial cells. Plasmin, known for a long time to activate the hemagglutinin of some influenza virus strains (Lazarowitz et al. 1973), is the prototype of these enzymes.

From the chick embryo, a frequently used model for studying the role of virus-activating proteases, an endoprotease has recently been isolated which specifically activates Sendai virus and avirulent NDV as well as human influenza A virus. It was demonstrated that this protease was identical with factor X, a vitamin-K-dependent serine protease in the prothrombin family which, in general, is synthesized in the liver and circulates as one of the plasma proteases essential for blood clotting (Gotoh et al. 1990). Examination of the distribution of this enzyme in the chick embryo tissues revealed that it was present in its active form only in the allantoic and amniotic fluid. Virus spread was confined to tissues in direct contact with these fluids. It was concluded that factor X is probably the major host determinant of paramyxovirus tropism in ovo (Ogasawara et al. 1992).

Another protease with similar substrate specificity has been isolated from rat lung. This enzyme is associated with the Clara cells of the bronchiolar epithelia and has been called tryptase Clara. It consists of a 30-kD polypeptide, has an isoelectric point of pH 4.75, a pH optimum of 7.5, and a substrate specificity for the sequence Q/E-X-R at the cleavage site. The enzyme is strongly inhibited by aprotinin, diisopropyl-fluorophosphate, antipain, leupeptin, and Kunitz-type soybean inhibitor. Tryptase Clara does not require calcium ions, which differentiates it from factor X. The enzyme was shown to cleave the hemagglutinin and to activate the infectivity of the Aichi strain (H3) of influenza A virus (Kido et al. 1992). Tryptase Clara also activated the F protein of Sendai virus in vitro. Specific antibodies inhibited viral activation by the protease in vitro in lung block cultures, and in vivo in infected rats. These findings indicated that tryptase Clara is an activating protease for Sendai virus in rat lungs and therefore a cellular key determinant for pneumopathogenicity of this virus in rats (Tashiro et al. 1992b). The secretory cells producing tryptase Clara can be distinguished from the alveolar cells in which the virus replicates. Thus, it is clear that, in these cases, the glycoproteins are activated on released virus in the extracellular space (Fig. 3).

Other secreted proteases, such as acrosin (Garten et al. 1981), kallikrein, urokinase, plasmin, and thrombin (Scheiblauer et al. 1992), also activate influenza A viruses. Some of these proteases are major participants in the reaction cascades of coagulation, fibrinolysis, and the complement system, all involved in inflammation. It should be noted, however, that these proteases have been found to cleave the hemag-

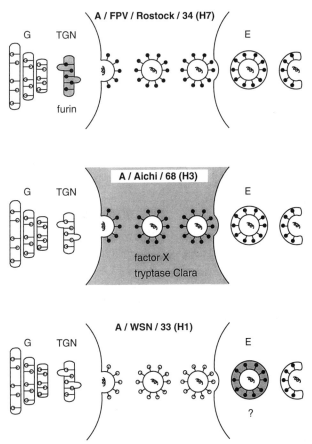

Figure 3 Stages of glycoprotein activation in the replication cycle. Three different compartments have been identified in which viral glycoprotein activation occurs. This is illustrated here on three influenza A virus strains. The hemagglutinin of strain A/FPV/Rostock/34 (H7) is activated on the exocytotic transport route in the TGN by furin. The hemagglutinin of strain A/Aichi/68 (H3) is activated on virions released into the extracellular space by secreted proteases, such as factor X or tryptase Clara. The hemagglutinin of strain A/WSN/34 (H1) is cleaved in MDBK cells at the stage of virus entry, presumably in endosomes (E) by an as-yet-unidentified protease.

glutinin only under in vitro conditions. They have not been identified yet as activating enzymes in a natural setting.

It appears, however, that glycoproteins with a single arginine are not only cleaved by secretory proteases. It has been known for a long time that the WSN strain of influenza A virus (H1) contains uncleaved hemagglutinin when released from MDBK cells, yet is able to undergo multiple replication cycles in these cells without any exogenous protease being added (Lazarowitz et al. 1973). Evidence has now been obtained that the WSN hemagglutinin is activated in these cells after internalization of the infecting virus (Fig. 3). The nature of the activating enzymes which are presumably present in endosomes is not known yet (Boycott et al. 1994).

Endoproteinases Cleaving at Multibasic Cleavage Sites

The ubiquitous proteases responsible for cleavage at sequences of several arginine and lysine residues were not well understood until recently. It was known that the activating enzyme of the FPV hemagglutinin is calcium-dependent and has a neutral pH optimum (Klenk et al. 1984), and that it can be inhibited by specific peptidylchloroalkylketones (Garten et al. 1989). Such enzymes appeared also to be highly conserved, since the hemagglutinin of FPV is activated not only in virtually all mammalian and avian cells analyzed, but also in invertebrate cells (Kuroda et al. 1989). It was therefore interesting to find that a protease resembling these enzymes in its catalytic and other biochemical properties exists in the yeast *Saccharomyces cerevisiae*. This Kex2 protease is a membrane-bound (Julius et al. 1984), calcium-dependent (Fuller et al. 1989) enzyme that occurs in organelles corresponding to the Golgi apparatus of higher eukaryotic cells (Redding et al. 1991). It cleaves its natural substrates, pro-α-factor and pro-killer toxin, at R-R- and K-R sites, but it can also process mammalian hormone and neuropeptide precursors, such as pro-opiomelanocortin (Thomas et al. 1988), proinsulin (Thim 1986), and proalbumin (Bathurst et al. 1987). Kex2 became the prototype of a new family of enzymes that have structural homologies in their catalytic domains with subtilisin and are therefore called eukaryotic subtilisin-like endoproteases (Fig. 4) (Barr 1991; Steiner et al. 1992).

One of these Kex2 analogs is furin, the product of the *fur* gene that was discovered in the immediate upstream region of the human c-*fes/fps* proto-oncogene (Roebrock et al. 1986; Fuller et al. 1989; van den Ouweland et al. 1990; Wise et al. 1990). Furin has been cloned not only from human, but also from mouse (Hatsuzawa et al. 1990), rat (Misumi et al. 1990), bovine (Stieneke-Gröber et al. 1992), and *Drosophila* (Roebroek et al. 1992) tissues. It is expressed at high levels in liver and kidney; at low levels in brain, spleen, and thymus; and at very low levels in heart, lung, and testis (Schalken et al. 1987). Its apparently ubiquitous occurrence suggests that it is involved in protein processing in the constitutive exocytosis route (Barr 1991). Furin has a hydrophobic carboxy-terminal sequence, indicating that it is a type I membrane protein. It is

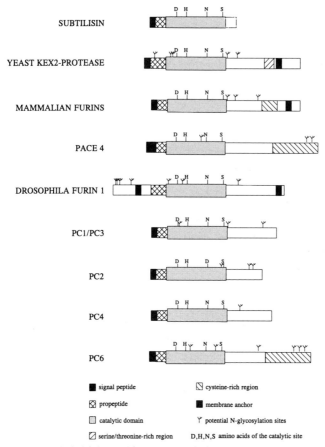

Figure 4 Subtilisin and its eukaryotic homologs.

calcium-dependent and has a neutral pH optimum. By overexpressing furin in different cell lines, its proteolytic activity could be assayed, and it has been shown to activate von Willebrand factor (Wise et al. 1990), ß-nerve growth factor (Bresnahan et al. 1990), renin (Hosaka et al. 1991), and factor C3 (Misumi et al. 1991).

Like the other subtilisin-like endoproteases, furin is activated by presumably autocatalytic removal of a pro-sequence at a R-T-K-R cleavage site (Leduc et al. 1992). Pro-peptide removal takes place in the *cis* Golgi region (M. Vey et al., in prep.). Addition of the endoplasmic reticulum retention signal KDEL to the carboxyl terminus of a truncated molecule resulted in intracellular retention of the protein and loss of activity, indicating that the endoplasmic reticulum is not an appropriate environment for pro-peptide processing (Rehemtulla et al. 1992). Activated furin accumulates in the *trans* Golgi network (TGN), which is the prime site of substrate cleavage, although a secretory form of furin has also been observed (Molloy et al. 1992, 1994; W. Schäfer et al., in prep.). The TGN localization of furin is in good agreement with the concept that viral glycoproteins containing the specific cleavage signal are activated in this compartment, too (Fig. 3).

The first viral glycoprotein found to be activated by furin was the hemagglutinin of FPV (Stieneke-Gröber et al. 1992). This conclusion was reached by two different approaches. First, it could be demonstrated that the FPV hemagglutinin was cleaved when it was coexpressed with human furin using vaccinia virus vectors. Second, bovine furin was identified as the endogenous protease responsible for cleavage activation of hemagglutinin in MDBK cells, a bovine kidney cell line allowing in vivo replication of FPV. It was, thus, not only shown that furin overexpressed from a foreign gene can activate the R-K-K-R cleavage site of the FPV hemagglutinin, but it was also demonstrated for the first time that the indigenous enzyme responsible for this type of proteolytic activation in a given cell is furin.

Several other viral glycoproteins that have similar cleavage sites as the FPV hemagglutinin have also shown to be activated by furin. These include the envelope glycoprotein gp160 of HIV-1 (Hallenberger et al. 1992; Decroly et al. 1994), the F protein of pathogenic strains of NDV (Gotoh et al. 1992; Moehring et al. 1993) and of human parainfluenza virus III (Ortmann et al. 1994), the PE2 protein of Sindbis virus (Moehring et al. 1993), and the gB protein of human cytomegalovirus (Vey et al. 1995).

The available evidence indicates that furin requires at its cleavage site, in addition to the paired basic residues in positions −1 and −2, an arginine in position −4. Thus, suitable substrates have tetrabasic sequences (R-K/R-K/R-R) or tribasic sequences (R-X-K/R-R), as is the case with all of the viral glycoproteins shown in Table 2. Interestingly, however, the basic residue at position −2 sometimes seems to be less critical. Studies on synthetic substrates have shown that an R-X-X-R motif still can act as a cleavage site, yet with 100 times lower efficiency than an R-X-K/R-R motif (Hatsuzawa et al. 1992). Thus, a mutation at the cleavage site of the F protein from R-T-K-R to R-T-E-R did not affect replication of human parainfluenza virus type 3 in a number of different host cells (Coelingh and Winter 1990), and a similar mutation at the cleavage site of an H5 hemagglutinin of influenza virus was still compatible with high cleavability (Kawaoka and Webster 1988). Furthermore, acquisition of pathogenicity of an avian H7 strain (Khatchikian et al. 1989) was found to result from insertion of the sequence R-T-A-R at the cleavage site (Morsy et al. 1994). The apathogenic NDV strain La

Sota also shows the motif R-X-X-R (Table 1), yet was found to be a poor substrate for furin (Gotoh et al. 1992). This observation can be explained by the presence of a hydrophobic aliphatic amino acid residue (L) in position +1 of this cleavage site, which has been shown to be not suitable for furin cleavage (Watanabe et al. 1992).

The other subtilisin-like endoproteases identified so far are PC4 (Nakayama et al. 1992), PC5/PC6 (Lusson et al. 1993; Nakagawa et al. 1993), PACE4 (Kiefer et al. 1991), PC1/PC3 (Seidah et al. 1991; Smeekens et al. 1991), and PC2 (Seidah et al. 1990; Smeekens and Steiner 1990). The latter two enzymes were thought to be constituents of only the regulated secretory pathway, since they are expressed in secretory vesicles of neuroendocrine cells and specifically activate prohormones at dibasic cleavage sites (K-K or K-R) (Thomas et al. 1991). However, recently, PC1/PC3 has also been found, together with furin, in a CD4-positive lymphocyte line and to activate the envelope glycoprotein of HIV-1 (Decroly et al. 1994). The cleavage capacity of PC2 and PC1/PC3 has also been tested on pathogenic and apathogenic NDV strains, but neither F protein with R-X-K/R-R consensus sequence nor F protein with a single arginine at the cleavage site was susceptible to these enzymes (Gotoh et al. 1992). However, F protein with the R-X-K/R-R cleavage site was cleaved by Kex2 (Nagai et al. 1991), as was the case with human parainfluenza virus III (Ortmann et al. 1994) and gp160 of HIV-1 (Moulard et al. 1994b). Although not as ubiquitous as furin, PC5/PC6 and PACE4 appear to be expressed in many tissues. This suggests that these enzymes are present in the constitutive secretory pathway. It will therefore be interesting to analyze their role as virus activation enzymes.

A protease not related to furin that cleaves gp160 of HIV-1 has also been isolated from lymphocytes (Kido et al. 1993). Furthermore, Lovo cells that have a defective furin gene are able to activate gp160, but not other viral glycoproteins with a R-X-K/R-R motif, such as the F protein of a pathogenic NDV strain (Ohnishi et al. 1994). These results indicate that some viral glycoproteins activated by furin can also be cleaved by other proteases that do not have to be members of the subtilisin family.

Proteases Activating at Nonbasic Cleavage Sites

A number of mutants have been isolated from Sendai virus in which the arginine at position 116 of the F protein has been exchanged for an isoleucine. This change at the cleavage site renders the mutants resistant to activation by trypsin but makes them sensitive to cleavage by elastase between Ile-116 and Phe-117 and by chymotrypsin between Gln-114 and

Ser-115 (Scheid and Choppin 1976; Tashiro and Homma 1983a,b; Hsu et al. 1987; Itoh et al. 1987; Tashiro et al. 1992a). Some of these protease activation mutants can undergo multiple replication cycles in chick embryos and MDCK cells, and sequence analysis has shown that the cleavage site at Ile-116 is used in these systems. Thus, it appears that MDCK cells and chick embryos contain elastase-like proteases that can activate these mutants (Tashiro et al. 1992a). In mouse lungs, infection by all mutants is restricted to a single replication cycle because activation does not occur (Tashiro and Homma 1983a, 1985; Mochizuki et al. 1988; Tashiro et al. 1988b, 1992a; Itoh et al. 1990). These results indicate that mouse lungs lack an elastase or chymotrypsin-like protease capable of activating the mutants. It has therefore been suggested that protease activation mutants may be used as live vaccines (Tashiro and Homma 1985; Tashiro et al. 1988a; Hsu et al. 1989).

Effect of Protease Inhibitors on Virus Replication

Several protease inhibitors have been described that block glycoprotein activation and therefore interfere with spread of infection. Cleavage of the hemagglutinin of the WSN strain of influenza A virus could be inhibited in vitro by ε-amino-*n*-caproic acid and by aprotinin (Zhirnov et al. 1982). Intraperitoneal administration of these inhibitors could suppress virus replication in the lungs of mice infected by a mouse-adapted strain of influenza virus (Zhirnov et al. 1984). ε-Amino-*n*-caproic acid, which is an analog of lysine, inhibits plasmin activity in vivo by competing for the interaction of fibrin, plasminogen, and plasminogen activator. Aprotinin is a well-known serine protease inhibitor with a relatively broad inhibitory spectrum that inhibits plasmin, kallikrein, trypsin, and chymotrypsin. Therefore, suppression of viral replication in mice by ε-amino-*n*-caproic acid and aprotinin might be due to inhibition of plasmin generation or of the action of plasmin itself. In any case, these inhibitors presumably interfere with replication of viruses that are activated by secreted proteases.

Peptidyl derivatives of chloroalkylketones are another type of inhibitor of serine proteases (Kettner and Shaw 1981). These compounds proved to be potent inhibitors of the intracellular protease furin. First it was shown that, unlike peptidyl chloromethylketones containing a single arginine, such compounds with paired basic amino acids inhibit cleavage activation of the FPV hemagglutinin and, thus, prevent multiple cycles of virus replication (Garten et al. 1989). When it became clear that the consensus sequence had an additional arginine four amino acids upstream of the cleavage site (Vey et al. 1992), peptidyl chloromethylketones with an arginine in this position were synthesized and tested for their activity to inhibit cleavage by furin in MDBK cells. Whereas the dibasic compounds decFAKR-CMK and decREIR-CMK inhibited at 1 mM concentrations, there was an increase in sensitivity by a factor of about 1000 when the new inhibitors showing the correct consensus sequence, such as decREKR-CMK, were used (Stieneke-Gröber et al. 1992). Peptidyl chloromethylketones also interfered with the biological activities of the FPV hemagglutinin. When polykaryocytosis in BHK 21-F cells induced by hemagglutinin at low pH was analyzed, complete inhibition of cell fusion was obtained again at micromolar concentrations of decREKR-CMK, whereas decFAKR-CMK and decRAIR-CMK had to be given at 100- to 1000-fold higher concentrations to see the same effect. It is therefore clear that the peptidyl chloromethylketones with the correct amino acid sequence, while not interfering with hemagglutination and thus receptor-binding, specifically block the cleavage-dependent fusion activity of the FPV HA (Stienecke-Gröber et al. 1992).

Peptidyl chloromethylketones also inhibit cleavage of the envelope glycoprotein of HIV-1 by endogenous furin present in human cells. This was shown by analyzing the effect of these compounds on HIV-1 glycoprotein expressed in BHK 21 cells by a vaccinia virus vector. In the presence of decREKR-CMK, cleavage was inhibited at 5 μM concentrations. In contrast, decRAIR-CMK and decFAKR-CMK inhibited cleavage only slightly or not at all. To elucidate the effects of the inhibitors on the fusion activity of the envelope glycoprotein, syncytium formation was analyzed in HeLa-CD4 cells, which are susceptible to fusion by the viral glycoprotein, since they contain the viral receptor. Again, there was a distinct effect when inhibitors with the correct consensus sequence (decRAKR-CMK and decREKR-CMK) were used, whereas inhibitors not showing this motif (decRAIR-CMK and decFAKR-CMK) did not inhibit fusion. By interfering with cleavage activation of gp160, decREKR-CMK and decRAKR-CMK also reduced the infectivity of HIV-1. They may therefore have a potential to arrest spread of infection in the organism (Hallenberger et al. 1992). A different type of inhibitor, a furin-directed α_1-antitrypsin variant, has also been shown to interfere with HIV-1 glycoprotein activation (Anderson et al. 1993).

Since furin is a calcium-dependent protease, depletion of calcium by the calcium-specific ionophore A23187 also interferes with glycoprotein cleavage by this enzyme. This was shown first with the FPV hemagglutinin (Klenk et al. 1984) and subsequently with the F protein of a number of paramyxoviruses (Kawahara et al. 1992), as well as the HIV-1 glycoprotein (Garten et al. 1994; Moulard et al. 1994a).

CONCLUSIONS

Many viral membrane proteins undergo posttranslational proteolytic cleavage by host enzymes. The data reviewed here indicate that these glycoproteins can be subdivided into two major groups according to their sensitivity to different types of proteases. One group, comprising the majority of the viral glycoproteins, is cleaved by ubiquitous proteases that recognize, in general, the consensus sequence R-X-K/R-R at the cleavage site. These enzymes, which are located in the Golgi apparatus or in the *trans* Golgi network, appear to be membrane-bound constituents of the nonregulated exocytotic pathway. Furin, a subtilisin-like eukaryotic endoprotease, is the prototype of these enzymes and has been identified as the cleavage enzyme of some of these viral glycoproteins. The other group contains viral glycoproteins that are cleaved, generally at sites consisting of isolated basic residues, by proteases available only in a few host systems. Since, according to the information available so far, these enzymes are soluble proteins secreted primarily from epithelial cells, cleavage takes place at the cell surface or in body fluids. Although the biological significance of cleavage is not fully understood with some viruses, in most instances, it has been found to be necessary for infectivity. This has been shown best with influenza viruses, paramyxoviruses, and HIV, which all have fusion proteins that are activated by proteolytic cleavage. Numerous studies indicate that the interplay of viral glycoproteins and cellular proteases may have a pivotal role in spread of infection, host range, and pathogenicity.

ACKNOWLEDGMENTS

We are greatly indepted to R. Rott, Justus-Liebig-Universität Giessen, and M. Tashiro, National Institute of Health, Tokyo, Japan, for many years of fruitful collaboration on cleavage activation of viral glycoproteins. We also thank our colleagues who were involved in the more recent studies, notably S. Hallenberger, M. and R. Ohuchi, A. Stieneke-Gröber, and M. Vey, all Philipps-Universität, Marburg, Germany, and E. Shaw and H. Angliker, Friedrich-Miescher-Institut, Basel, Switzerland. Finally, we acknowledge the expert secretarial help of S. Fischbach. Work by the authors was supported by grants from the Deutsche Forschungsgemeinschaft and the Bundesministerium für Forschung und Technologie.

REFERENCES

Akaike, T., A. Molla, M. Ando, S. Araki, and H. Maeda. 1989. Molecular mechanism of complex infection by bacteria and virus analyzed by a model using serratial protease and influenza virus in mice. *J. Virol.* **63**: 2252.

Anderson, E.D., L. Thomas, J.S. Hayflick, and G. Thomas. 1993. Inhibition of HIV-1 gp160-dependent membrane fusion by a furin-directed alpha 1-antitrypsin variant. *J Biol. Chem.* **268**: 24887.

Barr, P.J. 1991. Mammalian subtilisins: The long-sought dibasic processing endoproteases. *Cell* **66**: 1.

Barrett, T., D.K. Clarke, S.A. Evans, and B.K. Rima. 1987. The nucleotide sequence of the gene encoding the F protein of canine distemper virus: A comparison of the deduced amino acid sequence with other paramyxoviruses. *Virus Res.* **8**: 373.

Bathurst, I.C., S.O. Brennan, R.W. Carrell, L.S. Cousens, A.J. Brake, and P.J. Barr. 1987. Yeast KEX2 protease has the properties of a human proalbumin converting enzyme. *Science* **235**: 348.

Bedgood, R.M. and M.R. Stallcup. 1992. A novel intermediate in processing of murine leukemia virus envelope glycoproteins. Proteolytic cleavage in the late Golgi region. *J. Biol. Chem.* **267**: 7060.

Bosch, F.X., W. Garten, H.-D. Klenk, and R. Rott. 1981. Proteolytic cleavage of influenza virus hemagglutinins: Primary structure of the connecting peptide HA$_1$ and HA$_2$ determines proteolytic cleavability and pathogenicity of avian influenza virus. *Virology* **113**: 725.

Both, G.W., A.R. Bellamy, and D.B. Mitchell. 1994. Rotavirus protein structure and function. *Curr. Top. Microbiol. Immunol.* **185**: 67.

Boycott, R., H.-D. Klenk, and M. Ohuchi. 1994. Cell tropism of influenza A virus as dependent on proteolytic activation of the hemagglutinin at the stage of virus entry. *Virology* (in press).

Boyle, J.F., D.G. Weismiller, and K.V. Holmes. 1987. Genetic resistance to mouse hepatitis virus correlates with absence of virus-binding activity on target tissues. *J. Virol.* **61**: 185.

Bresnahan, P.A., R. Laude, L. Thomas, I. Thorner, H.L. Gibson, A.J. Brake, P.J. Barr, and G. Thomas. 1990. Human fur gene encodes a yeast Kex2-like endoprotein that cleaves pro-β-NGF *in vivo· J. Cell Biol.* **111**: 2851.

Brücher, K.H., W. Garten, H.-D. Klenk, E. Shaw, and K. Radsak. 1990. Inhibition of endoproteolytic cleavage of cytomegalovirus (HCMV) glycoprotein B by palmitoyl-peptidyl-chloromethyl ketone. *Virology* **178**: 617.

Buchmeier, M.J., R.M. Welsh, F.J. Dutko, and M.B.A. Oldstone. 1987. Site-specific antibodies define a cleavage site conserved among arenavirus GP-C glycoproteins. *J. Virol.* **61**: 982.

Castle, E., T. Nowak, U. Leidner, G. Wengler, and G. Wengler. 1985. Sequence analysis of the viral core protein and the membrane associated proteins V1 and NV2 of the flavivirus west nile virus and of the genome sequence for these proteins. *Virology* **145**: 227.

Cavanagh, D., P.J. Davis, D.J.C. Pappin, M.M. Binns, M.E.G. Boursnell, and T.D.K. Brown. 1986. Coronavirus IBV: Partial amino terminal sequencing of spike polypeptide S2 identifies the sequence Arg-Arg-Phe-Arg-Arg at the cleavage site of the spike precursor propolypeptide of IBV strains Beaudette and M41. *Virus Res.* **4**: 133.

Chambers, T.M., S. Yamnikova, Y. Kawaoka, D.K. Lvov, and R.G. Webster. 1989. Antigenic and molecular characterization of subtype H13 hemagglutinin of influenza virus. *Virology* **172**: 180.

Clegg, J.C.S. and G. Lloyd. 1983. Structural and cell-associated proteins of Lassa virus. *J. Gen. Virol.* **64**: 1127.

Coelingh, K.V.W. and C.C. Winter. 1990. Naturally occurring human parainfluenza type

3 viruses exhibit divergence in amino acid sequence of their fusion protein neutralizing epitopes and cleavage sites. *J. Virol.* **64:** 1329.

Coia, G., M.D. Parker, G. Speight, M.E. Byrne, and E.G. Westaway. 1988. Nucleotide and complete amino acid sequence of kunjin virus: Definitive gene order and characteristics of virus-specified proteins. *J. Gen. Virol.* **69:** 1.

Collins, A.R., R.L. Knobler, H. Powell, and M.J. Buchmeier. 1982. Monoclonal antibodies to murine hepatitis virus-4 (strain JHM) define the viral glycoprotein responsible for attachment and cell-cell fusion. *Virology* **119:** 358.

Collins P.L., Y.T. Huang, and G.W. Wertz. 1984. Nucleotide sequence of the gene encoding the fusion (F) glycoprotein of human respiratory syncytial virus. *Proc. Natl. Acad. Sci.* **81:** 7683.

Cranage, M.P., T. Kouzarides, A.T. Bankier, S. Satchwell, K. Weston, P. Tomlinson, B. Barrell, H. Hart, S.E. Bell, A.C. Minson, and G.L. Smith. 1986. Identification of the human cytomegalovirus glycoprotein B gene and induction of neutralizing antibodies via its expression in recombinant vaccinia virus. *EMBO J.* **5:** 3057.

Decroly, E., M. Vandenbranden, J.M. Ruysschaert, J. Cogniaux, G.S. Jacob, S.C. Howard, G. Marshall, A. Kompelli, A. Basak, F. Jean, C. Lazure, S. Benjannet, M. Chrétien, R. Day, and N.G. Seidah. 1994. The convertases furin and PC1 can both cleave the human immunodeficiency virus (HIV-1) envelope glycoprotein gp160 into gp160 (HIV-1 SU) and gp41 (HIV-1 TM). *J. Biol. Chem.* **269:** 12240.

de Curtis, I. and K. Simons. 1989. Isolation of exocytotic carrier vesicles from BHK cells. *Cell* **58:** 719.

Deregt, D., M. Sabara, and L.A. Babiuk. 1987. Structural proteins of bovine coronavirus and their intracellular processing. *J. Gen. Virol.* **68:** 2863.

Deshpande, K.L., V.A. Fried, M. Ando, and R.G. Webster. 1987. Glycosylation affects cleavage of an H5N2 influenza virus hemagglutinin and regulates virulence. *Proc. Natl. Acad. Sci.* **84:** 34.

Dong, J.Y., J.W. Dubay, L.P. Perez, and E. Hunter. 1992. Mutations within the proteolytic cleavage site of the Rous sarcoma virus glycoprotein define a requirement for dibasic residues for intracellular cleavage. *J. Virol.* **66:** 865.

Donis, R.O., W.J. Bean, Y. Kawaoka, and R.G. Webster. 1989. Distinct lineages of influenza virus H4 hemagglutinin genes in different regions of the world. *Virology* **169:** 408.

Feldmann, H., E. Kretzschmar, B. Klingeborn, R. Rott, H.-D. Klenk, and W. Garten. 1988. The structure of serotype H10 hemagglutinin of influenza A virus: Comparison of an apathogenic avian and a mammalian strain pathogenic for mink. *Virology* **165:** 428.

Fenouillet, E. and J.C. Gluckman. 1992. Immunological analysis of human immunodeficiency virus type 1 envelope glycoprotein proteolytic cleavage. *Virology* **187:** 825.

Frana, M.F., J.N. Behnke, L.S. Sturman, and K.V. Holmes. 1985. Proteolytic cleavage of the E2 glycoprotein of murine coronavirus: Host-dependent differences in proteolytic cleavage and cell fusion. *J. Virol.* **56:** 912.

Franze-Ferdinand, M.T., C. Zetina, S. Iapalucci, M.A. Lucero, C. Bouissou, R. Lopez, O. Rey, M. Daheli, G.N. Cohen, and M.M. Zahin. 1987. Molecular structure and early events in the replication of Tacaribe arenavirus S RNA. *Virus Res.* **7:** 309.

Freed, E.O. and D.J. Myers. 1992. Identification and characterization of fusion and processing domains of the human immunodeficiency virus type 2 envelope glycoprotein. *J. Virol.* **66:** 5472.

Fuller, R.S., A.J. Brake, and J. Thorner. 1989. Intracellular targeting and structural conservation of a prohormone-processing endoprotease. *Science* **246:** 482.

Garten, W. and H.-D. Klenk. 1983. Characterization of the carboxy peptidase involved in the proteolytic cleavage of the influenza hemagglutinin. *J. Gen. Virol.* **64:** 2127.

Garten, W., D. Linder, R. Rott, and H.-D. Klenk. 1982. The cleavage site of the hemagglutinin of fowl plague virus. *Virology* **122:** 186.

Garten, W., W. Berk, Y. Nagai, R. Rott, and H.-D. Klenk. 1980. Mutational changes of the protease susceptibility of glycoprotein F of Newcastle disease virus: Effects on pathogenicity. *J. Gen. Virol.* **50:** 135.

Garten, W., F.X. Bosch, D. Linder, R. Rott, and H.-D. Klenk. 1981. Proteolytic activation of the influenza hemagglutinin: The structure of the cleavage site and the enzymes involved in cleavage. *Virology* **115:** 361.

Garten, W., A. Stieneke, E. Shaw, P. Wikstrom, and H.-D. Klenk. 1989. Inhibition of proteolytic activation of influenza virus hemagglutinin by specific peptidyl chloroalkyl ketones. *Virology* **172:** 31.

Garten, W., K. Kuroda, W. Schuy, H. Naruse, C. Scholtissek, and H.-D. Klenk. 1985. Haemagglutinin transport mutants. *Vaccine* **3:** 227.

Garten, W., S. Hallenberger, D. Ortmann, W. Schäfer, M. Vey, H. Angliker, E. Shaw, and H.-D. Klenk. 1994. Processing of viral glycoproteins by the subtilisin-like endoprotease furin and its inhibition by specific peptidylchloromethylketones. *Biochimie* (in press).

Gething, M.-J., J. Henneberry, and J. Sambrook. 1989. Fusion activity of the hemagglutinin of influenza virus. *Curr. Top. Membr. Transp.* **13:** 339.

Gething, M.-J., J.M. White, and M.D. Waterfield. 1978. Purification of the fusion protein of Sendai virus: Analysis of the NH_2-terminal sequence generated during precursor activation. *Proc. Natl. Acad. Sci.* **75:** 2737.

Gething, M.-J., J. Bye, J. Skehel, and M. Waterfield. 1980. Cloning and DNA sequence of double-stranded copies of hemagglutinin genes from H2 and H3 strains elucidates antigenic shift and drift in human influenza virus. *Nature* **287:** 301.

Gotoh, D., T. Ogasawara, T. Toyoda, N.M. Inocencio, M. Hamaguchi, and Y. Nagai. 1990. An endoprotease homologous to the blood clotting factor X as a determinant of viral tropism in chick embryo. *EMBO J.* **9:** 4189.

Gotoh, B., Y. Ohnishi, N.M. Inocencio, E. Esaki, K. Nakayama, P.J. Barr, G. Thomas, and Y. Nagai. 1992. Mammalian subtilisin-related proteinases in cleavage-activation of the paramyxovirus fusion glycoprotein. Preference of furin/PACE over PC2 or PC1/PC3. *J. Virol.* **66:** 6391.

Günther, I., B. Glatthaar, G. Döller, and W. Garten. 1993. A H1 hemagglutinin of a human influenza A virus with a carbohydrate-modulated receptor binding site and an unusual cleavage site. *Virus Res.* **27:** 147.

Guo, H., F. di Marzo Verones, E. Tschachler, R. Pol, V.S. Kalyanaraman, R.C. Gallo, and M.S. Reitz. 1990. Characterization of an HIV-1 point mutant blocked in envelope glycoprotein cleavage. *Virology* **174:** 217.

Hakimi, J. and P.H. Atkinson. 1982. Glycosylation of intracellular Sindbis virus glycoproteins. *Biochemistry* **21:** 2140.

Hallenberger, S., V. Bosch, H. Angliker, E. Shaw, H.-D. Klenk, and W. Garten. 1992. Furin mediated cleavage activation of the HIV-1 glycoprotein and its inhibition by specific peptidyl-chloromethylketones. *Nature* **360:** 358.

Harnish, D.G., K. Dimock, D.H.L. Bishop, and W.E. Rawls. 1983. Gene mapping in Pichinde virus: Assignment of viral polypeptides to genomic L and S RNAs. *J. Virol.* **46:** 638.

Hatsuzawa, K., M. Nagahama, S. Takahashi, K. Takada, K. Murakami, and K. Nakayama. 1992. Purification and characterization of furin, a Kex2-like processing endoprotease, produced in Chinese hamster ovary cells. *J. Biol. Chem.* **23:** 16094.

Hatsuzawa, K., M. Hosaka, T. Nakagawa, M. Nagase, A. Shoda, K. Murakami, and K. Nakayama. 1990. Structure and expression of mouse furin, a yeast Kex2-related protease. *J. Biol. Chem.* **265:** 22075.

Herrler, G. and H.-D. Klenk. 1991. Structure and function of the HEF glycoprotein of influenza C virus. *Adv. Virus Res.* **40:** 213.

Hidaka, Y., T. Kanda, K. Iwasaki, A. Nomoto, T. Shioda, and H. Shibuta. 1984. Nucleotide sequence of a Sendai virus genome region covering the entire M gene and the 3 proximal 1013 nucleotides of the F gene. *Nucleic Acid Res.* **12:** 7965.

Hiti, A.L., A.R. Davis, and D.P. Nayak. 1981. Complete sequence shows that the hemagglutinin of the H0 and H2 subtypes of human influenza virus are closely related. *Virology* **111:** 113.

Homma, M. and M. Ohuchi. 1973. Trypsin action on the growth of Sendai virus in tissue culture cells. III. Structural difference of Sendai viruses grown in eggs and tissue culture cells. *J. Virol.* **12:** 1457.

Horimoto, T. and Y. Kawaoka. 1994. Reverse genetics provides direct evidence for a correlation of hemagglutinin cleavability and virulence of an avian influenza A virus. *J. Virol.* **68:** 3120.

Hosaka, M., M. Nagahama, W.-S. Kim, T. Watanabe, K. Hatsuzawa, J. Ikemizu, K. Murakami, and K. Nakayama. 1991. Arg-X-Lys/Arg-Arg motif as a signal for precursor cleavage catalyzed by furin within the constitutive secretory pathway. *J. Biol. Chem.* **266:** 12127.

Hsu, M.C., A. Scheid, and P.W. Choppin. 1987. Protease activation mutants of Sendai virus: Sequence analysis of the mRNA of the fusion (F) gene and direct identification of the cleavage site. *Virology* **156:** 84.

Hsu, M.C., M. Harbison, G. Reinhard, H. Grosz, and K.A. Davis. 1989. A model paramyxovirus vaccine: Protease activation mutants. In *Vaccines 89: Modern approaches to new vaccines including prevention of AIDS* (ed. R.A. Lerner et al.), p. 513. Cold Spring Harbor Laboratory, Cold Spring Harbor, New York.

Hu, X., R.W. Compans, Y. Matsuoka, and R. Ray. 1990. Molecular cloning and sequence analysis of the fusion glycoprotein gene of human parainfluenza virus type 2. *Virology* **179:** 915.

Huang, R.T.C., R. Rott, and H.-D. Klenk. 1981. Influenza viruses cause hemolysis and fusion of cells. *Virology* **110:** 243.

Itoh, M., H. Shibuta, and M. Homma. 1987. Single amino acid substituion of Sendai virus at the cleavage site of the fusion protein confers trypsin resistance. *J. Gen. Virol.* **68:** 2939.

Itoh, M., D.M. Tan, T. Hayashi, Y. Hochizuki, and M. Homma. 1990. Pneumopathogenicity of a Sendai virus protease-activation mutant, TCs, which is sensitive to trypsin and chymotrypsin. *J. Virol.* **64:** 5660.

Jain, S.K., S. DeCandido, and M. Kielian. 1991. Processing of the p62 envelope precursor protein of Semliki Forest virus. *J. Biol. Chem.* **266:** 5756.

Julius, D.A., A. Brake, L. Blair, R. Kunisawa, and J. Thorner. 1984. Isolation of the putative structural gene for the lysine-arginine cleaving endopeptidase required for processing of yeast prepro-α-factor. *Cell* **37:** 1075.

Kawahara, N., X.Z. Yang, T. Sakaguchi, K. Kiyotani, Y. Nagai, and T. Yoshida. 1992. Distribution and substrate specificity of intracellular proteolytic processing enzyme(s) for paramyxovirus fusion glycoproteins. *J. Gen. Virol.* **73:** 583.

Kawaoka, Y. and R.G. Webster. 1988. Sequence requirements for cleavage activation of influenza virus hemagglutinin expressed in mammalian cells. *Proc. Natl. Acad. Sci.*

85: 321.

————. 1989. Interplay between carbohydrate in the stalk and the length of the connecting peptide determines the cleavability of influenza virus hemagglutinin. *J. Virol.* **63:** 3296.

Kawaoka, Y., C.W. Naeve, and R.G. Webster. 1984. Is virulence of H5N2 influenza viruses in chickens associated with loss of carbohydrate from the hemagglutinin? *Virology* **139:** 303.

Kawaoka, Y., A. Nestorowicz, D.J. Alexander, and R.G. Webster. 1987. Molecular analyses of the hemagglutinin genes of H5 influenza viruses: Origin of a virulent turkey strain. *Virology* **158:** 218.

Kawaoka, Y., S. Yamnikova, T.M. Chambers, D.K. Lvov, and R.G. Webster. 1990. Molecular characterization of a new hemagglutinin, subtype H14, of influenza A virus. *Virology* **179:** 759.

Keller, P.M., A.J. Davidson, R.S. Lowe, C.D. Bennett, and R.W. Ellis. 1986. Identification and structure of the gene encoding gpII, a major glycoprotein of Varicella-Zoster virus. *Virology* **152:** 181.

Kettner, C. and E. Shaw. 1981. Inactivation of trypsin-like enzymes with peptides of arginine chloromethyl ketones. *Methods Enzymol.* **80:** 828.

Khatchikian, D., M. Orlich, and R. Rott. 1989. Increased viral pathogenicity after insertion of a 28S ribosomal RNA sequence into the haemagglutinin gene of an influenza virus. *Nature* **340:** 156.

Kido, H., K. Kamoshita, A. Fukutomi, and N. Katunuma. 1993. Processing protease for gp160 human immunodeficiency virus type I envelope glycoprotein precursor in human T4[+] lymphocytes: Purification and characterization. *J. Biol. Chem.* **268:** 13406.

Kido, H., Y. Yokogoshi, K. Sakai, M. Tashiro, Y. Kishino, A. Fukutomi, and N. Katunuma. 1992. Isolation and characterization of a novel trypsin-like protease found in rat bronchiolar epithelial Clara cells: A possible activator of the viral fusion glycoprotein. *J. Biol. Chem.* **267:** 13573.

Kiefer, M.C., J.E. Tucker, R. Joh, K.E. Landsberg, D. Saltman, and P.J. Barr. 1991. Identification of a second human subtilisin-like protease gene in the fes/fps region of chromosome 15. *DNA Cell Biol.* **10:** 757.

Kitame, F., K. Sugawara, K. Owada, and M. Homma. 1982. Proteolytic activation of hemolysis and fusion by influenza C virus. *Arch. Virol.* **73:** 357.

Klenk, H.-D. and R. Rott. 1988. The molecular biology of influenza virus pathogenicity. *Adv. Virus Res.* **34:** 247.

Klenk, H.-D., W. Garten, and R. Rott. 1984. Inhibition of proteolytic cleavage of the hemagglutinin of influenza virus by calcium-specific ionophore A23187. *EMBO J.* **3:** 2911.

Klenk, H.-D., R. Rott, M. Orlich, and J. Blödorn. 1975. Activation of influenza A viruses by trypsin treatment. *Virology* **68:** 426.

Klenk, H.-D., W. Wöllert, R. Rott, and C. Scholtissek. 1974. Association of influenza virus proteins with cytoplasmic fractions. *Virology* **57:** 28.

Koch, W., G. Hunsmann, and R. Friedrich. 1983. Nucleotide sequence of the envelope gene of Friend murine leukemia virus. *J. Virol.* **45:** 1.

Kowalski, M., J. Potz, L. Basiripour, T. Dorfman, W.C. Goh, E. Terwilliger, A. Dayton, C. Rosen, W. Haseltine, and J. Sodroski. 1987. Functional regions of the envelope glycoprotein of human immunodeficiency virus type 1. *Science* **237:** 1351.

Krystal, M., R.M. Elliott, E.W. Benz, J.F. Young, and P. Palese. 1982. Evolution of influenza A and B viruses. Conservation of structural features in the hemagglutinin genes. *Proc. Natl. Acad. Sci.* **79:** 4800.

Kuroda, K., A. Gröner, K. Frese, D. Drenckhahn, C. Hauser, R. Rott, W. Doerfler, and H.-D. Klenk. 1989. Synthesis of biologically active influenza virus hemagglutinin in insect larvae. *J. Virol.* **63:** 1677.

Lazarowitz, S.G. and P.W. Choppin. 1975. Enhancement of the infectivity of influenza A and B viruses by proteolytic cleavage of the hemagglutinin polypeptide. *Virology* **68:** 440.

Lazarowitz, S.G., R.W. Compans, and P.W. Choppin. 1971. Influenza virus structural and non-structural proteins in infected cells and their plasma membrane. *Virology* **46:** 830.

Lazarowitz, S.G., A.R. Goldberg, and P.W. Choppin. 1973. Proteolytic cleavage by plasmin of the HA polypeptide of influenza virus. Host cell activation of serum plasminogen. *Virology* **56:** 172.

Leduc, R., S.S. Molloy, B.A. Thorne, and G. Thomas. 1992. Activation of human furin precursor processing endoprotease occurs by an intramolecular autoproteolytic cleavage. *J. Biol. Chem.* **267:** 14304.

Li, S., M. Orlich, and R. Rott. 1990. Generation of seal influenza virus variants pathogenic for chickens because of hemagglutinin cleavage site changes. *J. Virol.* **64:** 3297.

Lobigs, M. and H. Garoff. 1990. Fusion function of the Semliki Forest virus spike is activated by proteolytic cleavage of the envelope glycoprotein p62. *J. Virol.* **64:** 1233.

Lobigs, M., J.M. Wahlber, and H. Garoff. 1990a. Spike protein oligomerization control of Semliki Forest virus fusion. *J. Virol.* **64:** 5214.

Lobigs, M., H. Zhao, and H. Garoff. 1990b. Function of Semliki Forest virus E3 peptide in virus assembly: Replacement of E3 with an artificial signal peptide abolishes spike heterodimerization and surface expression of E1. *J. Virol.* **64:** 4346.

Lusson, J., D. Vieau, J. Hamelin, R. Day, M. Chrétien, and N.G. Seidah. 1993. cDNA structure of the mouse and rat subtilisin/kexin-like PC5: A candidate proprotein convertase expressed in endocrine and nonendocrine cells. *Proc. Natl. Acad. Sci.* **90:** 6691.

Luytjes, W., L.S. Sturman, P.I. Bredenbeck, I. Chasite, B.A.M. van der Zeijst, M.C. Horzinek, and W.J.M. Spaan. 1987. Primary structure of the glycoprotein E2 of coronavirus MHV A59 and identification of the trypsin cleavage site. *Virology* **161:** 479.

Maeda, T. and S. Ohnishi. 1980. Activation of influenza virus by acidic media causes hemolysis and fusion of erythrocytes. *FEBS Lett.* **122:** 283.

McCune, J.M., L.B. Rabin, M.B. Feinberg, M. Lieberman, J.C. Kosek, G.R. Reyes, and I.L. Weissmann. 1988. Endoproteolytic cleavage of gp160 is required for the activation of human immunodeficiency virus. *Cell* **53:** 55.

Merkle, R.K., D.E. Helland, J.L. Welles, A. Shilatifard, W.A. Haseltine, and R.D. Cummings. 1991. gp160 of HIV-I synthesized by persistently infected Molt-3 cells is terminally glycosylated: Evidence that cleavage of gp160 occurs subsequent to oligosaccharide processing. *Arch. Biochem. Biophys.* **290:** 248.

Meyer, H., Y. Masuho, and M. Mach. 1990. The gp116 of the gp58/116 complex of human cytomegalovirus represents the amino-terminal part of the precursor molecule and contains a neutralizing epitope. *J. Gen. Virol.* **71:** 2443.

Middleton, Y., M. Tashiro, T. Thai, J. Oh, J. Seymour, E. Pritzer, H.-D. Klenk, R. Rott, and J.T. Seto. 1990. Nucleotide sequence analysis of the genes encoding the HN, M, NP, P and C proteins of two host range mutants of Sendai virus. *Virology* **176:** 656.

Misumi, Y., M. Sohda, and Y. Ikehara. 1990. Sequence of the cDNA encoding rat furin, a possible propeptide-processing endoprotease. *Nucleic Acids Res.* **18:** 6719.

Misumi, Y., K. Oda, T. Fujiwara, N. Takami, K. Tashiro, and Y. Ikehara. 1991. Functional expression of furin demonstrating its intracellular localization and endoprotease activity for processing of proalbumin and complement pro-C3. *J. Biol. Chem.* **266:** 16954.

Mochizuki, Y., M. Tashiro, and M. Homma. 1988. Pneumopathogenicity in mice of a Sendai virus mutant, TSrev-58, is accompanied by in vitro activation with trypsin. *J. Virol.* **62:** 3040.

Moehring, J.M., N.M. Innocencio, B.J. Robertson, and T.J. Moehring. 1993. Expression of mouse furin in a Chinese hamster cell resistant to *Pseudomonas* exotoxin A and viruses complements the genetic lesion. *J. Biol. Chem.* **268:** 2590.

Molloy, S.S., P.A. Bresnahan, K. Klimpel, L. Leppla, and G. Thomas. 1992. Human furin is a calcium-dependent serine endoprotease that recognizes the sequence Arg-X-X-Arg and efficiently cleaves anthrax toxin protective antigen. *J. Biol. Chem.* **267:** 16396.

Molloy, S.S., L. Thomas, J.K. Van Slyke, P.E. Stenberg, and G. Thomas. 1994. Intracellular trafficking and activation of the furin proprotein convertase: Localization to the TGN and recycling from the cell surface. *EMBO J.* **13:** 18.

Morrison, T.G., L.J. Ward, and A. Semerjian. 1985. Intracellular processing of the Newcastle disease virus fusion glycoprotein. *J. Virol.* **53:** 851.

Morsy, J., W. Garten, and R. Rott. 1994. Activation of an influenza virus A/turkey/Oregon/71 HA insertion variant by the subtilisin-like endoprotease furin. *Virology* (in press).

Moulard, M., L. Montagnier, and E. Bahroui. 1994a. Effects of calcium ions on proteolytic processing of HIV-1 gp160 precursor and on cell fusion. *FEBS letters* **338:** 281.

Moulard, M., T. Achstetter, M.P. Kieny, L. Montagnier, and E. Bahraoui. 1994b. Kex2p: A model for cellular endoprotease processing human immunodeficiency virus type 1 (HIV-1) envelope glycoprotein precursor. *Eur. J. Biochem.* (in press).

Munk, K., E. Pritzer, E. Kretzschmar, B. Gutte, W. Garten, and H.-D. Klenk. 1992. Carbohydrate masking of an antigenic epitope of influenza virus haemagglutinin independent of oligosaccharide size. *Glycobiology* **2:** 233.

Naeve, C.W. and R.G. Webster. 1983. Sequence of the hemagglutinin gene from influenza virus. *Virology* **129:** 298.

Nagai, Y., and H.-D. Klenk. 1977. Activation of precursors to both glycoproteins of Newcastle disease virus by proteolytic cleavage. *Virology* **77:** 125.

Nagai, Y., M. Hamaguchi, and T. Toyoda. 1989. Molecular Biology of Newcastle disease virus. *Prog. Vet. Microbiol. Immunol.* **5:** 16.

Nagai, Y., N.M. Inocencio, and B. Gotoh. 1991. Paramyxovirus tropism dependent on host proteases activating the viral fusion glycoprotein. *Behring Inst. Mitt.* **89:** 35.

Nagai, Y., H.-D. Klenk, and R. Rott. 1976a. Proteolytic cleavage of the viral glycoproteins and its significance for the virulence of Newcastle disease virus. *Virology* **72:** 494.

Nagai, Y., H. Ogura, and H.-D. Klenk. 1976b. Studies on the assembly of the envelope of Newcastle disease virus. *Virology* **69:** 523.

Nagai, Y., T. Yoshida, M. Hamaguchi, H. Naruse, M. Iinuma, K. Maeno, and T. Matsumoto. 1980. The pathogenicity of Newcastle disease virus isolated from migrating and domestic ducks and the susceptibility of the viral glycoproteins to proteolytic cleavage. *Microbiol. Immunol.* **24:** 173.

Nagai, Y., K. Shimokata, T. Yoshida, M. Hamaguchi, M. Iinuma, K. Maeno, T. Matsumoto, H.-D. Klenk, and R. Rott. 1979. The spread of a pathogenic and an apathogenic strain of Newcastle disease virus in the chick embryo as depending on the protease sensitivity of the virus glycoproteins. *J. Gen. Virol.* **45:** 263.

Nakagawa, T., M. Hosaka, S. Torii, T. Watanabe, K. Murakami, and K. Nakayama. 1993. Identification and functional expression of a new member of the mammalian Kex2-like processing endoprotease family: Its striking structural similarity to PACE4. *J. Biochem.* **113**: 132.

Nakayama, K., W.-S. Kim, S. Torii, M. Hosaka, T. Nakagawa, J. Ikemisu, T. Baba, and K. Murakami. 1992. Identification of the fourth member of the mammalian endo-protease family homologous to the yeast Kex protease. *J. Biol. Chem.* **267**: 5897.

Ogasawara, T., B. Gotoh, H. Suzuki, A. Jun-ichiro, K. Shimokata, R. Rott, and Y. Nagai. 1992. Expression of factor X and its significance for the determination of paramyxovirus tropism in the chick embryo. *EMBO J.* **11**: 467.

Ohnishi, Y., T. Shioda, K. Nakayama, S. Iwata, B. Gotoh, M. Hamaguchi, and Y. Nagai. 1994. A furin-defective cell line is able to process correctly the gp160 of human immunodeficiency virus type 1. *J. Virol.* **68**: 4075.

Ohuchi, M., R. Ohuchi, and K. Mifune. 1982. Demonstration of hemolytic and fusion activities of influenza C virus. *J. Virol.* **42**: 1076.

Ohuchi, M., M. Orlich, R. Ohuchi, B.E. Simpson, W. Garten, H.-D. Klenk, and R. Rott. 1989. Mutations at the cleavage site of the hemagglutinin alter the pathogenicity of influenza virus A/chick/Penn/83 (H5N2). *Virology* **168**: 274.

Ohuchi, R., M. Ohuchi, W. Garten, and H.-D. Klenk. 1991. Human influenza virus hemagglutinin with high sensitivity to proteolytic activation. *J. Virol.* **65**: 3530.

Orlich, M., D. Khatchikian, A. Teigler, and R. Rott. 1990. Structural variation occurring in the hemagglutinin of influenza virus A/Turkey/Oregon/71 during adaptation to different cell types. *Virology* **176**: 531.

Ortmann, D., M. Ohuchi, H. Angliker, E. Shaw, W. Garten, and H.-D. Klenk. 1994. Proteolytic cleavage of wild type and mutants of the F-protein of human parainfluenza virus type III by two subtilisin-like endoproteases, furin and Kex2. *J. Virol.* **64**: 2772.

Owens, R.J. and R.W. Compans. 1989. Expression of the human immunodeficiency virus envelope is restricted to basolateral surfaces of polarized epithelial cells. *J. Virol.* **63**: 978.

Paterson, R.G., T.J.R. Harris, and R.A. Lamb. 1984. Fusion protein of the paramyxovirus simian virus 5: Nucleotide sequence of mRNA predicts a highly hydrophobic glycoprotein. *Proc. Natl. Acad. Sci.* **81**: 6706.

Paterson, R.G., M.A. Shaughnessy, and R.A. Lamb. 1989. Analysis of the relationship between cleavability of a paramyxovirus fusion protein and length of the connecting peptide. *J. Virol.* **63**: 1293.

Pellett, P.E., M.D. Biggin, B. Barrell, and B. Roizman. 1985a. Epstein-Barr virus genome may encode a protein showing significant amino acid and predicted secondary structure homology with glycoprotein B of herpes simplex virus 1. *J. Virol.* **56**: 807.

Pellett, P.E., K.G. Kousoulas, L. Pereira, and B. Roizman. 1985b. Anatomy of the herpes simplex virus 1 strain F glycoprotein gB gene: Primary sequence and predicted protein structure of the wild-type and of monoclonal antibody-resistant mutants. *J. Virol.* **53**: 243.

Perez, L.G. and E. Hunter. 1987. Mutations within the proteolytic cleavage site of the Rous sarcoma virus glycoprotein that block processing to gp85 and gp37. *J. Virol.* **61**: 1609.

Pfeifer, J.B. and R.W. Compans. 1984. Structure of the influenza C glycoprotein gene as determined from cloned DNA. *Virus Research* **1**: 281.

Porter, A.G., C. Barber, N.H. Carey, R.A. Hallewell, G. Threlfall, and J.S. Emtage. 1979. Complete nucleotide sequence of an influenza virus hemagglutinin gene from cloned DNA. *Nature* **282**: 471.

Presley, J.F., J.M. Polo, R.E. Johnson, and D.T. Brown. 1991. Proteolytic processing of the Sindbis virus membrane protein precursor PE2 is nonessential for growth in vertebrate cells but is required for efficient growth in invertebrate cells. *J. Virol.* **65**: 1905.

Pritzer, E., K. Kuroda, W. Garten, Y. Nagai, and H.-K. Klenk. 1990. A host range mutant of Newcastle disease virus with an altered cleavage site for proteolytic activation of the F protein. *Virus Res.* **15**: 237.

Radsak, K., K.H. Brücher, W. Britt, H. Shiou, D. Schneider, and A. Kollert. 1990. Nuclear compartmentation of glycoprotein B of human cytomegalovirus. *Virology* **177**: 515.

Rasschaert, D. and H. Laude. 1987. The predicted primary structure of the peplomer protein E2 of the porcine coronavirus transmissible gastroenteritis virus. *J. Gen. Virol.* **68**: 1883.

Redding, K., C. Holcomb, and R.S. Fuller. 1991. Immunolocalization of Kex2 protease identifies a putative late Golgi compartment in the yeast *Saccharomyces cerevisiae. J. Cell Biol.* **113**: 527.

Rehemtulla, A., A.J. Dorner, and R.J. Kaufman. 1992. Regulation of PACE propeptide-processing activity: Requirement for a post-endoplasmic reticulum compartment and autoproteolytic activation. *Proc. Natl. Acad. Sci.* **89**: 8235.

Rice, C.M. and J.H. Strauss. 1981. Nucleotide sequence of the 26S mRNA of Sindbis virus and deduced sequence of the encoded virus structural proteins. *Proc. Natl. Acad. Sci.* **78**: 2062.

Rice, C.M., E.M. Lenches, S.R. Eddy, S.J. Shin, R.L. Sheets, and J.H. Strauss. 1985. Nucleotide sequence of yellow fever virus: Implications for flavivirus gene expression and evolution. *Science* **229**: 726.

Richardson, C., D. Hull, P. Greer, K. Hasel, A. Berkovich, G. Englund, W. Bellini, B. Rima, and R. Lazzerini. 1986. The nucleotide sequence of the mRNA encoding the fusion protein of measles virus (Edmonston strain): A comparison of fusion proteins from several different paramyxoviruses. *Virology* **155**: 508.

Robbins, A.K., D.J. Dorney, M.W. Wathen, M.E. Whealy, C. Gold, R.J. Watson, L.E. Holland, S.D. Weed, M. Levine, J.C. Glorioso, and L.W. Enquist. 1987. The pseudorabies virus II gene is closely related to the gB glycoprotein gene of herpes simplex virus. *J. Virol.* **61**: 2691.

Roebroek, A.J.M., J.A. Schalken, J.A.M. Leunissen, C. Onnekink, H.P.J. Bloemers, and W.J.M. van de Ven. 1986. Evolutionary conserved close linkage of the c-*fes/fps* protooncogene and genetic sequences encoding a receptor-like protein. *EMBO J.* **5**: 2197.

Roebroek, A.J.M., J.W.M. Creemers, I.G.L. Pauli, U. Kurzik-Dumke, M. Rentrop, E.A.F. Gateff, J.A.M. Leunissen, and W.J.M. van de Ven. 1992. Cloning and functional expression of Dfurin2, a subtilisin-like proprotein processing enzyme of *Drosophila melanogaster* with multiple repeats of a cysteine motif. *J. Biol. Chem.* **267**: 17208.

Ross, L.J.N., M. Sanderson, S.D. Scott, N.M. Binns, T. Doel, and B. Milne. 1989. Nucleotide sequence and characterization of the Marek's disease virus homologue of glycoprotein B of herpes simplex virus. *J. Gen. Virol.* **70**: 1789.

Rott, R. and H.-D. Klenk. 1988. Molecular basis of infectivity and pathogenicity of Newcastle disease virus. In *Newcastle disease: Developments in veterinary virology* (ed. D.J. Alexander), p. 98, Kluwer Academic, Boston.

Rott, R., M. Orlich, H.-D. Klenk, M.L. Wang, J.J. Skehel, and D.C. Wiley. 1984. Studies on the adaptation of influenza viruses to MDCK cells. *EMBO J.* **3**: 3328.

Salminen, A., J.M. Wahlberg, M. Lobigs, P. Liljeström, and H. Garoff. 1992. Membrane fusion process of Semliki Forest virus II: Cleavage-dependent reorganization of the spike protein complex controls virus entry. *J. Cell Biol.* **116:** 349.

Schalken, J.A., A.J.M. Roebroek, P.P.C.A. Oomen, S.S. Wagenaar, F.M.J. Debruyne, H.P.J. Bloemers, and W.J.M. van de Ven. 1987. *fur* gene expression as a discriminating marker for small cell and nonsmall cell lung carcinomas. *J. Clin. Invest.* **80:** 1545.

Scheiblauer, H., M. Reinacher, M. Tashiro, and R. Rott. 1992. Interactions between bacteria and influenza A virus in the development of influenza pneumonia. *J. Infect. Dis.* **166:** 783.

Scheid, A. and P.W. Choppin. 1974. Identification of biological activities of paramyxovirus glycoproteins. Activation of cell fusion, hemolysis, and infectivity by proteolytic cleavage of an inactive precursor protein of Sendai virus. *Virology* **57:** 470.

—————. 1976. Protease activation mutants of Sendai virus. Activation of biological properites by specific proteases. *Virology* **69:** 265.

Scheid, A., L.A. Caliguiri, R.W. Compans, and P.W. Choppin. 1972. Isolation of paramyxovirus glycoproteins. Association of both hemagglutinating and neuraminidase activities with the larger SV5 glycoprotein. *Virology* **50:** 640.

Scheid, A., M.C. Graves, S.M. Silver, and P.W. Choppin. 1978. Studies on the structure and function of paramyxovirus proteins. In *Negative strand viruses and the host cell* (ed. B.W.J. Mahy and R.D. Barry), p. 181. Academic Press, London.

Schlesinger, S. and M.I. Schlesinger. 1990. Replication of togaviridae and flaviviridae. In *Fields virology,* 2nd edition (ed. B.N. Fields and D.M. Knipe), vol. 1, p. 697. Raven Press, New York.

Schmidt, I., M. Skinner, and S. Siddell. 1987. Nucleotide sequence of gene encoding the surface projection glycoprotein of coronavirus MHV-JHM. *J. Gen. Virol.* **6:** 47.

Schultze, B., H.-J. Gross, R. Brossmer, and G. Herrler. 1991. The S protein of bovine coronavirus is a hemagglutinin recognizing 9-0-acetylated sialic acid as a receptor determinant. *J. Virol.* **65:** 6232.

Schuy, W., W. Garten, D. Linder, and H.-D. Klenk. 1984. The carboxyterminus of the hemagglutinin-neuraminidase of Newcastle disease virus is exposed at the surface of the viral envelope. *Virus Res.* **1:** 415.

Schwartz, D.E., R. Tizard, and W. Gilbert. 1983. Nucleotide sequence of Rous sarcoma virus. *Cell* **32:** 853.

Seidah, N.G., L. Gaspar, P. Mion, M. Marcinkiewicz, M. Mbikay, and M. Chrétien. 1990. cDNA sequence of two distinct pituitary proteins homologous to Kex2 and furin gene products: Tissue-specific mRNAs encoding candidates for pro-hormone processing proteinases. *DNA Cell Biol.* **9:** 415.

Seidah, N.G., M. Marcinkiewicz, S. Benjannet, L. Gaspar, G. Beaubien, M.G. Mattei, C. Lazure, M. Mbikay, and M. Chrétien. 1991. Cloning and primary sequence of a mouse candidate prohormone convertase PC1 homologous to PC2, furin, and Kex2: Distinct chromosomal localization and messenger RNA distribution in brain and pituitary compared to PC2. *Mol. Endocrinol.* **5:** 111.

Simons, K. and H. Garoff. 1980. The budding mechanisms of enveloped animal viruses. *J. Gen. Virol.* **50:** 1.

Skehel, J.J., P.M. Bayley, E.B. Brown, S.R. Martin, M.D. Waterfield, J.M. White, J.A. Wilson, and D.C. Wiley. 1982. Changes in the conformation of influenza virus hemagglutinin at the pH optimum of virus-mediated membrane fusion. *Proc. Natl. Acad. Sci.* **79:** 968.

Sleigh, M.J., G.W. Both, and G.G. Brownlee. 1979. The influenza virus haemagglutinin gene: Cloning and characterization of a double-stranded DNA copy. *Nucleic Acids Res.* **7:** 879.

Smeekens, S.P. and D.F. Steiner. 1990. Identification of a human insulinoma cDNA-encoding a novel mammalian protein structurally related to the yeast dibasic processing protease. *J. Biol. Chem.* **265:** 2997.

Smeekens, S.P., A.S. Avrruch, J. LaMendola, S.J. Chan, and D.F. Steiner. 1991. Identification of a cDNA encoding a second putative prohormone convertase related to PC2 in AtT20 cells and islets of Langerhans. *Proc. Natl. Acad. Sci.* **88:** 340.

Snijder, E.J., J.A. Den Boon, W.J.M. Spaan, M. Weiss, and M.C. Horzinek. 1990. Primary structure and post-translational processing of the Berne virus peplomer protein. *Virology* **178:** 355.

Sonigo, P., M. Alizon, K. Staskus, D. Klatzmann, S. Cole, O. Danos, E. Retzel, P. Tiollais, A. Haase, and S. Wain-Hobson. 1985. Nucleotide sequence of the visna lentivirus: Relationship to the AIDS virus. *Cell* **42:** 369.

Spaete, R.R., R.M. Thayer, W.S. Probert, F.R. Masiarz, S.H. Chamberlain, L. Rasmussen, T.C. Merigan, and C. Pachl. 1988. Human cytomegalovirus strain Towne glycoprotein B is processed by proteolytic cleavage. *Virology* **167:** 207.

Spaete, R.R., A. Sacena, P.I. Scott, G.J. Song, W.S. Probert, W.J. Britt, W.L. Gibson, L. Rasmussen, and C. Pachl. 1990. Sequence requirements for proteolytic processing of glycoprotein B of human cytomegalovirus strain Towne. *J. Virol.* **64:** 2922.

Spriggs, M.K., R.O. Olmsted, S. Venkatesan, J.E. Coligan, and P.L. Collins. 1986. Fusion glycoprotein of human parainfluenza virus type 3: Nucleotide sequence of the gene, direct identification of the cleavage-activation site and comparison with other paramyxoviruses. *Virology* **152:** 241.

Stauber, R., M. Pfleiderer, and S. Siddell. 1993. Proteolytic cleavage of the murine coronavirus surface glycoprotein is not required for fusion activity. *J. Gen. Virol.* **74:** 183.

Steiner, D.F., S.P. Smeekens, S. Ohagi, and S.J. Chan. 1992. The new enzymology of precursor processing endoproteases. *J. Biol. Chem.* **267:** 23435.

Stieneke-Gröber, A., M. Vey, H. Angliker, E. Shaw, G. Thomas, C. Roberts, H.-D. Klenk, and W. Garten. 1992. Influenza virus hemagglutinin with multibasic cleavage site is activated by furin, a subtilisin-like endoprotease. *EMBO J.* **11:** 2407.

Storz, J., R. Rott, and G. Kaluza. 1981. Enhancement of plaque formation and cell fusion of an enteropathogenic coronavirus by trypsin treatment. *Infect. Immun.* **31:** 1214.

Sturman, L.S., C.S. Ricard, and K.V. Holmes. 1985. Proteolytic cleavage of the E2 glycoprotein of murine coronavirus: Activation of cell-fusing activity of virions by trypsin and separation of two different 90K cleavage fragments. *J. Virol.* **56:** 904.

Sumiyoshi, H., K. Morita, C. Mori, I. Fuke, T. Shiba, Y. Sakaki, and A. Igarashi. 1986. Sequence of 3000 nucleotides at the 5′ end of Japanese encephalitis virus. *Gene* **48:** 195.

Tashiro, M. and M. Homma. 1983a. Pneumotropism of Sendai virus in relation to protease-mediated activation in mouse lungs. *Infect. Immun.* **39:** 879.

―――. 1983b. Evidence of proteolytic activation of Sendai virus in mouse lungs. *Arch. Virol.* **77:** 127.

―――. 1985. Protection of mice from wild-type Sendai virus infection by a trypsin-resistant mutant, TR-2. *J. Virol.* **53:** 228.

Tashiro, M., H.-D. Klenk, and R. Rott. 1987a. Inhibitory effect of a protease inhibitor, leupeptin, on the development of influenza pneumonia, mediated by concomitant bacteria. *J. Gen. Virol.* **68:** 2039.

Tashiro, M., Y. Fujii, K. Nakamura, and M. Homma. 1988a. Cell-mediated immunity induced in mice after vaccination with a protease activation mutant, TR-2, of Sendai virus. *J. Virol.* **62:** 2490.

Tashiro, M., K. Tobita, J.T. Seto, and R. Rott. 1989. Comparison of protective effects of serum antibody on respiratory and systemic infection of Sendai virus in mice. *Arch. Virol.* **107:** 85.

Tashiro, M., P. Ciborowski, H.-D. Klenk, G. Pulverer, and R. Rott. 1987b. Role of *staphylococcal* protease on the development of influenza pneumonia. *Nature* **325:** 536.

Tashiro, M., P. Ciborowski, M. Reinacher, G. Pulverer, H.-D. Klenk, and R. Rott. 1987c. Synergistic role of staphylococcal proteases in the induction of influenza virus pathogenicity. *Virology* **157:** 421.

Tashiro, M., J.T. Seto, S. Choosakul, H. Hegemann, H.-D. Klenk, and R. Rott. 1992a. Changes in specific cleavability of the Sendai virus fusion protein: Implications for pathogenicity in mice. *J. Gen. Virol.* **73:** 1575.

Tashiro, M., M. Yamakawa, K. Tobita, H.-D. Klenk, R. Rott, and J.T. Seto. 1990a. Organ tropism of Sendai virus in mice: Proteolytic activation of the fusion glycoprotein in mouse organs and budding site at the bronchial epithelium. *J. Virol.* **64:** 3627.

Tashiro, M., M. Yamakawa, K. Tobita, J.T. Seto, H.-D. Klenk, and R. Rott. 1990b. Altered budding site of a pantropic mutant of Sendai virus, F1-R, in the polarized epithelial cell. *J. Virol..* **64:** 4672.

Tashiro, M., Y. Yokogoshi, K. Tobita, J.T. Seto, R. Rott, and H. Kido. 1992b. Tryptase Clara an activating protease for Sendai virus in rat lungs that is involved in pneumopathogenicity. *J. Virol.* **66:** 7211.

Tashiro, M., I. James, S. Karri, K. Wahn, K. Tobita, H.-D. Klenk, R. Rott, and I.T. Seto. 1991. Pneumotropic revertants derived from a pantropic mutant, F1-R, of Sendai virus. *Virology* **184:** 227.

Tashiro, M., E. Pritzer, E.A. Koshnan, M. Yamakawa, K. Kuroda, H.-D. Klenk, R. Rott, and J.T. Seto. 1988b. Characterization of a pantropic variant of Sendai virus derived from a host range mutant. *Virology* **165:** 577.

Thim, L., M.T. Hansen, K. Norris, I. Hoegh, E. Boel, J. Forstrom, G. Ammerer, and N.P. Fiil. 1986. Secretion and processing of insulin precursors in yeast. *Proc. Natl. Acad. Sci.* **83:** 6766.

Thomas, G., B.A. Thorne, L. Thomas, R.G. Allen, D.E. Hruby, R. Fuller, and J. Thorner. 1988. Yeast kex2 endopeptidase correctly cleaves a neuroendocrine prohormone in mammalian cells. *Science* **241:** 226.

Thomas, L., R. Leduc, B.A. Thorne, S.P. Smeekens, D.F. Steiner, and G. Thomas. 1991. Kex2-like endoproteases PC2 and PC3 accurately cleave a model prohormone in mammalian cells: Evidence for a common core of neuroendocrine processing enzymes. *Proc. Natl. Acad. Sci.* **88:** 5297.

Toyoda, T., T. Sakaguchi, K. Imai, N.M. Inocencio, B. Gotoh, M. Hamaguchi, and Y. Nagai. 1987. Structural comparison of the cleavage-activation site of the fusion glycoprotein between virulent and avirulent strains of Newcastle disease virus. *Virology* **158:** 242.

Tsai, W.P. and S. Oroszlan. 1988. Novel glycosylation pathways of retroviral envelope proteins identified with avian reticuloendotheliosis virus. *J. Virol.* **62:** 3167.

Tsukiyama, K., Y. Yoshikawa, and K. Yamanouchi. 1988. Fusion glycoprotein (F) of rinderpest virus: Entire nucleotide sequence of the F mRNA, and several features of the F protein. *Virology* **164:** 523.

Ulmer, J.B. and G.E. Palade. 1991. Effects of brefeldin A on the processing of viral envelope glycoproteins in murine erythroleukemia cells. *J. Biol. Chem.* **266:** 9173.

van den Ouweland, A.M.W., H.L.P. Duijnhoven, G.D. Keizer, L.C.J. Dorssens, and W.J.M. van de Ven. 1990. Structural homology between the human fur gene product and the subtilisin-like protease encoded by yeast KEX2. *Nucleic Acids Res.* **18:** 664.

Vey, M., M. Orlich, S. Adler, H.-D. Klenk, R. Rott, and W. Garten. 1992. Hemagglutinin activation of pathogenic avian influenza viruses of serotype H7 requires the protease recognition motif R-X-K/R-R. *Virology* **188**: 408.

Vey, M., W. Schäfer, B. Reis, R. Ohuchi, W. Britt, W. Garten, H.-D. Klenk, and K. Radsak. 1995. Proteolytic processing of human cytomegalovirus glycoprotein B. *Virology* (in press).

Wahlberg, J.M., W.A. Boere, and H. Garoff. 1989. The heterodimeric association between the membrane proteins of Semliki Forest virus changes its sensitivity to mildly acidic pH during virus maturation. *J. Virol.* **63**: 4991.

Watanabe, T., N. Tsutoma, J. Ikemizu, M. Nagahama, K. Murakami, and K. Nakayama. 1992. Sequence requirements for precursor cleavage within the constitutive secretory pathway. *J. Biol. Chem.* **267**: 8270.

Watson, D.G. and J.M. Moehring. 1991. A mutant CHO-K1 strain with resistance to *Pseudomonas* exotoxin A and alphaviruses fails to cleave Sindbis virus glycoprotein PE2. *J. Virol.* **65**: 2332.

Waxham, M.N., A.C. Server, H.M. Goodman, and J.S. Wolinsky. 1987. Cloning and sequencing of the mumps virus fusion protein gene. *Virology* **159**: 381.

Whalley, J.M., G.R. Robertson, N.A. Scott, G.C. Hudson, C.W. Bell, and L.M. Woodworth. 1989. Identification and nucleotide sequence of a gene in equine herpesvirus 1 analogous to the herpes simplex virus gene encoding the major envelope glycoprotein gB. *J. Gen. Virol.* **70**: 383.

White, J.M. 1992. Membrane fusion. *Science* **258**: 917.

White, J.M., K. Matlin, and A. Helenius. 1981. Cell fusion by Semliki Forest influenza, and vesicular stomatitis viruses. *J. Cell. Biol.* **89**: 674.

Willey, R.C., J.S. Bonifacino, B.J. Potts, M.A. Martin, and R.D. Klausner. 1988. Biosynthesis cleavage, and degradation of the human immunodeficiency virus 1 envelope glycoprotein gp160. *Proc. Nat. Acad. Sci.* **85**: 9580.

Willey, R.C., T. Klimkeit, D.M. Frucht, J.S. Bonifacino, and M.A. Martin. 1991. Mutations within the human immunodeficiency virus tpye 1 gp160 envelope glycoprotein alter its intracellular transport and processing. *Virology* **184**: 319.

Wilson, J.A., J.J. Skehel, and D.C. Wiley. 1981. Structure of the haemagglutinin membrane glycoprotein of influenza virus at 3Å resolution. *Nature* **289**: 366.

Wise, R.J., P.J. Barr, P.A. Wong, M.C. Kiefer, A.J. Brake, and R.J. Kaufman. 1990. Expression of a human proprotein processing enzyme: Correct cleavage of the von Willebrand factor precursor at paired basic amino acid site. *Proc. Natl. Acad. Sci.* **87**: 9378.

WuDann, D. and P.G. Spear. 1989. Initial interaction of herpes simplex virus with cells is binding to heparan sulfate. *J. Virol.* **63**: 52.

Wünsch, M., A.S. Schulz, W. Koch, R. Friedrich, and G. Hunsmann. 1983. Sequence analysis of Gardner-Arnstein feline leukemia virus envelope gene reveals common structural properties of mammalian retroviral envelope gene. *EMBO J.* **2**: 2239.

Yoshida, T., Y. Nakayama, H. Nagura, T. Toyoda, K. Nishikawa, M. Hamaguchi, and Y. Nagai. 1986. Inhibition of the assembly of Newcastle disease virus by monensin. *Virus Res.* **4**: 179.

Yu, Q., P.J. Davis, T. Barrett, M.M. Binns, M.E.G. Boursnell, and D. Cavanagh. 1991. Deduced amino acid sequence of the fusion glycoprotein of turkey rhinotracheitis virus has greater identity with that of human respiratory syncytial virus, a pneumovirus, than that of paramyxoviruses and morbilliviruses. *J. Gen. Virol.* **72**: 75.

Zhirnov, O.P., A.V. Ovcharenka, and A.G. Bukrinskaya. 1982. Proteolytic activation of influenza WSN virus in culture cells is performed by homologous plasma enzymes. *J. Gen. Virol.* **63**: 469.

————.1984. Suppression of influenza virus replication in infected mice by protease inhibitors. *J. Gen. Virol.* **65:** 191.

15

Fusion of Influenza Virus in Endosomes: Role of the Hemagglutinin

Judith M. White
Department of Pharmacology
University of California
San Francisco, California 94143-0450

Influenza virus enters cells by receptor-mediated endocytosis. Consequently, the virus is delivered to mildly acidic intracellular organelles called endosomes (see Marsh and Pelchen-Matthews, this volume). The next step in the virus entry pathway is fusion between the viral membrane and the endosomal membrane, a process that provides a nondisruptive and efficient means for the virus to deliver its genome into the cytoplasm to initiate the replication cycle. Consistent with the intracellular site of genome penetration, the fusion activity of influenza virus is triggered by the mildly acidic pH of the endosomal lumen. Although the exact pH dependence for fusion differs for different strains of influenza, all strains demonstrate sharp pH profiles with midpoints in the pH 5 to pH 6 range. The low-pH-induced fusion reaction of influenza virus has been the object of much study and has served as a paradigm for the fusion reactions of other enveloped viruses that enter cells by receptor-mediated endocytosis.

The process of influenza virus fusion is mediated by its membrane fusion protein, the hemagglutinin (HA). HA is the product of a single gene. This fact, coupled with knowledge of the structure of HA to high resolution (Wilson et al. 1981), has attracted many investigators to study details of how the HA protein causes membrane fusion. The working model for HA-mediated membrane fusion entails three major steps: a low-pH-induced conformational change in HA, a hydrophobic interaction between HA and the target membrane, and the formation and opening of a fusion pore. During the last step, the lipids at the fusion site are rearranged.

It is clear from the preceding scenario that the fusion reaction is mediated by conformational changes *both* in the HA protein and in the

Present address: Department of Cell Biology, University of Virginia, Health Sciences Center, P.O. Box 439, Charlottesville, Virginia 22908.

lipids at the fusion site. Recent work has begun to dissect these transitions. There have been many recent comprehensive review articles on the subject of HA-mediated membrane fusion (Wiley and Skehel 1987; Stegmann et al. 1989; Steinhauer et al. 1992; White 1992; Bentz et al. 1993; Brunner and Tsurudome 1993; Clague et al. 1993; Doms 1993; Siegel 1993; Stegmann and Helenius 1993; Wilschut and Bron 1993). The purpose of this chapter is to highlight recent work on the conformational intermediates that form in the HA protein and in the lipids during the fusion reaction. In so doing, I aim to shed light on a major current challenge: to determine what conformation the HA protein is in during each stage of the lipid rearrangements that lead to the opening of the fusion pore.

CONFORMATIONAL CHANGES IN THE HA PROTEIN

Structure of the HA at Neutral pH

The hemagglutinin is a homotrimer. Each monomer contains two subunits, HA1 and HA2 (Fig. 1A). The HA1 subunits form the globular head domains which sit atop and largely shield the HA2 stem (Fig. 1A). The HA1 subunits contain both the receptor-binding sites, found near the top of the trimer, and the major antigenic determinants of the protein (Wiley and Skehel 1987; Wilson and Cox 1990). The HA2 subunits form the fibrous stem which is built around a coiled coil of three long (~70 Å) α helices, one from each monomer. Each HA2 subunit possesses two hydrophobic sequences that are critical for membrane fusion—the fusion peptide at the amino-terminal end and the transmembrane domain close to the carboxy-terminal end. The fusion peptide, residues 1–24 of the HA2 subunit (Fig. 1B), was postulated to play a key role in eliciting membrane fusion based on its similarity to the fusion peptide of Sendai virus in both location (amino-terminal) and composition (apolar). When the X-ray structure revealed that the fusion peptide is tucked in the interface of the native (pH 7) HA trimer, and when biological experiments revealed that fusion of influenza virus only occurs at low pH, a logical deduction was that low pH causes a conformational change in HA that liberates its fusion peptides for interaction with the target membrane. This prediction has proven to be true for all HAs studied to date.

Analysis of the Low-pH-induced Conformational Change

There are three major types (A, B, and C) and many subtypes of influenza virus (Murphy and Webster 1990). Conformational changes have been detected for HAs from all major types and for many subtypes

A   B   C   D

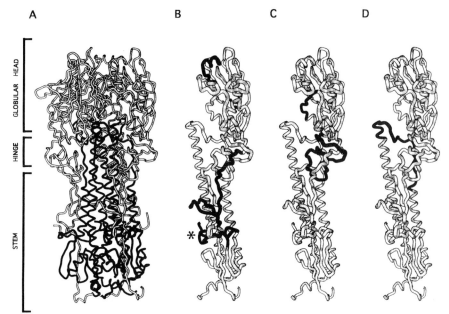

GLOBULAR HEAD

HINGE

STEM

Figure 1 Structure of the HA trimer (*A*) and the HA monomer (*B–D*). The thick black lines in *A* represent the HA2 subunits (Wilson et al. 1981; Wiley and Skehel 1987). The thick black lines in *B* and *C* represent segments of HA that change antibody reactivity during stage I and stage II of the low-pH-induced conformational change, respectively (White and Wilson 1987; Kemble et al. 1992). The asterisk in *B* is beside the fusion peptide. The thick black line in *D* represents a loop (HA2 residues 54–81) that adopts a helical configuration in response to low pH (Carr and Kim 1993; P.A. Bullough et al., pers. comm.).

(Doms 1993). These changes have been studied using a variety of biochemical (e.g., sensitivity to proteases and reducing agents, photo-chemical labeling, sedimentation analysis, changes in hydrophobicity), biophysical (e.g., circular dichroism and fluorescence spectroscopy), im-munological (e.g., altered antibody reactivity), and morphological (e.g., electron microscopy) techniques. Aspects of the conformational change have also been inferred from the selection and characterization of mutant HAs that display altered pH dependencies of fusion. A majority of the work on the conformational change has been performed on HA from the X:31 strain of influenza virus (type A; subtype H3), since the X:31 HA is the only HA whose structure is known to high resolution. Knowledge of the native (neutral pH; prefusogenic) structure has allowed meaningful interpretation of the biochemical, biophysical, and immunological con-sequences of exposure to low pH, as well as the phenotypes of mutant HAs. It is important to note that details of pH-, time-, and temperature-dependence, as well as the extent of conformational changes, differ for HAs from different virus types and subtypes (Ellens et al. 1990; Formanowski et al. 1990; Puri et al. 1990; Gutman et al. 1993). Unless otherwise stated, the ensuing discussion refers to the X:31 HA or to its close relative X:47 (type A; subtype H3).

The Conformational Change Occurs in Two Major Stages

Studies with antibodies against defined epitopes have suggested that the low-pH-induced conformational change in HA occurs in two major stages. In the first stage, alterations occur in the stem region of the molecule (White and Wilson 1987) and at the tips of the globular head domains (Kemble et al. 1992). Notably, these changes result in exposure of the fusion peptides. In the second stage, changes occur in the hinge and head regions of HA, suggesting a concerted and substantial dissociation of the globular head domains from each other (White and Wilson 1987). The first stage of the conformational change appears to be relatively temperature-independent, occurring over the same approximate time course at 25°C and at 37°C. In contrast, the second stage of the conformational change appears to be temperature-dependent: At 25°C, the change occurs considerably more slowly, and only after a substantial lag phase, than at 37°C (White and Wilson 1987). Examples of changes that occur during stage I and stage II of the conformational change are highlighted in Figure 1, B and C, respectively. A schematic view of these conformational intermediates is given in Figure 2.

Recent studies have supported the two-stage conformational change model. When X:31 and X:47 influenza viruses, among others, are acid-pretreated at 37°C in the *absence* of a target membrane, their previously rodlike HA spikes become wiry and disorganized as viewed in the electron microscope (Fig. 2) (Stegmann et al. 1987; Puri et al. 1990). Consistent with these changes, acid pretreatment at 37°C causes significant reductions in both the rotational (Junankar and Cherry 1986) and lateral (Gutman et al. 1993) mobility of HA in the plane of the membrane. However, if acid pretreatment is conducted at 0°C, the sturdy rod-like morphology of the HA spike is maintained (Stegmann et al. 1987), even though its fusion peptides have become exposed (Stegmann et al. 1990). These results are consistent with the hypothesis that HA progresses to a stage I- but not to a stage II-like conformation (Fig. 2) at 0°C.

In contrast to subtype H3 influenza A viruses (e.g., X:31 and X:47), the Japan strain of influenza (type A; subtype H2) is not rendered fusion-inactive by acid pretreatment at 37°C (at pH 5 for up to at least 15 min; Ellens et al. 1990; Puri et al. 1990). Moreover, even though its fusion

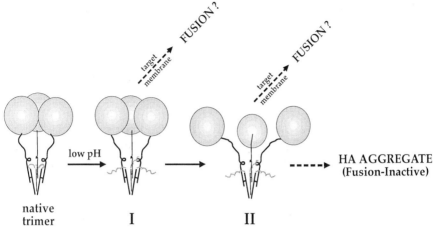

Figure 2   Stages in the low-pH-induced conformational change in HA (*horizontal arrows*) as they may relate to fusion (*angled dashed arrows*) and fusion-inactivation (*horizontal dashed arrow*). Gray segment in the stem represents the fusion peptide. In stage I, changes occur in the stem of the trimer and at the tips of the globular head domains, but the globular head domains do not dissociate substantially from each other (White and Wilson 1987; Kemble et al. 1992) and the spike maintains its sturdy rod-like morphology (Stegmann et al. 1987). In stage II, additional changes occur in the globular head domains, consistent with their substantial dissociation from one another (White and Wilson 1987). Stage II HA appears wiry and disorganized in the electron microscope (Stegmann et al. 1987). If X:31 HA is exposed to low pH in the absence of target membranes, it forms fusion-inactive aggregates (Stegmann et al. 1987; Ruigrok et al. 1988). (Adapted from Kemble et al. 1992.)

peptides are exposed by acid pretreatment, the gross morphology of the Japan HA spike is not altered (Puri et al. 1990), and it remains laterally mobile in the plane of the membrane (Gutman et al. 1993). These latter results suggest that when exposed to pH 5, even at 37°C, the Japan HA assumes a stage-I-like conformation but does not progress to a stage-II-like conformation.

What Is the Fusion-active Conformation of HA?

The native pH 7 conformation of HA is not fusogenic. As noted before, if X:31 influenza virus is acid-pretreated, the HA spike becomes disorganized as viewed in the electron microscope and relatively immobile in the plane of the membrane. Immobilization likely reflects aggregation through the exposed fusion peptides, as this occurs when the isolated HA ectodomain is acid-pretreated (Ruigrok et al. 1988). As a result of acid pretreatment, the fusion activity of X:31 HA is irreversibly inactivated.

Hence, the "end state" aggregated conformation of X:31 HA is not fusogenic (Fig. 2). A current challenge is to determine whether stage I or stage II HA more closely approximates the "fusion-active" conformation (Fig. 2).

The available evidence suggests that HA must progress at least as far as stage I (Fig. 2) in order to be fusogenic. If the fusion peptides are held in place by either small molecules (Bodian et al. 1993) or disulfide bonds engineered into the globular head domains (Godley et al. 1992; Kemble et al. 1992), the fusion activity of HA is greatly impaired. In addition, we have recently noted that some motion, consistent with a partial dissociation of the globular head domains, occurs during the first stage of the conformational change (Kemble et al. 1992). Since this motion is inhibited in the mutant HA with engineered disulfide bonds (Kemble et al. 1992), partial dissociation of the globular head domains is likely required to liberate the fusion peptides, and hence for HA to be fusogenic.

Studies with the disulfide-bonded mutant HA (Godley et al. 1992; Kemble et al. 1992) do not, however, indicate how far the globular head domains must dissociate in order for HA to be fusogenic. In other words, the question of whether HA must progress to (or toward) a stage-II-like conformation in order to be fusogenic is still open. Three lines of evidence suggest that major dissociation of the globular head domains (i.e., a stage-II-like conformation) is *not* required for X:31 HA to mediate a fusion reaction. First, fusion can occur at 0°C even though the globular head domains do not dissociate substantially from each other (Stegmann et al. 1990). Second, the time course for X:31 influenza virus fusion at 37°C, as assessed by a lipid mixing assay (Stegmann et al. 1986), more closely resembles that of the stage I, rather than the stage II, conformational changes (White and Wilson 1987). Third, there is a correlation between fusion-inactivation and stage II conformational changes (Junankar and Cherry 1986; Puri et al. 1990; Stegmann et al. 1990; Gutman et al. 1993). In the context of this discussion, it is also worth noting that the Japan HA (type A; subtype H2) appears to be fully fusogenic in a stage-I-like conformation (Puri et al. 1990).

There are two caveats to the previous suggestions that a stage-II-like conformation is not required to manifest the fusion activity of X:31 influenza virus. First, each fusion site (Fig. 3) uses only a small proportion of the HAs found on the virion surface (T. Danieli et al., in prep.). The biochemical, biophysical, and immunological assays that have been used to analyze the conformational change would not have detected changes in a few HA molecules clustered and sandwiched at the fusion site (Fig. 3). Second, most of the assays that have been used to describe the kinetics of fusion have monitored mixing between outer leaflet lipids,

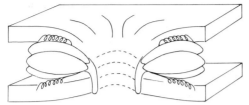

Figure 3 Schematic drawing of the HA fusion pore representing several conformationally altered (e.g., stage-I-like; Fig. 2) HA trimers at the fusion site. Note that if the membranes dimple more closely to one another (Chandler 1991; Wilschut and Bron 1993), the HA ectodomains need not tilt with respect to their transmembrane domains. (Adapted from White 1992.)

and hence only the *initiation* of the fusion reaction. From this initial "hemifusion" state (Kemble et al. 1994), a fusion pore (Fig. 3) must open and then dilate (Fig. 4). These later stages of the fusion reaction can only be assessed by electrophysiological techniques (Spruce et al. 1989, 1991) or by soluble content mixing assays (Sarkar et al. 1989). Hence, it is formally possible that a stage-II-like conformation is not required to initiate a fusion reaction (i.e., to form a hemifusion intermediate), but that it is required to complete the fusion process (i.e., to open or dilate the fusion pore). Arguing against this latter possibility, however, is an electron micrograph showing complete fusion between influenza virus and liposomes at 0°C, conditions under which stage II conformational changes were not detected (Stegmann et al. 1990).

Possible Role of a Low-pH-induced Loop-to-Helix Transition

A recent paper (Carr and Kim 1993) has focused attention on another part of HA that may play a role in the fusion reaction: HA2 residues 54–81. In the structure of X:31 HA at neutral pH, this segment forms a loop (highlighted in Fig. 1D) between the short α helix adjacent to the fusion peptide and the long α helix that forms the structural support for the HA trimer (Fig. 1A). Prior to the solution of the X-ray structure, it was predicted that HA2 residues 54–81 would be part of a longer α-helical coiled coil (Ward and Dopheide 1980). In this recent study (Carr and Kim 1993), synthetic peptides corresponding to this loop were shown to form a helical coiled coil, but only at low pH. More recent high-resolution structural studies have shown that this region is indeed in the form of an extended helical coiled coil in low-pH-treated HA devoid of the globular head domains and fusion peptides (P.A. Bullough et al. pers. comm.). Following this low-pH-dependent loop-to-helix transition, the fusion peptides are predicted to be at the top of the HA trimer.

Several questions remain regarding the low-pH-induced loop-to-helix transition of HA2 residues 54–81. For example, is dissociation of the globular head domains required for the extended coiled coil to form? If

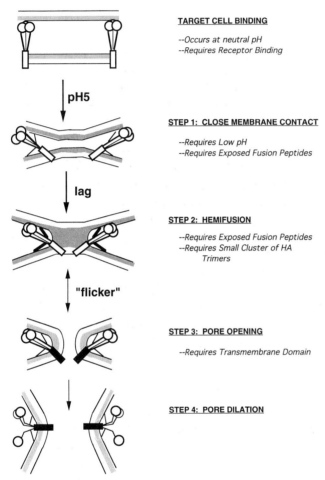

Figure 4 Steps in HA-mediated membrane fusion. Subsequent to membrane binding, mediated through receptor-binding sites located at the top of the trimer, and exposure to low pH, there are at least four steps involved in forming and opening a fusion pore: *step 1*, close membrane contact (Harter et al. 1989; Stegmann et al. 1990, 1991; Brunner et al. 1991); *step 2*, hemifusion (Kemble et al. 1994); *step 3*, pore opening; and *step 4*, pore dilation (Sarkar et al. 1989; Spruce et al. 1989, 1991). Proposed requirements for each step are indicated. HA is shown in a stage-I-like conformation (Fig. 2) in steps 1–3, as it remains an open question as to whether a stage-II-like conformation is required for any stage of the fusion reaction (see text). In step 4, HA is shown in a stage-II-like conformation (Fig. 2), as it assumes this conformation after fusion at 37°C (Stegmann et al. 1987). (Adapted from Kemble et al. 1994).

so, how much motion is required; does the loop-to-helix transition occur during the first or the second stage of the conformational change? Is this loop-to-helix transition relevant to fusion? If so, to what stage (Fig. 4) of the fusion reaction?

INTERACTION BETWEEN HA AND THE TARGET MEMBRANE

It has been known for some time that the low-pH-induced conformational changes in HA cause the HA ectodomain to become hydrophobic, as assessed by its binding to liposomes or its partitioning into the detergent TX-114 (Doms 1993). Photochemical labeling studies have suggested that this interaction occurs via the fusion peptides (Harter et al. 1989), although other parts of the trimer may be involved (Burger et al. 1991). The fusion peptide sequence is remarkably well conserved, especially among influenza A viruses (Bodian 1992). Its importance for fusion has been documented by the existence of fusion peptide mutants that are devoid of fusion activity (Gething et al. 1986) and by the recent demonstrations that preventing fusion peptide exposure abolishes fusion activity (Godley et al. 1992; Kemble et al. 1992; Bodian et al. 1993). Several issues should be considered in contemplating the role(s) of the fusion peptides in membrane fusion: (1) What is the conformation of HA when the fusion peptides bind to the target membrane (Fig. 2)? (2) When during the overall scheme of membrane fusion do the fusion peptides bind (Fig. 4)? (3) What is the structure of the fusion peptides as they bind to the target membrane? (4) At what angle with respect to the bilayer(s) do they bind? (5) Do the fusion peptides bind to the viral membrane as well as to the target membrane? Each issue is addressed briefly below.

What Is the Conformation of HA When the Fusion Peptides Bind to the Target Membrane?

Several lines of evidence suggest that exposure of the fusion peptides is an early event in the low-pH-induced conformational change of HAs from different influenza A subtypes (White and Wilson 1987; Puri et al. 1990). Recent studies (Brunner et al. 1991; Stegmann et al. 1991) have suggested that the hydrophobic association of the HA ectodomain with the target membrane is also an early event. Moreover, the time course for virus binding to liposomes mirrors the time course for exposure of the fusion peptides (Stegmann et al. 1990). Hence, our current picture is that a stage-I-like conformation (Fig. 2) is necessary and sufficient for HA to bind hydrophobically to target membranes.

When during the Overall Scheme of Membrane Fusion Do the Fusion Peptides Bind?

Shortly after exposure to low pH, the fusion peptides bind hydrophobically to the target membrane. This association probably brings the two opposed bilayers into close contact (Fig. 4; step 1). By conducting fusion reactions at 0°C, hydrophobic binding to the target membrane, taken here as a measure of close membrane contact, has been shown to occur well before the onset of outer leaflet lipid mixing (Stegmann et al. 1991), the next stage of the fusion reaction (Fig. 4; step 2). Hence, hydrophobic binding between HA and the target membrane appears to be necessary, but not sufficient, to induce membrane fusion.

In addition to their role in bringing membranes into close contact (Fig. 4; step 1), the fusion peptides play an active role in forming the postulated hemifusion intermediate (Fig. 4; step 2). This conclusion is based on the observations that mutations in the fusion peptide (Gething et al. 1986; Guy et al. 1992) or mutations that prevent fusion peptide exposure (Godley et al. 1992; Kemble et al. 1992) prevent outer leaflet lipid mixing. Notably, the fusion peptide mutant (Gly1 to Glu) shows no fusion activity (Gething et al. 1986; Guy et al. 1992), even though it can bind to target membranes, albeit more slowly and less efficiently than the wild type (Gething et al. 1986). Recent studies (Tsurudome et al. 1992) with HA from the PR8 strain of influenza virus (type A, subtype H1) have suggested that there might be an initial binding interaction involving a limited number of fusion peptides (e.g., Fig. 4; step 1), followed by the engagement of more fusion peptides coincident with the onset of lipid mixing (Fig. 4; step 2). However, bimodal fusion peptide interactions have not been observed for the X:31 HA (Stegmann et al. 1991).

What Is the Structure of the Fusion Peptides as They Bind to the Target Membrane?

In the native pH 7 structure of the influenza HA, the fusion peptides are in a coil with two tight turns (Fig. 1B). The possibility that the fusion peptides interact with the target membrane as a helix has been raised on the basis of several indirect lines of evidence: If modeled as an α helix, the fusion peptides conform to an α helix with one strongly hydrophobic face (see Fig. 1C in White 1992). A synthetic fusion peptide adopts a helical configuration at a membrane surface (Lear and DeGrado 1987; Rafalski et al. 1991). Photochemical labeling studies with the reagent [^{125}I]TID have suggested (Harter et al. 1989) that the fusion peptides of the isolated HA ectodomain interact with membranes through the hydrophobic face of the predicted α helix (but see also Gallaher et al. 1992). A synthetic fusion peptide, derived from a mutant HA (Gly1 to Glu) with no detectable fusion activity (Gething et al. 1986), shows a reduced tendency to form an α helix at a membrane interface (Rafalski et al. 1991). The reduced propensity of the mutant fusion peptide to form an α helix may correlate with its altered membrane-binding properties (Gething et al. 1986). Collectively, these studies suggest that the fusion peptides adopt a helical configuration at *some stage* of their interaction with the target membrane (Fig. 4). However, whether the fusion peptides of viral HA actually form a helix during the course of a fusion reaction, and precisely which residues of the fusion peptides bind to the target membrane, remain open questions (Gallaher et al. 1992; White 1992; Brunner and Tsurudome 1993). Even if the fusion peptides adopt a helical configuration at some stage of the fusion reaction, this would not preclude them from adopting a different conformation (e.g., β sheet, random coil) at a different stage of the fusion reaction (Rafalski et al. 1990).

At What Angle with Respect to the Bilayer(s) Do the Fusion Peptides Bind?

In an early model (White et al. 1986), the fusion peptides were envisioned to engage the target membrane perpendicular to the plane of the bilayer (i.e., like a dagger). Photochemical labeling studies with the isolated soluble HA ectodomain and asymmetrically labeled target bilayers suggested (Brunner 1989) that the fusion peptides bind parallel to the outer leaflet of the target bilayer. Hence, the first photochemical labeling studies appeared to rule out the early model. Due to limitations in using the soluble HA ectodomain, which can interact with target membranes in ways not accessible to membrane-anchored HA, this question has recently been reexamined using viral HA and radiolabeled phospholipid analogs of defined orientation (Stegmann et al. 1991). The recent results strongly suggest that, rather than interacting exclusively with the surface of the bilayer, the fusion peptides of viral HA engage the target bilayer more deeply, perhaps as originally envisioned (i.e., perpendicular to the plane of the bilayer), or perhaps at an oblique angle, as has been proposed for other viral fusion peptides (Brasseur et al. 1990). As it is possible that the fusion peptides play distinct roles at different stages of the fusion process (Stegmann et al. 1991; Guy et al. 1992; Schoch and Blumenthal 1993; Kemble et al. 1994), they may do so at different angles. In other words, a superficial interaction parallel to the plane of the bilayers may be followed by a more invasive interaction.

Do the Fusion Peptides Bind to the Viral Membrane as Well as to the Target Membrane?

It has been shown that the fusion peptides of viral HA interact with lipids in the target membrane (Harter et al. 1989; Stegmann et al. 1990, 1991). In addition, several current models (White 1992; Bentz et al. 1993; Stegmann and Helenius 1993) envision simultaneous interactions with the viral bilayer as well (Fig. 3). Interaction with the viral membrane was proposed previously, based on morphological observations of low-pH-treated HA (Ruigrok et al. 1986). Binding of fusion peptides from one HA trimer with both the viral and the target bilayers could serve to foster close membrane contact (Fig. 3; Fig. 4, step 1) (White 1992; Stegmann and Helenius 1993). Alternatively, the fusion peptides might serve as a surface for the mixing of viral and target lipids (Bentz et al. 1993). Experiments must now be designed to look for association between the fusion peptides and the viral membrane during the course of a fusion reaction.

FORMATION AND OPENING OF THE FUSION PORE

The low-pH-induced conformational alterations in HA and the resulting protein/lipid interaction disturb the lipids of the viral and target bilayers and ultimately lead to fusion. Fusion is now considered to proceed via the opening of a fusion pore. The concept of a fusion pore is derived largely from ultrastructural (Heuser and Reese 1981; Burger et al. 1988; Knoll et al. 1988; Chandler 1991; Curran et al. 1993) and electrophysiological (Spruce et al. 1989, 1991; Almers et al. 1991; Zimmerberg et al. 1991; Monck and Fernandez 1992) studies, many of regulated exocytosis. In a number of secretory systems, patch-clamp studies have monitored the increased membrane capacitance that accompanies vesicle fusion. The concurrent changes in membrane conductance are consistent with the opening of a narrow aqueous connection—a fusion pore—between the fusing compartments. Electrophysiological studies have suggested that a similar pore, approximately 1–2 nm in diameter, forms between HA-expressing cells and target cells (Spruce et al. 1989, 1991; Almers et al. 1991; White 1992). Freeze-fracture studies are consistent with the formation of an influenza virus fusion pore (Burger et al. 1988; Knoll et al. 1988).

Influenza virus binds at neutral pH to sialic acid-containing receptors on the host cell surface through binding sites located at the distal tip of the HA trimer (see Fig. 1A in White 1992). Subsequent to this initial binding interaction (Fig. 4, top panel) and the low-pH-induced conformational change, there are at least four steps involved in forming and opening a fusion pore: close membrane contact, formation of a hemifusion intermediate, opening a narrow fusion pore, and dilation of the pore (Fig. 4). Each step, with particular attention to possible roles for the HA protein, is considered below.

Step 1: Close Membrane Contact

Before membranes can fuse, they must come into close contact (Fig. 4; step 1). Combined ultrastructural and electrophysiological studies of cortical granule exocytosis have suggested that prior to fusion, the plasma membrane "dimples" toward the cortical granule membrane bringing the two bilayers into close apposition (Chandler 1991). The recent observation that exposure to low pH deforms influenza virus particles (Ruigrok et al. 1992) may reflect a related ability of the conformationally altered HA molecule to induce membrane curvature, perhaps due to binding of its exposed fusion peptides to the viral and/or target bilayers. In so doing, the two membranes would be brought into intimate contact. As assessed by hydrophobic binding of the virus to target membranes, close membrane contact occurs well before the onset of fusion (Stegmann et al. 1990).

Step 2: Hemifusion

The next step in the fusion reaction is thought to be formation of a hemifusion intermediate (Kemble et al. 1994). There are two aspects of this process that should be considered in view of recent results. The first is the need for several HAs to cluster to form a fusion site. The second is the geometry of the lipids in the hemifusion intermediate.

Clustering of HA Trimers

Several investigators have observed that following exposure to low pH, there is a lag phase before the onset of lipid mixing (Morris et al. 1989; Spruce et al. 1989; Stegmann et al. 1990; Clague et al. 1991). The lag phase has been revealed by conducting fusion reactions at suboptimal temperature or pH, with effector membranes that express a low surface density of HA, or with target membranes that lack a receptor. Indirect evidence (Doms and Helenius 1986; Morris et al. 1989; Spruce et al. 1989; Ellens et al. 1990) has suggested that the lag phase represents the time during which several HA trimers cluster to form a fusion site (Fig. 3). We have recently tested this hypothesis by analyzing the fusion activity of cell lines that express the Japan HA at nine different defined surface densities. This analysis revealed a sigmoidal dependence between the length of the lag phase (before the onset of lipid mixing) and HA surface density (T. Danieli et al., in prep.). A Hill plot analysis suggested that a minimum of three HA trimers is needed at the initial fusion site. Hence, it appears quite compelling that HAs must cluster, in a limited and orderly fashion, in the plane of the membrane before the onset of fusion. In support of this notion are the observations that HA must be rotationally (Junankar and Cherry 1986) and laterally (Gutman et al. 1993) mobile in the plane of the membrane for fusion to occur.

Structure of the Hemifusion Intermediate

For two membranes to fuse, their bilayers must go through a non-bilayer intermediate (Siegel 1993). Since HA-mediated fusion is not leaky, even to ions (Spruce et al. 1991), fusion is likely to involve a stage during which the outer, but not the inner, leaflets have joined and during which there is not yet mixing of the aqueous contents of the fusing compartments (Fig. 4; step 2). This state is defined as a hemifusion intermediate; it has been detected in pure lipid systems (Ellens et al. 1985; Leventis et al. 1986) and during electrically induced fusion of red blood cells (Song et al. 1991). We have recently observed that a genetically engineered HA (Kemble et al. 1993) that is anchored in the membrane by a lipid anchor instead of a proteinaceous transmembrane domain promotes hemifusion, but not complete fusion (Kemble et al. 1994). This finding suggests that the normal course of HA-mediated fusion is via a hemifusion intermediate. The nature of the lipids in the hemifusion intermediate has been debated. Although some models have invoked an inverted micellar configuration (Bentz et al. 1993), recent theoretical (Siegel 1993) and experimental (Stegmann 1993) work has suggested that the intermediate may be in the form of a lipid stalk (Kozlov et al. 1989). It should be noted that a functional (Gething et al. 1986; Guy et al. 1992) exposed (Godley et al. 1992; Kemble et al. 1992; Bodian et al. 1993) fusion peptide is required to form the hemifusion intermediate (Fig. 4; step 2).

Step 3: Opening of the Fusion Pore

The next stage of the fusion reaction is the opening of a narrow fusion pore. Electrophysiological measurements (Spruce et al. 1989, 1991) suggest that the initial pore is approximately 1–2 nm in diameter, has a variable initial conductance with a mean of about 150 pS, and has an initial opening time of approximately 100 μsec. The pore can "flicker"; that is, it will often open and close repeatedly before it becomes committed to further dilation. Hence, step 3 of the fusion reaction (Fig. 4) is *reversible.* The lipids in the initial fusion pore may be constrained, since fusion pore conductances have been detected before the onset of measurable lipid flow, as assessed by fluorescence microscopic techniques (Tse et al. 1993).

Step 4: Dilation of the Fusion Pore

The next stage of the fusion reaction (Fig. 4; step 4) involves the *irreversible* opening and progressive dilation of the fusion pore. Work with lipid-anchored HA, which promotes hemifusion, but not complete fusion, suggests that the transmembrane domain plays a critical role in this step (Kemble et al. 1994). The transmembrane domain may facilitate completion of the fusion process by stabilizing the aggregate of HA trimers at the fusion site (Guy et al. 1992), by ensuring proper orientation of the trimers at the fusion site (Wilschut and Bron 1993), by ensuring proper positioning of the fusion peptides with respect to the viral and target membranes (White 1992; Stegmann and Helenius 1993), by acting as a bilayer defect (Siegel 1993), or by filling hydrophobic voids created in the hemifusion intermediate (Siegel 1993). The fact that the pore suddenly opens irreversibly (Spruce et al. 1989, 1991) suggests that this stage (Fig. 4; step 4) of the fusion reaction may involve a different conformation of HA, perhaps its most stable conformation (Ruigrok et al. 1988), than does formation of the hemifusion intermediate. In other words, and highly speculatively, formation of the hemifusion intermediate may require a stage-I-like conformation, whereas a stage-II-like conformation (Fig. 2), and/or the loop-to-helix transition (Ward and Dopheide 1980; Carr and Kim 1993; P.A. Bullough et al., pers. comm.) of HA2 residues 54–81 (Fig. 1D), may be required to drive the irreversible opening of the fusion pore. The fusion peptides may also play a role in fusion pore dilation (Schoch and Blumenthal 1993).

PERSPECTIVES

In summary, HA-mediated fusion proceeds through a set of conformational intermediates in both the HA protein (Fig. 2) and in the lipids (Fig. 4) at the fusion site. A present challenge is to determine what conformation the HA protein is in during each stage of the fusion reaction. There are at least two areas in which such detailed analyses of HA-mediated fusion are valuable: in the design of antiviral agents and in elucidating the mechanisms of other fusion proteins.

Design of Novel Antiviral Agents

Two strategies have recently been suggested for interfering with the fusion activity of the influenza HA. The first involves targeting the vicinity of the fusion peptide directly. The idea of this strategy is to use small molecules to lock the fusion peptides in place. Toward this end, a potential small molecule binding site was found that subtends the fusion peptide. With the aid of a computer, a family of benzo- and hydroquinones was identified whose members could fit in the target site. These benzo- and hydroquinones prevent exposure of the fusion peptides and the fusion activity and infectivity of X:31 influenza virus in vitro (Bodian et al. 1993). The second strategy is based on the observation that engineered disulfide bonds (Godley et al. 1992) that lock the globular head domains of the HA trimer together prevent fusion peptide exposure and membrane fusion activity in vitro (Godley et al. 1992; Kemble et al. 1992). Bridging molecules that mimic the engineered disulfide bonds might prevent fusion. Thus, at least two regions of the HA protein have been identified as targets for the rational design of inhibitors of the fusion-inducing conformational change. As the conformational change involves sites throughout the length of the HA molecule (Godley et al. 1992; Kemble et al. 1992; Steinhauer et al. 1992; Yewdell et al. 1993), there are likely additional small molecule binding sites whose occupancy would have the same effect.

Relevance to Other Viral and to Cellular Fusion Proteins

A second area in which continued detailed analyses of HA-mediated membrane fusion will be profitable is in developing hypotheses and incisive experimental strategies with which to elucidate the fusion mechanisms of other viral fusion proteins. An important current challenge is to elucidate the fusion mechanisms of viruses (e.g., HIV and herpesviruses) that fuse at neutral pH. In addition, as many of the underlying principles of cellular fusion reactions appear to resemble those of viral fusion reactions (White 1992), ongoing studies into the fusion mechanism of the HA should continue to guide the emerging efforts to elucidate the mechanisms of proteins that mediate cell-cell fusion events (White and Blobel 1989; Blobel et al. 1992) and intracellular fusion events (Sollner et al. 1993).

ACKNOWLEDGMENTS

I thank all members of my laboratory, past and present, for their experimental and conceptual contributions to this work. I also thank Luke

Hoffman and Jason Rosé for preparing Figures 1 and 2; Helen Czerwonka for manuscript preparation; and Joanna Gilbert, Jill Hacker, and Luke Hoffman for critical reading of the manuscript. Work in my laboratory was supported by grants from the National Institutes of Health.

REFERENCES

Almers, W., L.J. Breckenridge, A. Iwata, A.K. Lee, A.E. Spruce, and F.W. Tse. 1991. Millisecond studies of single membrane fusion events. In *Calcium entry and action at the presynaptic nerve terminal* (ed. E.F. Stanley et al.), vol. 635, p. 318. New York Academy of Sciences, New York.

Bentz, J., H. Ellens, and D. Alford. 1993. Architecture of the influenza hemagglutinin fusion site. In *Viral fusion mechanisms* (ed. J. Bentz), p. 163. CRC Press, Boca Raton, Florida.

Blobel, C.P., T.G. Wolfsberg, C.W. Turck, D.G. Myles, P. Primakoff, and J.M. White. 1992. A potential fusion peptide and an integrin ligand domain in a protein active in sperm-egg fusion. *Nature* **356:** 248.

Bodian, D.L. 1992. "Structure-based design of an inhibitor of the conformational change of influenza hemagglutinin." Ph.D. thesis, University of California, San Francisco.

Bodian, D.L., R.B. Yamasaki, R.L. Buswell, J.F. Stearns, J.M. White, and I.D. Kuntz. 1993. Inhibition of the fusion-inducing conformational change of influenza hemagglutinin by benzoquinones and hydroquinones. *Biochemistry* **32:** 2967.

Brasseur, R., M. Vandenbranden, B. Cornet, A. Burny, and J.-M. Ruysschaert. 1990. Orientation into the lipid bilayer of an asymmetric amphipathic helical peptide located at the N-terminus of viral fusion proteins. *Biochim. Biophys. Acta* **1029:** 267.

Brunner, J. 1989. Testing topological models for the membrane penetration of the fusion peptide of influenza virus hemagglutinin. *FEBS Lett.* **257:** 369.

Brunner, J. and M. Tsurudome. 1993. Fusion protein membrane interactions as studied by hydrophobic photolabeling. In *Viral fusion mechanisms* (ed. J. Bentz), p. 67. CRC Press, Boca Raton, Florida.

Brunner, J., C. Zugliani, and R. Mischler. 1991. Fusion activity of influenza virus PR8/34 correlates with a temperature-induced conformational change within the hemagglutinin ectodomain detected by photochemical labeling. *Biochemistry* **30:** 2432.

Burger, K.N., G. Knoll, and A.J. Verkleij. 1988. Influenza virus-model membrane interaction. A morphological approach using modern cryotechniques. *Biochim. Biophys. Acta* **939:** 89.

Burger, K.N., S.A. Wharton, R.A. Demel, and A.J. Verkleij. 1991. Interaction of influenza virus hemagglutinin with a lipid monolayer. A comparison of the surface activities of intact virions, isolated hemagglutinins, and a synthetic fusion peptide. *Biochemistry* **30:** 11173.

Carr, C.M. and P.S. Kim. 1993. A spring-loaded mechanism for the conformational change of influenza hemagglutinin. *Cell* **73:** 823.

Chandler, D.E. 1991. Membrane fusion as seen in rapidly frozen secretory cells. *Ann. N.Y. Acad. Sci.* **635:** 234.

Clague, M.J., C. Schoch, and R. Blumenthal. 1991. Delay time for influenza virus hemagglutinin-induced membrane fusion depends on hemagglutinin surface density. *J. Virol.* **65:** 2402.

————. 1993. Toward a dissection of the influenza hemagglutinin-mediated membrane fusion pathway. In *Viral fusion mechanisms* (ed. J. Bentz), p. 113. CRC Press, Boca Raton, Florida.

Curran, M., F. Cohen, D. Chandler, P. Munson, and J. Zimmerberg. 1993. Exocytotic fusion pores exhibit semi-stable states. *J. Membr. Biol.* **133:** 61.

Doms, R.W. 1993. Protein conformational changes in virus-cell fusion. *Methods Enzymol.* **221:** 61.

Doms, R.W. and A. Helenius. 1986. Quaternary structure of influenza virus hemagglutinin after acid treatment. *J. Virol.* **60:** 833.

Ellens, H., J. Bentz, and F.C. Szoka. 1985. H^+- and Ca^{2+}-induced fusion and destabilization of liposomes. *Biochemistry* **24:** 3099.

Ellens, H., J. Bentz, D. Mason, F. Zhang, and J.M. White. 1990. Fusion of influenza hemagglutinin-expressing fibroblasts with glycophorin-bearing liposomes: Role of hemagglutinin surface density. *Biochemistry* **29:** 9697.

Formanowski, F., S.A. Wharton, L.J. Calder, C. Hofbauer, and H. Meier-Ewert. 1990. Fusion characteristics of influenza C viruses. *J. Gen. Virol.* **71:** 1181.

Gallaher, W.R., J.P. Segrest, and E. Hunter. 1992. Are fusion peptides really "sided" insertional helices? (Letter to the editor). *Cell* **70:** 531.

Gething, M.-J., R.W. Doms, D. York, and J.M. White. 1986. Studies on the mechanism of membrane fusion: Site-specific mutagenesis of the hemagglutinin of influenza virus. *J. Cell Biol.* **102:** 11.

Godley, L., J. Pfeifer, D. Steinhauer, B. Ely, G. Shaw, R. Kaufmann, E. Suchanek, C. Pabo, J.J. Skehel, D.C. Wiley, and S. Wharton. 1992. Introduction of intersubunit disulfide bonds in the membrane-distal region of the influenza hemagglutinin abolishes membrane fusion activity. *Cell* **68:** 635.

Gutman, O., T. Danieli, J.M. White, and Y.I. Henis. 1993. Effects of exposure to low pH on the lateral mobility of influenza hemagglutinin expressed at the cell surface. *Biochemistry* **32:** 101.

Guy, H.R., S.R. Durell, C. Schoch, and R. Blumenthal. 1992. Analyzing the fusion process of influenza hemagglutinin by mutagenesis and molecular modeling. *Biophys. J.* **62:** 95.

Harter, C., P. James, T. Bächi, G. Semenza, and J. Brunner. 1989. Hydrophobic binding of the ectodomain of influenza hemagglutinin to membranes occurs through the "fusion peptide." *J. Biol. Chem.* **264:** 6459.

Heuser, J.E. and T.S. Reese. 1981. Structural changes after transmitter release at the frog neuromuscular junction. *J. Cell Biol.* **88:** 564.

Junankar, P.R. and R.J. Cherry. 1986. Temperature and pH dependence of the haemolytic activity of influenza virus and of the rotational mobility of the spike glycoproteins. *Biochim. Biophys. Acta* **854:** 198.

Kemble, G.W., T. Danieli, and J.M. White. 1994. Lipid-anchored influenza hemagglutinin promotes hemifusion, not complete fusion. *Cell* **76:** 383.

Kemble, G.W., Y. Henis, and J.M. White. 1993. GPI- and transmembrane-anchored influenza hemagglutinin differ in structure and receptor binding activity. *J. Cell Biol.* **122:** 1253.

Kemble, G.W., D.L. Bodian, J. Rosé, I.A. Wilson, and J.M. White. 1992. Intermonomer disulfide bonds impair the fusion activity of influenza virus hemagglutinin. *J. Virol.* **66:** 4940.

Knoll, G., K.N.J. Burger, R. Bron, G. van Meer, and A.J. Verkleij. 1988. Fusion of liposomes with the plasma membrane of epithelial cells: Fate of incorporated lipids as followed by freeze fracture and autoradiography of plastic sections. *J. Cell Biol.* **107:**

2511.

Kozlov, M.M., S.L. Leikin, L.V. Chernomordik, V.S. Markin, and Y.A. Chizmadzhev. 1989. Stalk mechanism of vesicle fusion. Intermixing of aqueous contents. *Eur. Biophys. J.* **17:** 121.

Lear, J.D. and W.F. DeGrado. 1987. Membrane binding and conformational properties of peptides representing the NH2 terminus of influenza HA-2. *J. Biol. Chem.* **262:** 6500.

Leventis, R., J. Gagne, N. Fuller, R.R. Rand, and J.R. Silvius. 1986. Divalent cation induced fusion and lipid lateral segregation in phosphatidylcholine-phosphatidic acid vesicles. *Biochemistry* **25:** 6978.

Monck, J.R. and J.M. Fernandez. 1992. The exocytotic fusion pore. *J. Cell Biol.* **119:** 1395.

Morris, S., D. Sarkar, J. White, and R. Blumenthal. 1989. Kinetics of pH-dependent fusion between 3T3 fibroblasts expressing influenza hemagglutinin and red blood cells. Measurement by dequenching of fluorescence. *J. Biol. Chem.* **264:** 3972.

Murphy, B.R. and R.G. Webster. 1990. Orthomyxoviruses. In *Virology* (ed. B.N. Fields et al.) p. 1091. Raven Press, New York.

Puri, A., F.P. Booy, R.W. Doms, J.M. White, and R. Blumenthal. 1990. Conformational changes and fusion activity of influenza virus hemagglutinin of the H2 and H3 subtypes: Effects of acid pretreatment. *J. Virol.* **64:** 3824.

Rafalski, M., J.D. Lear, and W.F. DeGrado. 1990. Phospholipid interactions of synthetic fusion peptides representing the N-terminus of HIV gp41. *Biochemistry* **29:** 7917.

Rafalski, M., A. Ortiz, A. Rockwell, L.C. van Ginkel, J.D. Lear, W.F. DeGrado, and J. Wilschut. 1991. Membrane fusion activity of the influenza virus hemagglutinin: Interaction of HA2 N-terminal peptides with phospholipid vesicles. *Biochemistry* **30:** 10211.

Ruigrok, R.W.H., E.A. Hewat, and R.H. Wade. 1992. Low pH deforms the influenza virus envelope. *J. Gen. Virol.* **73:** 995.

Ruigrok, R.W.H., N.G. Wrigley, L.J. Calder, S. Cusack, S.A. Wharton, E.B. Brown, and J.J. Skehel. 1986. Electron microscopy of the low pH structure of influenza virus haemagglutinin. *EMBO J.* **5:** 41.

Ruigrok, R.W.H., A. Aitken, L.J. Calder, S.R. Martin, J.J. Skehel, S.A. Wharton, W. Weis, and D.C. Wiley. 1988. Studies on the structure of the influenza virus haemagglutinin at the pH of membrane fusion. *J. Gen. Virol.* **69:** 2785.

Sarkar, D.P., S.J. Morris, O. Eidelman, J. Zimmerberg, and R. Blumenthal. 1989. Initial stages of influenza hemagglutinin-induced cell fusion monitored simultaneously by two fluorescent events: Cytoplasmic continuity and membrane mixing. *J. Cell Biol.* **109:** 113.

Schoch, C. and R. Blumenthal. 1993. Role of fusion peptide sequence in initial stages of influenza hemagglutinin-induced cell fusion. *J. Biol. Chem.* **268:** 9267.

Siegel, D.P. 1993. Modeling protein-induced fusion mechanisms: Insights from the relative stability of lipidic structures. In *Viral fusion mechanisms* (ed. J. Bentz), p. 475. CRC Press, Boca Raton, Florida.

Sollner, T., S.W. Whiteheart, M. Brunner, H. Erdjument-Bromage, S. Geromanos, P. Tempst, and J.E. Rothman. 1993. SNAP receptors implicated in vesicle targeting and fusion. *Nature* **362:** 318.

Song, L., Q.F. Ahkong, D. Georgescauld, and J.A. Lucy. 1991. Membrane fusion without cytoplasmic fusion (hemifusion) in erythrocytes that are subjected to electrical breakdown. *Biochim. Biophys. Acta* **1065:** 54.

Spruce, A.E., A. Iwata, and W. Almers. 1991. The first milliseconds of the pore formed by a fusogenic viral envelope protein during membrane fusion. *Proc. Natl. Acad. Sci.*

88: 3623.

Spruce, A.E., A. Iwata, J.M. White, and W. Almers. 1989. Patch clamp studies of single cell-fusion events mediated by a viral fusion protein. *Nature* **342:** 555.

Stegmann, T. 1993. Influenza hemagglutinin-mediated membrane fusion does not involve inverted phase lipid intermediates. *J. Biol. Chem.* **268:** 1716.

Stegmann, T. and A. Helenius. 1993. Influenza virus fusion: From models toward a mechanism. In *Viral fusion mechanisms* (ed. J. Bentz), p. 89. CRC Press, Boca Raton, Florida.

Stegmann, T., F.P. Booy, and J. Wilschut. 1987. Effects of low pH on influenza virus. Activation and inactivation of the membrane fusion capacity of the hemagglutinin. *J. Biol. Chem.* **262:** 17744.

Stegmann, T., R.W. Doms, and A. Helenius. 1989. Protein-mediated membrane fusion. *Annu. Rev. Biophys. Biophys. Chem.* **18:** 187.

Stegmann, T., J.M. White, and A. Helenius. 1990. Intermediates in influenza-induced membrane fusion. *EMBO J.* **9:** 4231.

Stegmann, T., J.M. Delfino, F.M. Richards, and A. Helenius. 1991. The HA2 subunit of influenza hemagglutinin inserts into the target membrane prior to fusion. *J. Biol. Chem.* **266:** 18404.

Stegmann, T., D. Hoekstra, G. Scherphof, and J. Wilschut. 1986. Fusion activity of influenza virus: A comparison between biological and artificial target membrane vesicles. *J. Biol. Chem.* **261:** 10966.

Steinhauer, D.A., N.K. Sauter, J.J. Skehel, and D.C. Wiley. 1992. Receptor binding and cell entry by influenza viruses. *Semin. Virol.* **3:** 91.

Tse, F.W., A. Iwata, and W. Almers. 1993. Membrane flux through the pore formed by a fusogenic viral envelope protein during cell fusion. *J. Cell Biol.* **121:** 543.

Tsurudome, M., R. Glück, R. Graf, R. Falchetto, U. Schaller, and J. Brunner. 1992. Lipid interactions of the hemagglutinin HA2 NH_2-terminal segment during influenza virus-induced membrane fusion. *J. Biol. Chem.* **267:** 20225.

Ward, C.W. and T.A. Dopheide. 1980. Influenza virus haemagglutinin. Structural predictions suggest that the fibrillar appearance is due to the presence of a coiled-coil. *Aust. J. Biol. Sci.* **33:** 449.

White, J.M. 1992. Membrane fusion. *Science* **258:** 917.

White, J.M. and C.P. Blobel. 1989. Cell-to-cell fusion. *Curr. Opin. Cell Biol.* **1:** 934.

White, J.M. and I.A. Wilson. 1987. Anti-peptide antibodies detect steps in a protein conformational change: Low-pH activation of the influenza virus hemagglutinin. *J. Cell Biol.* **105:** 2887.

White, J., R. Doms, M.-J. Gething, M. Kielian, and A. Helenius. 1986. Viral membrane fusion proteins. In *Virus attachment and entry into cells* (ed. R.L. Crowell and K. Lonberg-Holm), p. 54. American Society for Microbiology, Washington, D.C.

Wiley, D.C. and J.J. Skehel. 1987. The structure and function of the hemagglutinin membrane glycoprotein of influenza virus. *Annu. Rev. Biochem.* **56:** 365.

Wilschut, J. and R. Bron. 1993. The influenza virus hemagglutinin: Membrane fusion activity in whole virions and reconstituted virosomes. In *Viral fusion mechanisms* (ed. J. Bentz), p. 133. CRC Press, Boca Raton, Florida.

Wilson, I.A. and N.J. Cox. 1990. Structural basis of immune recognition of influenza virus hemagglutinin. *Annu. Rev. Immunol.* **8:** 737.

Wilson, I.A., J.J. Skehel, and D.C. Wiley. 1981. Structure of the haemagglutinin membrane glycoportein of influenza virus at 3 Å resolution. *Nature* **289:** 366.

Yewdell, J.W., A. Taylor, A. Yellen, A. Caton, W. Gerhard, and T. Bachi. 1993. Mutations in or near the fusion peptide of the influenza virus hemagglutinin affect an antigenic site in the globular region. *J. Virol.* **67:** 933.

Zimmerberg, J., M. Curran, and F.S. Cohen. 1991. A lipid/protein complex hypothesis for exocytotic fusion pore formation. *Ann. N.Y. Acad. Sci.* **635:** 307.

16

The Influenza A Virus M2 Ion Channel Protein and Its Role in the Influenza Virus Life Cycle

Robert A. Lamb,[1,2] **Leslie J. Holsinger,**[2]
and Lawrence H. Pinto[3]
[1]Howard Hughes Medical Institute
[2]Department of Biochemistry, Molecular Biology and Cell Biology
[3]Department of Neurobiology and Physiology
Northwestern University, Evanston, Illinois 60208-3500

The influenza virus M2 protein has an ion channel activity that permits ions to enter the virion during uncoating and also acts to modulate the pH of intracellular compartments. In this review, we discuss the structure of the M2 protein; the observations concerning the effect of the antiviral drug amantadine on influenza virus replication which led to the notion that the M2 protein could affect intracellular pH; the direct evidence indicating that the M2 protein has an ion channel activity that is blocked by amantadine; and properties of the M2 protein's ion channel activity.

STRUCTURE OF THE M2 PROTEIN

The influenza A virus envelope contains three integral membrane proteins, hemagglutinin (HA), neuraminidase (NA), and the M2 protein. Contained inside the viral envelope are the ribonucleoprotein (RNP) structures, which consist of one of the eight genomic RNA segments encapsidated with nucleocapsid protein (NP) and the associated RNA transcriptase protein complex. The influenza virus membrane protein (M1) is a peripheral membrane protein that is thought to associate with both the RNPs and the lipid bilayer (for review, see Lamb 1989). The M2 integral membrane protein (97 amino acids) is encoded by a spliced mRNA derived from genome RNA segment 7 (Lamb and Choppin 1981; Lamb et al. 1981). The M2 protein is abundantly expressed at the plasma membrane of virus-infected cells but is greatly underrepresented in virions, as only a few (on average 20–60) molecules are incorporated into virus particles (Lamb et al. 1985; Zebedee et al. 1985; Zebedee and Lamb 1988).

Cellular Receptors of Animal Viruses
© 1994 Cold Spring Harbor Laboratory Press 0-87969-429-7/94 $5 + .00

In polarized cells, as for the surface for budding of influenza virus particles, the M2 protein is expressed at the apical cell surface (Hughey et al.
1992). The M2 protein spans the membrane once and, by using domain-
specific antibodies and specific proteolysis, it has been shown that M2
protein is oriented such that it has 24 amino-terminal extracellular
residues, a 19-residue transmembrane (TM) domain, and a 54-residue
cytoplasmic tail (Lamb et al. 1985). The presence of an amino-terminal
extracellular domain in the absence of a cleavable signal sequence indicates M2 is a model type III integral membrane protein (nomenclature of
von Heijne and Gavel 1988) that is dependent on the signal recognition
particle for cotranslational insertion into the endoplasmic reticulum
membrane (Hull et al. 1988).

The native form of the M2 protein is minimally a homotetramer consisting of a pair of either disulfide-linked dimers or disulfide-linked
tetramers (Fig. 1) (Holsinger and Lamb 1991; Sugrue and Hay 1991;
Panayotov and Schlesinger 1992). In studies with chemical cross-linking
reagents, a small amount of a large complex (150–180 kD) has been
identified that appears to contain only M2 molecules and thus may
represent a higher-order structure of 10–12 M2 molecules (Holsinger and
Lamb 1991), but the significance of this species is presently unclear.

EFFECTS OF ANTIBODIES TO THE M2 PROTEIN ON
INFLUENZA VIRUS GROWTH

An indication of the function of the M2 protein in the influenza virus life
cycle came from studies with a monoclonal antibody (14C2) specific for
the amino-terminal domain of M2. When this antibody was included in
an agarose overlay of a standard plaque assay titration, it was found to
restrict the size of plaque growth of a variety of influenza A virus strains
(Zebedee and Lamb 1988). Variant viruses resistant to the antibody were
isolated, and they were found to have compensating changes in the
cytoplasmic tail of M2 as well as in the amino-terminal domain of the
M1 protein (Zebedee and Lamb 1989a), suggesting that the antibody
may be interfering with critical M1/M2 interactions during virus assembly and budding. Alternatively, the M2 antibody may prevent virus particles released by one cell from successfully penetrating neighboring cells.
Although it is now known that the influenza virus M2 protein has ion
channel activity, as described below, it seems possible that the M2
protein is multifunctional and its cytoplasmic tail forms protein-protein
interactions.

Although it was known that the basic structure of the M2 protein is
relatively conserved among a variety of strains (Lamb 1989; Zebedee

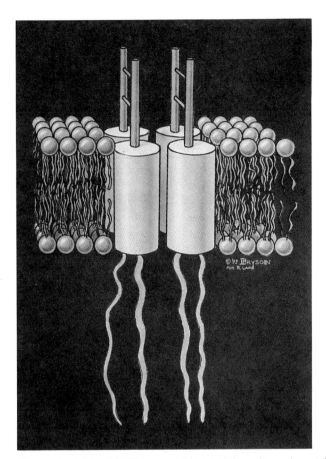

Figure 1 Schematic diagram of the M2 ion channel protein oligomer in a lipid bilayer. For a description of the protein, see the text. (Copyright held by Mary K. Bryson 1993.)

and Lamb 1989b), and that an M2-specific antibody restricts virus growth, M2 might have represented a protein to which a protective antibody response was direct. Passively transferred 14C2 monoclonal antibody to M2 reduced the level of virus replication in mice challenged with influenza A virus (Treanor et al. 1990), but no response in humans to the M2 protein after an influenza virus infection has been reported.

THE INFLUENZA VIRUS LIFE CYCLE AND THE EFFECT OF THE ANTIVIRAL DRUG AMANTADINE

Biosynthesis of HA

The HA polypeptide chain is synthesized on membrane-bound ribosomes and is translocated into the endoplasmic reticulum. Core carbohydrate chains are added cotranslationally, and HA oligomerizes to form a trimer ($t_{1/2} \approx$ 7–10 min) (Gething et al. 1986). As HA is transported through the exocytotic pathway to the plasma membrane, its carbohydrate chains are trimmed. By the time of transport of HA to the *medial* Golgi apparatus, some carbohydrate chains are terminally glycosylated (for review, see Lamb 1989). HA is synthesized as a precursor, HA0, that is proteolytically cleaved to form the disulfide-linked subunits HA1 and HA2. This cleavage event is the first step in the pathway that permits HA to undergo its conformational change at low pH, converting native HA to its fusogenic forms. Thus, cleavage of HA is a key determinant of infectivity and pathogenicity (Klenk et al. 1975; Lazarowitz and Choppin 1975). For those influenza virus subtypes that contain the appropriate multibasic amino acids at the cleavage site (largely H5 and H7 avian and equine subtypes) (Kawaoka and Webster 1988; Ohuchi et al. 1989), the HA0 precursor is cleaved in the *trans* Golgi network (TGN) by fusion, a subtilisin-like endoprotease (Steineke-Gröber et al. 1992). On the other hand, human strains of influenza virus contain a single basic residue in the cleavage site and when grown in tissue culture or in ovo, cleavage of HA occurs after HA is expressed at the cell surface.

Virus Entry into Cells and HA Fusion

Influenza virus particles are internalized into cells by receptor-mediated endocytosis. After exposure of virions to the low-pH environment found in endosomal compartments, the HA undergoes a low-pH-induced conformational change that releases the hydrophobic fusion peptide, and this domain mediates the fusion of the viral membrane with the endosomal membrane (for review, see Lamb 1989; White 1990). The consequence of this membrane fusion event is that the viral RNPs are released into the cytoplasm and then the RNPs are transported to the nucleus to begin mRNA transcription. A schematic illustration of the life cycle of the virus is shown in Figure 2.

Early Effects of Amantadine on Influenza Virus Replication

Amantadine (1-aminoadamantane hydrochloride) and its structural analog rimantadine are antiviral drugs, which at micromolar concentrations specifically inhibit influenza A virus replication (Davies et al. 1964). The M2 protein was implicated in having an essential role in the life cycle of influenza virus during studies with the drug. Mutants were isolated that were resistant to the effect of the drug, and both genetic and sequencing studies indicated that these mutants contained changes that mapped pre-

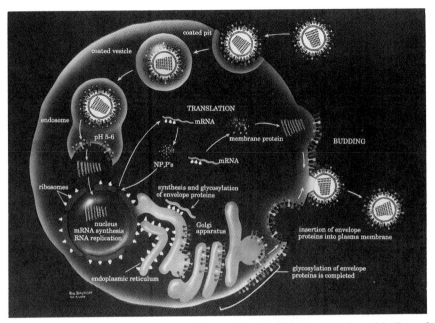

Figure 2 Schematic diagram of the life cycle of influenza virus from binding of the virus to the host cell plasma membrane to exit of the virus by budding at the plasma membrane. (Copyright held by Mary K. Bryson 1993.)

dominantly to the M2 transmembrane domain (Lubeck et al. 1978; Hay et al. 1979, 1985; Scholtissek and Faulkner 1979). For all influenza strains, the amantadine block to virus replication occurs at an early stage between the steps of virus penetration and uncoating (Skehel et al. 1978; Bukrinskaya et al. 1982). It has been found that in the presence of amantadine, the M1 protein fails to dissociate from the RNPs (Bukrinskaya et al. 1982; Martin and Helenius 1991), and the transport of the RNP complex to the nucleus does not occur (Martin and Helenius 1991).

Late Effects of Amantadine on Influenza Virus Replication

In addition to the "early" effect of amantadine, the drug has a second "late" effect on the replication of some subtypes of avian influenza viruses which have an HA that is cleaved intracellularly and which have a high pH optimum of fusion (e.g., fowl plague virus [FPV]). A large body of data indicates that addition of amantadine to virus-infected cells causes a premature conformational change in HA as the HA molecules are transported through the TGN (Sugrue et al. 1990; Ciampor et al. 1992a,b; Grambas and Hay 1992; Grambas et al. 1992). By immunological and biochemical criteria, this form of HA is indistinguishable from the low-pH-induced form of HA. The low-pH conformational transition in HA is thought to occur because the intraluminal pH of the TGN compartment has been lowered below the threshold needed to induce the acid-pH transition of HA (Skehel et al. 1982; for review, see Wiley and Skehel 1987). This "late" effect of amantadine can be reversed by addition of the sodium ionophore monensin (Sugrue et al. 1990). Moreover, alterations in HA which either increase or decrease the pH at which the HA conformational change occurs also influence susceptibility to drug action (Steinhauer et al. 1991). The consequence of the irreversible conformational change in HA, which brings about the extrusion of the fusion peptide at the wrong time in the infectious cycle and in the wrong subcellular compartment, is that the HA oligomers aggregate and viral budding is greatly restricted (for review, see Wiley and Skehel 1987; Ruigrok et al. 1991).

RATIONALE FOR THE INFLUENZA VIRUS M2 PROTEIN HAVING ION CHANNEL ACTIVITY

Taken together, the above summarized data led to the hypothesis that the function of the influenza virus M2 protein is to act as an ion channel that modulates the pH of the intracellular compartment (Sugrue and Hay 1991; Hay 1992). The M2 protein was speculated to keep the pH of the TGN lumen above the threshold for the low-pH conformational change. When the M2 ion channel is blocked by amantadine, the TGN luminal pH is predicted to be lowered, and this causes HA to undergo its low-pH transition (Fig. 3). As the same mutations in the M2 protein transmembrane domain abolish susceptibility to both the "early" and "late" effects of amantadine, a rational explanation is that the M2 protein in virions and the M2 protein in virus-infected cells have the same function. It is generally believed that once the virion particle has been endocytosed, the ion channel activity of the virion-associated M2 protein permits the flow of ions from the endosome into the virion interior to disrupt protein-protein interactions and free the RNPs from the M1 protein (Fig. 4) (for review, see Hay 1992; Helenius 1992; Marsh 1992; Skehel 1992). An attractive feature of this hypothesis for virus uncoating is that the low pH of endosomes where uncoating occurs, in contrast to the neutral pH at the plasma membrane where assembly occurs, would push the equilibrium of the disassembly/assembly process in favor of uncoating. In addition to the data discussed above which indicate that amantadine blocks the separation of the M1 protein from the RNAs, some data from an in vitro analysis of virion disruption are probably re-

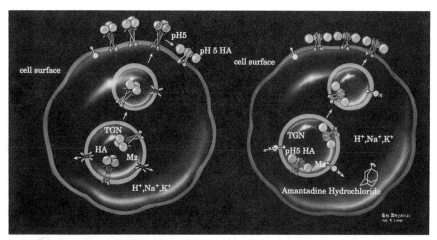

Figure 3 Schematic diagram to illustrate the proposed function of the M2 protein ion channel in the TGN to maintain the intraluminal pH above the threshold for the conformational transition of HA. When the M2 ion channel is blocked by amantadine, HA undergoes its low-pH transition. (Copyright held by Mary K. Bryson 1993.)

lated to natural uncoating. To solubilize the M1 protein from purified virions, it has become customary to use detergent and high salt concentrations.

Interestingly, Zhirnov (1990) reported that if the pH of the detergent buffer was lowered to pH 5.5, there was no need to add nonphysiological salt concentrations to achieve M1 protein solubilization. In addition, recent electron microscopic observations on low-pH-treated virus indicated a destabilization and malformation of the viral membrane following acid treatment, and it was suggested that this might be a consequence of the acid-induced dissociation of M1 from the membrane and RNP complexes (Ruigrok et al. 1992). Another consequence of the M2 ion channel activity in virions during the uncoating process may be to prepare HA for the fusion process. Bron and colleagues (1993) found that fusion of influenza virus with liposomes was slowed down in the presence of amantadine; this effect was not seen with viruses containing an M2 protein-specific amantadine-resistant mutation. The fusion inhibition by amantadine was reversed by addition of the proton-ionophore monensin. It was suggested that intraviral low pH facilitates influenza virus fusion, possibly by weakening interactions of the cytoplasmic tail of HA with the M1 protein and/or nucleocapsid (Bron et al. 1993). Similar data to those obtained by Bron and colleagues have also been obtained by Wharton et al. (1994). Although there is no direct evidence for an interaction between HA and M1 or the nucleocapsid, it has been

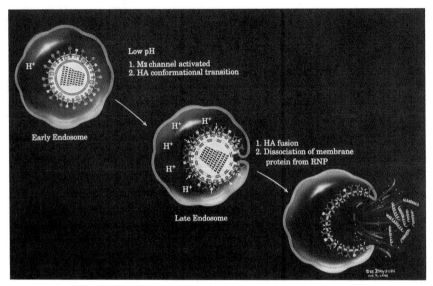

Figure 4 Schematic diagram of the proposed role of the M2 ion channel activity in virus entry, facilitating the flow of ions from the lumen of the endosome into the virion interior and bringing about dissociation of protein-protein interactions between the HA cytoplasmic tail and M1 and/or RNPs and M1 from the RNPs. For details, see the text. (Copyright held by Mary K. Bryson 1993.)

found that alterations to the cytoplasmic tail of HA, specifically truncations, affect viral infectivity (Simpson and Lamb 1992).

EVIDENCE THAT THE M2 PROTEIN ALTERS INTRACELLULAR pH

To obtain direct evidence that the M2 protein could alter the pH of intracellular compartments in the absence of an influenza virus infection, the effect of expressing M2 on the biogenesis of HA was examined (Ohuchi et al. 1994; Takeuchi and Lamb 1994). In setting up a system to reconstruct the effect of M2 protein expression on HA maturation, it was necessary to use an HA that is cleaved intracellularly, as cleavage is a prerequisite for the change to the low-pH (acid) conformational form, which possesses fusion activity. This requirement was not mitigated by the ability of uncleaved HA to undergo limited acid-induced conformational changes when cells are treated at pH 5 (Boulay et al. 1987). Normally, in an influenza virus infection, structural changes in uncleaved HA do occur on exit from the Golgi complex (Copeland et al. 1986), but these do not lead to the production of low-pH HA. A second criterion for the experimental test system was that HA must have a high pH of transition to the acid pH form. In the absence of an influenza virus infection to lower intracellular pH, the ability of HA to undergo its conformational change would depend solely on the effect of M2 on the pH of the TGN, if the assumption is made that the vector system employed has no effect on the TGN luminal pH. Thus, the FPV Rostock HA was chosen for study because it is cleaved intracellularly, it has a high pH of transition (pH 5.9), and its conformational forms have been studied extensively in influenza virus-infected cells treated with amantadine, as described above (Ohuchi et al. 1994; Takeuchi and Lamb 1994).

When FPV HA was expressed from cDNA in CV1 cells and HeLa T4 cells, it was found using biochemical assays that the majority of the HA molecules were in a form indistinguishable from the low-pH form of HA (Takeuchi and Lamb 1994). In addition, the fusion capacity of the FPV HA expressed from cDNA was greatly diminished (Ohuchi et al. 1994). The lysosomaltropic agent, ammonium chloride, stabilized the accumulation of HA in its native form (Takeuchi and Lamb 1994) and increased its fusion ability (Ohuchi et al. 1994). Coexpression of HA and the FPV M2 protein stabilized the accumulation of HA in its pH-neutral (native) form, indicating that expression of M2 affects intracellular pH and that amantadine prevented the rescue of HA in its native form (Ohuchi et al. 1994; Takeuchi and Lamb 1994). Thus, these data lend strength to the hypothesis that the M2 ion channel activity is required in the TGN to maintain HA in its native form.

MEASUREMENT OF THE M2 PROTEIN ION CHANNEL ACTIVITY

Direct evidence that the M2 protein has ion channel activity was obtained by expressing the M2 protein in oocytes of *Xenopus laevis* and measuring membrane currents (Pinto et al. 1992). The M2 ion channel activity was found to be blocked by amantadine, thereby providing direct evidence for the mechanism of action of the drug (Pinto et al. 1992; Wang et al. 1993). Altered M2 proteins containing changes in the TM domain, when found in virus, lead to resistance to amantadine; when these proteins were expressed in oocytes, they exhibited ion channel activities that were not affected by the drug (Pinto et al. 1992). The ion selectivity of the M2 ion channel activity was investigated and was found to be permeable to Na^+ ions. It is likely that this monovalent cation conductance also extends to protons (Pinto et al. 1992). Specific changes in the M2 protein TM domain alter the kinetics and ion selectivity of the channel, providing strong evidence that the M2 TM domain constitutes the pore of the channel (Pinto et al. 1992). This notion is supported by the finding that when a peptide corresponding to the M2 protein TM domain was incorporated into planar membranes, a proton translocation susceptible to block by amantadine could be detected (Duff and Ashley 1992).

It is important to note that the M2 ion channel could not succeed in acidifying the interior of the virion if it were permeable only to protons. Since M2 is the only ion channel found in virions, no other path exists for the flow of ions to neutralize the electrical charge carried by protons. This charge could be carried either by co-influx of anions or efflux of cations. Since the M2 ion channel does not seem to conduct anions (Pinto et al. 1992), the observed conductance to alkali ions is consistent with the proposed role in acidification.

REGULATION OF THE M2 PROTEIN ION CHANNEL ACTIVITY BY pH

In mammalian cells infected with influenza virus, approximately 10^6–10^7 molecules of M2 protein accumulate at the cell surface (Zebedee et al. 1985); if these were all active channels, it seems likely that the continuous ion flux through the channel would be extremely deleterious to the cell. Two observations indicate that the conductance of the ion channel in oocytes expressing the wild-type M2 protein is not activated by changes in membrane voltage: The current-voltage relationship was linear throughout the range of membrane voltages that were applied, and the current amplitude did not change with time (Pinto et al. 1992). Many ion channels are regulated by ligand interactions, but there is no known ligand for which M2 protein acts as a receptor, and in any case, the small size of the M2 protein extracellular domain (24 residues) makes an unknown ligand interaction unlikely.

These considerations led to an investigation of other means of activation of the wild-type M2 protein-associated conductance. Because the intracellular sites of action of the M2 protein are the endosome and the TGN compartments, both of which are acidic, it seemed possible that M2 protein ion conductance would be regulated by changes in pH. When the sensitivity of the M2 protein-associated ion channel activity was tested using the oocyte expression system, it was found that the currents increased monotonically with decreasing pH, and a change from pH 7.4 to pH 5.4 increased the inward current seven- to tenfold (Pinto et al. 1992). Further support for the notion that if the M2 channel were active at the cell surface it would be deleterious to the cell is the observation that oocytes expressing the M2 protein and held at pH 6.2 can be readily distinguished from oocytes expressing M2 protein and held at pH 6.2 in the presence of the ion channel blocker amantadine. In those oocytes ex-

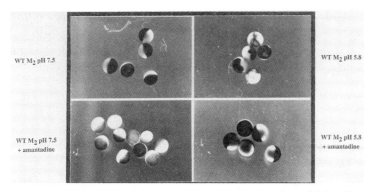

Figure 5   Oocytes expressing wild-type M2 protein exhibit pH-sensitive cell death. Oocytes expressing the wild-type M2 protein were incubated for 24 hr in ND96 (pH 7.5) followed by a 24-hr incubation in ND96 at the pH indicated, with or without amantadine.

pressing the activated M2 ion channel, there was a significant alteration of the morphology of the oocytes at the animal and vegetative pole interface, a sign of impending oocyte death (Fig. 5).

CHARACTERIZATION OF THE AMANTADINE BLOCK

The amino acid sequence of the M2 protein transmembrane domain is fairly well conserved in human, swine, equine, and avian strains. Nonetheless, there are some amino acid differences, and it seems likely that these could lead to altered properties of the channel. For example, in tissue culture cells, different strains of influenza virus show a difference in susceptibility to inhibition of virus growth by amantadine: Influenza A/chicken/Germany/34 (FPV Rostock) is less sensitive to amantadine than A/chicken/Germany/27 (FPV Weybridge). Studies on the nature of the amantadine block of the ion channel activity of the M2 protein of subtypes FPV Rostock, FPV Weybridge, and A/Udorn/72, when expressed in oocytes of *X. laevis,* indicated that amantadine is effective as a closed state blocker and less effective once the channel has been activated by lowered pH (Wang et al. 1993). The forward rate constant for the three M2 proteins was Udorn>Weybridge>Rostock.

Because amantadine block is nearly irreversible, it is not practical to measure an equilibrium constant. However, by making measurements of the ion channel activity of oocytes expressing the M2 protein with amantadine after a fixed time (2 min) of exposure to amantadine, it was possible to calculate the isochronic apparent inhibitory constant, appK_i, and it was found that Udorn<Weybridge<Rostock (Wang et al. 1993). These data are consistent with the observed difference in susceptiblity of the FPV subtypes to inhibition of virus growth by amantadine, with Weybridge being more sensitive than Rostock (Hay et al. 1985).

PREDICTED STRUCTURE OF THE M2 TRANSMEMBRANE DOMAIN AND THE ROLE OF SPECIFIC RESIDUES IN ION CHANNEL ACTIVITY AND AMANTADINE BLOCK

It has been suggested from theoretical modeling studies (Sugrue and Hay 1991; Sansom and Kerr 1993), and from circular dichroism measurements of the M2 TM domain peptide obtained in the presence of lipids (Duff et al. 1992), that the M2 protein TM domain adopts an α-helical secondary structure. When the TM domain is modeled as an α helix (Fig. 6), residues 27, 30, 31, 34, 37, 38, and 41 are found to be located on the same face of the α helix, and specific changes at residues 27, 30, 31, and 34 lead to an ion channel that is resistant to block by amantadine (Hay et al. 1985; Grambas et al. 1992; Pinto et al. 1992; Wang et al. 1993). In addition, it has been shown that the change $H_{37}A$ results in channel activity that is not pH-activated (Pinto et al. 1992) and that the change $L_{38}F$ in the FPV Rostock M2 protein results in a channel activity that is activated by pH but is largely resistant to amantadine block (Wang et al. 1993). Taken together, the data concerning these point mutations indicate that changing any residue on this face of the putative α helix of the M2 TM domain alters properties of the M2 ion channel (Holsinger et al. 1994). In modeling the M2 TM domain as an α helix, there are a few observations that need to be taken into consideration. First, an amantadine-resistant influenza virus has been isolated that contains the M2 TM domain change of $A_{30}P$ (Hay et al. 1985), and a proline can be (but is not necessarily) a helix-breaking residue. Second, the insertion of an amino acid into the putative α helix has the potential to disrupt the conformation of the protein, yet a mutant M2+V, $A_{30}T$, which contains an additional valine residue in the TM domain as well as a change leading to amantadine resistance, retains ion channel activity (Pinto et al. 1992). Thus, it is clearly of importance to determine the structure of the TM domain within the context of the complete M2 macromolecular complex.

Although the observation that amantadine-resistant mutations occur within the outer leaflet of the transmembrane domain (Hay et al. 1985) and the theoretical modeling studies indicate amantadine could fit in the center of four M2 α-helical TM domains (Sansom and Kerr 1993), no experimental data indicate that amantadine binds to the pore region of

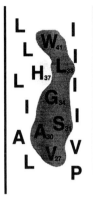

Figure 6 Helical net projection of the postulated α helix of the M2 protein membrane-spanning domain. Amino acid residues 25–43 are shown beginning at the bottom of the helix and winding upward. Residues that lie on one face of the α helix and which affect either ion channel activity or amantadine sensitivity are darkened. The histidine residue involved in modulation of channel activity by pH is shown lightly shaded. (Reprinted, with permission, from Holsinger et al. 1994.)

the M2 ion channel. Amantadine is a hydrophobic molecule and can penetrate lipid bilayers (Epand et al. 1987), and even if radioactively labeled drug of sufficiently high specific activity could be obtained, drug-binding studies with M2 protein in a lipid bilayer would be difficult to interpret. Indirect evidence for the manner by which amantadine blocks the M2 ion channel has been obtained by using electrophysiological methods. The Hill coefficient for amantadine block (0.91 ± 0.02) was calculated, and it indicates that one amantadine molecule blocks each functional M2 ion channel complex. Although this is compatible with the drug blocking the pore region of a tetrameric M2 protein channel, it is still possible that amantadine binds elsewhere on the molecule but modifies the pore region upon binding. Generally, for blockers that bind to the pore region, one of the following two characteristics is often observed: (1) the appK_i for the blocker is lower for the open pore or (2) for charged blockers such as amantadine, the current-voltage relationship of the blocked channel is nonlinear and often shows easier passage of current in one direction (for review, see Hille 1992). These characteristics of the M2 ion channel activity were tested, but the data obtained were not those expected for amantadine binding to the pore. The appK_i was higher for the open channel of each of the three subtypes, and the current-voltage relationship in the presence of amantadine was linear (Wang et al. 1993). Thus, two of the characteristics generally associated with a blocker that binds to the pore region were not found. A third characteristic often observed in blockers that bind rapidly to the pore region is that the currents of single open channels show rapid closures in the presence of the blocker (Neher and Steinback 1978), but these measurements await to be determined. From the data obtained to date, a possibility that cannot be eliminated is that amantadine acts as an "allosteric" blocker which binds to a part of the channel protein that is not in the pore-forming region, but upon binding, the drug causes a conformational change in the pore-forming region.

M2 ION CHANNELS FROM DIFFERENT INFLUENZA VIRUS
SUBTYPES HAVE DIFFERENT LEVELS OF ACTIVITY

For the Udorn M2 protein, the TM domain changes $V_{27}A$, $V_{27}S$, $V_{27}T$, $S_{31}N$, and $G_{34}E$ were found to yield channel activities with pH activation curves that could not be distinguished from wild-type M2, and all showed a quasi-linear slope of activation to pH 5.4, the lowest pH the oocytes could tolerate and give reversibly low currents upon return to pH 7.5 (Holsinger et al. 1994). Mutations in the Udorn M2 protein TM domain of $A_{30}P$ and $W_{41}A$ effectively abolished meaningful channel activity at both pH 7.5 and pH 6.2, even though $M2\text{-}A_{30}P$ and $M2\text{-}W_{41}A$ form tetramers that are expressed at the oocyte plasma membrane (Holsinger et al. 1994). Interestingly, one naturally occurring mutant, $M2\text{-}A_{30}T$, was found that exhibited a small pH activation response which was distinct from all the other mutants tested (Holsinger et al. 1994). When the $A_{30}T$ mutation was found in FPV Rostock, virus growth was impaired, and when the virus was passaged in the absence of amantadine, the $A_{30}T$ mutation readily reverted to wild type (Grambas et al. 1992). Thus, these in vivo observations suggest pH activation is of great importance to the ion channel function in the influenza virus life cycle.

It has been observed that oocytes expressing the mutant M2 ion channels have differing membrane currents (Pinto et al. 1992; Wang et al. 1993; Holsinger et al. 1994). In addition to a varying pH activation response, a difference in the total cell-surface currents of oocytes expressing the M2 proteins could be due to different levels of expression. As all the point mutants that have been examined to date can be readily detected at the oocyte plasma membrane, the assumption was made that the total M2 protein accumulation in oocytes, as determined by a quantitative immunoblot, directly reflected the surface expression levels (Holsinger et al. 1994). Calculation of the specific activity of these M2 ion channel activities (μA/ng M2) indicated that in comparison to wild-type M2, the M2-S_{31}N mutation had a neutral effect, whereas M2 molecules containing the changes V_{27}A, V_{27}S, V_{27}T, and G_{34}E had a 2.5-fold increase in activity over wild-type M2. In contrast, M2-A_{30}T, which is only weakly pH activated, had a specific activity 2.5-fold lower than wild-type M2 (Holsinger et al. 1994). The calculation of the specific activity of the M2 ion channels is a useful measurement; however, until single channel recordings are made, it cannot be distinguished whether the channel currents vary in activity due to changes in ion flux or due to changes in the fraction of time that each individual channel spends in the open state, or due to changes in the fraction of molecules that do not enter into an active ion channel complex.

The activities of the FPV Rostock, FPV Weybridge, and Udorn M2 proteins have been evaluated in mammalian cells using as an assay the M2-mediated alteration in the conformational form of HA (either low-pH or native form) (Grambas and Hay 1992; Grambas et al. 1992; Takeuchi and Lamb 1994). The data obtained indicate that the ion channel activity of FPV Rostock M2 is greater than that of either the FPV Weybridge or Udorn M2 proteins. In addition, when FPV Rostock and FPV Weybridge viruses containing M2 TM domain point mutations that confer amantadine resistance were investigated, using as an assay their effect on the percentage native FPV HA that could be identified, it was found that the primary structure of the whole M2 TM domain influenced the consequence of specific residue changes. For example, the change G_{34}E in FPV Rostock M2 protein was found to diminish M2 protein activity, whereas the G_{34}E change in FPV Weybridge M2 protein was found to increase the M2 protein activity (Grambas et al. 1992). Estimates of ion channel specific activity made by measuring the whole-cell currents of oocytes expressing M2 proteins with changes in the TM domain as a function of M2 protein expression levels (Holsinger et al. 1994), lend further support to the notion that the relationship of the role of a specific residue at a particular position in the M2 ion channel to the overall molecular architecture of the M2 ion channel is complex. For example, in both FPV Rostock and FPV Weybridge, the change S_{31}N lowers M2 protein activity, but with Udorn M2 protein, it leads to amantadine resistance with little change in ion channel specific activity. In contrast, the change A_{30}P in FPV Weybridge leads to a viable virus (Hay et al. 1985), whereas the change A_{30}P in Udorn M2 protein effectively abolishes ion channel activity (Holsinger et al. 1994). In addition, when M2 residue 27 in FPV Rostock is threonine, it leads to amantadine resistance (Hay et al. 1985), whereas the presence of threonine in the equivalent position in Udorn M2 protein leads to channel activity that is amantadine-sensitive (Holsinger et al. 1994).

COMPARISON OF THE INFLUENZA VIRUS M2 PROTEIN ION
CHANNEL STRUCTURE WITH THAT OF OTHER
KNOWN CHANNELS

In addition to the influenza virus M2 ion channel protein, the only other known ion channel that has a single TM domain is the 130-residue I_{SK} (min K) K$^+$ channel (Takumi et al. 1988; Folander et al. 1990; Pragnell et al. 1990; Sugimoto et al. 1990; Goldstein and Miller 1991). Interestingly, I_{SK}, like the M2 protein, is thought to be a type III integral membrane protein. Thus, in comparison to ion channels cloned having a multiple membrane-spanning domain architecture with their pore thought to be formed by larger oligomeric complexes that share similar structural elements (for review, see Jan and Jan 1989; Miller 1992), the influenza virus M2 protein is a minimalistic or primitive ion channel.

ACKNOWLEDGMENTS

Research in the authors' laboratories was supported by U.S. Public Health Service research grants AI-20201 (R.A.L.) and AI-31882 (L.H.P.) from the National Institute of Allergy and Infectious Diseases. R.A.L. is an Investigator of the Howard Hughes Medical Institute.

REFERENCES

Boulay, F., R.W. Doms, I. Wilson, and A. Helenius. 1987. The influenza hemagglutinin precursor as an acid-sensitive probe of the biosynthetic pathway. *EMBO J.* **6:** 2643.

Bron, R., A.P. Kendal, H.-D. Klenk, and J. Wilschut. 1993. Role of the M2 protein in influenza virus membrane fusion: Effects of amantadine and monensin on fusion kinetics. *Virology* **195:** 808.

Bukrinskaya, A.G., N.K. Vorkunova, G.V. Kornilayeva, R.A. Narmanbetova, and G.K. Vorkunova. 1982. Influenza virus uncoating in infected cells and effects of rimantadine. *J. Gen. Virol.* **60:** 49.

Ciampor, F., C.A. Thompson, S. Grambas, and A.J. Hay. 1992a. Regulation of pH by the M2 protein of influenza A viruses. *Virus Res.* **22:** 247.

Ciampor, F., P.M. Bayley, M.V. Nermut, E.M.A. Hirst, R.J. Sugrue, and A.J. Hay. 1992b. Evidence that the amantadine-induced, M2-mediated conversion of influenza A virus hemagglutinin to the low pH conformation occurs in an acidic trans Golgi compartment. *Virology* **188:** 14.

Copeland, C.S., R.W. Doms, E.M. Bolzau, R.G. Webster, and A. Helenius. 1986. Assembly of influenza hemagglutinin trimers and its role in intracellular transport. *J. Cell Biol.* **103:** 1179.

Davies, W.L., R.R. Grunert, R.F. Haff, J.W. McGahen, E.M. Neumayer, M. Paulshock, J.C. Watts, T.R. Wood, E.C. Herrmann, and C.E. Hoffmann. 1964. Antiviral activity of I-adamantanamine (amantadine). *Science* **144:** 862.

Duff, K.C. and R.H. Ashley. 1992. The transmembrane domain of influenza A M2 protein forms amantadine-sensitive proton channels in planar lipid bilayers. *Virology*

190: 485.

Duff, K.C., S.M. Kelly, N.C. Price, and J.P. Bradshaw. 1992. The secondary structure of influenza A M2 transmembrane domain: A circular dichroism study. *FEBS Lett.* **311:** 256.

Epand, R.M., R.F. Epand, and R.C. McKenzie. 1987. Effects of viral chemotherapeutic agents on membrane properties: Studies of cyclosporin A, benzlooxycarbonyl-D-Phe-L-Phe-Gly and amantadine. *J. Biol. Chem.* **262:** 1526.

Folander, K., J. Smith, J. Antanavage, C. Bennett, R.B. Stein, and R. Swanson. 1990. Cloning and expression of the delayed rectifier I_{SK} channel from neonatal rat heart and diethylstilbestrol-primed rat uterus. *Proc. Natl. Acad. Sci.* **87:** 2975.

Gething, M.-J., K. McCammon, and J. Sambrook. 1986. Expression of wild-type and mutant forms of influenza hemagglutinin: The role of folding in intracellular transport. *Cell* **46:** 939.

Goldstein, S.A.N. and C. Miller. 1991. Site-specific mutations in a minimal voltage-dependent K^+ channel alter ion selectivity and open-channel block. *Neuron* **7:** 403.

Grambas, S. and A.J. Hay. 1992. Maturation of influenza A virus hemagglutinin— Estimates of the pH encountered during transport and its regulation by the M2 protein. *Virology* **190:** 11.

Grambas, S., M.S. Bennett, and A.J. Hay. 1992. Influence of amantadine resistance mutations on the pH regulatory function of the M2 protein of influenza A viruses. *Virology* **191:** 541.

Hay, A.J. 1992. The action of adamantanamines against influenza A viruses: Inhibition of the M2 ion channel protein. *Semin. Virol.* **3:** 21.

Hay, A.J., N.C.T. Kennedy, J.J. Skehel, and G. Appleyard. 1979. The matrix protein gene determines amantadine-sensitivity of influenza viruses. *J. Gen. Virol.* **42:** 189.

Hay, A.J., A. Wolstenholme, J.J. Skehel, and M.H. Smith. 1985. The molecular basis of the specific anti-influenza action of amantadine. *EMBO J.* **4:** 3021.

Helenius, A. 1992. Unpacking the incoming influenza virus. *Cell* **69:** 577.

Hille, B. 1992. *Ionic channels of excitable membranes.* Sinauer Associates, Sunderland, Massachusetts.

Holsinger, L.J. and R.A. Lamb. 1991. Influenza virus M2 integral membrane protein is a homotetramer stabilized by formation of disulfide bonds. *Virology* **183:** 32.

Holsinger, L.J., D. Nichani, L.H. Pinto, and R.A. Lamb. 1994. Influenza A virus M_2 protein: A structure-function analysis. *J. Virol.* **68:** 1551.

Hughey, P.G., R.W. Compans, S.L. Zebedee, and R.A. Lamb. 1992. Expression of the influenza A virus M2 protein is restricted to apical surfaces of polarized epithelial cells. *J. Virol.* **66:** 5542.

Hull, J.D., R. Gilmore, and R.A. Lamb. 1988. Integration of a small integral membrane protein, M2, of influenza virus into the endoplasmic reticulum: Analysis of the internal signal-anchor domain of a protein with an ectoplasmic NH2 terminus. *J. Cell Biol.* **106:** 1489.

Jan, L.Y. and Y.N. Jan. 1989. Voltage-sensitive ion channels. *Cell* **56:** 13.

Kawaoka, Y. and R.G. Webster. 1988. Sequence requirements for cleavage activation of influenza virus hemagglutinin expressed in mammalian cells. *Proc. Natl. Acad. Sci.* **85:** 324.

Klenk, H.D., R. Rott, M. Orlich, and J. Blodorn. 1975. Activation of influenza A viruses by trypsin treatment. *Virology* **68:** 426.

Lamb, R.A. 1989. Genes and proteins of the influenza viruses. In *The influenza viruses* (ed. R.M. Krug), p. 1. Plenum Press, New York.

Lamb, R.A. and P.W. Choppin. 1981. Identification of a second protein (M2) encoded by

RNA segment 7 of influenza virus. *Virology* **112:** 729.

Lamb, R.A., C.-J. Lai, and P.W. Choppin. 1981. Sequences of mRNAs derived from genome RNA segment 7 of influenza virus: Colinear and interrupted mRNAs code for overlapping proteins. *Proc. Natl. Acad. Sci.* **78:** 4170.

Lamb, R.A., S.L. Zebedee, and C.D. Richardson. 1985. Influenza virus M2 protein is an integral membrane protein expressed on the infected-cell surface. *Cell* **40:** 627.

Lazarowitz, S.G. and P.W. Choppin. 1975. Enhancement of the infectivity of influenza A and B viruses by proteolytic cleavage of the hemagglutinin polypeptide. *Virology* **68:** 440.

Lubeck, M.D., J.L. Schulman, and P. Palese. 1978. Susceptibility of influenza A viruses to amantadine is influenced by the gene coding for the M protein. *J. Virol.* **28:** 710.

Marsh, M. 1992. Keeping the viral coat on. *Curr. Biol.* **2:** 379.

Martin, K. and A. Helenius. 1991. Nuclear transport of influenza virus ribonucleoproteins: The viral matrix protein (M1) promotes export and inhibits import. *Cell* **67:** 117.

Miller, C. 1992. Hunting for the pore of voltage-gated channels. *Curr. Biol.* **2:** 573.

Neher, E. and J.H. Steinback. 1978. Local anaesthetics transiently block currents through single acetylcholine-receptor channels. *J. Physiol.* **277:** 153.

Ohuchi, M., A. Cramer, M. Vey, R. Ohuchi, and H.-D. Klenk. 1994. Rescue of vector expressed fowl plague virus hemagglutinin in biologically active form by acidotropic agents and co-expressed M2 protein. *J. Virol.* **68:** 920.

Ohuchi, M.M., R. Orlich, B.E. Ohuchi, B.E.J. Simpson, W. Garten, H.-D. Klenk, and R. Rott. 1989. Mutations at the cleavage site of the hemagglutinin effect the pathogenicity of influenza virus A/Chick/Penn/83 (H5N2). *Virology* **168:** 274.

Panayotov, P.P. and R.W. Schlesinger. 1992. Oligomeric organization and strain- specific proteolytic modification of the virion M2 protein of influenza A H1N1 viruses. *Virology* **186:** 352.

Pinto, L.H., L.J. Holsinger, and R.A. Lamb. 1992. Influenza virus M2 protein has ion channel activity. *Cell* **69:** 517.

Pragnell, M., K.J. Snay, J.S. Trimmer, N.J. MacLusky, F. Naftolin, L.K. Kaczmerek, and M.B. Boyle. 1990. Estrogen induction of a small, putative K^+ channel mRNA in rat uterus. *Neuron* **4:** 807.

Ruigrok, R.W.H., E.A. Hewat, and R.H. Wade. 1992. Low pH deforms the influenza virus envelope. *J. Gen. Virol.* **73:** 995.

Ruigrok, R.W.H., E.M.A. Hirst, and A.J. Hay. 1991. The specific inhibition of influenza A virus maturation by amantadine: An electron microscopic examination. *J. Gen. Virol.* **72:** 191.

Sansom, M.S.P. and I.D. Kerr. 1993. Influenza virus M2 protein: A molecular modelling study of the ion channel. *Protein Eng.* **6:** 65.

Scholtissek, C. and G.P. Faulkner. 1979. Amantadine-resistant and sensitive influenza A strains and recombinants. *J. Gen. Virol.* **44:** 807.

Simpson, D.A. and R.A. Lamb. 1992. Alterations to influenza virus hemagglutinin cytoplasmic tail modulate virus infectivity. *J. Virol.* **66:** 790.

Skehel, J.J. 1992. Influenza virus. Amantadine blocks the channel. *Nature* **358:** 110.

Skehel, J.J., A.J. Hay, and J.A. Armstrong. 1978. On the mechanism of inhibition of influenza virus replication by amantadine hydrochloride. *J. Gen. Virol.* **38:** 97.

Skehel, J.J., P. Bayley, E. Brown, S. Martin, M.D. Waterfield, J. White, J. Wilson, and D.C. Wiley. 1982. Changes in the conformation of influenza virus hemagglutinin at the pH optimum of virus-mediated membrane fusion. *Proc. Natl. Acad. Sci.* **79:** 968.

Steineke-Gröber, A.M., M. Vey, H. Angliker, E. Shaw, G. Thomas, C. Roberts, H.-D. Klenk, and W. Garten. 1992. Influenza virus hemagglutinin with a multibasic cleavage site is activated by furin, a subtilisin-like protease. *EMBO J.* **11:** 2407.

Steinhauer, D.A., S.A. Wharton, J.J. Skehel, D.C. Wiley, and A.J. Hay. 1991. Amantadine selection of a mutant influenza virus containing an acid-stable hemagglutinin glycoprotein: Evidence for virus-specific regulation of the pH of glycoprotein transport vesicles. *Proc. Natl. Acad. Sci.* **88:** 11525.

Sugimoto, T., Y. Tanabe, R. Shigemoto, M. Iwai, T. Takumi, H. Ohkubo, and S. Nakanishi. 1990. Immunohistochemical study of a rat membrane protein which induces a selective potassium permeation: Its localization in the apical membrane portion of epithelial cells. *J. Membr. Biol.* **113:** 39.

Sugrue, R.J. and A.J. Hay. 1991. Structural characteristics of the M2 protein of influenza A viruses: Evidence that it forms a tetrameric channel. *Virology* **180:** 617.

Sugrue, R.J., G. Bahadur, M.C. Zambon, M. Hall-Smith, A.R. Douglas, and A.J. Hay. 1990. Specific structural alteration of the influenza haemagglutinin by amantadine. *EMBO J.* **9:** 3469.

Takeuchi, K. and R.A. Lamb. 1994. Influenza virus M2 protein ion channel activity stabilizes the native form of fowl plague virus hemagglutinin during intracellular transport. *J. Virol.* **68:** 911.

Takumi, T., H. Ohkubo, and S. Nakanishi. 1988. Cloning of a membrane protein that induces a slow voltage-gated potassium current. *Science* **242:** 1042.

Treanor, J.J., E.L. Tierney, S.L. Zebedee, R.A. Lamb, and B.R. Murphy. 1990. Passively transferred monoclonal antibody to the M2 protein inhibits influenza A virus replication in mice. *J. Virol.* **64:** 1375.

von Heijne, G. and Y. Gavel. 1988. Topogenic signals in integral membrane proteins. *Eur. J. Biochem.* **174:** 6711.

Wang, C., K. Takeuchi, L.H. Pinto, and R.A. Lamb. 1993. The ion channel activity of the influenza A virus M2 protein: Characterization of the amantadine block. *J. Virol.* **67:** 5585.

Wharton, S.A., R.B. Belshe, J.J. Skehel, and A.J. Hay. 1994. Role of virion M2 protein in influenza virus uncoating: Specific reduction in the rate of membrane fusion between virus and liposomes by amantadine. *J. Gen. Virol.* **75:** 945.

White, J.M. 1990. Viral and cellular membrane fusion proteins. *Annu. Rev. Physiol.* **52:** 675.

Wiley, D.C. and J.J. Skehel. 1987. The structure and function of the hemagglutinin membrane glycoprotein of influenza virus. *Annu. Rev. Biochem.* **56:** 365.

Zebedee, S.L. and R.A. Lamb. 1988. Influenza A virus M2 protein: Monoclonal antibody restriction of virus growth and detection of M2 in virions. *J. Virol.* **62:** 2762.

————. 1989a. Growth restriction of influenza A virus by M2 protein antibody is genetically linked to the M1 protein. *Proc. Natl. Acad. Sci.* **86:** 1061.

————. 1989b. Nucleotide sequences of influenza A virus RNA segment 7: A comparison of five isolates. *Nucleic Acids Res.* **17:** 2870.

Zebedee, S.L., C.D. Richardson, and R.A. Lamb. 1985. Characterization of the influenza virus M2 integral membrane protein and expression at the infected-cell surface from cloned cDNA. *J. Virol.* **56:** 502.

Zhirnov, O.P. 1990. Solubilization of matrix protein M1/M from virions occurs at different pH for orthomyxo- and paramyxoviruses. *Virology* **176:** 274.

17

Expression of Viral Receptors and the Vectorial Release of Viruses in Polarized Epithelial Cells

Simon P. Tucker
Infectious Disease Research
Searle Research and Development
c/o Monsanto Company
St. Louis, Missouri 63198

Eckard Wimmer
Department of Microbiology
State University of New York
Stony Brook, New York 11794

Richard W. Compans
Emory University School of Medicine
Department of Microbiology and Immunology
Atlanta, Georgia 30322

The external surfaces of the body are lined with epithelial cells, which act as the primary barrier to virus infection and to dissemination of progeny virus from the infected host. Individual cells in an epithelial layer are joined by junctional complexes that restrict the diffusion of molecules across the cell layer. In addition, the junctional complexes serve to restrict the lateral diffusion of membrane components between the apical and basolateral domains, which, in combination with differential targeting of membrane components, serves to maintain the apical and basolateral surfaces as distinct domains containing different sets of lipids and proteins (Simons and van Meer 1988; Simons and Wandinger-Ness 1990; Compans and Srinivas 1991; Rodriguez-Boulan and Powell 1992). There are several mechanisms employed by viruses to traverse the epithelial barrier (Tucker and Compans 1993), and in many cases the epithelial cells comprising the barrier can serve as sites of virus infection.

In 1978, Rodriguez-Boulan and Sabatini reported the polarized budding of several enveloped viruses from either the apical or the basolateral surfaces of Madin-Darby canine kidney (MDCK) cells. Subsequently, a great deal of interest has developed in studies of virus-infected epithelial cells. Studies of the intracellular transport and surface expression of viral proteins have provided important information about the mechanisms by which membrane proteins are targeted to specific plasma membrane domains of epithelial cells. In addition, the restriction of virus entry or release to specific membrane domains has significant implications for the pathogenesis of viral infections. Many of these studies have involved the growth of epithelial cell lines in culture, which has provided a powerful tool for investigators interested in the mechanisms of cell polarization, the regulation of epithelial transport processes, and interactions with pathogenic microorganisms. In general, epithelial cell lines that undergo differentiation in culture exhibit features which, to varying degrees, correspond to those of the tissue of origin. The cultured cells form organized epithelial layers when grown to confluence, in which each cell exhibits junctional complexes and defined apical (facing the culture media) and basolateral (facing the culture dish) domains. Epithelial cell lines are frequently grown on porous supports (Michalopoulos and Pitot 1975; Misfeldt et al. 1976; Cereijido et al. 1978), which facilitates increased cell differentiation (Shannon and Pitelka 1981; vanMeer and Simons 1982; Handler et al. 1984) and provides the investigator with ready access to both the apical and basolateral surfaces. As a result of the comparative simplicity of these systems, much of the recent data generated on the interactions of viruses with epithelial surfaces are derived from studies using continuous cell lines grown on porous supports. In this chapter, we summarize some of the more recent findings concerning virus entry and release from polarized epithelial cells and briefly discuss some practical limitations of the techniques currently employed.

GROWTH OF EPITHELIAL CELL LINES ON POROUS SUPPORTS

To facilitate access to the basolateral surface for relatively large ligands, such as bacteria or viruses, epithelial cells have often been grown on filters containing 3.0-μm pores (see, e.g., Fuller et al. 1984; Finlay et al. 1988; Rodriguez et al. 1991; Svensson et al. 1991). In the course of our studies on virus/epithelial cell interactions, we have observed that various epithelial cell lines exhibit the ability to migrate through the pores and grow on the opposing face of filter membranes containing such comparatively large pores (Tucker et al. 1992). These observations have obvious and significant implications for studies involving the growth of cells on filter membrane substrates of large pore size. During electron microscopic studies involving the growth of Vero C1008 (a polarized epithelial cell line derived from the African green monkey), Caco-2 (a polarized human intestinal epithelial cell line), and MDCK epithelial cell lines on filter membrane substrates containing 3.0-μm pores, we observed that numerous sections revealed the growth of cells on both faces of the filter (Fig. 1). The amount of cell growth on the lower surface appeared cell-type-dependent, since the number of sections containing MDCK cells on the lower face was significantly less than observed for filters seeded with Caco-2 or Vero C1008 cells. Interestingly, the Caco-2 and Vero C1008 cells that established colonies on the lower filter face appeared to have a more flattened morphology with fewer and smaller microvilli than the cells growing on the upper face of the filter (Fig. 1). However, cell populations on both filter surfaces exhibited junctional complexes. Electron microscopic observations of cells infected with influenza virus or vesicular stomatitis virus (VSV) revealed that cells growing on the lower filter face exhibited the same polarity of virus release as the cells on the upper face of the filter. Thus, influenza virus was observed at the apical surface and VSV at the basolateral surface of the invasive cell types (Tucker et al. 1992). The cells growing on the lower filter surface are therefore polarized by these criteria. The implication of this observation for studies involving the interaction of viruses with epithelial cells is significant. Because the epithelial cells growing on the lower filter surface remain polarized, a microorganism applied to the

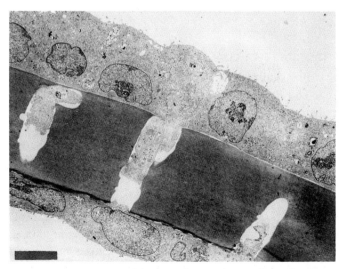

Figure 1 Epithelial cell penetration and growth on the lower surface of filter membranes containing 3.0-μm pores. Transwell tissue culture inserts (Costar Co., Cambridge, Massachuestts) were seeded with 2 x 10^6 Vero C1008 cells and analyzed by transmission electron microscopy at 7 days postseeding. Similar observations were made of filter membranes seeded with Caco-2 or MDCK cells (not shown). Bar, 4 μm.

basal side of the filter may predominantly encounter apical membranes if the cell sheet on this surface has grown sufficiently. Obviously, the potential for such an interaction complicates the interpretation of any data generated from this type of experiment.

Other workers have recently reported the migration of human umbilical vein endothelial cells through filter membranes containing 3.0-μm pores and the establishment of confluent monolayers on both sides of the filter (Virji et al. 1991), suggesting that this is a relatively common occurrence. Initial studies suggest three potential solutions to this problem. If not constrained by other limitations, the utilization of a cell line which does not significantly migrate through 3.0-μm pores or grow on the lower face of the filter is indicated. Alternatively, appropriate selective procedures may yield a less invasive variant of the original cell line. The latter approach may be feasible for some cell lines since the cells which invaded the filter in our studies exhibited morphological and physiological differences from the parent cell line, and these differences were retained upon multiple serial passages (Tucker et al. 1992). Finally, filter membrane substrates with pores sufficiently large to allow microorganisms access but small enough to prevent cellular migration may be used. Studies with the highly invasive Vero C1008 cell type grown on filter membranes containing pores of various sizes suggest that a pore size of 1.0 μm would be suitable (Tucker et al. 1992).

VIRUS ENTRY IN POLARIZED EPITHELIAL CELLS

The differential expression of host cell receptors is a major determinant of viral host-range and tissue tropism. In the context of virus infection of epithelial cells, the polarity of host cell receptor distribution defines the domain from which infection may be mediated. Thus, VSV entry is restricted to the basolateral surface of MDCK cells (Fuller et al. 1984), whereas SV40 infection only occurs following binding to the apical plasma membrane domain (Clayson and Compans 1988). In most cases studied, the characteristics of entry appear to be similar for various epithelial cell types (Tucker and Compans 1993). Some viruses exhibit a marked restriction of binding/entry to a specific membrane domain, whereas others exhibit little preference. Since some viruses may bind to more than a single type of host cell receptor molecule, the possibility exists that infection by viruses in the latter category is mediated by binding to a different receptor population on each membrane domain. Indeed, this appears to be the mechanism by which herpes simplex viruses enter epithelial cells via either surface. Recent evidence indicates that the infectious route of a glycoprotein-C (gC)-deficient herpes simplex virus 1

(HSV-1) mutant is restricted to the basolateral surface of MDCK cells (Sears et al. 1991). Since wild-type HSV-1 was able to infect MDCK cells following adsorption to either the apical or basolateral surfaces, it was concluded that HSV-1 infection is mediated by two different host cell receptor molecules; one expressed on the apical domain that must interact with gC to mediate infection, and a second located on the basolateral surface that binds to viral attachment proteins other than gC (Sears et al. 1991). Nonpolarized entry may also be mediated by binding to a single class of receptor molecules that is expressed on both cell surfaces. Influenza virus is therefore able to bind and initiate infection at both the apical and basolateral domains, since membrane glycoproteins on both surfaces contain sialic acid residues, which serve as receptors for the viral hemagglutinin. Virus/epithelial cell interactions involving identified cellular proteins as virus receptors have been less clearly defined. However, recent studies have shown that poliovirus, which has a comparatively well characterized receptor, binds and initiates infection at both the apical and basolateral surfaces of polarized epithelial cells (Tucker et al. 1993a).

Early studies on the interaction of poliovirus with nonsusceptible cell lines (Kaplan 1955; McLaren et al. 1959) and the demonstration that virus replication can occur in nonprimate cells following the introduction of poliovirus RNA (DeSomer et al. 1959; Holland et al. 1959) indicated that, at least in cultured cells, host range can be determined by mechanisms controlling viral entry. Later studies involving the transfection of nonsusceptible mouse L cells with human DNA clones showed that susceptibility to all three poliovirus serotypes is conferred by expression of a polypeptide with a predicted molecular weight between 43 kD and 45 kD (Mendelsohn et al. 1986; 1989). Expression of the cloned cDNA from a recombinant vaccinia virus vector resulted in the synthesis of a major 65-kD protein product and a polypeptide of approximately 46 kD at significantly lower levels (Zibert et al. 1991). It is likely that the 65-kD polypeptide represents glycosylation intermediates of the smaller species. It has been found more recently that the mature poliovirus receptor molecules expressed at the surface of a variety of human cells have a molecular weight of >80 kD (Bernhardt et al. 1994). The predicted amino acid sequence indicates that the poliovirus receptor has eight potential N-glycosylation sites and represents a new member of the immunoglobulin superfamily (Mendelsohn et al. 1989; Zibert et al. 1991). Several monoclonal antibodies that block poliovirus infection have been isolated. One of these, D171, which binds only to poliovirus-susceptible cells and blocks infection of all three poliovirus serotypes (Nobis et al. 1985), was used as an additional screen for the L-cell transformants described above and therefore reacts with the identical receptor molecule. Since poliovirus host range appears to be regulated largely by the expression of an identified receptor molecule, it seemed likely that, in the event that the receptor was expressed on a particular plasma membrane domain of polarized epithelial cells, poliovirus entry would be similarly restricted. In addition, because poliovirus is transmitted via the fecal/oral route and must traverse gut epithelial cells to initiate an infection, such a restriction of viral entry in polarized epithelial cells is likely to be of considerable significance to viral pathogenesis.

We have investigated the localization of the poliovirus receptor on plasma membranes of polarized epithelial cells by measuring the adsorption of purified, radiolabeled poliovirus to either the apical or basolateral surfaces of cells grown on filter membranes containing 0.4-μm pores. Approximately equivalent levels of purified poliovirus were found to adsorb to the apical and basolateral surfaces of either polarized Caco-2 or Vero C1008 cell monolayers, and binding to both surfaces was inhibited by monoclonal antibody D171 (Tucker et al. 1993a). This suggests that the receptor is expressed at similar levels on both surfaces. Such a lack of polarization is in contrast to the cell-surface expression of many cell-surface proteins, which are characteristically expressed either on the apical or basolateral plasma membranes of polarized epithelial cells (Fujita et al. 1973; Richardson and Simmons 1979; Lisanti et al. 1989; Sargiacomo et al. 1989).

To determine whether infectious entry is mediated by the same receptor on both the apical and basolateral surfaces, each surface was incubated with increasing concentrations of monoclonal D171 prior to the adsorption of virus. Infection via either surface of Caco-2 and Vero C1008 cells, as measured by poliovirus-specific polypeptide synthesis, was significantly reduced by D171 antibody treatment (Fig. 2). This result is consistent with the poliovirus binding data discussed above and indicates that infection is mediated by binding to the same receptor molecule or epitope expressed on both the apical and basolateral surfaces. This result is of interest because the finding of the same protein species on both the apical and basolateral surfaces is unusual and therefore may suggest the existence of forms of the poliovirus receptor on each plasma membrane domain differing, for example, at the level of posttranslational modifications.

VIRUS RELEASE FROM INFECTED POLARIZED EPITHELIAL CELLS

In 1978, Rodriguez-Boulan and Sabatini reported that enveloped RNA viruses are released from MDCK cells in a polar fashion; VSV budded predominantly from the basolateral plasma membrane, whereas Sendai

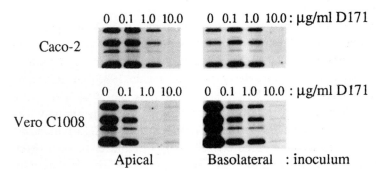

Figure 2 Poliovirus infectious entry of Caco-2 and Vero C1008 cells occurs at the apical and basolateral surfaces and is mediated by the same receptor on both domains. Monolayers of Caco-2 and Vero C1008 cells grown on Transwell tissue culture inserts (0.4-µm pore size) were incubated for 2 hr at 4°C with 0–10 µg/ml of monoclonal antibody D171 applied to either the basolateral or apical surfaces. Following aspiration of the antibody, the monolayers were infected with poliovirus (moi = 10 pfu/cell) via the same plasma membrane incubated with the antibody. Cells were radiolabeled at 8 hpi, and immunoprecipitated poliovirus proteins were analyzed by SDS-PAGE and fluorography.

and influenza virions were released exclusively from the apical domain. Type C retroviruses were also observed to be shed preferentially from the basolateral membrane of polarized epithelial cells (Roth et al. 1983a). More detailed analysis revealed that the envelope glycoproteins of these viruses, which assemble at the plasma membrane, accumulate on the same membrane domain from which budding occurs (Rodriguez-Boulan and Pendergast 1980; Roth et al. 1983a,b) and are directionally transported to this surface when expressed in the absence of other virus-specific polypeptides (Roth et al. 1983b; Jones et al. 1985; Stephens et al. 1986). These observations have led to the hypothesis that the site of insertion of the envelope glycoprotein(s) determines the site of viral assembly. A recent report on the assembly of HIV particles in polarized epithelial cells supports this hypothesis (Owens et al. 1991). Infection of epithelial cells with a recombinant vaccinia virus expressing the HIV-1 *gag* (core) polyprotein in the absence of the envelope glycoprotein resulted in the assembly and release of HIV-like particles in approximately equivalent amounts from both apical and basolateral domains. In contrast, coexpression of *gag* and *env* genes resulted in targeting of 94–97% of the particles to the basolateral domain. Since the envelope glycoprotein exhibited an almost exclusive distribution to this domain when expressed from a recombinant vector (Owens and Compans 1989), it is reasonable to conclude that the envelope glycoprotein is the only targeted component and that its interaction with *gag* defines the domain from which virus is selectively released. It is not clear whether a similar situation exists with other viruses. For example, a VSV temperature-sensitive mutant (ts045), which exhibited a defect in the transport of its envelope glycoprotein, G, at the restrictive temperature, still budded from the basolateral domain (Bergmann and Fusco 1988). In this case, preferential transport of the M protein to the basolateral plasma membrane was reported, suggesting that M protein may be targeted similarly to G. However, the spikeless particles produced by the ts045 mutant are known to contain the membrane anchor region of the G protein (Metsikko and Simons 1986), and this may play an essential role in determining the maturation site of the virus particles produced by this mutant. In some cases, more than a single component of the virus exhibits targeted transport. Thus the HA, NA, and M_2 proteins of influenza virus are independently transported to the apical domain in the absence of other influenza virus gene products (Roth et al. 1983b; Jones et al. 1985; Hughey et al. 1992).

Several enveloped viruses which assemble at intracellular membranes are also asymmetrically released from polarized epithelial cells. Herpes simplex viruses (HSV) -1 and -2 which assemble and bud at the inner nuclear membrane (Darlington and Moss 1968) are preferentially released at the basolateral plasma membrane (Srinivas et al. 1986). Since herpesviruses bud into the lumen of the nuclear envelope, which is continuous with the endoplasmic reticulum, the virions are presumably transported by the same mechanism responsible for the delivery of soluble, secreted polypeptides by these cells. The basolateral release of HSV suggests that the virions express targeting signals recognized in a luminal context, or that an interaction occurs between virions and a targeted membrane-bound factor(s). In this respect, the virions may resemble endogenous secretory products which are released in a directional fashion. Bunyaviruses and coronaviruses, which are also assembled at intracellular membranes, use a similar transport pathway. Most bunyavirus assembly occurs in the Golgi complex, and budding occurs at smooth-surfaced membranes in this region (Murphy et al. 1973; Smith and Pifat 1982), after which virus is transported to the cell surface. Punta Toro virus, a member of the sandfly fever group of bunyaviruses, was released virtually exclusively from the basolateral surface of polarized epithelial cells following assembly in the Golgi complex (Chen et al. 1991). Immunoelectron microscopic analysis of hepatocytes infected with another bunyavirus, Rift Valley fever virus, also revealed an apparent selective release from the basolateral domain (Anderson and Smith 1987). Since in the latter example direct virus budding at the basolateral plasma membrane was also observed in some sections, at least one of the components of Rift Valley fever virus contains the appropriate signals to direct vectorial transport prior to virion assembly.

The vectorial transport and release of nonenveloped viruses has been less widely investigated. However, studies using SV40 and poliovirus have indicated that nonenveloped viruses may also be targeted for release at a particular plasma membrane domain. SV40 is a nonenveloped virus that is assembled in the nucleus of infected cells. Clayson et al. (1989) reported an almost exclusive release of SV40 from the apical surface of polarized Vero C1008 and primary African green monkey kidney epithelial cells. The authors also noted that treatment of infected cells with the sodium ionophore monensin, which serves as an inhibitor of vesicular transport, resulted in the inhibition of SV40 release but had no effect on virus-specific protein synthesis or the assembly of infectious virus. Since extensive virus release was observed prior to detectable cell lysis, the vectorial transport and release of SV40 may therefore be mediated by a vesicular transport mechanism in these cell types. Consistent with this hypothesis, cytoplasmic virions have been observed to be enclosed within membranous vesicular compartments during the period of virus release (Clayson et al. 1989). Since the SV40 receptor is expressed on the apical surface (Clayson and Compans 1988), it is possible that targeting of progeny virions to this domain is mediated by intracellular association with receptor molecules.

Recent studies involving poliovirus-infected epithelial cells have revealed a marked polarization in the pattern of virus release exhibited by some epithelial cell types (Tucker et al. 1993b). Extracellular poliovirus was almost exclusively detected in the apical media overlying monolayers of infected Caco-2 cells, irrespective of the membrane domain inoculated (Fig. 3). The latter result suggests that poliovirus release may be mediated by a vectorial transport mechanism in polarized human intestinal epithelial cells. Interestingly, comparatively high titers of poliovirus were detected in culture media prior to significantly apparent cytopathology (Tucker et al. 1993b). Although it is difficult to exclude the possibility of individual cell lysis, these results are at least consistent with the possibility of a nonlytic release mechanism at early times postinfection. Although nonenveloped viruses, such as poliovirus and SV40, are generally considered to be released by lysis of the infected cell, several apparently nonlytic release processes have also been described that are likely to involve some form of vesicular transport (Dunnebacke et al. 1969; Bienz et al. 1973; Clayson et al. 1989). Such a vesicular transport mechanism would account for the directional release of poliovirus by utilization of the currently accepted mechanism for the vectorial delivery of endogenous and exogenous membrane-bound and secretory proteins. The process by which poliovirions might become en-

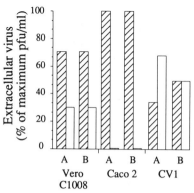

Figure 3   Release of poliovirus from polarized and nonpolarized cells. Monolayers of polarized Caco-2 and Vero C1008 epithelial cells and non-polarized CV1 cells grown on Transwell filters (0.4-μm pore size) were infected with poliovirus (moi 1 pfu/cell) via either the basolateral (B) or apical (A) surfaces. At 16 hpi, media were collected from the apical (*hatched bars*) and basal (*open bars*) chambers, and the titer of extracellular virus was determined by plaque assay. The titer of residual inoculum virus was determined by plaque assay of media collected at 2 hpi and was found to be less than 10 pfu/ml in each case. This value was deducted from the titer obtained at 16 hpi. Virus titers are expressed as a percentage of the maximal virus titer measured in the apical and basolateral media for each cell line and route of inoculum.

closed in, or associated with, vesicles bearing targeting signals remains to be elucidated. However, there is considerable evidence that poliovirus replication complexes are associated with host membranes, which are most likely derived from the rough endoplasmic reticulum (Takegami et al. 1983a,b; Tershak 1984; Takeda et al. 1986; Irurzan et al. 1992). Poliovirus-infected cells also characteristically exhibit a highly vesiculated cytoplasm, and continuous phospholipid biosynthesis to form membranes of defined composition appears essential for viral RNA synthesis (Guinea and Carrasco 1990, 1991). Since polarized epithelial cells also transport lipids in a vectorial fashion (Simons and van Meer 1988), poliovirus transport to the apical plasma membrane may be a consequence of interaction with these, or similar, membranes. Alternatively, the vectorial transport of poliovirus may be mediated by an as-yet-uncharacterized process involving the recognition of targeting signals contained within the virion structure. We are also unable to exclude the possibility that vectorial lysis and/or extrusion of infected cells prior to lysis contribute to vectorial release.

The vectorial release of poliovirus may be restricted to epithelial cells of intestinal origin, because our results indicate that another polarized epithelial cell line derived from the African green monkey kidney (Vero

C1008 cells) released virus in an essentially nondirectional manner comparable to the pattern of release from nonpolarized CV1 cells (Fig. 3). However, it is noteworthy that the transepithelial resistance values for Vero C1008 cell layers are approximately an order of magnitude lower than those achieved by Caco-2 cell monolayers, and a more significant degree of preferential release of poliovirus into the apical compartment was apparent in some experiments involving Vero C1008 cells. These observations suggest that Vero C1008 cell monolayers may be more intrinsically "leaky"; a property likely to be exacerbated by poliovirus-induced cytopathology.

We have considered several possibilities for the mechanism involved in the vectorial release of poliovirus from polarized epithelial cells. It is possible that virus particles are contained within vesicles which are transported to, and fuse with, the intact apical plasma membrane. Alternatively, virus may be transported as aggregates that are expelled through the apical plasma membrane. Additional possible mechanisms for the apical release of poliovirus from Caco-2 cells include the directional lysis of virus-infected cells or the extrusion of infected cells from the monolayer, followed by lysis in the apical chamber. Structures consistent with the first two possibilities, vectorial vesicle and aggregate transport, were observed by transmission electron microscopy (Tucker et al. 1993b). Additional studies with monensin and ammonium chloride revealed that both of these inhibitors of vesicular transport mechanisms had some limited selective effect on poliovirus release from Caco-2 cells (Tucker et al. 1993b). However, because the effects of both compounds were more manifest on the levels of virus detected in the basolateral media than in the apical media, the mechanisms involved in the polarized release of the large majority of poliovirus from the apical domain of Caco-2 cells do not involve a monensin- or ammonium chloride-sensitive step. This result is in contrast to the reported inhibitory effect of monensin upon the polarized release of SV40 from the apical domain of African green monkey kidney epithelial cells (Clayson et al. 1989), suggesting that different processes are involved in the vectorial targeting of these nonenveloped viruses.

During the course of this work, we observed a significant inhibition of poliovirus replication mediated by the fungal metabolite brefeldin A (BFA). Experiments with this compound were initiated because of its effects on the Golgi complex, the organelle responsible for sorting proteins into distinct sets of vesicles prior to transport to either the apical or basolateral surface. Since BFA is reported to have an effect on polarized transport processes (Hunziker et al. 1991; Low et al. 1991), we reasoned that poliovirus release from Caco-2 cells might be affected by BFA in the event that similar sorting mechanisms were involved. The polarized release of poliovirus was not selectively inhibited by BFA treatment at early or late times postinfection, and, because removal of BFA did not

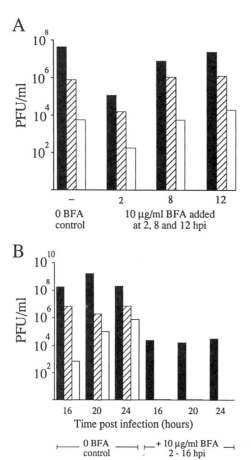

Figure 4 (*A*) Effect of BFA on poliovirus release at early and late times postinfection. Monolayers of Caco-2 cells grown on Transwell filters (0.4-μm pore size) were infected with poliovirus (moi 1 pfu/cell) at their apical surface. At 2, 8, or 12 hpi, BFA was added to give a concentration of 10 μg/ml. At 16 hpi, the titers of cell-associated (*solid bars*), apical extracellular (*hatched bars*), and basolateral extracellular (*open bars*) virus were determined. (*B*) Effect of removal of a BFA block on poliovirus replication and virus release. Monolayers of Caco-2 cells were grown and infected as described above. At 2 hpi, media were exchanged for media containing 0 or 10 μg/ml of BFA. At 16 hpi, the monolayers were washed, and incubation was continued in the absence of BFA. The titers of cell-associated (*solid bars*), apical extracellular (*hatched bars*), and basolateral extracellular (*open bars*) virus were determined at the times indicated.

result in a burst of progeny virus at later times postinfection, it is unlikely that BFA has an effect on the assembly and release of infectious virus (Fig. 4). However, BFA was found to markedly inhibit the production of infectious progeny by interfering with poliovirus biosynthetic processes (Fig. 4) (Irurzan et al. 1992; Maynell et al. 1992; Tucker et al. 1993b), an observation which supports the notion that portions of the exocytic transport pathway are involved in poliovirus replication. It has been suggested that BFA effects are mediated by dissociation of a protein known as β-COP from membranes of the Golgi complex (Klausner et al. 1992). It is possible that the association of poliovirus replication complexes with host membranes occurs via a similar mechanism, perhaps involving β-COP.

Our findings that the poliovirus receptor is present on both surfaces of a human intestinal epithelial cell line, allowing infection to be mediated by adsorption to either surface, and that poliovirus release occurs almost exclusively at the apical surface of this cell type, provide interesting implications for viral pathogenesis. A simple model for poliovirus infection and dissemination from the human gut may therefore be proposed. On the basis of published observations, it can be concluded that lymphoid structures (such as Peyer's patches) located in the gastrointestinal epithelium comprise the initial replication site and are probably the portal of entry (Bodian 1956; Sabin 1956). Traversal of the epithelium at these sites may be M-cell-mediated (Sicinski et al. 1990) or may occur following necrosis of the epithelial barrier. The results presented above suggest that, in the absence of extensive necrosis, the M-cell-mediated route may be preferred, since only a small proportion of virus may be released at the basolateral surface of the infected epithelial cell. During the later stages of infection, dissemination of progeny virus into the gut may be mediated by infection of intestinal wall epithelial cells via their basolateral surface, followed by the vectorial release of virus from these cells into the apical or luminal environment. A similar mechanism was proposed by Rubin et al. and was based on these authors' observations of reovirus-infected epithelial cells (Wolf et al. 1981; Rubin et al. 1985). The current studies provide further evidence in support of this model of viral pathogenesis and suggest that studies using epithelial cell lines grown on porous supports provide an excellent model for epithelial surfaces lining the gut.

CONCLUSIONS

The demonstration that virus entry and release are often restricted to specific plasma membrane domains of polarized epithelial cells has stimulated a great deal of interest concerning the cell biology of virus infection and its relationship to viral pathogenesis. Polarized epithelial cells in culture, which can be grown on permeable supports, provide excellent systems for investigating the events in virus entry and release at the cellular level, and much information is being obtained using such systems. The information obtained using such "in vitro" systems is enhancing our knowledge of pathogenic mechanisms, and it is anticipated that future studies will begin to correlate "in vitro" and "in vivo" observations.

The polarized expression of receptor molecules has obvious significance for viruses that infect epithelial cells. If the receptor molecule is localized to the basolateral surface, it is evident that the barrier presented by the epithelium is more significant than if the receptor is expressed on the apical surface or is nonpolarized. In addition, since a virus that is specifically released from the apical surface of an epithelial cell is targeted to the lumen and away from underlying tissues, the resulting infection should have an increased likelihood of being localized to the epithelial surface. Conversely, basolateral release should favor the establishment of a systemic infection. Indeed, a mutant of Sendai virus was recently described that produces a systemic infection and is released bidirectionally from polarized epithelial cells in tissue culture, in contrast to the wild-type virus, which is released apically and produces an infection localized to the respiratory tract (Tashiro et al. 1990). It is anticipated that further study will provide insights into the mechanisms involved in the polarized entry and release of viruses from epithelial cells and lead to a more complete understanding of viral pathogenesis.

ACKNOWLEDGMENTS

The authors' research was supported by research grants CA-18611 and CA-28146 from the National Cancer Institute and AI-2680 and AI-28147.

REFERENCES

Anderson, G.W.J. and J.F. Smith. 1987. Immunoelectron microscopy of Rift Valley fever viral morphogenesis in primary rat hepatocytes. *Virology* **161:** 91.

Bergmann, J.E. and P.J. Fusco. 1988. The M protein of vesicular stomatitis virus associates specifically with the basolateral membranes of polarized epithelial cells independently of the G protein. *J. Cell Biol.* **107:** 1707.

Bernhardt, G., J.A. Bibb, J. Bradley, and E. Wimmer. 1994. Molecular characterization of the cellular receptor for poliovirus. *Virology* **199:** 105.

Bienz, K., D. Egger, and D.A. Wolff. 1973. Virus replication, cytopathology, and lysosomal enzyme response of mitotic and interphase Hep-2 cells infected with poliovirus. *J. Virol.* **11:** 565.

Bodian, D. 1956. Poliovirus in chimpanzee tissues after virus feeding. *Am. J. Hyg.* **64:** 181.

Cereijido, M., E.S. Robbins, W.J. Dolan, C.A. Rotunno, and D.D. Sabatini. 1978. Polarized monolayers formed by epithelial cells on a permeable and translucent support. *J. Cell Biol.* **77:** 853.

Chen, S.-Y., Y. Matsuoka, and R.W. Compans. 1991. Assembly and polarized release of punta toro virus and the effects of brefeldin A. *J. Virol.* **65:** 1427.

Clayson, E.T. and R.W. Compans. 1988. Entry of simian virus 40 is restricted to the apical surfaces of polarized epithelial cells. *Mol. Cell. Biol.* **8:** 3391.

Clayson, E.T., L.V.J. Brando, and R.W. Compans. 1989. Release of SV40 virions from epithelial cells is polarized and occurs without cell lysis. *J. Virol.* **63:** 2278.

Compans, R.W. and R.V. Srinivas 1991. Protein sorting in polarized epithelial cells. *Curr. Top. Microbiol. Immunol.* **170:** 141.

Darlington, R.W. and L.J.I. Moss. 1968. Herpesvirus envelopment. *J. Virol.* **2:** 48.

DeSomer, P., A. Pruzie, and E. Schonne. 1959. Infectivity of poliovirus RNA for embryonated eggs and unsusceptible cell lines. *Nature* **184:** 652.

Dunnebacke, T.H., J.D. Levinthal, and R.C. Williams. 1969. Entry and release of poliovirus as observed by electron microscopy of cultured cells. *J. Virol.* **4:** 505.

Finlay, B.B., B. Gumbiner, and S. Falkow. 1988. Penetration of Salmonella through a polarized Madin-Darby canine kidney epithelial cell monolayer. *J. Cell Biol.* **107:** 221.

Fuller, S., C.-H. von Bonsdorff, and K. Simons. 1984. Vesicular stomatitis virus infects and matures only through the basolateral surface of the polarized epithelial cell line, MDCK. *Cell* **38:** 65.

Fujita, M., K. Kawai, S. Asano, and N. Nakao. 1973. Protein components of two different regions of an intestinal plasma epithelial cell membrane. *Biochim. Biophys. Acta* **307:** 141.

Guinea, R. and L. Carrasco. 1990. Phospholipid biosynthesis and poliovirus genome replication, two coupled phenomena. *EMBO J.* **9:** 2011.

――――. 1991. Effects of fatty acids on lipid synthesis and viral RNA replication in poliovirus-infected cells. *Virology* **185:** 473.

Handler, J.S., A.S. Preston, and R.E. Steele. 1984. Factors affecting the differentiation of epithelial transport and responsiveness to hormones. *Fed. Proc.* **43:** 2221.

Holland, J.J., L.C. Mclaren, and J.T. Syverton. 1959. The mammalian cell virus relationship. III. Production of infectious poliovirus by non-primate cells exposed to poliovirus ribonucleic acid. *Proc. Soc. Exp. Biol. Med.* **100:** 843.

Hughey, P.G., R.W. Compans, S.L. Zebedee, and R.A. Lamb. 1992. Expression of the influenza A virus M2 protein is restricted to apical surfaces of polarized epithelial cells. *J. Virol.* **66:** 5542.

Hunziker, W., J.A. Whitney, and I. Mellman. 1991. Selective inhibition of transcytosis by Brefeldin A in MDCK cells. *Cell* **67:** 617.

Irurzan, A., L. Perez, and L. Carrasco. 1992. Involvement of membrane traffic in the replication of poliovirus genomes: Effects of brefeldin A. *Virology* **191:** 166.

Jones, L.V., R.W. Compans, A.R. Davis, T.J. Bos, and D.P. Nayak. 1985. Surface expression of the influenza neuraminidase, an amino-terminally anchored viral membrane glycoprotein, in polarized epithelial cells. *Mol. Cell. Biol.* **5:** 2181.

Kaplan, A.S. 1955. Comparison of susceptible and resistant cells to infections with poliomyelitis virus. *Ann. N.Y. Acad. Sci.* **61:** 830.

Klausner, R.D., J.G. Donaldson, and J. Lippincott-Schwartz. 1992. Brefeldin A: Insights into the control of membrane traffic and organelle structure. *J. Cell Biol.* **116**: 1071.

Lisanti, M.P., A. Le Bivic, M. Sargiacomo, and E. Rodriguez-Boulan. 1989. Steady-state distribution and biogenesis of endogenous Madin-Darby canine kidney glycoproteins: Evidence for intracellular sorting and polarized cell surface delivery. *J. Cell Biol.* **109**: 2145.

Low, S.H., S.H. Wong, B.L. Tang, P. Tan, V.N. Subramaniam, and W. Hong. 1991. Inhibition by brefeldin A of protein secretion from the apical cell surface of Madin-Darby canine kidney cells. *J. Cell Biol.* **266**: 17729.

Maynell, L.A., K. Kirkegaard, and M.W. Klymkowsky. 1992. Inhibition of poliovirus RNA synthesis by Brefeldin A. *J. Virol.* **66**: 1985.

McLaren, L.C., J.J. Holland, and J.T. Syverton. 1959. The mammalian cell-virus relationship. I. Attachment of poliovirus to cultivated cells of primate and non-primate origin. *J. Exp. Med.* **109**: 475.

Mendelsohn, C., E. Wimmer, and V.R. Racaniello. 1989. Cellular receptor for poliovirus: Molecular cloning, nucleotide sequence and expression of a new member of the immunoglobulin superfamily. *Cell* **56**: 855.

Mendelsohn, C., B. Johnson, K.A. Lionetti, P. Nobis, E. Wimmer, and V.R. Racaniello. 1986. Transformation of a human poliovirus receptor gene into mouse cells. *Proc. Natl. Acad. Sci.* **83**: 7845.

Metsikko, K. and K. Simons. 1986. The budding mechanism of spikeless vesicular stomatitis virus particles. *EMBO J.* **5**: 1913.

Michalopoulos, G.H. and H.C. Pitot. 1975. Primary culture of parenchymal liver cells on collagen membranes. *Exp. Cell Res.* **94**: 70.

Misfeldt, D.S., S.T. Hamamoto, and D.R. Pitelka. 1976. Transepithelial transport in cell culture. *Proc. Natl. Acad. Sci.* **73**: 1212.

Murphy, F.A., A.K. Harrison, and S.G. Whitfield. 1973. Bunyaviridae: Morphologic and morphogenetic similarities of Bunyamwera serologic serogroup viruses and several other arthropod-borne viruses. *Intervirology* **1**: 297.

Nobis, P., R. Zibirre, G. Meyer, J. Kuhne, G. Warnecke, and G. Koch. 1985. Production of a monoclonal antibody against an epitope on HeLa cells that is the functional poliovirus binding site. *J. Gen. Virol.* **6**: 2563.

Owens, R.J. and R.W. Compans. 1989. Expression of the HIV envelope glycoprotein is restricted to the basolateral surfaces of polarized epithelial cells. *J. Virol.* **63**: 978.

Owens, R.J., J.W. Dubay, E. Hunter, and R.W. Compans. 1991. Human immunodeficiency virus envelope protein determines the site of virus release in polarized epithelial cells. *Proc. Natl. Acad. Sci.* **75**: 5071.

Richardson, J.C.W. and N.L. Simmons. 1979. Demonstration of protein asymmetries in the plasma membrane of cultured renal (MDCK) epithelial cells by lactoperoxidase-mediated iodination. *FEBS Lett.* **105**: 201.

Rodriguez, D., J.-R. Rodriguez, G.K. Ojakian, and M. Esteban. 1991. Vaccinia virus preferentially enters polarized epithelial cells through the basolateral surface. *J. Virol.* **65**: 494.

Rodriguez-Boulan, E. and M. Pendergast. 1980. Polarized distribution of envelope proteins in the plasma membrane of infected epithelial cells. *Cell* **20**: 45.

Rodriguez-Boulan, E. and S.K. Powell. 1992. Polarity of epithelial and neuronal cells. *Annu. Rev. Cell Biol.* **8**: 395.

Rodriquez-Boulan, E. and D.D. Sabatini. 1978. Asymmetric budding of viruses in epithelial monoloayers. A model system for the study of epithelial polarity. *Proc. Natl. Acad. Sci.* **75**: 5071.

Roth, M.G., R.V. Srinivas, and R.W. Compans. 1983a. Basolateral maturation of retrovirus in polarized epithelial cells. *J. Virol.* **45:** 1065.

Roth, M.G., R.W. Compans, L. Guisti, A.R. Davis, D.P. Nayak, M.J. Gething, and J. Sambrook. 1983b. Influenza virus hemagglutinin expression is polarized in cells infected with recombinant SV40 viruses carrying cloned hemagglutinin DNA. *Cell* **33:** 435.

Rubin, D.H., M.L. Kornstein, and A.O. Anderson. 1985. Reovirus serotype 1 intestinal infection: A novel replicative cycle with ileal disease. *J. Virol.* **53:** 391.

Sabin, A.B. 1956. Pathogenesis of poliomyelitis. *Science* **123:** 1151.

Sargiacomo, M., M. Lisanti, L. Graeve, A. Le Bivic, and E. Rodriguez-Boulan. 1989. Integral and peripheral protein composition of the apical and basolateral membrane domains in MDCK cells. *J. Membr. Biol.* **107:** 277.

Sears, A.E., B. McGwuire, and B. Roizman. 1991. Two asymmetrically distributed cell receptors interact with different viral proteins. *Proc. Natl. Acad. Sci.* **88:** 5087.

Shannon, J.M. and D.R. Pitelka. 1981. The influence of cell shape on the induction of functional differentiation in mouse mammary cells in vitro. *In Vitro* **17:** 1016.

Sicinski, P., J. Rowinski, J.B. Warchol, Z. Jarzabek, W. Gut, B. Szczygiel, K. Bielecki, and G. Koch. 1990. Poliovirus type 1 enters the human host through intestinal M cells. *Gastroenterology* **98:** 56.

Simons, K. and A. Wandinger-Ness. 1990. Polarized sorting in epithelia. *Cell* **62:** 207.

Simons, K. and G. van Meer. 1988. Lipid sorting in epithelial cells. *Biochemistry* **27:** 6197.

Smith, J.F. and D.Y. Pifat. 1982. Morphogenesis of sandfly fever viruses (Bunyaviridae family). *Virology* **121:** 61.

Srinivas, R.V., N. Balachandran, F.V. Alonso-Caplen, and R.W. Compans. 1986. Expression of herpes simplex virus glycoproteins in polarized epithelial cells. *J. Virol.* **58:** 689.

Stephens, E.B., R.W. Compans, P. Earl, and B. Moss. 1986. Surface expression of viral glycoproteins in polarized epithelial cells using vaccinia virus vectors. *EMBO J.* **5:** 237.

Svensson, L., B.B. Finlay, D. Bass, H.B. von Bonsdorff, and H.B. Greenberg. 1991. Symmetric infection of rotavirus on polarized human intestinal epithelial cells (CaCo-2). *Virology* **65:** 4190.

Takeda, N., R.J. Kuhn, C.F. Yang, T. Takegami, and E. Wimmer. 1986. Initiation of poliovirus plus-strand RNA synthesis in a membrane complex of infected HeLa cells. *J. Virol.* **60:** 43.

Takegami, T., R.J. Kuhn, C.W. Anderson, and E. Wimmer. 1983a. Membrane-dependent uridylylation of the genome-linked protein VPg of poliovirus. *Proc. Natl. Acad. Sci.* **80:** 7447.

Takegami, T., B.L. Semler, C.W. Anderson, and E. Wimmer. 1983b. Membrane fractions active in poliovirus RNA replication contain VPg precursor polypeptides. *Virology* **128:** 33.

Tashiro, M., M. Yamakawa, K. Tobita, J.T. Seto, H.-D. Klenk, and R. Rott. 1990. Altered budding site of a pantropic mutant of Sendai virus, F1-R in polarized epithelial cells. *J. Virol.* **64:** 4672.

Tershak, D.R. 1984. Association of poliovirus proteins with the endoplasmic reticulum. *J. Virol.* **52:** 777.

Tucker, S.P. and R.W. Compans. 1993. Virus infection of polarized epithelial cells. *Adv. Virus Res.* **42:** 187.

Tucker, S.P., L.R. Melsen, and R.W. Compans. 1992. Migration of polarized epithelial cells through permeable membrane substrates of defined pore size. *Eur. J. Cell Biol.* **58:** 280.

Tucker, S.P., C.L. Thornton, R.W. Compans, and E. Wimmer. 1993a. Bi-directional entry of poliovirus into polarized epithelial cells. *J. Virol.* **67:** 29.

Tucker, S.P., C.L. Thornton, E. Wimmer, and R.W. Compans. 1993b. Vectorial release of poliovirus from polarized human intestinal epithelial cells. *J. Virol.* **67:** 4274.

vanMeer, G. and K. Simons. 1982. Viruses budding from either the apical or basolateral plasma membrane domains of MDCK cells have unique phospholipid compositions. *EMBO J.* **7:** 847.

Virji, M., D.J.P. Kayhty, C. Ferguson, E. Alexandrescu, and R. Moxon. 1991. Interaction of *Haemophilus influenzae* with cultured endothelial cells. *Microbiol. Pathol.* **10:** 231.

Wolf, J.L., D.H. Rubin, R. Finberg, R.S. Kauffman, A.H. Sharpe, J.S. Trier, and B. N. Fields. 1981. Intestinal M cells: A pathway for entry of reovirus into the host. *Science* **212:** 471.

Zibert, A., H. Selinka, O. Elroy-Stein, B. Moss, and E. Wimmer. 1991. Vaccinia virus-mediated expression and identification of the human poliovirus receptor. *Virology* **182:** 250.

18

Early Steps in Reovirus Infection of Cells

Max L. Nibert
Institute for Molecular Virology and Department of Biochemistry
University of Wisconsin
Madison, Wisconsin 53706

Bernard N. Fields
Department of Microbiology and Molecular Genetics
and Shipley Institute of Medicine
Harvard Medical School
and Department of Medicine, Brigham and Women's Hospital
Boston, Massachusetts 02115

When an animal virus is introduced to a cell which it can infect, a series of ordered steps commences. These steps involve particular virus/cell interactions and, depending on the type of virus, can include binding by viral attachment proteins to receptors on the cell surface, endocytosis and uptake of viral particles into cellular vacuoles, interaction of viral proteins with a cellular membrane, penetration of the membrane so that components of the viral particle enter the cytoplasm, localization of viral components to particular sites within the cell interior, and initiation of the viral genetic program. A striking relationship can be seen between the structure, or *form*, of a virus and its activity, or *function*, at particular steps in the entry process. In general, the early steps in infection are linked to a series of structural changes in the infecting viral particle. These structural changes are sometimes characterized by the terms *uncoating* and *disassembly*; however, these terms seem too passive and limited in scope to describe the complex structural transitions that occur at these steps.

In this chapter, we discuss how different structural forms of the mammalian reoviruses interact with mammalian cells at different early steps in infection (for another review of this subject, see Nibert et al. 1991a). We begin by characterizing three forms of reovirus particles—virions, ISVPs, and cores—that mediate three discrete functions in the initiation of infection and by describing dramatic structural transitions that distinguish these particle forms. We then discuss the individual steps of attachment to cell-surface receptors, activational proteolysis in endocytic

Cellular Receptors for Animal Viruses
© 1994 Cold Spring Harbor Laboratory Press 0-87969-429-7/94 $5 + .00

vacuoles, interaction with cellular membranes, and initiation of transcription of the viral mRNAs. Last, we suggest a broadened relevance to understanding the early steps in infection by describing a relationship between the maintenance of persistent reovirus infections and viral and cellular mutations that affect early steps. For a discussion of the early steps in reovirus infection of host animals, which includes some interesting analogies to the material discussed here, the reader is directed to Georgi and Fields (this volume).

THREE ESTABLISHED FORMS OF REOVIRUS PARTICLES AND THEIR FUNCTIONS

Reoviruses are prototype members of the family Reoviridae and infect a variety of mammalian and avian hosts. Like that of other family members (rotaviruses, orbiviruses, and coltiviruses are other Reoviridae that infect mammals), the reovirus genome is segmented and formed from double-stranded (ds)RNA. The ten reovirus gene segments are currently defined to encode 12 primary translation products (segments S1 and M3 encode 2 products each), 8 of which are incorporated into fully assembled viral particles, or *virions*. The eight structural proteins of reoviruses are associated with two concentric capsid layers, each of which possesses icosahedral symmetry (Fig. 1). Among nonenveloped viruses, this multicapsid organization of structural proteins appears unique to members of the Reoviridae. For reoviruses, our current understanding is that the icosahedral protein lattices on which the inner and outer capsids are based comprise two proteins each: $\lambda 2$ and $\mu 1$ in the outer capsid and $\lambda 1$ and $\sigma 2$ in the inner capsid. Other proteins associate with these primary lattice-forming proteins to complete each capsid layer: $\sigma 1$ and $\sigma 3$ in the outer capsid and $\lambda 3$ and $\mu 2$ in the inner capsid (for more information about reovirus structure and replication, see Schiff and Fields 1990).

Outer capsid components can be progressively removed from reovirus virions when exposed to a variety of proteases in vitro. The results of protease treatments are two distinct types of subvirion particles, infectious subvirion particles (ISVPs) and cores, which primarily differ from each other and from virions by the particular outer capsid proteins that they lack (Fig. 1). Structural features of the different reovirus particles are discussed below, especially as informed by recent studies involving cryoelectron microscopy and image reconstructions to approximately 3-nm resolution (Dryden et al. 1993). Also discussed are the unique biological properties of the different particle forms, which suggest that they are interesting not only from a structural perspective, but also be-

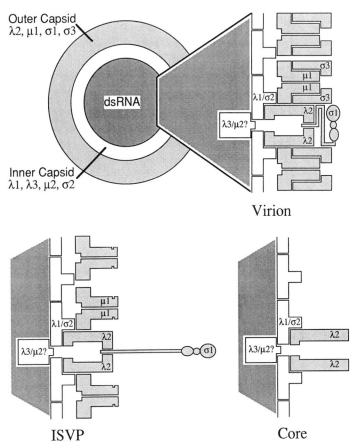

Figure 1 Organization of proteins in the outer and inner capsids of reovirus particles. Reoviruses possess two concentric protein capsid layers (outer and inner) surrounding the centrally located dsRNA genome. In intact virions, four species of proteins are assigned to each layer, as schematized in more detail in the regional blow-up. The organization of σ1 in virions, shown here as folded against the virion surface, remains poorly defined. Proteins λ2 and σ1, and perhaps proteins λ3 and μ2 as well, are localized to sites of fivefold symmetry in the capsid icosahedra. Subvirion particle forms—ISVPs and cores—can be derived from virions by proteolysis in vitro and are distinguished by structural changes in their outer capsids. ISVPs have lost protein σ3, have an endoproteolytically cleaved form of protein μ1 (notched polygon), and have a conformationally altered, extended form of cell-attachment protein σ1. Cores have additionally lost proteins μ1 and σ1 and have a conformationally altered form of protein λ2.

cause they play specific and essential roles during the early steps in reovirus infection (Fig. 2).

Virions

Virions represent the fully assembled particle form that accumulates within infected cells and is obtained by purification procedures routinely yielding reovirus particles for experimental work. The outer icosahedral lattice exhibits T=13(*laevo*) symmetry and is formed primarily by protein $\mu1$ (600 copies per virion, encoded by the M2 gene segment). The $\mu1$ protein undergoes an apparent autoproteolytic cleavage during viral assembly so that in virions it is represented by its amino- and carboxy-

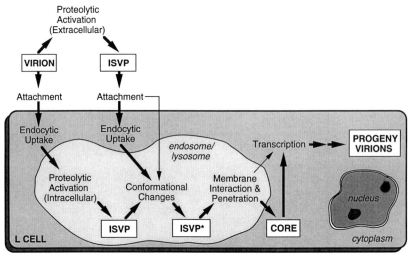

Figure 2   Early steps in reovirus infection of cells. Roles of the three established particle forms of reoviruses—virions, ISVPs, and cores—are highlighted (as well as those of a putative fourth form, the ISVP* (Nibert 1993). As indicated, both virions and ISVPs can attach to cells and initiate productive infection. ISVPs can be generated by proteolysis in both extra- and intracellular locations. The ISVP is proposed to give rise to a related particle form, the ISVP*, via conformational changes in its outer capsid. It is the ISVP* which is thought to interact with and then penetrate a cellular membrane (probably that of an endosome or lysosome, but possibly the plasma membrane in some cases [*thin arrow*]). The ISVP* may undergo further uncoating to form a core particle: Cores can mediate transcription of viral mRNAs in vitro and are also thought to do so within the cytoplasm of cells undergoing infection. Alternatively, the ISVP* or a related particle distinct from cores may mediate transcription within cells (*thin arrow*).

terminal fragments, μ1N and μ1C (Nibert et al. 1991b). The μ1 and μ1N polypeptides are amino-terminally myristoylated so that although reoviruses are nonenveloped, they contain a large number of myristoyl (saturated C14 fatty acyl) groups in their outer capsids (Nibert et al. 1991b). The μ1 lattice is substituted around the icosahedral fivefold axes by a pentameric complex of another outer capsid protein, λ2 (60 copies per virion, encoded by L2). Two other outer capsid proteins associate with the μ1-λ2 lattice. The σ3 protein (600 copies per virion, encoded by S4) forms a 1:1 complex with μ1 (Jayasuriya et al. 1988; Dryden et al. 1993). It is a metalloprotein that binds approximately one Zn^{++} ion per molecule so that there is also a large amount of zinc in the reovirus outer capsid (Schiff et al. 1988). Protein σ1 (36–48 copies, encoded by S1) serves as the receptor-recognition protein of reoviruses and occurs as a homo-oligomer (trimer or tetramer) at each of the icosahedral vertices (Fraser et al. 1990; Strong et al. 1991). It is thought to assume conformations in viral particles that differ as to the degree of extension of σ1 from the particle surface (Furlong et al. 1988). The extended σ1 oligomer has a head-and-tail morphology, which has been correlated with protein sequences, suggesting that the tail domain is formed from alternating regions of α-helical coiled-coil and cross-β sandwich motifs of super-secondary structure involving the amino-terminal two-thirds of σ1 sequence (Fraser et al. 1990; Nibert et al. 1990). The structure of the reovirus inner capsid appears to be shared by all three particle types as discussed with respect to cores below.

The diameter of virions approaches 85 nm, making reoviruses among the largest nonenveloped viruses. As seen in image reconstructions (Fig. 3) (Dryden et al. 1993), a prominent feature on the surface of virions consists of 60 tetrameric and 60 hexameric clusters of radially extended, fingerlike subunits, corresponding to protein σ3. The clusters surround 120 solvent channels, which extend the full thickness of the outer capsid layer but do not penetrate the inner capsid. Each tetrameric complex is in fact arranged as a partial hexamer, interrupted by one subunit from a pentameric, star-like aggregate of λ2 that substitutes the outer lattice around each axis of fivefold symmetry. Twelve potential channels at the fivefold sites are closed off in virions by virtue of an outer region of λ2 that is folded over and pointing toward the fivefold axis, where it and its pentameric neighbors appear to grasp the base of the σ1 fiber protein (Fig. 4). In virions, σ1 is thought generally to assume a folded conformation atop the λ2 pentamers, but this form of σ1 has been poorly visualized to date. Only a portion of protein μ1 is exposed on the surface of virions in regions left vacant by σ3 and λ2.

Virions appear to be designed for maximum stability in environments

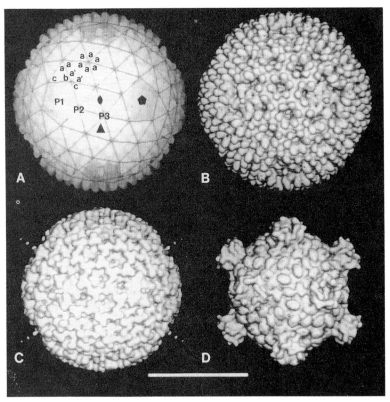

Figure 3 Image reconstructions of reovirus particles after cryoelectron microscopy. Surface representations of virions (*B*), ISVPs (*C*), and cores (*D*) of
serotype 1 reovirus strain Lang are shown. Beaded fibers of protein $\sigma1$ projecting from the surface of ISVPs and pentagonal turrets of protein $\lambda2$ projecting
from the surface of cores are especially evident. Tetrameric and hexameric arrays of protein $\sigma3$ can be seen on the surface of virions, and trimeric arrays of
protein $\mu1$ can be seen on the surface of ISVPs. Star-like, pentameric arrays of
$\lambda2$ can be seen on the surface of both virions and ISVPs. The diagram of a
T=13(*laevo*) lattice (*A*) is labeled with the positions of channels (P1, P2, P3),
distinct types of $\sigma3$ subunits (a, a′, b, and c), and axes of symmetry (oval [2],
triangular [3], and pentagonal [5] symbols). Bar, 50 nm. (Reprinted, by
copyright permission of the Rockefeller University, from Dryden et al. 1993.)

outside cells, but also to be capable of undergoing activation for infection
upon encountering a target cell. The primary determinant of virion
stability may be the $\sigma3$ protein, via its interactions with all three of the
other outer capsid proteins $\mu1$, $\lambda2$, and $\sigma1$. Current thinking is that $\sigma3$ interacts with $\mu1$ and $\lambda2$ to interlock the outer capsid lattice and prevent $\mu1$
and $\lambda2$ from prematurely experiencing their penetration- and transcrip-

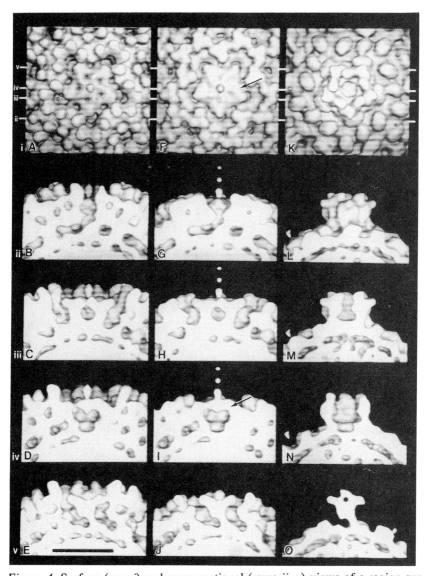

Figure 4 Surface (row *i*) and cross-sectional (rows *ii–v*) views of a region surrounding a fivefold axis of symmetry in reovirus particles. Views of virions (*A–E*), ISVPs (*F–J*), and cores (*K–O*) of serotype 1 reovirus strain Lang are shown. Cross-sectional views in row *iv* pass directly through the fivefold axis. Changes in the conformation of cell attachment protein σ1 (fiber) between virions and ISVPs and in penton protein λ2 (core spike, or turret; *arrows*) between ISVPs and cores can be inferred from these images. Bar, 20 nm. (Reprinted, by copyright permission of the Rockefeller University, from Dryden et al. 1993.)

tion-related changes in conformation (see below). In addition, an interaction between σ3 and σ1 may be important for retaining σ1 in its more folded conformation within virions. Nonextended σ1 seems likely to represent a more stably particle-associated form of this protein whose activity, receptor binding, is essential for infection.

ISVPs

When a reovirus virion enters a proteolytic environment, such as the small intestinal lumen of a mammalian host (Bodkin et al. 1989), the lumen of a late endosome or lysosome within a cell undergoing infection (Sturzenbecker et al. 1987), or a test tube containing protease in vitro, it undergoes dramatic structural alterations to generate a subvirion particle called the ISVP. This transition involves loss of the 600 σ3 subunits from the outer capsid via a stepwise process of proteolytic degradation. In addition, the 600 μ1/μ1C subunits in the outer lattice undergo a conservative endoproteolytic cleavage such that a large amino-terminal fragment, δ, and a smaller carboxy-terminal fragment, φ, are generated and remain particle-bound (Nibert and Fields 1992). A further alteration occurs in the vertex-associated σ1 protein in that it changes from a poorly visualized, presumably compact conformation in virions into an extended, flexible fiber that projects as much as 45 nm out from the surface of ISVPs (Furlong et al. 1988).

ISVPs are about 80 nm in diameter, not including the extended σ1 fibers (the latter could extend the diameter to >160 nm!). As seen in image reconstructions (Fig. 3) (Dryden et al. 1993), prominent features are 200 trimeric aggregates representing protein μ1, which are linked via local twofold interactions over much of the ISVP surface. The interactions between individual μ1 subunits appear to change significantly at different radii within the outer capsid so that an interlocking structure is formed. The μ1 lattice is percolated with solvent channels, the largest of which are the 120 radially directed ones evident in virions and accentuated in ISVPs by the loss of σ3. Structural consequences have yet to be attributed to the endoproteolytic cleavage of μ1 that occurs during the generation of ISVPs. In fact, the structure of μ1 in virions and ISVPs appears quite similar, except for a small rotational difference noted at intermediate radii within the outer capsid. In addition to increasing dramatically the portions of μ1 subunits exposed to the particle surface, the loss of σ3 increases the exposure of the λ2 pentamers at each icosahedral vertex. Only minor changes in λ2 are seen between virions and ISVPs, and the potential fivefold channels remain closed in ISVPs by proteins λ2 and σ1 (Fig. 4). In ISVPs, the bottom portion of an extended σ1 fiber is visualized projecting out to 11 nm above each fivefold axis. The flexibility of these fibers is the probable cause of their not being better seen, but the absence of the projecting densities in virions is the best evidence to date that σ1 has a less extended form in virions than in ISVPs.

ISVPs appear best designed of the three reovirus particles to carry out several of the virus/cell interactions early in infection. Although the relative activities of nonextended and extended σ1 in binding to cell-surface receptors remain undefined, the extended form of σ1 in ISVPs seems better suited due to increased exposure and projection from the particle surface of putative receptor-binding regions of the protein (Furlong et al. 1988; Dermody et al. 1990; Nibert et al. 1990). One idea is that σ1 extension is not always needed but contributes importantly to binding in certain settings or to certain cell types within host animals. The extension of σ1 might also enhance the capacity of viral particles to mediate multivalent attachment to receptors as a prelude to endocytic uptake from the cell surface. Loss of σ3 appears to be the primary distinguishing feature of ISVPs. ISVPs are unique among reovirus particles in exhibiting a capacity to interact with lipid bilayers, which is thought to reflect an interaction between viral components and a cellular membrane that must occur during penetration (Lucia-Jandris et al. 1993; Nibert 1993; Tosteson et al. 1993). Our current model is that loss of σ3 from the outer capsid is necessary to relieve steric hindrance and to provide mobility to regions of μ1 so that they may change conformation and migrate into the membrane bilayer (see below). ISVPs are thus proposed to be metastable precursors to a conformationally related particle form (the ISVF* suggested in Fig. 2) that directly mediates penetration (Nibert 1993). The conformational flexibility of the outer capsid components in ISVPs may explain why protein σ3 is needed to stabilize the outer capsid in virions until a target cell is approached.

Cores

Under certain proteolytic conditions in vitro, and possibly inside cells that are undergoing infection as well, a reovirus ISVP can undergo additional alterations to its outer capsid so as to generate a second subvirion form, the core. The transition from ISVP to core primarily involves proteolytic degradation and loss of the 600 μl (or μ1N and μ1C) subunits. We now know that cores are also characterized by having lost the 12 homo-oligomeric fibers of protein σ1. The remaining outer capsid component λ2 is retained by cores but was recently determined to have undergone a large change in conformation from that in virions and ISVPs (see below). We note here that λ2 acts as the reovirus guanylyltrans-ferase, involved in forming the 5' cap at the end of each viral mRNA (Seliger et al. 1987; Mao and Joklik 1991), and has been proposed to provide in addition one or both of the two methyltransferase activities in-volved in forming the final reovirus cap structure (Seliger et al. 1987).

Cores continue to contain a full complement of the reovirus inner cap-sid proteins. Current understanding is that the inner lattice proper is formed by proteins λ1 (120 copies, encoded by gene segment L3) and σ2 (120–180 copies, encoded by S2). Both these proteins exhibit a capacity to bind dsRNA in vitro, which may be important for viral assembly and/or RNA synthesis (Schiff et al. 1988; Dermody et al. 1991). Protein λ1, like σ3 in the outer capsid, appears to be a metalloprotein that might bind one Zn^{++} ion per molecule (Bartlett and Joklik 1988; Schiff et al. 1988). It also contains sequences reminiscent of an ATP-binding motif, which may indicate that it has enzymatic activity. Also associated with the inner capsid are the two minor proteins λ3, the putative catalytic sub-unit of the reovirus dsRNA-dependent RNA polymerase (Starnes and Joklik 1993), and μ2 (~12 copies each; encoded by L1 and M1, respec-tively). Their low copy number in viral particles has led to a proposal that λ3 and μ2 are localized to the icosahedral vertices of the inner cap-sid, and recent image reconstructions from cryoelectron micrographs of empty reovirus particles are consistent with this notion (K.A. Dryden et al., in prep.). The ten segments of dsRNA comprising the reovirus genome are located in the core interior, surrounded by the inner capsid. Several studies, including recent cryoelectron microscopy (Dryden et al. 1993), suggest that the dsRNA is mostly packed as a nematic liquid crys-tal, in which dsRNA helices occur in locally parallel arrays, and not within ribonucleoprotein complexes.

As again seen in image reconstructions (Fig. 3) (Dryden et al. 1993), dominant features on the surface of cores are pentameric turrets, project-ing upward around the fivefold axes and formed by protein λ2. The tur-rets extend to give cores an outer diameter of 80 nm, similar to ISVPs. During the conversion of ISVPs to cores, an outer region of each λ2 sub-unit, which folds over and points toward the fivefold axis in virions and ISVPs, undergoes a large structural transition (Fig. 4). This region of λ2 apparently rotates about a swivel type of hinge such that its tip, which previously contacted the base of the σ1 fiber, is moved upward and out-ward from the fivefold axis by as much as 3-nm translation in each direc-tion. It is this translation which generates the turret-like structure and opens a channel of 8-nm diameter through the turret at each fivefold axis. The loss of σ1 from cores is probably attributable to this change in λ2, since a pentavalent binding site for the base of the σ1 fiber is destroyed in the process. Whether the ISVP-to-core transition initiates with the change in λ2 or with a preceding change in μ1 conformation remains to be determined. The inner capsid to which the λ2 turrets attach at their bases has a diameter of only 65 nm. It is substantially thinner than the outer capsid, but appears more solid in that it is not penetrated by solvent channels, except perhaps within a region surrounded by λ2 at each fivefold axis. Besides the turrets, the surface of cores displays 150 nodules that merge with the solid inner shell (Fig. 3). It is presently difficult to assign these nodules and other features of the inner capsid to individual core components, but proteins λ1 and σ2 must make the major contributions.

Of the three recognized reovirus particles, cores are the only non-infectious form. This is consistent with their having lost both the cell attachment protein σ1 and protein μ1, which is thought to mediate interaction with the lipid bilayer during penetration (see below). Cores have, however, gained an essential activity in that they are capable of synthesizing the ten full-length viral mRNAs. This activity is latent in virions and ISVPs: Despite the fact that the latter particles can reiteratively synthesize small initiator oligonucleotides, they are not capable of extending these into complete transcripts as are cores (Yamakawa et al. 1982). An implication is that the ISVP-to-core transition includes a structural alteration that relieves a block to transcript elongation. It is generally considered that the core is the particle form introduced into the cytoplasm by the penetration process so that it can initiate transcription, but this fact is poorly evidenced in the literature (see, e.g., Borsa et al. 1981). Reovirus mRNAs do not have poly(A) tails, but they do have a doubly methylated 5' cap structure that is entirely synthesized by enzymatic components of the core. One published model for how transcription might be effected within the core involves moving dsRNA templates past enzymatic sites fixed within the inner capsid, possibly at the base of each λ2 pentamer so that a nascent mRNA can be extruded from the core through the channel of the λ2 turret (Joklik 1983; Shatkin and Kozak 1983). The opening of the turret channels in cores alone, correlating with transcriptase activation, is consistent with this (Fig. 4) (Dryden et al. 1993). Which aspects of the ISVP-to-core transition are most relevant to transcriptase activation and which to penetration remain to be determined.

A SERIES OF EARLY INTERACTIONS BETWEEN REOVIRUSES AND CELLS

Having introduced the reovirus structural proteins, the positions that they occupy within virions and subvirion particles, the structural changes involved in the transitions between particle forms, and the roles of the different particles in infection (Fig. 2), we now consider the early steps in reovirus infection, as they are currently understood, in order and in somewhat greater detail.

Attachment to Cell-surface Receptors and Endocytosis

A variety of genetic and biochemical studies have shown that protein σ1 plays the key role in binding reoviruses to cells in culture and tissues in vivo. Early genetic studies suggested that σ1 is the viral hemagglutinin and also the predominant type-specific neutralization antigen (for review, see Tyler and Fields 1990). Other genetic studies suggested that the σ1 protein determines tissue tropism and the pathway of spread within host animals (for review, see Tyler and Fields 1990). This variety of functions of σ1 almost certainly relates to its function in receptor binding. Studies by Lee and colleagues (e.g., Leone et al. 1992) in particular have provided firm biochemical evidence that σ1 protein, as isolated from virions, infected cells, or cells or bacteria expressing σ1 from cloned S1 genes, is unique among reovirus proteins in its capacity to attach with high affinity to cells in culture.

The nature of the receptor(s) for reoviruses on cell surfaces has received considerable attention (for review, see Sauve et al. 1992). There is strong evidence that one minimal receptor for serotype 3 reoviruses is an α-linked, terminal sialic acid residue, as found on many glycoproteins and glycolipids (Paul et al. 1989). For example, attachment to sialic acid, primarily as found on the surface protein glycophorin A, appears to be the basis for serotype 3 reoviruses binding and agglutinating erythrocytes (Paul and Lee 1987). Other reports have suggested that a 68-kD protein, related to but distinct from the β-adrenergic receptor, can serve as a receptor for serotype 3 reoviruses (Co et al. 1985). It may be that binding to sialic acid and binding to one or more specific protein receptors are separate activities of the reovirus σ1 protein. Alternatively, it may be that the "true" receptor for reoviruses on cells is a specific sialylated protein, to which σ1 binds through interactions with both sialic acid and specific protein sequences to effect high-affinity attachment. The relevant importance of particular reovirus receptors may also vary from cell to cell (Rubin et al. 1992), and there may be important differences in receptor binding by reovirus strains from the three serotypic groups. Additional work is needed to resolve these issues.

Studies of reovirus receptors are intimately linked to studies of the regions of σ1 active in attachment. Sequences in the carboxy-terminal half of σ1 are implicated in receptor binding by several studies involving deletion mutants of expressed protein (Nagata et al. 1987), fragmentation of σ1 by proteases (Yeung et al. 1989), and identification of sequences recognized by neutralizing antibodies (Bassel-Duby et al. 1986). Coupled with knowledge of the tail-and-head morphology of σ1 and predictions for morphology/sequence correlations (Furlong et al. 1988; Fraser et al. 1990; Nibert et al. 1990), a model identifying the σ1 head as an important receptor-recognition domain has arisen. Other work, however, has shown that the capacity of σ1 or modifications thereof to bind either to cells or to sialic acid do not always correlate. Moreover, recent work identified sequences within a middle region of σ1, near residue 200, as determining differences in the capacity of different reovirus strains to hemagglutinate (Dermody et al. 1990). According to the current morphology/sequence correlations, these hemagglutination-determining sequences occur not within the σ1 head, but within the tail, in a domain predicted to be formed by a cross-β-sheet motif (Dermody et al. 1990). Thus, a simple idea is that this region represents a sialic-acid-binding domain that is distinct from another receptor-binding region within the σ1 head. Alternatively, this portion of the σ1 tail may be important for determining the oligomeric structure and binding activities of the σ1 head.

A number of questions remain about the roles of σ1 in cell attachment. These include which sequences and structural regions of σ1 are directly involved, what roles are played by different conformers of σ1, and what specific cellular moieties can serve as receptors. In addition, little is understood about the relationship between attachment by reoviruses to receptors on the cell surface and endocytic uptake resulting in productive infection. One or more different receptor-binding activities of σ1 may, for example, be required for instigating endocytosis of reovirus particles (Choi 1994). There also remain possibilities for σ1 binding to receptors to play roles in infection after endocytic uptake, such as in directing reovirus particles into particular endocytic vacuoles where subsequent steps in infection, including proteolysis and penetration, must occur.

Proteolytic Activation within Endocytic Vacuoles

Original observations regarding the proteolysis of reovirus outer capsid proteins were that it occurred when virions were exposed to most proteases in vitro and also within cells undergoing infection. The reproducible nature of these cleavages was intriguing, as was the fact that they did not involve complete degradation of viral particles, but rather proteolysis of only certain outer capsid components (Fig. 1). For example, when radiolabeled virions were used to infect cells, cleavage and loss of protein σ3 and conversion of protein μ1C protein to its cleaved product δ were seen to occur very early in infection. The timing of these cleavages correlated with the accumulation of infecting particles into cellular vacuoles resembling lysosomes. Thus, the explanation arose that input virions undergo cleavage by proteases within lysosomes to generate particles similar or identical to ISVPs that are generated by proteolysis in vitro (for a review of this early literature, see Zarbl and Millward 1983).

The first direct evidence for proteolysis as an *essential* step in reovirus infections originated with an observation that these infections are subject to inhibition by the weak base ammonium chloride (Canning and Fields 1983). Weak bases were known to be concentrated within acidic cellular vacuoles by ion trapping and consequently to raise the pH within those compartments; furthermore, they had been shown to inhibit the growth of other viruses that require exposure to acid pH within endocytic vacuoles as an early step in their infections. Sturzenbecker et al. (1987) pursued the original reovirus observation and showed convincingly that infections initiated by virions, but not by ISVPs, are subject to inhibition with ammonium chloride. Moreover, certain experiments showed that ammonium chloride acts very early (within the first hour) in the viral replication cycle and that the degree to which viral growth is inhibited after infection in the presence of ammonium chloride correlates with the degree to which cleavages of proteins σ3 and μ1C in input virions are blocked. These findings were proposed to indicate most simply that ammonium chloride acts to raise the pH within endocytic vacuoles including lysosomes, thereby to inhibit the activity of acidic proteases residing in those compartments, and thus to block a required proteolytic conversion of virions to ISVPs. ISVPs were thought to escape this block because they had already undergone proteolysis in vitro. In fact, other interpretations of these observations are possible, but recent studies using a variety of inhibitors directed at cellular proteases have supported the original model. Those studies have also suggested that specific endocytic proteases are required for converting virions to ISVPs within cells (M.L. Nibert et al., in prep.). Other remaining questions involve the precise cellular compartment(s) in which this proteolysis occurs: Although lysosomes represent the most hydrolytic of endocytic vacuoles, active proteases are also found in endosomes (especially late endosomes) and the *trans* Golgi network.

The capacity of ISVPs to be generated outside cells, prior to attachment and endocytosis, has also been demonstrated. The one setting in which this clearly occurs is when newborn mice are given virions by the peroral route. In that case, current evidence indicates that proteolysis to generate ISVPs occurs within the small intestinal lumen, presumably mediated by secreted pancreatic serine proteases present in high concentration (Bodkin et al. 1989), and is required as a first step for efficient infection of mouse tissues via that route (Bass et al. 1990). For additional details, see Georgi and Fields (this volume).

Interaction with and Penetration of the Vacuolar Membrane

Like all viruses, reoviruses face the challenge of crossing a cellular membrane to gain access to the cytoplasm as an early step in infection (Fig. 2). This is a biophysically demanding feat, since it involves passage of viral components, which are often large and polar in character, from an aqueous through a lipid and back into an aqueous environment. Changes in viral surface characteristics are clearly required, presumably accomplished in most cases by conformational changes in viral surface proteins, at least the one(s) which interacts directly with the membrane bilayer. As nonenveloped viruses, reoviruses cannot use a generalized fusion mechanism to accomplish this task, and our experimental challenge is to determine what mechanism they do use. We have begun to address this problem by considering it in two parts: How do reoviruses first interact with a lipid bilayer and then how do they introduce viral components across it?

We have recently developed three assays by which to study the interaction between reovirus particles and lipid bilayers. The first of these assays was first utilized for reoviruses by Borsa and colleagues and involves the capacity of viral particles to release ^{51}Cr from preloaded L cells (Borsa et al. 1979). We have extended work with this assay as described below. More recent studies have demonstrated a capacity of reovirus particles to induce channels with variable conductances in artificial planar bilayers (Fig. 5) (Tosteson et al. 1993). Finally, we have succeeded in developing hemolysis as an assay for reovirus/membrane interactions, whereby reovirus particles interact with the plasma membrane of erythrocytes to cause release of hemoglobin (Nibert 1993; M.L. Nibert and B.N. Fields, in prep.). To our knowledge, the latter represents the first time that hemolysis has been demonstrated for a nonenveloped virus.

One of the most important facts that we have learned from these assays is that the capacity to interact with membranes is restricted to the ISVP form of reoviruses; virions and cores do not exhibit the activity. This finding is consistent with the model that ISVPs are essential intermediates in the process of reovirus entry into cells (Fig. 2). We have also exploited the ease of reovirus genetics to gain insight into a particular

A.   PE:PS

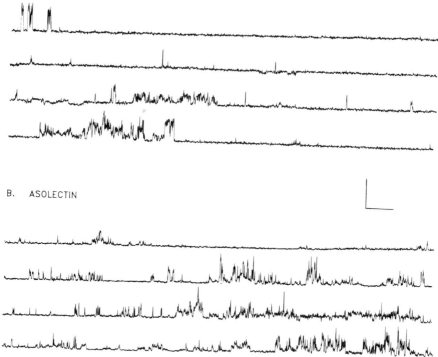

B.   ASOLECTIN

Figure 5 Bilayer channels induced by reovirus ISVPs. When ISVPs are applied to planar lipid bilayers, formed from either phosphatidyl ethanolamine: phosphatidyl serine (PE:PS; *A*) or asolectin (*B*) in these examples, they induce the formation of ion-permeant channels. These channels have variable conductances and exhibit rapid openings and closings. Such activity is unique to ISVPs among reovirus particles and is thought to reflect the membrane interaction that must occur as part of the penetration process early in infection. Each trace here represents a continuous, 3-sec record. Markers: conductance (vertical), 0.4 nanoSiemens (*A*) and 0.2 nanoSiemens (*B*); time (horizontal), 200 milliseconds (*A* and *B*).

viral gene/protein that determines activity in the assays for membrane interaction. For example, we determined that individual strains of reoviruses differ in the capacity of their ISVPs to release ^{51}Cr from L cells: The serotype 1 strain Lang is less efficient than the serotype 3 strain Abney at causing Cr release under particular conditions (Lucia-Jandris et al. 1993). Using reassortant viruses containing mixtures of genes from these two strains, we found that behavior in the Cr release assay segregated with the M2 gene segment, which encodes the major outer capsid protein μ1 (Lucia-Jandris et al. 1993). Protein μ1 is present in cleaved form (fragments μ1N, δ, and ϕ) as the primary protein on the surface of ISVPs and is implicated by these findings as playing a role, either direct or indirect, in reovirus/membrane interactions.

Several features of the μ1 protein are consistent with its role in membrane interaction being a direct one. As described above, μ1 is found in purified virions primarily in the form of two fragments, μ1N and μ1C, resulting from the assembly-related cleavage of μ1 after residue 42 in its sequence. The finding of a potential N-myristoylation sequence at the amino terminus of μ1 led to a demonstration that μ1 and its aminoterminal fragment μ1N are in fact modified by a myristoyl group (Nibert et al. 1991b). In other viruses containing myristoylated structural proteins, these fatty acyl groups have been proposed to play roles in membrane interaction, both during assembly and early in infection, and we have made the same proposal for reoviruses. During the proteolytic conversion of ISVPs to virions, the μ1C fragment is cut into two smaller fragments, δ and ϕ, via a cleavage near residue 580 in the μ1 sequence (Nibert and Fields 1992). Both δ and ϕ remain attached to ISVPs in stoichiometric quantities. An analysis of sequences surrounding the δ/ϕ cleavage junction suggests another structural basis for the putative function of μ1 in interacting with membranes; in particular, this junction is flanked by a predicted pair of long α helices which are strongly amphipathic in character (Nibert and Fields 1992). Similar amphipathic α helices have been implicated in the membrane-binding activities of a variety of proteins, including toxins and viral fusion proteins. Thus, we would propose that these α helices, together with the myristoyl group at the extreme amino terminus of μ1/μ1N, are involved in interacting directly with a cellular membrane bilayer during penetration by reoviruses. Future studies are needed to test this hypothesis. A conformational change in μ1 expected to precede its interaction with membranes (associated with formation of the ISVP* suggested in Fig. 2) is the subject of current intensive study.

At present, we have little insight into the steps that follow membrane interaction and permit reovirus components to penetrate into the cytoplasm. It is conceivable that the result of reovirus/membrane interaction is a local disruption of the bilayer such that virus accesses the cytoplasm directly through a large breach. Alternatively, a more precise structure may be formed by viral proteins within the membrane such that viral components can enter the cytoplasm. One of many possibilities is that protein μ1 interacts with the membrane and then extrudes the core into the cytoplasm through an expanding pore, similar to fusion by enveloped viruses. Another possibility is that a reovirus particle never completely enters the cytoplasm, but only sticks one or more of its λ2 spikes across the membrane so that viral mRNAs are extruded into the cytoplasm. Future studies will attempt to define the mechanism of reovirus penetration, including the structure that viral proteins form within the membrane. Other remaining questions concern the specific cellular location(s) at which penetration occurs in infections initiated by either virions or ISVPs. Although the current model favors penetration from one or another endocytic vacuole, this remains unproven.

Switch-on of Viral mRNA Synthesis

Most of the available information about how transcription-related enzymes within an infecting reovirus particle are activated early in infection was discussed with regard to cores above. Important remaining questions concern the particular type of viral particle (core or conformationally altered ISVP) from which viral transcription first occurs (Fig. 2), as well as the specific site within cells (cytoplasm or modified endocytic vacuole) at which it occurs. Future studies must also address the structural basis for the arrest of transcript elongation in virions and ISVPs and how this arrest has been relieved in transcribing particles.

PERSISTENT VERSUS LYTIC INFECTIONS: AN EARLY STEP IN INFECTION IS A NIDUS FOR VIRAL AND CELLULAR MUTATIONS DURING THE MAINTENANCE OF PERSISTENT REOVIRUS INFECTIONS

Some reovirus strains, after they are subjected to passage at a high multiplicity of infection, are effective at establishing and maintaining persistent infections in L cells. In one study, the capacity of high-passage reovirus stocks to establish persistent infections was attributed to viruses with mutations in their S4 genes (σ3 proteins), which arise and undergo amplification during high-multiplicity passage (Ahmed and Fields 1982). The mechanism by which mutations in S4 support the establishment of persistent infections is unknown. Additional mutations in viral as well as cellular genes are selected during the maintenance of persistent infections in L cells. This is highlighted by the observation that cells cured of persistent reovirus infection support significantly better growth of viruses isolated from the persistent culture before curing (designated PI viruses) than of wild-type (wt) viruses (Ahmed et al. 1981). One study identified mutations in the viral S1 gene (σ1 and σ1s proteins) as determinants of the enhanced capacity of PI viruses to replicate in cured cells (Kauffman et al. 1983), but as with S4 and establishment, the mechanism by which mutations in S1 affect the maintenance of persistent reovirus infections is unknown.

Observations led us to predict recently that cellular mutations important for the maintenance of persistent reovirus infections are related to early steps in the viral replication cycle (Dermody et al. 1993). To test this hypothesis, we studied the capacity of wt viruses to grow in cured cells, but in this case we used either of the two infectious forms of wt viruses—virions and ISVPs—to initiate infection. The rationale was that if cured cells are altered in their capacity to effect the virion-to-ISVP conversion, which as noted above is an essential early step in reovirus infection, then wt virions and ISVPs might differ in their capacities to initiate infection of these cells. Experimental findings indicated that wt ISVPs are in fact not subject to interference with growth in cured cells as are wt virions, consistent with the hypothesis that cured cells are mutant in their capacity to convert virions to ISVPs. Future studies will attempt to pinpoint these cellular mutations, but possible candidates include cellular factors involved in the acidification of endocytic vacuoles and specific lysosomal acidic proteases that are required for converting virions to ISVPs.

Since intact virions of PI viruses can efficiently initiate infections of cured cells, thus differing from wt virions, we made another, correlative prediction that PI viruses, like cured cells, are mutant in regard to virion-to-ISVP conversion (Dermody et al. 1993). To test this prediction, we compared PI viruses to wt viruses in their capacity to initiate infection in the presence of the weak base ammonium chloride (Fig. 6). As discussed above, ammonium chloride is thought to inhibit the growth of reoviruses after infection with wt virions by raising the pH within acidic cellular vacuoles, including lysosomes, and thereby blocking the activity of cellular acidic proteinases that convert virions to ISVPs (Sturzenbecker et al. 1987). Consistent with this model, infections initiated by wt ISVPs are not subject to inhibition with this agent (Sturzenbecker et al. 1987). We hypothesized that virions of PI viruses might also show reduced sensitivity to having infection blocked by ammonium chloride, and this hypothesis was supported by the experimental findings (Fig. 6) (Dermody et al. 1993). The molecular basis of this effect is the subject of ongoing work.

In sum, our recent studies suggest that both cured cells and PI viruses contain mutations that affect some early step in the reovirus replication cycle. This step seems to represent a nidus for virus-cell coevolution during the maintenance of persistent reovirus infections. The involvement of an early step in infection in the long-term maintenance of a persistent infection may appear paradoxical but has suggested to us that the persistent

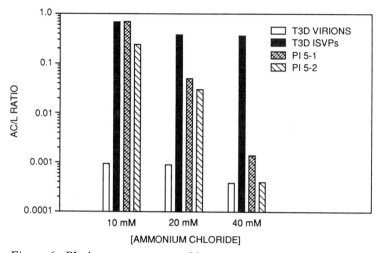

Figure 6   PI viruses are mutant with respect to an early step in infection. Infections initiated by virions, but not ISVPs, of serotype 3 reovirus strain Dearing (T3D) are subject to inhibition by ammonium chloride (AC) at concentrations between 10 and 40 mM. This is reflected by a decrease in yield of viral progeny after 24-hr growth in the presence, as compared to in the absence, of ammonium chloride (AC/L ratio). Viruses, presumably in the form of virions, obtained from long-term persistently infected cultures (PI viruses 5-1 and 5-2 here) resist the effects of low concentrations of ammonium chloride but are inhibited by higher concentrations. This behavior suggests that PI viruses are mutant with respect to proteolytic activation or some other acid-dependent step in infection. (Reprinted, with permission, from Dermody et al. 1993.)

reovirus infections which we have studied require continuing transmission of viruses between cells in the culture (horizontal transmission) to be maintained. This is consistent with a notion that these persistent infections are best described as carrier cultures. Our findings argue that carrier cultures involving other types of viruses and cells might be useful sources of both viral and cellular mutants altered with respect to the early steps in viral infections. In addition, our findings indicate that virus/cell interactions occurring near the outset of a replication cycle can be determinants of the outcome of infection: persistent versus lytic.

SUMMARY

Reoviruses are among the largest nonenveloped viruses, and, because of their double-capsid morphology, they are expected to exhibit some unique features in the way they invade cells. In this chapter, we have described the three generally recognized forms of reovirus particles—virions, ISVPs, and cores—as well as a putative fourth form, the ISVP*. We have also discussed the roles they play in the early steps in infection. The existence of these different particle forms reflects a series of complex structural alterations that occur within the reovirus outer capsid as the virus initiates infection of a cell. These structural alterations include not only losses of proteins by proteolyic degradation and elution, but also conservative endoproteolytic cleavages and conformational changes in proteins that remain particle-bound. All four of the reovirus outer capsid proteins —$\lambda2$, $\mu1$, $\sigma1$, and $\sigma3$—are affected by these structural changes, and knowledge of these effects has contributed greatly toward understanding the functions of individual proteins in the early steps in infection as they are currently defined: attachment to cell-surface receptors and endocytosis ($\sigma1$), proteolytic activation within endocytic vacuoles ($\mu1$ and $\sigma3$), interaction with and penetration of the vacuolar membrane ($\mu1$), and switch-on of viral mRNA synthesis ($\mu1$ and $\lambda2$). Future studies will try to define more precisely the molecular and cell biological mechanisms of these early reovirus/cell interactions.

ACKNOWLEDGMENTS

Our thanks to the many recent members of the Fields laboratory for helpful discussions and encouragement and to Marcia Kazmierczak for assistance in preparing the manuscript. This work was supported by U.S. Public Health Service grants R-37AI-13178 and NS-16998. B.N.F. is additionally supported by the Shipley Institute of Medicine. M.L.N. is supported by an award to the Institute for Molecular Virology, University of Wisconsin-Madison, from the Lucille P. Markey Charitable Trust and by a Steenbock Career Development Award from the Department of Biochemistry, University of Wisconsin-Madison.

REFERENCES

Ahmed, R. and B.N. Fields. 1982. Role of the S4 gene in the establishment of persistent reovirus infection in L cells. *Cell* **28**: 605.

Ahmed, R., W.M. Canning, R.S. Kauffman, A.H. Sharpe, J.V. Hallum, and B.N. Fields. 1981. Role of the host cell in persistent viral infection: Coevolution of L cells and reovirus during persistent infection. *Cell* **25**: 325.

Bartlett, J.A. and W.K. Joklik. 1988. The sequence of the reovirus serotype 3 L3 genome segment which encodes the major core protein $\lambda1$. *Virology* **167**: 31.

Bass, D.M., D. Bodkin, R. Dambrauskas, J.S. Trier, B.N. Fields, and J.L. Wolf. 1990. Intraluminal proteolytic activation plays an important role in replication of type 1 reovirus in the intestines of neonatal mice. *J. Virol.* **64**: 1830.

Bassel-Duby, R., D.R. Spriggs, K.L. Tyler, and B.N. Fields. 1986. Identification of attenuating mutations on the reovirus type 3 S1 double-stranded RNA segment with a rapid sequencing technique. *J. Virol.* **60:** 64.

Bodkin, D.K., M.L. Nibert, and B.N. Fields. 1989. Proteolytic digestion of reovirus in the intestinal lumen of neonatal mice. *J. Virol.* **63:** 4767.

Borsa, J., M.D. Sargent, P.A. Lievaart, and T.P. Copps. 1981. Reovirus: Evidence for a second step in the intracellular uncoating and transcriptase activation process. *Virology* **111:** 191.

Borsa, J., B.D. Morash, M.D. Sargent, T.P. Copps, P.A. Lievaart, and J.G. Szekely. 1979. Two modes of entry of reovirus particles into L cells. *J. Gen. Virol.* **45:** 161.

Canning, W.M. and B.N. Fields. 1983. Ammonium chloride prevents lytic growth of reovirus and helps to establish persistent infection in mouse L cells. *Science* **219:** 987.

Choi, A.H.C. 1994. Internalization of virus binding proteins during entry of reovirus into K562 erythroleukemia cells. *Virology* **200:** 301.

Co, M.S., G.N. Gaulton, A. Tominaga, C.J. Homcy, B.N. Fields, and M.I. Greene. 1985. Structural similarities between the mammalian beta-adrenergic receptor and reovirus type 3 receptors. *Proc. Natl. Acad. Sci.* **82:** 5315.

Dermody, T.S., M.L. Nibert, R. Bassel-Duby, and B.N. Fields. 1990. A σ1 region important for hemagglutination by serotype 3 reovirus strains. *J. Virol.* **64:** 5173.

Dermody, T.S., M.L. Nibert, J.D. Wetzel, X. Tong, and B.N. Fields. 1993. Cells and viruses with mutations affecting viral entry are selected during persistent infection of L cells by mammalian reoviruses. *J. Virol.* **67:** 2055.

Dermody, T.S., L.A. Schiff, M.L. Nibert, K.M. Coombs, and B.N. Fields. 1991. S2 gene nucleotide sequences of prototype strains of the three reovirus serotypes: Characterization of core protein σ2. *J. Virol.* **65:** 5721.

Dryden, K.A., G. Wang, T.S. Baker, M.A. Yeager, M.L. Nibert, K.M. Coombs, D.B. Furlong, and B.N. Fields. 1993. Early steps in reovirus infection are associated with dramatic changes in supramolecular structure and protein conformation: Analysis of virions and subviral particles by cryoelectron microscopy and three-dimensional image analysis. *J. Cell Biol.* **122:** 1023.

Fraser, R.D.B., D.B. Furlong, B.L. Trus, M.L. Nibert, B.N. Fields, and A.C. Steven. 1990. Molecular structure of the cell-attachment protein of reovirus: Correlation of computer-processed electron micrographs with sequence-based predictions. *J. Virol.* **64:** 2990.

Furlong, D.B., M.L. Nibert, and B.N. Fields. 1988. Sigma 1 protein of mammalian reoviruses extends from the surfaces of viral particles. *J. Virol.* **62:** 246.

Jayasuriya, A.K., M.L. Nibert, and B.N. Fields. 1988. Complete nucleotide sequence of the M2 gene segment of reovirus serotype 3 Dearing and analysis of its protein product μ1. *Virology* **163:** 591.

Joklik, W.K. 1983. The reovirus particle. In *The reoviridae* (ed. W.K. Joklik), p. 9. Plenum Press, New York.

Kauffman, R.S., R. Ahmed, and B.N. Fields. 1983. Selection of a mutant S1 gene during reovirus persistent infection: Role in maintenance of the persistent state. *J. Virol.* **131:** 79.

Leone, G., L. Maybaum, and P.W.K. Lee. 1992. The reovirus cell attachment protein possesses two independently active trimerization domains: Basis of dominant negative effects. *Cell* **71:** 479.

Lucia-Jandris, P., J.W. Hooper, and B.N. Fields. 1993. Reovirus M2 gene is associated with chromium release from mouse L cells. *J. Virol.* **67:** 5339.

Mao, Z. and W.K. Joklik. 1991. Isolation and characterization of protein λ2, the reovirus guanylyltransferase. *Virology* **185:** 377.

Nagata, L., S.A. Masri, R.T. Pon, and P.W.K. Lee. 1987. Analysis of functional domains on reovirus cell attachment protein σ1 using cloned S1 gene deletion mutants. *Virology* **160**: 162.

Nibert, M.L. 1993. "Structure and function of reovirus outer capsid proteins as they relate to early steps in infection." Ph.D. thesis, Harvard University, Cambridge, Massachusetts.

Nibert, M.L. and B.N. Fields. 1992. A carboxy-terminal fragment of protein μ1/μ1C is present in infectious subvirion particles of mammalian reoviruses and is proposed to have a role in penetration. *J. Virol.* **66**: 6408.

Nibert, M.L., T.S. Dermody, and B.N. Fields. 1990. Structure of the reovirus cell-attachment protein: A model for the domain organization of σ1. *J. Virol.* **64**: 2976.

Nibert, M.L., D.B. Furlong, and B.N. Fields. 1991a. Mechanisms of viral pathogenesis: Distinct forms of reoviruses and their roles during replication in cells and host. *J. Clin. Invest.* **88**: 727.

Nibert, M.L., L.A. Schiff, and B.N. Fields. 1991b. Mammalian reoviruses contain a myristoylated structural protein. *J. Virol.* **65**: 1960.

Paul, R.W. and P.W.K. Lee. 1987. Glycophorin is the reovirus receptor on human erythrocytes. *Virology* **159**: 94.

Paul, R.W., A.H.C. Choi, and P.W.K. Lee. 1989. The α-anomeric form of salic acid is the minimal receptor determinant recognized by reovirus. *Virology* **172**: 382.

Rubin, D.H., J.D. Wetzel, M.V. Williams, T.A. Cohen, C. Dworkin, and T.S. Dermody. 1992. Binding of type 3 reovirus by a domain of the σ1 protein important for hemagglutination leads to infection of murine erythroleukemia cells. *J. Clin. Invest.* **90**: 2536.

Sauve, G.J., H.U. Saragovi, and M.I. Greene. 1992. Reovirus receptors. *Adv. Virus Res.* **42**: 323.

Schiff, L.A. and B.N. Fields. 1990. Reoviruses and their replication. In *Fields virology* (ed. B.N. Fields and D.M. Knipe), p. 1275. Raven Press, New York.

Schiff, L.A., M.L. Nibert, M.S. Co, E.G. Brown, and B.N. Fields. 1988. Distinct binding sites for zinc and double-stranded RNA in the reovirus outer capsid protein σ3. *Mol. Cell. Biol.* **8**: 273.

Seliger, L.S., K. Zheng, and A.J. Shatkin. 1987. Complete nucleotide sequence of reovirus L2 gene and deduced amino acid sequence of viral mRNA guanylyltransferase. *J. Biol. Chem.* **262**: 16289.

Shatkin, A.J. and M. Kozak. 1983. Biochemical aspects of reovirus transcription and translation. In *The reoviridae* (ed. W.K. Joklik), p. 9. Plenum Press, New York.

Starnes, M.C. and W.K. Joklik. 1993. Reovirus protein λ3 is a poly(C)-dependent poly(G) polymerase. *Virology* **193**: 356.

Strong, J.E., G. Leone, R. Duncan, R.K. Sharma, and P.W.K. Lee. 1991. Biochemical and biophysical characterization of the reovirus cell attachment protein σ1: Evidence that it is a homotrimer. *Virology* **184**: 23.

Sturzenbecker, L.J., M. Nibert, D. Furlong, and B.N. Fields. 1987. Intracellular digestion of reovirus particles requires a low pH and is an essential step in the viral infectious cycle. *J. Virol.* **61**: 2351.

Tosteson, M.T., M.L. Nibert, and B.N. Fields. 1993. Ion channels induced in lipid bilayers by subvirion particles of the nonenveloped mammalian reoviruses. *Proc. Natl. Acad. Sci.* **90**: 10549.

Tyler, K.L. and B.N. Fields. 1990. Reoviruses. In *Fields virology* (ed. B.N. Fields and D.M. Knipe), p. 1307. Raven Press, New York.

Yamakawa, M., Y. Furuichi, and A.J. Shatkin. 1982. Reovirus transcriptase and capping enzymes are active in intact virions. *Virology* **118**: 157.

Yeung, M.C., D. Lim, R. Duncan, M.S. Shahrabadi, L.W. Cashdollar, and P.W.K. Lee.

1989. The cell attachment proteins of type 1 and type 3 reovirus are differentially susceptible to trypsin and chymotrypsin. *Virology* **170:** 62.

Zarbl, H. and S. Millward. 1983. The reovirus multiplication cycle. In *The reoviridae* (ed. W.K. Joklik), p. 79. Plenum Press, New York.

19

Early Events in Human Herpesvirus Infection of Cells

Neil R. Cooper
Department of Immunology, IMM 19
The Scripps Research Institute
La Jolla, California 92037

Herpesviruses are large, highly complex enveloped viruses containing linear double-stranded DNA. Following primary infection, which is frequently inapparent, the intact viral genome persists in host cells for the life of the individual. Since the presence of the viral genome does not significantly impair normal cellular functions, herpesvirus latent infections are largely asymptomatic. Latently infected cells also escape destruction by the immune system, in part because few viral proteins that can be recognized and targeted by the immune system are produced during latency. In addition, some herpesviruses have evolved specific strategies that interfere with immune recognition. Many, if not all, latent herpesvirus infections are interrupted by periods of reactivation induced by trauma, stress, infection, immunosuppression, or other processes. With reactivation, herpesviruses enter the productive phase of the viral life cycle, and viral particles are produced. Virus production leads to death of the host cell. Furthermore, virus-producing cells are targeted for destruction by the immune system. Destruction of cells and immune processes lead to inflammation with its associated symptomatology.

Most of the herpesviruses are ubiquitous pathogens. For example, more than 90% of individuals worldwide have been exposed to herpes simplex virus type 1 (HSV-1) and Epstein-Barr virus (EBV) by adulthood. The other human herpesviruses, which include cytomegalovirus (HCMV), varicella zoster virus (VZV), herpes simplex virus type 2 (HSV-2), and herpesviruses 6, 7, and 8 (or 6A, 7, and 6B) are also quite prevalent in most populations. Herpesviruses have been found in many species. Marek's disease in chickens, Aujeszky's disease in pigs, and infectious bovine rhinotracheitis in cattle, all caused by herpesviruses, represent serious veterinary problems.

Cellular Receptors for Animal Viruses
© 1994 Cold Spring Harbor Laboratory Press 0-87969-429-7/94 $5 + .00

The immune system appears to play a critical role in preventing herpesvirus reactivation and resulting disease, despite its inability to eliminate latent infections. This has become evident as a result of the use of immunosuppressive regimens to treat certain diseases and to prepare individuals for organ and bone marrow transplants, the careful study of individuals with genetic immunodeficiencies, and the increasing prevalence of AIDS, an immunosuppressive disease. Reactivation of latent herpesvirus genomes, particularly HSV-1, EBV, and HCMV, occurs frequently in such individuals, with serious and occasionally fatal results.

The types of diseases produced by herpesviruses are extremely diverse, as they are dependent on the cell type(s) targeted, the site(s) of latency and reactivation, and the nature of the immune responses, which differ for each of the viruses. In some instances, such as EBV, the viral receptor is a major determinant of tropism, although this is probably not the case for most of the other herpesviruses. Some enter cells by fusion with the plasma membrane, others by endocytosis. In this review, I summarize current understanding of the early events in human herpesvirus entry into cells.

HERPES SIMPLEX VIRUS

HSV types 1 and 2 cause a variety of human diseases, including lesions on the oral and genital mucosal surfaces, eye lesions, and encephalitis. They replicate in numerous sites and cell types in vivo and possess a similar promiscuity for multiple cell types in vitro. Following initial infection and replication in epithelial cells, HSV becomes latent in neuronal cells in ganglia. Recurrent infection is associated with movement of the virus through nerve axons, followed by replication in epithelial cells.

On the basis of biological behavior and other characteristics, HSV is classified as an α herpesvirus. HSV encodes 10 known viral envelope glycoproteins: gB, gC, gD, gE, gG, gH, gI, gJ, gK, and gL. Of these, gC, gE, gG, gI, and gJ are not essential for HSV infection of, and replication in, epithelial cells in culture. In contrast, viral glycoproteins gB, gD, and gH cannot be deleted from the viral genome; such information is not yet available for gK and gL. Despite its nonessential role for infection in vitro, evidence exists that gC plays a role in virus adherence to epithelial cells (see below), a finding that emphasizes the importance of interpreting in vitro studies with mutants and cell lines with caution. Of the HSV glycoproteins, only homologs of gB and gH are found in other herpesviruses.

Cellular Receptors for HSV

The initial step in HSV infection of cells is binding to heparan sulfate proteoglycan molecules on the surface of cells (WuDunn and Spear 1989). HSV directly binds to heparin, a glycosaminoglycan (GAG) related to heparin, and heparin inhibits virus attachment to epithelial cell lines in vitro. Agents that bind to heparan sulfate also block HSV absorption. Enzymatic removal of cell-surface heparan sulfate reduces binding and infectivity of subsequently added HSV, whereas digestion of other cell-surface GAGs is without effect. Finally, HSV binds poorly to mutant cell lines defective in various aspects of GAG synthesis, and such cell lines are also resistant to HSV infection (Shieh et al. 1992). Comparable results are obtained with both HSV-1 and HSV-2. The involvement of a cell-surface heparin-like molecule in HSV binding has been confirmed by several laboratories (Lycke et al. 1991; Yura et al. 1992).

Although attachment to cell-surface heparan sulfate mediates initial contact of HSV with the cell, subsequent interactions of the virus with cell membrane components are required for the virus to penetrate the cellular plasma membrane. Some evidence for a cell-surface receptor for viral gD has been presented (Johnson and Ligas 1988; Johnson et al. 1990; Kuhn et al. 1990). Although this interaction is not inhibited by heparin (Johnson et al. 1990), the nature of the gD cellular receptor has not been elucidated. HSV gD is required for viral entry into cells, but it is not needed for attachment, since HSV devoid of gD binds well to cells (Ligas and Johnson 1988), and certain monoclonal antibodies (MAbs) to gD reduce infectivity but do not impair binding of HSV to cells (Fuller and Spear 1987). Therefore, the membrane constituent to which gD binds is likely to be involved in an entry step which occurs subsequent to attachment.

HSV wild-type strains have been demonstrated to attach to both the apical and the basal surfaces of polarized epithelial cells in tissue culture (Sears et al. 1991). However, gC mutant strains only attach to the basal surface of such cells. These findings indicate that there are at least two HSV-binding moieties on the surface of polarized epithelial cells in culture; these receptors have not been further characterized.

It has been reported that the high-affinity basic fibroblast growth factor (bFGF) receptor mediates HSV-1 attachment to, and penetration of, cells (Kaner et al. 1990) and that HSV-1 binds bFGF (Baird et al. 1990). However, recent studies by several laboratories using multiple approaches clearly demonstrate that the high-affinity bFGF receptor is not the HSV receptor (Kaner et al. 1991; Mirda et al. 1992; Muggeridge et al. 1992). Most likely, bFGF blocks HSV binding and infection by competing for cell-surface heparan sulfate.

HSV Entry into Cells

HSV enters cells by pH-independent direct fusion of the viral envelope with the plasma membrane of the cell. Evidence from this conclusion came initially from the demonstration that viral envelope proteins appear on the cell surface shortly after binding (Para et al. 1980; Jennings et al. 1987) and from the finding that lipid vesicles containing HSV glycoproteins fuse with cell membranes (Johnson et al. 1984). Subsequent studies have directly demonstrated fusion by electron microscopy (Fuller and Spear 1987; Fuller et al. 1989; Fuller and Lee 1992) and have shown that the entry process is pH-independent (Wittels and Spear 1990).

HSV Glycoproteins Involved in Attachment and Infection

Of the HSV glycoproteins, both gB and gC bind to heparin-Sepharose, although HSV gC appears to represent the major heparin-binding glycoprotein, since significantly fewer gC-negative HSV virions bind to cells than do gB-negative or wild-type virions (Herold et al. 1991). In addition, HSV with mutant gC penetrates cells more slowly and possesses only 5–10% of the infectivity of wild-type HSV. Finally, monoclonal and polyclonal antibodies to gC interfere with absorption to cells (Fuller and Spear 1985; Kuhn et al. 1990; Svennerholm et al. 1991). Thus, gC appears to play an important role in viral attachment to cells, although it is not absolutely required for HSV infectivity in vitro, as noted above. In addition, as described earlier, gC-containing and gC-negative HSV virions both bind to polarized epithelial cells (Sears et al. 1991). Presumably, gB mediates viral attachment to heparin-specific proteoglycans (HSPGs) on cells in the absence of gC. Independent evidence also favors a role for gB in viral attachment to cells (Johnson et al. 1984; Kuhn et al. 1990).

HSV glycoproteins gB, gD, and gH are essential for HSV replication in tissue culture (Little et al. 1981; Cai et al. 1988; Desai et al. 1988; Johnson and Ligas 1988). However, virions lacking any one of these glycoproteins absorb to cells (Cai et al. 1988; Desai et al. 1988; Ligas and Johnson 1988; Forrester et al. 1992) and MAbs to each fail to block attachment of wild-type virions to cells, although they do greatly reduce infectivity (Fuller and Spear 1987; Highlander et al. 1987, 1988; Fuller et al. 1989). It appears, therefore, that these glycoproteins function primarily in steps occurring after initial attachment, i.e., stabilization of binding, changes in envelope and nucleocapsid structure, de-envelopment, penetration, etc. Recent attempts to sequence these events and the involvement of the various glycoproteins of HSV have revealed discernible structural changes in the envelope and tegument of HSV during the attachment and penetration processes (Fuller and Lee 1992).

The precise roles of the essential glycoproteins, gB, gD, and gH, in the entry process are not clear. Although gB may play a role in attachment to HSPGs as noted above, it also functions subsequently, possibly during the fusion step, since HSV deleted in gB fails to fuse with cells (Cai et al. 1988). However, HSV mutants lacking gD and gH also fail to fuse with cells (Ligas and Johnson 1988; Forrester et al. 1992). Other approaches using monoclonal antibodies, virosomes, and viral mutants have also implicated gB, gD, and gH in fusion and entry (Deluca et al. 1982; Bzik et al. 1984; Fuller and Spear 1987; Highlander et al. 1987; Desai et al. 1988; Fuller et al. 1989; Forrester et al. 1992; Navarro et al. 1992). Some evidence suggests that gH functions after gD (Forrester et al. 1992; Fuller and Lee 1992) and that gD stabilizes viral building required for the initiation of fusion (Fuller and Lee 1992). Viral gB, gD, and gH function independently, since gB extracted from cells is not associated with other glycoproteins (Claesson-Welsh and Spear 1986), and gB and gD (and also gC) are located on morphologically distinguishable spikes on the viral envelope (Stannard et al. 1987).

An additional glycoprotein, gL, has also been implicated in virus-induced cell fusion (Little et al. 1981). Recent studies indicate that this protein forms a complex with gH and is required for cell-surface expression of gH (Hutchinson et al. 1992b). Recent studies suggest that yet another HSV glycoprotein, gK, previously implicated in fusion between HSV-infected cells (syncytia) (Bond and Person 1984), is likely also involved in cell fusion and, thus, may play a role in HSV entry into cells (Hutchinson et al. 1992a).

Entirely analogous results to those obtained for HSV have been obtained for two other α herpesviruses, pseudorabies virus (PRV) and bovine herpesvirus type 1 (BHV-1). Both of these herpesviruses bind to a heparin-like molecule on cell surfaces via their gC homologs, which have heparin-binding activity (Mettenleiter et al. 1990; Sawitzky et al. 1990; Okazaki et al. 1991; Zsak et al. 1991). The gB homolog of both viruses has also been reported to possess heparin-binding ability (Sawitzky et al. 1990; Okazaki et al. 1991). A role for the gB and gD homologs of PRV and BHV in viral entry has also been demonstrated (Liang et al. 1991; Peeters et al. 1992b), and gH of PRV has been implicated (Peeters et al. 1992a).

Summary

HSV entry into cells is a complex multistep process involving distinct, presumably sequential interactions between several viral glycoproteins and distinct membrane constituents. Infection appears to be initiated by the attachment of HSV, via gC and potentially also gB, to ubiquitously distributed HSPG moieties on the cell surface. Subsequent steps include attachment of gD to unidentified cell-surface receptors, and interactions of gB, gD, gH, and possibly gK and gL with membrane constituents, leading to penetration of the nucleocapsid into the cell by direct fusion with the external cellular membrane. Considerable additional study is required to elucidate the initial steps in HSV entry into cells.

HUMAN CYTOMEGALOVIRUS

HCMV is responsible for disease in the fetus, newborn, children, and adults. Infection in utero is associated with a high frequency of developmental and nervous system defects. Although infection of children and adults is frequently inapparent, infectious mononucleosis and serious systemic disease may result. Most serious, however, are HCMV infections in individuals with congenital or acquired immunodeficiencies, including recipients of organ and bone marrow grafts, and patients with AIDS. HCMV-induced interstitial pneumonia is a serious, frequently fatal complication of organ transplantation in man. The HCMV genome can be found in a number of cell types in vivo including epithelial, endothelial, monocytoid, and lymphoid cells; however, the major site(s) of infection and latency is not known.

HCMV is classified as a β herpesvirus. The virus encodes three prominent disulfide-linked envelope glycoprotein complexes termed gC-I (55 and 130 kD), gC-II (47–52 kD), and gC-III (86 and 145 kD). Of these, gp 55/130 and gp 86 are homologs of HSV gB and gH, respectively. The gB and gH homologs are necessary for growth of HCMV in tissue culture, whereas gC-II is dispensable.

Cellular Receptors for HCMV

Recent studies indicate that the first step in HCMV infection, like that of the α herpesvirus HSV, is binding to a heparin-like molecule, undoubtedly an HSPG(s), on cell surfaces (Kari and Gehrz 1992; Neyts et al. 1992; Compton et al. 1993). Heparin, but not other major GAGs, inhibits HCMV attachment and infectivity, and treatment of cells with heparin-cleaving enzymes, but not other GAG-cleaving enzymes, impairs HCMV binding and infectivity (Neyts et al. 1992; Compton et al. 1993). In addition, HCMV does not bind to mutant cells either lacking HSPGs or bearing deficient HSPGs (Neyts et al. 1992; Compton et al.

1993). Finally, HCMV binds to heparin agarose (Kari and Gehrz 1992; Neyts et al. 1992; Compton et al. 1993).

Although initial binding of HCMV to HSPGs on cells is readily dissociable by heparin or high salt, viral attachment rapidly becomes nondissociable and, thus, converts to higher-affinity binding (Compton et al. 1993). These data suggest that HCMV interacts sequentially with cell-surface HSPGs and subsequently with a high-affinity binding site or receptor. The observation that it takes 90 minutes to saturate HCMV binding to cells (Taylor and Cooper 1989), whereas heparin-dissociable binding converts within minutes to heparin-resistant binding, suggests that the heparin-binding step is rate-limiting in HCMV absorption to cells. Steady-state heparin- and NaCl-resistant binding likely correspond to the high affinity (K_d = 1.1 nM) HCMV binding observed earlier (Taylor and Cooper 1989). In addition, it has been reported that HCMV virions specifically bind to a 34-kD membrane glycoprotein present in detergent extracts of a variety of cell types including cells of endothelial, epithelial, lymphoid, fibroblastic, and monocytoid origins (Adlish et al. 1990; Taylor and Cooper 1990; Nowlin et al. 1991). HCMV attachment to these various cell types correlates with the distribution and relative abundance of the 34-kD membrane protein (Nowlin et al. 1991). Very recent studies suggest that the 34-kD HCMV-binding molecule is annexin II, a widely distributed protein implicated in cellular adhesion reactions and in binding plasminogen and plasminogen activator (Wright et al. 1994).

Additional cellular components have been implicated in HCMV attachment and entry. A 92.5-kD membrane protein reactive with an anti-idiotypic (AbId) MAb generated by immunization with a neutralizing MAb to the gH homolog of HCMV has been described (Keay et al. 1989). The AbId MAb does not impair virus binding to the cells but does block viral fusion and infection (Keay and Baldwin 1991), suggesting that the 92.5-kD cellular molecule functions at the fusion step.

It was suggested that an MHC class I antigen may function as an HCMV receptor (Grundy et al. 1987b), since HCMV was observed to bind β_2-microglobulin (β_2m) (Grundy et al. 1987a). It was postulated that HCMV with bound β_2m interacts with cell-surface HLA class I molecules after displacing β_2m molecules normally bound to the histocompatibility antigen (Grundy et al. 1987b). The ability to bind β_2m has been attributed to the presence of an MHC class I homolog in the virus (Beck and Barrell 1988), which is capable of binding β_2m (Browne et al. 1990). However, HCMV does not bind to purified HLA class I antigen (Taylor and Cooper 1990); furthermore, HCMV binds to (Taylor and Cooper 1990; Nowlin et al. 1991) and infects MHC class I negative cells (Nowlin et al. 1991). Therefore, MHC class I molecules do not represent a necessary HCMV receptor.

HCMV Entry into Cells

A variety of genetic, biochemical, and morphological criteria indicate that HCMV penetrates cells by pH-independent fusion with the plasma membrane (Compton et al. 1992). HCMV infects epithelial cells that are defective in endosome acidification. Similarly, HCMV infectivity is unaffected by various agents that impair either endocytosis or endosomal acidification. Finally, electron microscopic studies have provided direct evidence of fusion of the viral envelope with the plasma membrane.

HCMV Glycoproteins Involved in HCMV Attachment and Infection

HCMV glycoproteins gB and gC-II both possess the ability to bind heparin (Kari and Gehrz 1992; Compton et al. 1993). It is not known which of these glycoproteins is the primary ligand. Thus, HCMV, a β herpesvirus, like the α herpesviruses HSV, BHV, and PRV, possesses two heparin-binding envelope glycoproteins. The gB homolog of both classes of herpesviruses functions in this capacity. The second HSPG-binding protein, gC for HSV and gC-II for HCMV, is unique for each type of herpesvirus.

As described earlier, AbId MAbs generated against a neutralizing MAb to gH detect a 92.5-kD membrane protein (Keay et al. 1989; Keay and Baldwin 1991), a finding which implicates gH in binding to this cell-surface molecule. These AbId MAbs inhibit viral fusion with the cell membrane, but not viral attachment (Keay and Baldwin 1991), indicating that the gH/92.5-kD interaction pertains to the fusion step. The recently identified gL homolog of HCMV, which complexes with gH and is required for membrane expression of gH (Kaye et al. 1992), could also be involved in fusion. These observations are quite similar to those described for HSV (Hutchinson et al. 1992b) and potentially EBV (see below).

Summary

HCMV binds initially to HSPG moieties on the cell surface via gB and gC-II. This initial low-affinity interaction converts rapidly to high-affinity binding. The identity of the high-affinity receptor is not known, but an unidentified 34-kD membrane protein has been implicated in binding of HCMV to multiple cell types. In addition, for HCMV to penetrate cells, which is accomplished by direct fusion with the plasma membrane, an interaction between viral gH and an unidentified 92.5 membrane protein is also required. These events are schematically depicted in Figure 1. Thus, HCMV entry into cells involves sequential interactions between several viral glycoproteins and distinct cellular components.

EPSTEIN-BARR VIRUS

EBV is also a ubiquitous virus, as more than 90% of individuals worldwide have been exposed to the virus by adulthood and carry the virus for life in latent form. EBV is the causative agent of infectious mononucleosis, a benign lymphoproliferative disease, and it is strongly associated with a number of human malignancies of lymphoid and epithelial cell origins such as nasopharyngeal carcinoma, Burkitt's lymphoma, most subtypes of Hodgkin's disease, and many non-Hodgkins lymphomas of B- and T-cell origins. In patients with primary or secondary immunodeficiencies, EBV-induced disease is a major problem. EBV-associated lymphomas and lymphoproliferative disease represent common, frequently fatal complications of allogeneic bone marrow and organ transplants in iatrogenically immunosuppressed patients.

EBV is classified as a γ herpesvirus. The EBV genome is found in a small proportion of circulating B lymphocytes and in epithelial cells from the oropharynx (Henle et al. 1967; Pope et al. 1968; Lemon et al. 1977; Sixbey et al. 1984; Wolf et al. 1984). The site of latency is likely

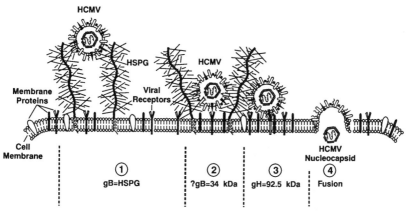

Figure 1 Schematic representation of the early events in HCMV entry into cells.

to be the B lymphocyte, since the immunosuppressive regimen used to prepare patients for bone marrow transplants ablates latent infection (Gratama et al. 1988).

The most abundant EBV envelope proteins are gp350 and gp220, which are encoded by the same viral gene (Dolyniuk et al. 1976; Thorley-Lawson and Edson 1979; Beisel et al. 1985), and p140 (Dolyniuk et al. 1976; Edson and Thorley-Lawson 1981). Additional viral envelope proteins include gp85, the homolog of gH in HSV (Heineman et al. 1988), and two recently described glycoproteins, gp43 (Sanchez-Pinel et al. 1991) and gp 78/55 (Mackett et al. 1990). The homolog of HSV gB, gp110, although present in infected cells, is not detectable in the virus (Pellett et al. 1985; Emini et al. 1987; Gong et al. 1987; Gong and Kieff 1990).

Cellular Receptors for EBV

Selective binding of EBV to B lymphocytes was first demonstrated 20 years ago (Jondal and Klein 1973). Numerous studies during the next 10 years suggested that the EBV receptor on B cells was a complement receptor, since both receptors cocapped together and independently of other surface proteins, and they exhibited the same distribution on multiple cell lines. Antibodies to either ligand blocked binding of the other (Cooper et al. 1988). The complement receptor implicated in these studies was later shown to be the receptor for the C3dg fragment of C3, or CR2. With the development of MAbs directed against CR2, the molecule was characterized as a 145-kD B-cell-specific glycoprotein (Iida et al. 1983). Although the initially developed MAbs failed to directly block virus, or complement binding, they did so in the presence of a second antibody to immunoglobulin, and immune precipitates formed with these MAbs bound C3dg or EBV (Fingeroth et al. 1984; Weis et al. 1984). Subsequently, an MAb to CR2 that directly blocks EBV and C3dg binding to cells and EBV infection of cells in the absence of a second antibody was identified (Nemerow et al. 1985). CR2, purified by affinity chromatography, binds both ligands in a dose-related manner, definitively showing that CR2, now designated CD21, is the B-cell EBV receptor (Nemerow et al. 1986). Subsequent studies with recombinant CD21 (Moore et al. 1989) and with cells transfected with CR2 cDNA (Ahearn et al. 1988; Carel et al. 1989) confirm the dual binding specificity of CD21.

Molecular cloning of CD21 reveals that the extracellular domain of the molecule is composed of 15 or 16 tandem repeating elements, termed short consensus repeats (SCRs) of 60–75 amino acids each. This structural motif, identified by four highly conserved cysteine residues and several other partially conserved amino acids, is found in more than 30 eukaryotic and prokaryotic molecules. Although many of these are complement-regulatory molecules and complement proteins, other SCR-containing molecules such as the IL-2 receptor and the selectins, are not. The three-dimensional structure of an SCR, solved by two-dimensional NMR (Norman et al. 1991), reveals it to be a β-sheet structure with two antiparallel β strands opposing three antiparallel β strands connected by loops. The amino and carboxyl termini are at opposite ends of the molecule in alignment, an arrangement that accounts for the extended flexible "string of pearls" appearance of CD21 in high-resolution electron microscopic studies (Moore et al. 1989). Studies with chimeric CR2 and recombinant CR2 molecules indicate that the binding site for EBV and C3dg is in the two amino-terminal SCRs (Lowell et al. 1989; Carel et al. 1990; Moore et al. 1991) and that homologous primary sequence epitopes mediate attachment, as further discussed below and as depicted in Figure 2. Recent studies using several approaches indicate that the determinants in CD21 to which EBV and C3dg bind are primarily conformational in nature (Martin et al. 1991; Molina et al. 1991). Although binding of EBV to CD21 is the first step in infection, viral binding alone does not assure infection of B cells. This is clearly shown by the extremely low levels of infection achieved by incubating EBV with cells expressing high levels of the receptor following transfection with CR2 cDNA (Ahearn et al. 1988; Carel et al. 1989).

EBV readily infects normal B cells in culture, and many B-cell lymphomas and tumors are EBV positive, particularly those occurring in immunocompromised individuals. Although EBV-bearing T-cell lym-

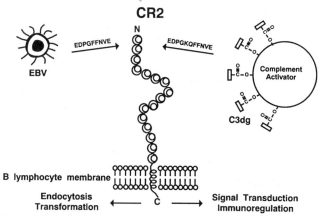

Figure 2 Schematic representation of CD21, its ligands, and functions.

phomas are being reported with increasing frequency, the EBV receptor on T cells that initiates infection has not been clearly identified. EBV does not readily infect normal T cells, despite the reported presence of low levels of CR2 (identified with MAbs) which is able to bind EBV (Fisher et al. 1991). An EBV-binding moiety on some normal T cells unrelated to CR2 has also been reported (Sauvageau et al. 1990). Some T-cell lines also bear CD21 (identified by amino acid sequencing) (Fingeroth et al. 1988). In addition, a T-cell line that lacks CR2 (lack of reactivity with MAbs) has been reported to bind EBV and to be infectible by the virus, possibly via a distinct EBV-binding molecule genetically related to CD21 (by hybridization), which the cell line bears (Hedrick et al. 1992). Immature thymocytes also bear CD21 (identified with MAbs) (Watry et al. 1991), which binds EBV leading to infection (Münch et al. 1992).

Epithelial cells can be infected with EBV since the viral genome is found in the epithelial tumor cells of nasopharyngeal carcinoma (zur Hausen et al. 1970) and in epithelial lesions in oral hairy leukoplakia (Greenspan et al. 1985). As with EBV infection of T cells, however, the identity of the receptor used by EBV to infect epithelial cells is not clear. Furthermore, a number of apparently contradictory findings have been published. EBV has been reported to bind to primary explant cultures of epithelial cells and some epithelial cell lines (Sixbey et al. 1987; Birkenbach et al. 1992) and fresh patient isolates of EBV to infect primary epithelial cells in vitro (Sixbey et al. 1983). Certain MAbs, notably HB-5, directed against B-cell CR2, react with sections of freshly obtained epithelial tissue and some epithelial cell lines (Young et al. 1986, 1989a,b; Cooper et al. 1990; Birkenbach et al. 1992). However, other MAbs directed against CD21, notably OKB-7, which reacts close to the EBV-binding site, fail to react (Young et al. 1989b). HB-5 has also been shown to immunoprecipitate a 200-kD molecule from freshly obtained epithelial tissues and some epithelial cell lines (Young et al. 1989b; Birkenbach et al. 1992); however, the 200-kD molecule is not reactive with OKB-7 or with gp350/220 (Young et al. 1989b; Birkenbach et al. 1992) and, thus, is unlikely to play a role in EBV infection of epithelial cells. Low levels of authentic CD21, verified by nucleotide sequencing and reactivity with gp350/220, were also identified in an epithelial cell line (Birkenbach et al. 1992). However, it remains to be determined whether CD21 generally mediates EBV absorption to, and infection of, epithelial cells, since most epithelial cells and cell lines lack detectable CD21. Epithelial cells transfected with CD21 cDNA are readily infectible with EBV (Li et al. 1992), demonstrating that CD21 can serve as a functional EBV receptor if expressed on epithelial cells.

EBV Entry into Cells

Electron microscopic studies indicate that EBV enters normal B cells by endocytosis into large thin-walled endocytic vesicles followed by de-envelopment within the low-pH environment of the vesicle, fusion of the viral envelope with the vesicle membrane, and entry of the nucleocapsid into the cytoplasm (Nemerow and Cooper 1984a). These observations have been confirmed using biophysical techniques (Miller and Hutt-Fletcher 1992). The membrane components involved in endocytosis, de-envelopment, and fusion have not yet been identified, although a calmod-ulin-dependent process has been implicated in EBV endocytosis (Nemerow and Cooper 1984b; Miller and Hutt-Fletcher 1992). CR2 is also internalized during viral entry, since additional EBV binds poorly to B cells (Inghirami et al. 1988), and B cells die when incubated with EBV together with a protein synthesis inhibitor coupled to anti-CR2 (Tedder et al. 1986). CD21 is associated with several proteins in the B-cell membrane including CD19, TAPA-1, and Leu-13 (Matsumoto et al. 1991; Bradbury et al. 1992), as schematically indicated in Figure 3. Although these molecules likely represent components of a signal transducing complex, the possibility that they facilitate entry into B lymphocytes has not yet been examined.

Interestingly, EBV enters lymphoblastoid cells by pH-independent direct fusion with the plasma membrane (Nemerow and Cooper 1984a; Miller and Hutt-Fletcher 1992). The reasons for this fundamental difference with the mechanism of entry into normal B cells is not known.

Studies using biophysical techniques indicate that EBV also enters freshly explanted epithelial cells by direct fusion with the plasma mem-

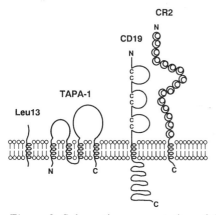

Figure 3 Schematic representation of CD21 and its associated molecules in the membrane of a normal B cell.

brane (Miller and Hutt-Fletcher 1992). It is not known whether specific plasma membrane molecules are involved in this process.

EBV Glycoproteins Involved in Attachment and Infection

EBV gp350/220 is the ligand for CD21 (Wells et al. 1982; Nemerow et al. 1987; Tanner et al. 1987). The evidence for this conclusion includes binding of the purified proteins to each other, binding of beads coated with purified recombinant gp350/220 to CR2 on B cells followed by capping of CR2 and blocking of EBV absorption to, and infection of, cells (Nemerow et al. 1987; Tanner et al. 1987, 1988). Furthermore, CD21 is the only B-cell membrane protein that binds to gp350/220 (Tanner et al. 1987).

Comparison of the amino acid sequence of gp350/220 with that of C3dg, the natural ligand for CR2, reveals two short regions of sequence similarity, as shown in Figure 4 (Nemerow et al. 1987; Sim et al. 1987; Tanner et al. 1987). The first of these regions, which is located at or near the amino terminus of gp350/220, overlaps the sequence in C3dg previously implicated in the binding of this peptide to CR2 (Fig. 1) (Lambris et al. 1985); the second region corresponds to the region in C3dg involved in the unusual thiolester bond in this molecule (Tack et al. 1980). Studies using synthetic peptides, coupled with other approaches, indicate that the first region of sequence similarity, EDPGFFNVE, mediates EBV binding to CR2 (Nemerow et al. 1989). The evidence includes the finding that peptides corresponding to this region bind to purified CR2 and to CR2-positive, but not CR2-negative, cells and block CR2 binding to immobilized EBV. Slight changes in sequence abrogate binding. Multimeric forms of the viral peptide inhibit both gp350/220 and C3dg bind-

Primary Sequence Similarities between C3dg and gp 350/220

C3dg   1211 L T T A K D K N R W E D P G K Q L Y N V E A T S Y A 1236

gp 350/220 T I Q S L I H L T G E D P G - - F F N V E I P E F P
            11   34

C3dg   1002 H L I V T P S G C G E Q N M I 1016

gp 350/220 L T S G T P S G C E N I S G A
            368   382

Figure 4 Homologous amino acid sequences in the CD21 ligands, EBV glycoprotein gp350/220, and the C3dg fragment of C3.

ing to B cells. Finally, and most importantly, multimeric conjugates of the peptide also block EBV infection of B cells at extremely low concentration. The other peptide possesses none of these properties. Thus, EBV uses a C3dg-like primary sequence epitope to attach to and infect B cells.

In addition to mediating attachment, the interaction of gp350/220 with CR2 plays a role in the endocytic process that initiates infection, since beads coated with recombinant gp350/220 undergo polar endocytosis into large, thin-walled vesicles, a process morphologically indistinguishable from that used by intact virus to enter cells (Nemerow and Cooper 1984a; Tanner et al. 1987). The mechanisms involved have not yet been elucidated.

The gH glycoprotein of EBV, gp85, is involved in viral envelope fusion since an MAb to this molecule inhibits fusion but not attachment (Miller and Hutt-Fletcher 1988). Furthermore, lipid vesicles containing incorporated EBV proteins (virosomes) bind and fuse with CR2-positive, but not-negative, B-lymphoblastoid cells; virosomes lacking gH bind to, but fail to fuse with, the B-cell lines (Haddad and Hutt-Fletcher 1989). It is not known whether cellular proteins interact with viral gH during the fusion process.

Summary

EBV initiates infection of B lymphocytes by binding to CD21, also known as the C3dg receptor, and CR2. Although EBV also infects some T cells and epithelial cells, the cell-surface receptor responsible for initiating infection of these cell types has not been clearly identified. EBV binds to a 9-amino-acid, C3dg-like primary sequence epitope located at or very near the amino terminus of the major glycoprotein of EBV, gp350/220. Viral attachment, as well as C3dg attachment, is to a conformationally determined epitope(s) located in the two amino-terminal SCRs of CD21. In normal B cells, this interaction is followed by endocytosis of EBV into large, thin-walled endocytic vesicles; viral deenvelopment; and entry of the viral nucleocapsid into the cytoplasm of the cell. The viral entry process involves an unidentified cellular calmodulin-dependent process. For viral fusion from within endocytic vesicles in B cells, EBV gH is also required. CD21 is noncovalently associated with several other proteins in the B-cell membrane. It is not known whether these or other membrane proteins play a role in the entry process. Thus, EBV entry into B cells involves multiple interactions between distinct viral glycoproteins and cellular constituents.

COMMENT

Recent studies using contemporary techniques of protein chemistry and molecular and cell biology indicate that delivery of herpesvirus genomes in infectious form into the cytoplasm of potentially infectible cells depends on successful completion of a series of highly specific interactions between distinct viral and cellular constituents. These reactions not only mediate firm, stable viral attachment to the appropriate cell type, but they are also likely to be responsible for the changes in cell membrane structure that permit fusion of the viral and cellular lipid bilayer membranes. They undoubtedly also initiate and perhaps sustain the changes in viral envelope and nucleocapsid structure, such as de-envelopment, fusion, and uncoating, which are required for entry of the viral genome into the cell in an infectious form.

The success of viruses as human pathogens stems from their ability to elude intrinsic and immune-based host defense mechanisms. As obligate intracellular parasites, viruses also depend on rapid entry into a susceptible cell for their survival. The cell-surface molecules and cellular processes selected through evolution by herpesviruses for attachment and entry likely facilitate rapid targeting of the virus to the appropriate cell type. In addition, the cellular molecules subverted by herpesviruses for attachment and entry may subserve normal cellular functions, such as channel formation, pinocytosis, endocytosis, internalization of signaling molecules or nutrients, antigen processing, and signal transduction, which may facilitate not only viral entry but also subsequent stages of infection.

The selected molecules can also interfere with effective immune recognition of the virus-infected cell. Examples of all of these have been described for various viruses, and some pertain to herpesvirus infection. For example, the EBV receptor facilitates internalization of its ligands into normal endocytic vesicles and their penetration into the cytoplasm. It also is a signaling molecule that modulates B-cell activation and proliferation, functions which likely facilitate EBV infection. HCMV encodes proteins related to channel-forming proteins which may facilitate entry, an MHC homolog, and other molecules which may interfere with effective antigen presentation and/or immune recognition.

Current knowledge only permits the description of the early events in herpesvirus infection of cells in outline form. Advances in this area, which are likely to be rapidly forthcoming, will permit the description of these processes in molecular terms. Such knowledge is likely to increase the understanding of normal cellular processes, as has been amply shown for a number of viral proteins involved in later stages of multiple viral infections. It is also anticipated that detailed studies of the early events in virus infection will identify novel possible targets for antiviral agents able to prevent or modify herpesvirus infections.

ACKNOWLEDGMENTS

This is publication 7797-IMM from the Department of Immunology of The Scripps Research Institute. I thank Catalina Hope for assistance with the manuscript. Work from the laboratory was supported by National Institutes of Health grants CA-52241, CA-14692, and AI-25016.

REFERENCES

Adlish, J.D., R.S. Lahijani, and S.C. St. Jeor. 1990. Identification of a putative cell receptor for human cytomegalovirus. *Virology* **176:** 337.

Ahearn, J.M., S.D. Hayward, J.C. Hickey, and D.T. Fearon. 1988. Epstein-Barr virus (EBV) infection of murine L cells expressing recombinant human EBV/C3d receptor. *Proc. Natl. Acad. Sci.* **85:** 9307.

Baird, A., R.Z. Florkiewicz, P.A. Maher, R.J. Kaner, and D.P. Hajjar. 1990. Mediation of virion penetration into vascular cells by association of basic fibroblast growth factor with herpes simplex virus type 1. *Nature* **348:** 344.

Beck, S. and B.G. Barrell. 1988. Human cytomegalovirus encodes a glycoprotein homologous to MHC class-I antigens. *Nature* **331:** 269.

Beisel, C., J. Tanner, T. Matsuo, D. Thorley-Lawson, F. Kezdy, and E. Kieff. 1985. Two major outer envelope glycoproteins of Epstein-Barr virus are encoded by the same gene. *J. Virol.* **54:** 665.

Birkenbach, M., X. Tong, L.E. Bradbury, T.F. Tedder, and E. Kieff. 1992. Characterization of an Epstein-Barr virus receptor on human epithelial cells. *J. Exp. Med.* **176:** 1405.

Bond, V.C. and S. Person. 1984. Fine structure physical map locations of alterations that affect cell fusion in herpes simplex virus type 1. *Virology* **132:** 368.

Bradbury, L.E., G.S. Kansas, S. Levy, R.L. Evans, and T.F. Tedder. 1992. The CD19/CD21 signal transducing complex of human B lymphocytes includes the target of antiproliferative antibody-1 and Leu-13 molecules. *J. Immunol.* **149:** 2841.

Browne, H., G. Smith, S. Beck, and T. Minson. 1990. A complex between the MHC class I homologue encoded by human cytomegalovirus and β_2 microglobulin. *Nature* **347:** 770.

Bzik, D.J., B.A. Fox, N.A. Deluca, and S. Person. 1984. Nucleotide sequence of a region of the herpes simplex virus type 1 gB glycoprotein gene: Mutations affecting rate of virus entry and cell fusion. *Virology* **137:** 185.

Cai, W., B. Gu, and S. Person. 1988. Role of glycoprotein B of herpes simplex virus type 1 in viral entry and cell fusion. *J. Virol.* **62:** 2596.

Carel, J.C., B. Frazier, T.J. Ley, and V.M. Holers. 1989. Analysis of epitope expression and the functional repertoire of recombinant complement receptor 2 (CR2/CD21) in mouse and human cells. *J. Immunol.* **143:** 923.

Carel, J.C., B.L. Myones, B. Frazier, and V.M. Holers. 1990. Structural requirements for C3d,g/Epstein-Barr virus receptor (CR2/CD21) ligand binding, internalization and viral infection. *J. Biol. Chem.* **265:** 12293.

Claesson-Welsh, L. and P.G. Spear. 1986. Oligomerization of herpes simplex virus glycoprotein B. *J. Virol.* **60:** 803.

Compton, T., R. Nepomuceno, and D. Nowlin. 1992. Human cytomegalovirus penetrates host cells by pH independent fusion at the cell-surface. *Virology* **191:** 387.

Compton, T., D.M. Nowlin, and N.R. Cooper. 1993. Initiation of human cytomegalovirus infection requires initial interaction with cell-surface heparan sulfate. *Virology* **193:** 834.

Cooper, N.R., M.D. Moore, and G.R. Nemerow. 1988. Immunobiology of CR2, the B lymphocyte receptor for Epstein-Barr virus and the C3d complement fragment. *Annu. Rev. Immunol.* **6:** 85.

Cooper, N.R., B.M. Bradt, J.S. Rhim, and G.R. Nemerow. 1990. CR2 complement receptor. *J. Invest. Dermatol.* **94:** 112S.

Deluca, N., D.J. Bzik, V.C. Bond, S. Person, and W. Snipes. 1982. Nucleotide sequences of herpes simplex virus type 1 (HSV-1) affecting virus entry, cell fusion, and production of glycoprotein gB (VP7). *Virology* **122:** 411.

Desai, P.J., P.A. Schaffer, and A.C. Minson. 1988. Excretion of non-infectious virus particles lacking glycoprotein H by a temperature-sensitive mutant of herpes simplex virus type 1: Evidence that gH is essential for virion infectivity. *J. Gen. Virol.* **69:** 1147.

Dolyniuk, M., R. Pritchett, and E.D. Kieff. 1976. Proteins of Epstein-Barr virus I. Analysis of the polypeptides of purified enveloped Epstein-Barr virus. *J. Virol.* **17:** 935.

Edson, C.M. and D.A. Thorley-Lawson. 1981. Epstein-Barr virus membrane antigens: Characterization, distribution, and strain differences. *J. Virol.* **39:** 172.

Emini, E.A., J. Luka, M.E. Armstrong, P.M. Keller, R.W. Ellis, and G.R. Pearson. 1987. Identification of an Epstein-Barr virus glycoprotein which is antigenically homologous to the Varicella-Zoster virus glycoprotein II and the herpes simplex virus glycoprotein B. *Virology* **157:** 552.

Fingeroth, J.D., M.L. Clabby, and J.D. Strominger. 1988. Characterization of a T-lymphocyte Epstein-Barr virus/C3d receptor (CD21). *J. Virol.* **62:** 1442.

Fingeroth, J.D., J.J. Weiss, T.F. Tedder, J.L. Strominger, P.A. Bird, and D. T. Fearon. 1984. Epstein-Barr virus receptor of human B lymphocytes is the C3d receptor CR2. *Proc. Natl. Acad. Sci.* **81:** 4510.

Fisher, E., C. Delibrias, and M.D. Kazatchkine. 1991. Expression of CR2 (the C3dg/EBV receptor CD21) on normal human peripheral blood T cells. *J. Immunol.* **146:** 865.

Forrester, A., H. Farrell, G. Wilkinson, J. Kaye, N. Davis-Poynter, and T. Minson. 1992. Construction and properties of a mutant of herpes simplex virus type 1 with glycoprotein H coding sequences deleted. *J. Virol.* **66:** 341.

Fuller, A.O. and W.-C. Lee. 1992. Herpes simplex virus type 1 entry through a cascade of virus-cell interactions requires different roles of gD and gH in penetration. *J. Virol.* **66:** 5002.

Fuller, A.O. and P.G. Spear. 1985. Specificities of monoclonal and polyclonal antibodies that inhibit adsorption of herpes simplex virus to cells and lack of inhibition by potent neutralizing antibodies. *J. Virol.* **55:** 475.

———. 1987. Anti-glycoprotein D antibodies that permit adsorption but block infection of herpes simplex virus 1 prevent virion-cell fusion at the cell surface. *Proc. Natl. Acad. Sci.* **84:** 5454.

Fuller, A.O., R.E. Santos, and P.G. Spear. 1989. Neutralizing antibodies specific for glycoprotein H of herpes simplex virus permit viral attachment to cells but prevent penetration. *J. Virol.* **63:** 3435.

Gong, M. and E. Kieff. 1990. Intracellular trafficking of two major Epstein-Barr virus glycoproteins, gp350/220 and gp110. *J. Virol.* **64:** 1507.

Gong, M., T. Ooka, T. Matsuo, and E. Kieff. 1987. Epstein-Barr virus glycoprotein homologous to herpes simplex virus gB. *J. Virol.* **61**: 499.

Gratama, J.W., M.A. Oosterveer, F.E. Zwaan, J. Lepoutre, G. Klein, and I.Ernberg. 1988. Eradication of Epstein-Barr virus by allogeneic bone marrow transplantation: Implications for sites of viral latency. *Proc. Natl. Acad. Sci.* **85**: 8693.

Greenspan, J.S., D. Greenspan, E.T. Lennette, D.I. Abrams, M.A. Conant, V. Petersen, and U.K. Freese. 1985. Replication of Epstein-Barr virus within the epithelial cells of oral "hairy" leukoplakia, an AIDS-associated lesion. *N. Engl. J. Med.* **313**: 1564.

Grundy, J.E., J.A. McKeating, and P.D. Griffiths. 1987a. Cytomegalovirus strain of AD169 binds β_2-microglobulin in vitro after release from cells. *J. Gen. Virol.* **68**: 777.

Grundy, J.E., J.A. McKeating, P.J. Ward, A.R. Sanderson, and P.D. Griffiths. 1987b. β_2-microglobulin enhances infectivity of cytomegalovirus and when bound to virus enables class I HLA molecules to be used as a virus receptor. *J. Gen. Virol.* **68**: 793.

Haddad, R.S. and L.M. Hutt-Fletcher. 1989. Depletion of glycoprotein gp85 from virosomes made with Epstein-Barr virus proteins abolishes their ability to fuse with virus receptor-bearing cells. *J. Virol.* **63**: 4998.

Hedrick, J.A., D. Watry, C. Speiser, P. O'Donnell, J.D. Lambris, and C.D. Tsoukas. 1992. Interaction between Epstein-Barr virus and a T cell line (HSB-2) via a receptor phenotypically distinct from complement receptor type 2. *Eur. J. Immunol.* **22**: 1123.

Heineman, T., M. Gong, J. Sample, and E. Kieff. 1988. Identification of the Epstein-Barr virus gp85 gene. *J. Virol.* **62**: 1101.

Henle, W., V. Diehl, G. Kohn, H. zur Hausen, and G. Henle. 1967. Herpes-type virus and chromosome marker in normal leukocytes after growth with irradiated Burkitt cells. *Science* **157**: 1064.

Herold, B.C., D. WuDunn, N. Soltys, and P.G. Spear. 1991. Glycoprotein C of herpes simplex virus type 1 plays a principal role in the adsorption of virus to cells and in infectivity. *J. Virol.* **65**: 1090.

Highlander, S.L., W. Cai, S. Person, M. Levine, and J.C. Glorioso. 1988. Monoclonal antibodies define a domain on herpes simplex virus glycoprotein B involved in virus penetration. *J. Virol.* **62**: 1881.

Highlander, S.L., S.L. Sutherland, P.J. Gage, D.C. Johnson, M. Levine, and J. C. Glorioso. 1987. Neutralizing monoclonal antibodies specific for herpes simplex virus glycoprotein D inhibit virus penetration. *J. Virol.* **61**: 3356.

Hutchinson, L., K. Goldsmith, D. Snoddy, H. Ghosh, F.L. Graham, and D.C. Johnson. 1992a. Identification and characterization of a novel herpes simplex virus glycoprotein, GK, involved in cell fusion. *J. Virol.* **66**: 5603.

Hutchinson, L., H. Browne, V. Wargent, N. Davis-Poynter, S. Primorac, K. Goldsmith, A.C. Minson, and D.C. Johnson. 1992b. A novel herpes simplex virus glycoprotein, gL, forms a complex with glycoprotein H (gH) and affects normal folding and surface expression of gH. *J. Virol.* **66**: 2240.

Iida, K., L. Nadler, and V. Nussenzweig. 1983. Identification of the membrane receptor for the complement fragment C3d by means of a monoclonal antibody. *J. Exp. Med.* **158**: 1021.

Inghirami, G., M. Nakamura, J.E. Balow, A.L. Notkins, and P. Casali. 1988. Model for studying virus attachment: Identification and quantitation of Epstein-Barr virus-binding cells using biotinylated virus in flow cytometry. *J. Virol.* **62**: 2453.

Jennings, S.R., P.A. Lippe, K.J. Pauza, P.G. Spear, L. Pereira, and S.S. Tevethia. 1987. Kinetics of expression of herpes simplex virus type 1-specific glycoprotein species on the surfaces of infected murine, simian, and human cells: Flow cytometric analysis. *J. Virol.* **61**: 104.

Johnson, D.C. and M.W. Ligas. 1988. Herpes simplex viruses lacking glycoprotein D are unable to inhibit virus penetration: Quantitative evidence for virus-specific cell-surface receptors. *J. Virol.* **62:** 4605.

Johnson, D.C., R.L. Burke, and T. Gregory. 1990. Soluble forms of herpes simplex virus glycoprotein D bind to a limited number of cell-surface receptors and inhibit virus entry into cells. *J. Virol.* **64:** 2569.

Johnson, D.C., M. Wittels, and P.G. Spear. 1984. Binding to cells of virosomes containing herpes simplex virus type 1 glycoproteins and evidence for fusion. *J. Virol.* **52:** 238.

Jondal, M. and G. Klein. 1973. Surface markers on human B and T lymphocytes. II. The presence of Epstein-Barr virus receptors on B lymphocytes. *J. Exp. Med.* **138:** 1365.

Kaner, R.J., A. Baird, R.Z. Florkiewicz, A. Mansukhani, C. Basilico, and D.P. Hajjar. 1991. Response to: Fibroblast growth factor receptor: Does it have a role in the binding of herpes simplex virus? (Shieh, M.T. and P.G. Spear) *Science* **253:** 208.

Kaner, R.J., A. Baird, A. Mansukhani, C. Basilico, B.D. Summers, R.Z. Florkiewicz, and D.P. Hajjar. 1990. Fibroblast growth factor receptor is a portal of cellular entry for herpes simplex virus type 1. *Science* **248:** 1410.

Kari, B. and R. Gehrz. 1992. A human cytomegalovirus glycoprotein complex designated gC-II is a major heparin-binding component of the envelope. *J. Virol.* **66:** 1761.

Kaye, J.F., U.A. Gompels, and A.C. Minson. 1992. Glycoprotein H of human cytomegalovirus (HCMV) forms a stable complex with the HCMV UL115 gene product. *J. Gen. Virol.* **73:** 2693.

Keay, S. and B. Baldwin. 1991. Anti-idiotype antibodies that mimic gp86 of human cytomegalovirus inhibit viral fusion but not attachment. *J. Virol.* **65:** 5124.

Keay, S., T.C. Merigan, and L. Rasmussen. 1989. Identification of cell surface receptors for the 86-kilodalton glycoprotein of human cytomegalovirus. *Proc. Natl. Acad. Sci.* **86:** 10100.

Kuhn, J., M.D. Kramer, W. Willenbacher, U. Wieland, E.U. Lorentzen, and R.W. Braun. 1990. Identification of herpes simplex virus type 1 glycoproteins interacting with the cell-surface. *J. Virol.* **64:** 2491.

Lambris, J.D., V.S. Ganu, S. Hirani, H.J. Muller-Eberhard, and G.C. Tsokos. 1985. Mapping of the C3d receptor (CR2) binding site and a neoantigenic site in the C3d domain of the third component of complement. *Proc. Natl. Acad. Sci.* **82:** 4235.

Lemon, S.M., L.M. Hutt, J.E. Shaw, J.-L. Li, and J.S. Pagano. 1977. Replication of EBV in epithelial cells during infectious mononucleosis. *Nature* **268:** 268.

Li, Q.X., L.S. Young, G. Niedobitek, C.W. Dawson, M. Birkenbach, F. Wang, and A.B. Rickinson. 1992. Epstein-Barr virus infection and replication in a human epithelial cell system. *Nature* **356:** 347.

Liang, X., L.A. Babiuk, S. van Drunen Littel-van den Hurk, D.R. Fitzpatrick, and T.J. Zamb. 1991. Bovine herpesvirus 1 attachment to permissive cells is mediated by its major glycoproteins gI, gIII, and gIV. *J. Virol.* **65:** 1124.

Ligas, M.W. and D.C. Johnson. 1988. A herpes simplex virus mutant in which glycoprotein D sequences are replaced by β-galactosidase sequences binds to but is unable to penetrate into cells. *J. Virol.* **62:** 1486.

Little, S.P., J.T. Jofre, R.J. Courtney, and P.A. Schaffer. 1981. A virion-associated glycoprotein essential for infectivity of herpes simplex virus type 1. *Virology* **115:** 149.

Lowell, C.A., L.B. Klickstein, R.H. Carter, J.A. Mitchell, D.T. Fearon, and J. M. Ahearn. 1989. Mapping of the Epstein-Barr virus and C3dg binding sites to a common domain on complement receptor type 2. *J. Exp. Med.* **170:** 1931.

Lycke, E., M. Johansson, B. Svennerholm, and U. Lindahl. 1991. Binding of herpes simplex virus to cellular heparan sulphate, an initial step in the adsorption process. *J. Gen. Virol.* **72:** 1131.

Mackett, M., M.J. Conway, J.R. Arrand, R.S. Haddad, and L.M. Hutt-Fletcher. 1990. Characterization and expression of a glycoprotein encoded by the Epstein-Barr virus *Bam*HI I fragment. *J. Virol.* **64:** 2545.

Martin, D.R., A. Yuryev, K.R. Kalli, D.T. Fearon, and J.M. Ahearn. 1991. Determination of the structural basis for selective binding of Epstein-Barr virus to human complement receptor type 2. *J. Exp. Med.* **174:** 1299.

Matsumoto, A.K., J. Kopicky-Burd, R.H. Carter, D.A. Tuveson, T.F. Tedder, and D.T. Fearon. 1991. Intersection of the complement and immune systems: A signal transduction complex of the B lymphocyte-containing complement receptor type 2 and CD19. *J. Exp. Med.* **173:** 55.

Mettenleiter, T.C., L. Zsak, F. Zukerman, N. Sugg, H. Kern, and T. Ben-Porat. 1990. Interaction of glycoprotein gcIII with a cellular heparinlike substance mediates adsorption of pseudorabies virus. *J. Virol.* **64:** 278.

Miller, N. and L.M. Hutt-Fletcher. 1988. A monoclonal antibody to glycoprotein gp85 inhibits fusion but not attachment of Epstein-Barr virus. *J. Virol.* **62:** 2366.

———. 1992. Epstein-Barr virus enters B cells and epithelial cells by different routes. *J. Virol.* **66:** 3409.

Mirda, D.P., D. Navarro, P. Paz, P.L. Lee, L. Pereira, and L.T. Williams. 1992. The fibroblast growth factor receptor is not required for herpes simplex virus type 1 infection. *J. Virol.* **66:** 448.

Molina, H., C. Brenner, S. Jacobi, J. Gorba, J.C. Carel, T. Kinoshita, and V. M. Holers. 1991. Analysis of Epstein-Barr virus-binding sites on complement receptor type 2 (CR2/CD21) using human-mouse chimeras and peptides. *J. Biol. Chem.* **266:** 12173.

Moore, M.D., R.G. DiScipio, N.R. Cooper, and G.R. Nemerow. 1989. Hydrodynamic, electron microscopic and ligand binding analysis of the Epstein-Barr virus/C3dg receptor (CR2). *J. Biol. Chem.* **264:** 20576.

Moore, M.D., M.J. Cannon, A. Sewall, M. Finlayson, M. Okimoto, and G.R. Nemerow. 1991. Inhibition of Epstein-Barr virus infection in vitro and in vivo by soluble CR2 (CD21) containing two short consensus repeats. *J. Virol.* **65:** 3559.

Muggeridge, M.I., G.H. Cohen, and R.J. Eisenberg. 1992. Herpes simplex virus infection can occur without involvement of the fibroblast growth factor receptor. *J. Virol.* **66:** 824.

Münch, K., M. Messerle, B. Plachter, and U.H. Koszinowski. 1992. An acidic region of the 89K murine cytomegalovirus immediate early protein interacts with DNA. *J. Gen. Virol.* **73:** 499.

Navarro, D., P. Paz, and L. Pereira. 1992. Domains of herpes simplex virus I glycoprotein B that function in virus penetration, cell-to-cell spread, and cell fusion. *Virology* **186:** 99.

Nemerow, G.R. and N.R. Cooper. 1984a. Early events in the infection of human B lymphocytes by Epstein-Barr virus: The internalization process. *Virology* **132:** 186.

———. 1984b. Infection of B lymphocytes by a human herpes virus Epstein-Barr virus is blocked by calmodulin antagonists. *Proc. Natl. Acad. Sci.* **81:** 4955.

Nemerow, G.R., M.F.E. Siaw, and N.R. Cooper. 1986. Purification of the Epstein-Barr virus/C3d complement receptor of human B lymphocytes: Antigenic and functional properties of the purified protein. *J. Virol.* **58:** 709.

Nemerow, G.R., R.A. Houghten, M.D. Moore, and N.R. Cooper. 1989. Identification of the epitope in the major envelope protein of Epstein-Barr virus that mediates viral binding to the B lymphocyte EBV receptor (CR2). *Cell* **56:** 369.

Nemerow, G.R., R. Wolfert, M.E. McNaughton, and N.R. Cooper. 1985. Identification and characterization of the Epstein-Barr virus receptor on human B lymphocytes and its relationship to the C3d complement receptor. *J. Virol.* **55**: 347.

Nemerow, G.R., C. Mold, V. Keivens-Schwend, V. Tollefson, and N.R. Cooper. 1987. Identification of gp350 as the viral glycoprotein mediating attachment of Epstein-Barr virus (EBV) to the EBV/C3d receptor of B cells: Sequence homology of gp350 and C3 complement fragment C3d. *J. Virol.* **61**: 1416.

Neyts, J., R. Snoeck, D. Schols, J. Balzarini, J.D. Esko, A. Van Schepdael, and E. De Clercq. 1992. Sulfated polymers inhibit the interaction of human cytomegalovirus with cell-surface heparan sulfate. *Virology* **189**: 48.

Norman, D.G., P.N. Barlow, M. Baron, A.J. Day, R.B. Sim, and I. Campbell. 1991. Three-dimensional structure of a complement control protein module in solution. *J. Mol. Biol.* **219**: 717.

Nowlin, D.M., N.R. Cooper, and T. Compton. 1991. Expression of a human cytomegalovirus receptor correlates with infectibility of cells. *J. Virol.* **65**: 3114.

Okazaki, K., T. Matsuzaki, Y. Sugahara, S. Okada, M. Hasebe, Y. Iwamura, M. Ohnishi, T. Kanno, M. Shinizu, and E. Honda. 1991. BHV-1 adsorption is mediated by the interaction of glycoprotein III with heparinlike moiety on the cell-surface. *Virology* **181**: 666.

Para, M.F., R.B. Bauke, and P.G. Spear. 1980. Immunoglobin G(Fc)-binding receptors on virions of herpes simplex virus type 1 and transfer of these receptors to the cell-surface by infection. *J. Virol.* **34**: 512.

Peeters, B., N. deWind, R. Broer, A. Gielkens, and R. Moormann. 1992a. Glycoprotein H of pseudorabies virus is essential for entry and cell-to-cell spread of the virus. *J. Virol.* **66**: 3888.

Peeters, B., N. de Wind, M. Hooisma, F. Wagenaar, A. Gielkens, and R. Moormann. 1992b. Pseudorabies virus envelope glycoproteins gp50 and gII are essential for virus penetration, but only gII is involved in membrane fusion. *J. Virol.* **66**: 894.

Pellett, P.E., M.D. Biggin, B. Barrell, and B. Roizman. 1985. Epstein-Barr virus genome may encode a protein showing significant amino acid and predicted secondary structure homology with glycoprotein B of herpes simplex virus 1. *J. Virol.* **56**: 807.

Pope, J.H., M.K. Horne, and W. Scott. 1968. Transformation of foetal human leukocytes in vitro by filtrates of a human leukaemic cell line containing herpes-like virus. *Int. J. Cancer* **3**: 857.

Sanchez-Pinel, A., J. Bernad, H. Rives, L. Lapchine, J. Icart, and J. Didier. 1991. Identification of a novel EBV-induced membrane glycoprotein of 43 kDa with H667 MAb. *Virology* **180**: 31.

Sauvageau, G., R. Stocco, S. Kasparian, and J. Menezes. 1990. Epstein-Barr virus receptor expression on human CD8$^+$ (cytotoxic/suppressor) T lymphocytes. *J. Gen. Virol.* **71**: 379.

Sawitzky, D., H. Hampl, and K.-O. Habermehl. 1990. Comparison of heparin-sensitive attachment of pseudorabies virus (PRV) and herpes simplex virus type 1 and identification of heparin-binding PRV glycoproteins. *J. Gen. Virol.* **71**: 1221.

Sears, A.E., B.S. McGwire, and B. Roizman. 1991. Infection of polarized MDCK cells with herpes simplex virus 1: Two asymmetrically distributed cell receptors interact with different viral proteins. *Proc. Natl. Acad. Sci.* **88**: 5087.

Shieh, M.-T., D. WuDunn, R.I. Montgomery, J.D. Esko, and P.G. Spear. 1992. Cell-surface receptors for herpes simplex virus are heparan sulfate proteoglycans. *J. Cell Biol.* **116**: 1273.

Sim, R.B., V. Malhotra, A.J. Day, and A. Erdei. 1987. Structure and specificity of complement receptors. *Immunol. Lett.* **14**: 183.

Sixbey, J.W., J.G. Nedrud, N. Raab-Traub, R.A. Hanes, and J.S. Pagano. 1984. Epstein-Barr virus replication in oropharyngeal epithelial cells. *N. Engl. J. Med.* **310**: 1225.

Sixbey, J.W., D.D. Davis, L.S. Young, L. Hutt-Fletcher, T.F. Tedder, and A.B. Rickinson. 1987. Human epithelial cell expression of an Epstein-Barr virus receptor. *J. Gen. Virol.* **68**: 805.

Sixbey, J.W., E.H. Vesterinen, J.G. Nedrud, N. Raab-Traub, L.A. Walton, and J.S. Pagano. 1983. Replication of Epstein-Barr virus in human epithelial cells infected *in vitro. Nature* **306**: 480.

Stannard, L.M., A.O. Fuller, and P.G. Spear. 1987. Herpes simplex virus glycoproteins associated with different morphological entities projecting from the virion envelope. *J. Gen. Virol.* **68**: 715.

Svennerholm, B., S. Jeansson, A. Vahlne, and E. Lycke. 1991. Involvement of glycoprotein C (gC) in adsorption of herpes simplex virus type 1 (HSV-1) to the cell. *Arch. Virol.* **120**: 273.

Tack, B., R. Harrison, J. Janatova, M. Thomas, and J. Prahl. 1980. Evidence for presence of an internal thiolester bond in third component of human complement. *Proc. Natl. Acad. Sci.* **77**: 5764.

Tanner, J., J. Weis, D. Fearon, Y. Whang, and E. Kieff. 1987. Epstein-Barr virus gp350/220 binding to the B lymphocyte C3d receptor mediates adsorption, capping and endocytosis. *Cell* **50**: 203.

Tanner, J., Y. Whang, J. Sample, A. Sears, and E. Kieff. 1988. Soluble gp350/220 and deletion mutant glycoproteins block Epstein-Barr virus adsorption to lymphocytes. *J. Virol.* **62**: 4452.

Taylor, H.P. and N.R. Cooper. 1989. Human cytomegalovirus binding to fibroblasts is receptor mediated. *J. Virol.* **63**: 3991.

———. 1990. Human cytomegalovirus receptor on fibroblasts is a 30 kDa membrane protein. *J. Virol.* **64**: 2484.

Tedder, T.F., V.S. Goldmacher, J.M. Lambert, and S.F. Schlossman. 1986. Epstein-Barr virus binding induces internalization of the C3d receptor: A novel immunotoxin delivery system. *J. Immunol.* **137**: 1387.

Thorley-Lawson, D.A. and C.M. Edson. 1979. Polypeptides of the Epstein-Barr virus membrane antigen complex. *J. Virol.* **32**: 458.

Watry, D., J.A. Hedrick, S. Siervo, G. Rhodes, J.J. Lamberti, J.D. Lambris, and C.D. Tsoukas. 1991. Infection of human thymocytes by Epstein-Barr virus. *J. Exp. Med.* **173**: 971.

Weis, J.J, T.F. Tedder, and D.T. Fearon. 1984. Identification of a 145,000 M_r membrane protein as the C3d receptor (CR2) of human B lymphocytes. *Proc. Natl. Acad. Sci.* **81**: 881.

Wells, A., N. Koide, and G. Klein. 1982. Two large virion envelope glycoproteins mediate Epstein-Barr virus binding to receptor-positive cells. *J. Virol.* **41**: 286.

Wittels, M. and P.G. Spear. 1990. Penetration of cells by herpes simplex virus does not require a low pH-dependent endocytic pathway. *Virus Res.* **18**: 271.

Wolf, H., M. Haus, and E. Wilmes. 1984. Persistence of Esptein-Barr virus in the parotid gland. *J. Virol.* **51**: 795.

Wright, J.F., A. Kurosky, and S. Wasi. 1994. An endothelial cell-surface form of annexin II binds human cytomegalovirus. *Biochem. Biophys. Res. Commun.* **198**: 983.

WuDunn, D. and P.G. Spear. 1989. Initial interaction of herpes simplex virus with cells is binding to heparin sulfate. *J. Virol.* **63**: 52.

Young, L.S., D. Clark, J.W. Sixbey, and A.B. Rickinson. 1986. Epstein-Barr virus receptors on human pharyngeal epithelia. *Lancet* I: 240.

Young, L.S., C.W. Dawson, and A.B. Rickinson. 1989a. Epstein-Barr virus/complement receptor and epithelial cells. *Lancet* 2: 448.

Young, L.S., C.W. Dawson, K.W. Brown, and A.B. Rickinson. 1989b. Identification of a human epithelial cell surface protein sharing an epitope with the C3d/Epstein-Barr virus receptor molecule of B lymphocytes. *Int. J. Cancer* **43:** 786.

Yura, Y., H. Iga, Y. Kondo, K. Harada, H. Tsujimoto, T. Yanagawa, H. Yoshida, and M. Sato. 1992. Heparan sulfate as a mediator of herpes simplex virus binding to basement membrane. *J. Invest. Dermatol.* **98:** 494.

Zsak, L., N. Sugg, T. Ben-Porat, A.K. Robbins, M.E. Whealy, and L.W. Enquist. 1991. The gIII glycoprotein of pseudorabies virus is involved in two distinct steps of virus attachment. *J. Virol.* **65:** 4317.

zur Hausen, H., H. Schulte-Holthausen, G. Klein, W. Henle, G. Henle, P. Clifford, and L. Santesson. 1970. EB-virus DNA in biopsies of Burkitt tumors and anaplastic carcinomas of the nasopharynx. *Nature* **288:** 1056.

20

Interaction of Reovirus with Eukaryotic Host: Pathogenesis and Host Immune Response

Ann B. Georgi and Bernard N. Fields
Department of Microbiology and Molecular Genetics
Harvard Medical School
Boston, Massachusetts 02115

To achieve productive infection, microbial pathogens must first overcome several host protective barriers. To accomplish this, pathogens have developed varied strategies to gain entry into host permissive tissue, replicate, spread within the host, and/or shed back into the environment while overcoming host defense mechanisms. For enteric viruses such as poliomyelitis, coxsackieviruses, and reovirus, entry through the alimentary tract requires that the virus particles be resistant to gut proteases and that they possess a mechanism for crossing the mucosal surface of the intestine to gain access to permissive tissue. Mammalian reoviruses have proven useful for the study of pathogenesis of enteric virus infection.

The molecular structure of reovirus (described by Nibert and Fields, this volume) has been well characterized. Briefly, the virion consists of a double icosahedral protein shell encapsulating a segmented double-stranded RNA genome. In recent years, much has been learned about specific gene products and their contributions to reovirus pathogenesis.

Three distinct serotypes of the mammalian reoviruses (designated types 1, 2, and 3) have been defined by hemagglutination-inhibition and neutralization analyses. Genetic reassortment of gene segments between serotypes occurs following mixed infection. The genetic contributions of each of the parental serotypes can be determined by differences in electrophoretic mobility of the genes on SDS gels (Ramig et al. 1977).

Phenotypic differences in pathways of spread and tissue tropism between the different reovirus serotypes and the property of genetic reassortment make reovirus a useful model for the study of mechanisms of molecular pathogenesis in enteric viruses.

Cellular Receptors for Animal Viruses
© 1994 Cold Spring Harbor Laboratory Press 0-87969-429-7/94 $5 + .00

VIRAL ENTRY INTO THE HOST

Although the mechanism of spread following reovirus infection in mice and rats has been examined using several routes of entry (primarily peroral, intracerebral, intratracheal, and intramuscular inoculation), one natural route of entry into the host is via the alimentary tract. Once reovirus has been ingested, it is subjected to proteolytic digestion by enzymes present in the lumen of the intestine (Bodkin et al. 1989). During this proteolytic step, the virus outer capsid protein, $\sigma 3$, is removed from the virion and a second outer capsid protein, $\mu 1c$, is cleaved to form δ and a small fragment, ϕ (Joklik 1972; Nibert et al. 1991). These cleavage events produce a structurally altered form of the virus called an intermediate subviral particle (ISVP). Electron microscopic examination of ISVPs shows that $\sigma 1$, the cell-attachment protein which is folded up on the intact virion, is fully extended on ISVPs (Furlong et al. 1988).

Primary replication of virus in the lumen is inhibited by pretreatment of animals with protease inhibitors to block virus conversion to ISVPs. If mice are inoculated with ISVPs, protease treatment has no effect on primary replication but does reduce virus production in subsequent rounds of replication (Bass et al. 1990). Rather than being inactivated by proteolysis, the virus requires this structural conversion event in order to gain entry into host tissue (Fig. 1) (Bodkin et al. 1989).

Although reovirus serotype 1 Lang is found in several different tissues following peroral inoculation in newborn or adult mice, it does not produce lethal infection in these animals. Type 1 virions are found specifically associated with the apical surface of M (microfold) cells in the dome epithelial layer overlying Peyer's patches within 30 minutes following peroral inoculation into 9-day-old suckling or adult mice. No other intestinal epithelial cell type shows any virus association. No binding to the apical surface of absorptive or goblet cells lining the Peyer's patch or adjacent villi has been observed with type 1 virus (Wolf et al. 1981, 1983, 1987; Bass et al. 1988).

The virus is transcytosed in endosomes through M cells and delivered to the mononuclear lymphocytes and monocytes of the Peyer's patch. Virions are subsequently found on the surface of mononuclear cells and in the intercellular space beneath the basal lamina of M cells. Entry of virus into the absorptive and crypt cells occurs from the basal surface (Wolf et al. 1981, 1983, 1987; Bass et al. 1988).

Viral factories indicative of replication have been found within 6 hours in mononuclear cells of the Peyer's patch, which appears to be the site of primary replication for type 1 virus (Bass et al. 1988). Experiments with type 1 poliovirus show that it too is selectively bound and endocytosed by M cells in the intestinal lumen. Virus subsequently ap-

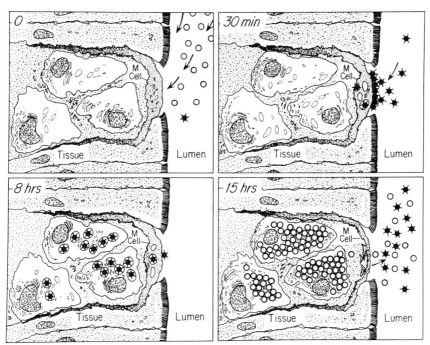

Figure 1 Diagram showing temporal stages of reovirus infection in the intestine. Intact virus particles (open circles) are proteolytically processed to ISVPs (closed hexagons with protrusions representing extended σ1 proteins) in the lumen (time 0). ISVPs are taken up by M cells (30 min) and transcytosed to the underlying mononuclear cells where replication occurs (8 hr). Some replicated virus is shed back into the lumen and proteolytically converted to ISVPs (15 hr). (Reprinted, with permission, from Bodkin et al. 1989.)

pears in Peyer's patches, where it replicates (Bodian 1955; Melnick 1990; Sicinski et al. 1990). Evidence for localization of coxsackievirus in Peyer's patches has also been reported (Melnick 1990). This process may allow delivery of enteric viruses to the host lymphatic system (Bodian 1955; Wolf et al. 1981, 1987).

Reovirus type 3 Dearing is also found on the surface and in endosomes in M cells. However, unlike type 1 Lang, type 3 Dearing virus binds to the apical surfaces and is internalized by absorptive cells, goblet cells, and tuft cells of the intestinal epithelial layer in 9-day-old or adult mice. Virus is observed in lysosome-like structures only in the apical half of these cells, indicating that like type 1, type 3 is transcytosed only by M cells. The specificity of attachment to M cells by type 1 is conferred by the S1 gene product, σ1 (Wolf et al. 1983), the viral attachment protein (Weiner et al. 1977, 1980b; Lee et al. 1981). The S1 gene also encodes a small nonstructural polypeptide, σNS, which is not associated with the particle capsid and is not known to influence virus/host interaction. The type 3 σ1 protein may recognize binding sites on other intestinal cell types as well as those on M cells. By 24 hours postinoculation, both type 1 and type 3 virions are found in mesenteric lymph nodes. However, only type 1 virus is found in the spleen by 48 hours after infection (Kauffman et al. 1983). This indicates that the early mechanism of spread of the two serotypes is most likely by different routes; type 1 Lang spreads more readily by the hematogenous route (see below) (Wolf et al. 1983).

These experiments in 9-day-old suckling and adult mice have been extremely useful in describing the route of entry of different reovirus isolates across the mucosal surface of the intestinal lumen. However, neither type 1 Lang nor type 3 Dearing causes lethality by this route of inoculation. Lethal infection by a serotype 3 murine field isolate, clone 9, however, does occur following peroral inoculation in mice up to 5 days old. Clone 9 is a highly neurotropic virus that produces a fatal encephalitis in neonatal mice. Survival of neonates increases substantially during the first 70 hours after birth following infection with type 3 clone 9 virus. When 1.5×10^6 pfu/mouse is administered within 30–40 hours after birth, survival rates are quite low, between 0 and 20%. However, when the same inoculum is given to animals 50–70 hours old, survival increases to 55–75% (L. Morrison, unpubl.). Several explanations are consistent with this observation, including the development of the nervous system, changes in receptors on the developing neurons, and the development of M cells and the maturation of the Peyer's patches in neonates.

Wolf et al. (1987) have studied the development of M cells in neonatal mice and the ability of these cells to take up reovirus type 1 for delivery to the lymphoid follicles of maturing Peyer's patches. They found aggregates of lymphoid cells in the small intestine that most likely correspond to immature Peyer's patches. These immature patches are overlaid by epithelial cells, only 1% of which are differentiated M cells in 2-day-old mice. The percentage of these differentiated cells steadily increases over the next 7 days until by day 9, approximately 7.4% are mature M cells. In contrast to the results with mice older than 9 days, type 1 virus is found to be nonselectively adherent to the undifferentiated epithelial cells overlying the immature Peyer's patches in 2-day-old mice. However, no evidence of viral transcytosis has been observed in these undifferentiated cells. As the number of differentiated M cells increases, the binding of type 1 virus becomes more selective for M cells. Virus is transcytosed across the differentiated M cells into immature Peyer's patches. One explanation for the increased lethality of type 3 clone 9 virus in neonates is that immature Peyer's patches may produce inadequate immune response, allowing more prolific production of virus.

Concomitant with reovirus uptake and transcytosis through M cells is a fourfold reduction in M-cell number during the first 3 days of infection in 10-day-old mice. This M-cell depletion may cause the mucosal surface of the lumen to be more susceptible to opportunistic infections by other microbial organisms and may compromise the ability of host cells to mount appropriate immune responses to reovirus infection. Six days after infection, the number of M cells increases twofold and by 13 days after infection, the M-cell numbers are the same as in uninfected mice (Bass et al. 1988).

A second natural route of entry for reovirus is through the respiratory tract. Electron microscopy of lung tissue following intratracheal inoculation of reovirus type 1 Lang in neonatal rats shows virus particles binding specifically to pulmonary M cells. Similar to intestinal reovirus infection, the virus is endocytosed by M cells overlying bronchus-associated lymphoid tissue (BALT) and transcytosed to the basal lamina (Fig. 2). This result provides further evidence that reovirus crosses the mucosal surface of host tissue via M-cell transcytosis for entry to permissive cells (Morin 1993).

PRIMARY REPLICATION AND SPREAD

The spread of reovirus throughout the host has been studied extensively using several different routes of inoculation. Serotype 1 and serotype 3 show different mechanisms of spread; type 1 is primarily hematogenous, whereas serotype 3 spreads through neurons to the central nervous system (CNS) (Tyler et al. 1986). Early experiments that followed the spread of virus injected intracerebrally clearly demonstrate serotypic differences. Type 1 virus appears rapidly in the eye but not in neuronal cells, indicating spread by a nonneuronal route. Type 3, however, is found only in retinal ganglion cells, suggesting that spread of this serotype is via neuronal pathways. Monoreassortants specific for S1 show clearly that it is the sole genetic determinant of the route of spread in these experiments (Tyler et al. 1985).

Tyler et al. (1986) have reported that both type 1 Lang and type 3 Dearing reovirus spread to the CNS following hindlimb footpad inoculation of 1-day-old mice. The pathway of spread, however, shows serotypic differences. If the sciatic nerve of the infected hindlimb is transsected or the animals are treated with colchicine, a potent inhibitor of fast axonal transport, type 1 virus still spreads to the spinal cord, whereas type 3 spread is inhibited. This result suggests that although type 3 virus spreads via fast axonal transport along the sciatic nerve, type 1

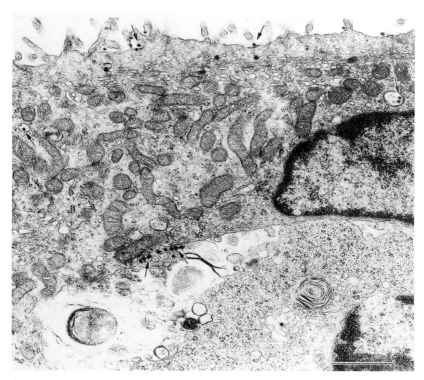

Figure 2 Electron micrograph of a pulmonary M cell showing reovirus type 1 Lang particles (*arrows*) attached to the surface, internalized in membrane-bound vesicles, and on the basal surface within BALT. Bar, 1 μm. (Courtesy of M. Morin.)

spread is hematogenous. Genetic mapping using type 1 and type 3 reassortant viruses confirms that different pathways of spread are determined once again by the S1 gene product, σ1 (Tyler et al. 1986).

Further studies by Flamand et al. (1991) show that type 1 virus is taken up by sensory neurons following footpad inoculation but confirm that the primary spread of this serotype is hematogenous. A few motor neurons are positive for viral antigen by 45 hours postinoculation with type 1 Lang, but these cells may be infected via the sensory neurons. No evidence has been found for direct penetration of type 1 at the periphery of motor neurons. Type 3 Dearing virus, however, appears in both sensory and motor neurons of the spinal cord by 19 hours after inoculation. By this time also, extensive infection of connective tissue in the footpad is found with both serotypes, indicating that primary replication of the virus occurs in this tissue. By 2–4 days following type 3 infection, virus is detected histochemically in several hundred motor and sensory neurons of the spinal cord, whereas type 1 virus is found primarily in the endothelium of blood vessels and in the meninges. Viral titers in the blood of type 1 infected animals are significantly higher than titers of type 3 infected animals. It appears, therefore, that although type 1 is able to penetrate and move along neurons, it does not amplify in these cells. The primary pathway of type 1 spread to the CNS is via the bloodstream. In contrast, type 3 virus moves through the motor and sensory neurons to the spinal cord (Flamand et al. 1991).

Recent preliminary experiments designed to examine the early steps of spread from the site of hindlimb injection indicate that virus is taken up by macrophages at the site of inoculation and rapidly appears in the sciatic nerve. The significance of this finding is not yet clear (M. Mann, unpubl.).

Studies of reovirus spread from the intestine (one of the natural routes of reovirus infection) show again that type 1 Lang and type 3 Dearing utilize different pathways. Type 1 replicates well in intestinal tissue, and high-titer virus can be recovered up to 8 days following peroral inoculation. Thus, it appears that the primary site of replication of type 1 virus is in the intestinal tract when virus is administered orally. In contrast, type 3 Dearing is not detected in intestinal tissue 4 days after peroral inoculation. This effect has been genetically mapped to both the S1 and L2 genes. The S1 gene contribution is more significant to growth in the intestine, but both genes are involved (Bodkin and Fields 1989). The S1 gene product, σ1, has already been described as the viral attachment protein. The L2 gene product, λ2, is a core spike protein that extends to the surface of the virion and may interact with σ1, anchoring it to the virus particle. Biochemical studies indicate that type 1 Lang σ1 is considerably more resistant to proteolytic digestion than type 3 Dearing σ1. The λ2/σ1 protein interaction may provide different accessibility to a cleavage site on σ1, making type 1 virus more resistant to degradation in the intestine (Bodkin and Fields 1989).

The spread of reovirus type 3 clone 9 from the gastrointestinal tract to the brain of neonatal mice has been described by Morrison et al. (1991). Following peroral inoculation, type 3 clone 9 virus enters the Peyer's patch via M-cell transcytosis. By 2–3 days postinoculation, antigen can be found in mononuclear cells in Peyer's patches. By 3 days after infection, virus appears in the neurons of the myenteric plexus. Within 4–5 days postinfection, clone 9 virus is found in the dorsal motor nucleus of the vagus. No viral antigen can be detected in endothelial cells, meninges, choroid plexus, hypothalamus, or area postrema, which are accessible to the bloodstream, indicating that the spread of type 3 clone 9 to

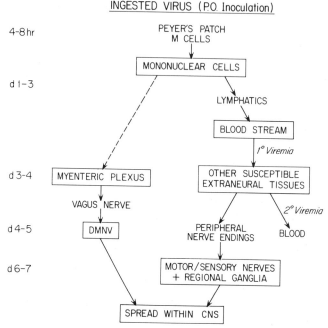

Figure 3 Schematic diagram of type 3 clone 9 reovirus pathogenesis following peroral inoculation in neonatal mice. Temporal progression from 4 hr through 7 days is indicated on left side of diagram. (Reprinted, with permission, from Morrison et al. 1991.)

the CNS occurs through parasympathetic neurons innervating the intestinal tract (Fig. 3) (Morrison et al. 1991). These findings with clone 9 are consistent with experiments showing that the spread of type 3 Dearing from the footpad is primarily through neurons, whereas spread of type 1 Lang is primarily hematogenous (Tyler et al. 1986; Flamand et al. 1991).

TROPISM

Intracerebral inoculation of type 1 or type 3 virus into 1-day-old animals shows that the two serotypes have different patterns of infection. Type 3 infects primarily neurons, causing a lethal necrotizing encephalitis; type 1 infects ependymal cells lining the ventricles, causing hydrocephalus which is not usually fatal. Examination of type 1 and type 3 reassortant viruses shows definitively that the distribution of viral antigen (tropism) is determined by the S1 gene. The S1 gene product is σ1, the viral attachment protein. This result raises the possibility that there may be different receptors on neurons and ependymal cells with different specificities for type 1 or type 3 σ1 recognition (Weiner et al. 1977, 1980b).

Reovirus strain type 3 (H/Ta) has been shown to have attenuated growth in neurons. The tissue distribution is identical to type 3 Dearing, indicating that the S1 gene tropic determinants are the same. However, the growth of type 3 (H/Ta) in neuronal tissue is reduced. Although both type 3 Dearing and (H/Ta) strains grow well in cultured mouse fibroblasts, viral titers in the brain 7 days following intracerebral inoculation of (H/Ta) are only 1% of type 3 Dearing titers. Similarly, the LD_{50} (lethal dose 50) of Dearing is 1000-fold higher than that of (H/Ta). This phenotype has been genetically mapped to the M2 gene. The M2 gene product is $\mu1$, an outer capsid protein. These results demonstrate that whereas tissue specificity may be determined by the S1 gene, virus growth is a multigenic property with the M2 gene playing an essential role in virulence (Hrdy et al. 1982).

The specificity of reovirus serotype 3 for neurons and serotype 1 for epithelial cells in the intestine and ependymal cells in the brain has been discussed above. These tissue specificities are defined by the S1 gene-encoded viral capsid protein, $\sigma1$. Other serotypic differences in tissue tropism exist. Studies of viral clearance from the blood following intravenous injection of type 1 Lang and type 3 Dearing demonstrate these differences. Both types are cleared from the blood within 10 minutes following intravenous inoculation. However, whereas type 3 becomes concentrated in the liver, type 1 is found in both the liver and lungs. Genotypic mapping using viral reassortants shows that the tropic determinant for uptake by the lungs is the type 1 S1 gene product $\sigma1$ (Verdin et al. 1988).

Although $\sigma1$ is considered the main tropic determinant in the CNS, other viral proteins can affect tissue specificity, particularly outside the CNS. The M1 gene encodes a core protein, $\mu2$, whose exact function is not known, although it is believed to play a role in RNA synthesis. This gene is linked to myocarditis following footpad inoculation in neonates. The presence of myocarditis genetically maps to a variant type 1 M1 gene (Sherry and Fields 1989; Sherry et al. 1989). The cytopathic effect in virus-infected cultured murine myocytes, but not cardiac fibroblasts, parallels the genetic mapping of reovirus-induced myocarditis (Baty and Sherry 1993). In addition, reovirus type 1 Lang replicates well in bovine aortic endothelial cells, whereas type 3 Dearing grows poorly. This difference is determined by the M1 gene (Matoba 1993).

HOST IMMUNE RESPONSE

One important reason for understanding the pathogenesis of virus infection is to develop antiviral strategies. Studies of cytotoxic T lymphocytes

(CTL), T cells, and monoclonal antibodies to reovirus outer capsid proteins have all contributed to understanding mechanisms of host response to viral infection.

Reovirus-induced CTLs are produced in the spleens of mice following intraperitoneal injection of either serotype 1 or 3. Spleen cells harvested from infected animals up to 8 weeks after inoculation can be stimulated by syngeneic cells infected with the same virus serotype in vitro. These stimulated CTLs are able to recognize and lyse reovirus-infected target macrophages in culture. The cytotoxic activity of the reovirus-induced CTLs is mediated by dual specificities of virus serotype and histocompatibility antigen expression on the surface of the target cells (Finberg et al. 1979; Zinkernagel and Doherty 1979). The neutralization epitope of the reovirus σ1 is a viral antigen recognized by CTLs on target cells.

In vivo experiments demonstrate the ability of T cells to modify reovirus infection. Adoptive transfer of spleen cells from reovirus-immune adult mice protects neonates from infection following footpad inoculation of type 3 Dearing, peroral inoculation of type 3 clone 9, or intracerebral inoculation of type 1 Lang. However, these adoptively transferred spleen cells are not able to prevent lethal infection of type 3 Dearing following intracerebral inoculation. Both CD4 and CD8 cells have been shown to be involved in protection from reovirus infection by T cells. These cells appear to abrogate infection by interfering with primary replication of the virus (Virgin and Tyler 1991).

Another component of T-cell response to reovirus infection is the inflammatory response associated with delayed hypersensitivity following challenge to primed animals. When 8- to 10-week-old animals are challenged with virus in the footpad 7 days after subcutaneous immunization on the dorsal flanks, a measurable swelling of the footpad is observed. This effect can be adoptively transferred by removing the inguinal and axillary lymph nodes of immunized animals and injecting cell suspensions made from these nodes into unimmunized mice. Furthermore, the response appears to be T-cell-mediated, since anti-Thy 1.2 plus guinea pig complement treatment of the dissociated cells from lymph nodes of immunized mice reduces the inflammatory response. Measurable swelling of the footpad is observed with both serotype 1 Lang and type 3 Dearing. The response has dual specificity; it is determined both by virus serotype and identity at the MHC H2 locus. Serotype specificity is determined by the S1 gene (Weiner et al. 1980a).

In contrast to the action of T cells, monoclonal antibodies to σ1 capsid protein appear to block spread of the virus to the CNS while having only limited effect on primary replication. Anti-σ1 monoclonal antibody

G5 (MAbG5), administered intraperitoneally either before, at the same time as, or after footpad inoculation of type 3 Dearing, does not prevent viral replication in skeletal muscle of the footpad but is able to prevent lethal infection by blocking spread of the virus to the CNS. Spread of the virus to the superior spinal cord is almost completely blocked under all three experimental conditions. It appears that MAbG5 is able to block spread of the virus from the muscle (footpad) to the CNS despite nearly normal replication of the virus (Tyler et al. 1989).

Intracerebral inoculation of type 3 Dearing, followed by intraperitoneal treatment with MAbG5 24 hours later, shows similar blocking of viral spread to neurons of the brain and retina. Neuropathology in these animals shows no significant neuronal necrosis by day 10 postinfection. Control animals (without MAbG5) are generally moribund by day 9–10 and have extensive perivascular and meningeal inflammation in the cortex, hippocampus, and thalamus. By day 16–17 postinoculation, antibody-treated animals still have no tissue necrosis or viral inclusions. However, these animals do show an inflammatory response to infection in the hippocampus and thalamus (Tyler et al. 1989).

The effect of MAbG5 on type 3 clone 9 administered perorally again demonstrates the ability of this antibody to prevent spread to the CNS. Clone 9 normally causes lethal infection when given perorally to newborn mice. However, when MAbG5 is administered intraperitoneally either before or up to 24 hours following inoculation of clone 9, primary viral replication in intestine is only slightly affected, and spread to the spinal cord and brain is almost completely blocked (Tyler et al. 1989). These results parallel results from experiments with poliovirus which show that although IgG does not inhibit viral replication in the intestine, systemic disease is prevented (Ogra 1984).

A panel of monoclonal antibodies raised against reovirus capsid proteins, $\sigma 1$, 3, and $\mu 1$, as well as the core spike, $\lambda 2$, all demonstrate protection from viral infection under specific conditions. Each of the monoclonal antibodies acts by a different mechanism and at different stages of pathogenesis. Data from experiments suggest that some monoclonal antibodies inhibit primary replication; some prevent entry, replication, and spread in the CNS; and still others prevent hematogenous spread (Tyler et al. 1989. 1993; Virgin et al. 1991).

SUMMARY

In this chapter, we have discussed viral entry, replication in host tissue, spread and tropism, clearance, and host immune response to infection. Studies of reovirus are advantageous because the contribution of specific viral genes to different stages of pathogenesis can be defined by genetic

Table 1 Molecular determinants of reovirus pathogenesis

Gene	Protein	Location	Function
S1	σ1	outer capsid	hemagglutination and serotypic determinant cell attachment tropism route of spread NT monoclonal antibody epitope[a] delayed hypersensitivity
S4	σ3	outer capsid	protective monoclonal antibody[a]
M1	μ2	core	myocarditis growth in cultured bovine aortic endothelial cells
M2	μ1	outer capsid (ISVP)	modification of T3 neurovirulence protective monoclonal antibody[a] penetration of cell membrane
L2	λ2	core to capsid	growth in intestine (with σ1) protective monoclonal antibody[a]

[a]Important in pathogenesis, although not a function of the viral gene.

reassortants (Table 1). This property has allowed us to begin to understand the molecular basis of pathogenesis of enteric and neurotropic viruses. Similarly, genes involved in the host's immune responses can be separated and examined individually. The fact that reovirus enables us to separate both the steps of viral pathogenesis and host immune response makes it a valuable tool for developing antiviral strategies in the future.

ACKNOWLEDGMENTS

The authors thank Mary Anne Mann, Marybeth Morin, and Lynda Morrison for careful review of the manuscript. Support for this work was received from U.S. Public Health Service grant 5R37AI-13178, National Institute of Neurological and Communicative Disorders and Stroke program project grant 5P50 NS-16998, and the Shipley Institute of Medicine.

REFERENCES

Bass, D.M., J.S. Trier, R. Dambrauskas, and J.L. Wolf. 1988. Reovirus type 1 infection of small intestinal epithelium in suckling mice and its effect on M cells. *Lab. Invest.* **55**: 226.

Bass, D.M., D. Bodkin, R. Dambrauskas, J.S. Trier, B.N. Fields, and J.L. Wolf. 1990. Intraluminal proteolytic activation plays an important role in replication of type 1 reovirus in the intestines of neonatal mice. *J. Virol.* **64:** 1830.

Baty, C.J. and B. Sherry. 1993. Cytopathogenic effect in cardiac myocytes but not in cardiac fibroblasts is correlated with reovirus-induced acute myocarditis. *J. Virol.* **67:** 6295.

Bodian, D. 1955. Emerging concept of poliomyelitis infection. *Science* **122:** 105.

Bodkin, D.K. and B.N. Fields. 1989. Growth and survival of reovirus in intestinal tissue: Role of the L2 and S1 genes. *J. Virol.* **63:** 1188.

Bodkin, D.K., M.L. Nibert, and B.N. Fields. 1989. Proteolytic digestion of reovirus in the intestinal lumens of neonatal mice. *J. Virol.* **63:** 4676.

Finberg, R., H.L. Wiener, B.N. Fields, B. Benacerraf, and S.J. Burakoff. 1979. Generation of cytolytic T lymphocytes after reovirus infection: Role of S1 gene. *Proc. Natl. Acad. Sci.* **76:** 442.

Flamand, A., J.-P. Gagner, L.A. Morrison, and B.N. Fields. 1991. Penetration of the nervous systems of suckling mice by mammalian reoviruses. *J. Virol.* **65:** 123.

Furlong, D.B., M.L. Nibert, and B.N. Fields. 1988. Sigma 1 protein of mammalian reoviruses extends from the surface of viral particles. *J. Virol.* **62:** 246.

Hrdy, D.B., D.H. Rubin, and B.N. Fields. 1982. Molecular basis of reovirus neurovirulence: Role of the M2 gene in avirulence. *Proc. Natl. Acad. Sci.* **79:** 1298.

Joklik, W.K. 1972. Studies on the effect of chymotrypsin on reovirions. *Virology* **49:** 700.

Kauffman, R.S., J.L. Wolf, R. Finberg, J.S. Trier, and B.N. Fields. 1983. The σ1 protein determines the extent of spread of reovirus from the gastrointestinal tract of mice. *Virology* **124:** 403.

Lee, P.W.K., E.C. Hayes, and W.K. Joklik. 1981. Protein σ1 is the reovirus attachment protein. *Virology* **108:** 156.

Matoba, Y., W.S. Colucci, B.N. Fields, and T.W. Smith. 1993. The reovirus M1 gene determines the relative capacity of growth of reovirus in cultured bovine aortic endothelial cells. *J. Clin. Invest.* **92:** 2883.

Melnick, J.L. 1990. Enteroviruses: Polioviruses, coxsackie viruses. echoviruses, and newer enteroviruses. In *Virology,* 2nd edition (ed. B.N. Fields et al.), p. 549. Raven Press, New York.

Morin, M.J. 1993. "Pathogenesis of reovirus infection in the lungs." Ph.D. thesis, Harvard University, Cambridge, Massachusetts.

Morrison, L.A., R.L. Sidman, and B.N. Fields. 1991. Direct spread of reovirus from the intestinal lumen to the central nervous system through vagal autonomic nerve fibers. *Proc. Natl. Acad. Sci.* **88:** 3852.

Nibert, M.L., D.B. Furlong, and B.N. Fields. 1991. Mechanisms of viral pathogenesis. *J. Clin. Invest.* **88:** 727.

Ogra, P.L. 1984. Mucosal immune response to poliovirus vaccines in childhood. *Rev. Infect. Dis.* (suppl. 2) **6:** 5361.

Ramig, R.F., R.K. Cross, and B.N. Fields. 1977. Genome RNAs and polypeptides of reovirus serotypes 1, 2, and 3. *J. Virol.* **22:** 726.

Sherry, B. and B.N. Fields. 1989. The reovirus M1 gene, encoding a viral core protein, is associated with the myocardic phenotype of a reovirus variant. *J. Virol.* **63:** 4850.

Sherry, B., F.J. Schoen, E. Wenske, and B.N. Fields. 1989. Derivation and characterization of an efficiently myocardic reovirus variant. *J. Virol.* **63:** 4840.

Sicinski, P., J. Rowinski, J.B. Warchol, Z. Jarzabek, W. Gut, B. Szczygiel, K. Bielecki, and G. Koch. 1990. Poliovirus type 1 enters the human host through intestinal M cells.

Gastroenterology **98:** 56.

Tyler, K.L., D.A. McPhee, and B.N. Fields. 1986. Distinct pathways of viral spread in the host determined by reovirus S1 gene segment. *Science* **233:** 770.

Tyler, K.L., R.T. Bronson, K.B. Byers, and B.N. Fields. 1985. Molecular basis of viral neurotropism: Experimental reovirus infection. *Neurology* **35:** 88.

Tyler, K.L., M.A. Mann, B.N. Fields, and H.W. Virgin IV. 1993. Protective anti-reovirus monoclonal antibodies and their effects on viral pathogenesis. *J. Virol.* **67:** 3446.

Tyler, K.L., H.W. Virgin IV, R. Bassel-Duby, and B.N. Fields. 1989. Antibody inhibits defined stages in the pathogenesis of reovirus serotype 3 infection of the central nervous system. *J. Exp. Med.* **170:** 887.

Verdin, E.M., S.P. Lynn, B.N. Fields, and E. Maratos-Flier. 1988. Uptake of reovirus serotype 1 by the lungs from the bloodstream is mediated by the viral hemagglutinin. *J. Virol.* **62:** 545.

Virgin, H.W., IV, and K.L. Tyler. 1991. Role of immune cells in protection against and control of reovirus infection in neonatal mice. *J. Virol.* **65:** 5157.

Virgin, H.W., IV, M.A. Mann, B.N. Fields, and K.L. Tyler. 1991. Monoclonal antibodies to reovirus reveal structure/function relationships between capsid proteins and genetics of susceptibility to antibody action. *J. Virol.* **65:** 6772.

Weiner, H.L., M.I. Greene, and B.N. Fields. 1980a. Delayed hypersensitivity in mice infected with reovirus I. Identification of host and viral gene products responsible for the immune response. *J. Immunol.* **125:** 278.

Weiner, H.L., L.M. Powers, and B.N. Fields. 1980b. Absolute linkage of virulence and central nervous system cell tropism of reoviruses to viral hemagglutinin. *J. Infect. Dis.* **141:** 609.

Weiner, H.L., D. Drayna, D.R. Averill, Jr., and B.N. Fields. 1977. Molecular basis of reovirus virulence: Role of the S1 gene. *Proc. Natl. Acad. Sci.* **74:** 5744.

Wolf, J.L., R. Dambrauskas, A.H. Sharpe, and J.S. Trier. 1987. Adherence to and penetration of the intestinal epithelium by reovirus type 1 in neonatal mice. *Gastroenterology* **92:** 82.

Wolf, J.L., R.S. Kauffman, R. Finberg, R. Dambrauskas, B.N. Fields, and J.S. Trier. 1983. Determinants of reovirus interaction with the intestinal M cells and absorptive cells of murine intestine. *Gastroenterology* **85:** 291.

Wolf, J.L., D.H. Rubin, R. Finberg, R.S. Kauffman, A.H. Sharpe, J.S. Trier, and B.N. Fields. 1981. Intestinal M cells: A pathway for entry of reovirus into the host. *Science* **212:** 471.

Zinkernagel, R.M. and P.C. Doherty. 1979. MHC-restricted cytotoxic T cells: Studies on the biological role of polymorphic major transplantation antigens determining T cell restriction-specificity function and responsiveness. *Adv. Immun.* **27:** 51.

21

Specificity of Coronavirus/Receptor Interactions

Kathryn V. Holmes and Gabriela S. Dveksler
Department of Pathology
Uniformed Services University of the Health Sciences
Bethesda, Maryland 20814-4799

CORONAVIRUS

Coronavirus Glycoproteins That Bind to Cell Membranes

Coronaviruses are large, enveloped, plus-strand RNA viruses that cause epidemic diseases of man and domestic animals (Wege et al. 1982; Spaan et al. 1988; Holmes 1989; Lai 1990; Moestl 1990). Coronaviruses generally have limited host ranges and infect only a limited number of tissues. One factor that determines the host range is that the viral attachment glycoproteins may recognize species-specific determinants on the receptor glycoproteins. Recently, receptors for four coronaviruses have been identified (Table 1) (Dveksler et al. 1991, 1993b; Williams et al. 1991; Delmas et al. 1992; Schultze and Herrler 1992; Yeager et al. 1992; Yokomori and Lai 1992a,b; Nedellec et al. 1994). These receptors include glycoproteins in the immunoglobulin superfamily (MHVR, Bgp), metalloproteases (pAPN and hAPN), and a carbohydrate moiety (9-*O*-acetylated neuraminic acid). The diversity of receptors and their interactions with different virus strains provide fascinating insight into the importance of virus receptors in virus pathogenesis.

Two coronavirus envelope glycoproteins have the capacity to bind to receptors on cell membranes (Fig. 1) (Holmes 1989). All coronaviruses encode a 180–200-kD glycoprotein, S, which forms the large, petal-shaped spikes that make up the characteristic corona around the virion. In addition to S, the group of coronaviruses serologically related to mouse hepatitis virus (MHV) (Hogue et al. 1984) encodes a glycoprotein, HE, that has hemagglutinating and esterase activities. The characteristics of these two viral envelope glycoproteins, their mutations and the variable levels of their expression, are important determinants of coronavirus species specificity and virulence. We discuss the S and HE glycoproteins, describe how they interact with specific receptors, and consider the biological implications of the interactions between viral glycoproteins and receptors.

Cellular Receptors for Animal Viruses
© 1994 Cold Spring Harbor Laboratory Press 0-87969-429-7/94 $5 + .00

Table 1 Binding and receptor specificities of mammalian coronaviruses

Coronavirus	Host	Binds to BBM[a] of	Receptor[b]
MHV-A59	mouse	mouse (not SJL)	MHVR and other CEA-related glycoproteins of rodents
TGEV	pig	pig, dog, human, cat	porcine aminopeptidase N (pAPN)
HCV-229E	human	pig, dog, human, cat	human aminopeptidase N (hAPN)
BCV	cow	many species	9-*O*-acetylated neuraminic acid, and possibly glycoprotein

[a]BBM indicates purified apical brush border membranes from small intestine of species indicated (Compton 1988).

[b]Characterization of receptors is described in the text and in the following references: Dveksler et al. (1991, 1993b); Williams et al. (1991); Delmas et al. (1992, 1994); Schultz and Herrler (1992); Yeager et al. (1992); Yokomori and Lai (1992a,b); Nedellec et al. (1994).

Spike Glycoprotein

The large spikes of coronaviruses are oligomers, probably trimers (Delmas and Laude 1990), of the spike glycoprotein S, held together by noncovalent bonds. There are approximately 200 spikes per virion, and the spikes are approximately 20 nm long and 7 nm wide. The genes encoding the S glycoproteins of infectious bronchitis virus (IBV) (Cavanagh et al. 1988), bovine coronavirus (BCV) (Abraham et al. 1990), transmissible gastroenteritis virus of swine (TGEV) (Rasschaert and Laude 1987), porcine respiratory coronavirus (PRCV) (Rasschaert et al. 1990), feline infectious bronchitis virus (de Groot et al. 1989), human coronaviruses HCV-229E (Raabe et al. 1990) and HCV-OC43 (Mounir and Talbot 1993), and many strains of MHV (Luytjes et al. 1987; Schmidt et al. 1987) have been cloned and sequenced, and the cloned cDNAs have been expressed in eukaryotic cells. The S glycoproteins have numerous potential sites for N-linked glycosylation. Analysis of the amino acid sequences predict that the S glycoprotein has four domains. The amino-terminal domain, a peptide called S1, comprises about one half of the molecule. It appears to have a globular structure composed of numerous β sheets connected by loops of varying lengths. The S2 peptide is acylated and contains three domains, a stalk domain that includes two α helices in a coiled-coil arrangement, a transmembrane domain, and a cytoplasmic domain characterized by numerous cysteine residues.

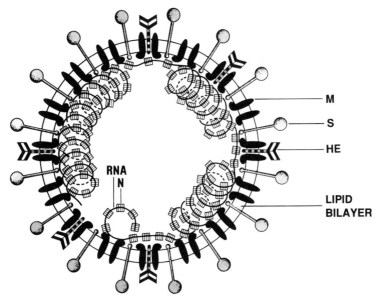

Figure 1 Model of the structure of coronavirus virions. The envelopes of all coronaviruses contain the membrane glycoprotein (M), which may play a role in virus assembly, and the spike glycoprotein (S), which binds to glycoprotein receptors on cell membranes. Some coronaviruses in the MHV/HCV-OC43 serogroup also contain the hemagglutinin-esterase glycoprotein (HE), which binds to 9-*O*-acetylated neuraminic acid moieties on cell membranes and causes hemagglutination. The nucleocapsid protein (N) and the viral genomic RNA from within the virions are released into the cell after S and/or HE bind to specific receptors, initiating penetration. (Reprinted, with permission, from Sturman and Holmes 1983.)

There is considerable diversity in the amino acid sequences of the S1 glycoproteins of different coronaviruses. In many coronaviruses, including MHV-A59, BCV, and IBV, the junction between S1 and S2 includes a short sequence of basic amino acids that can be cleaved by host-dependent trypsin-like proteases in the Golgi. The percent of virion-associated S cleaved to S1 and S2 varies considerably depending on the virus strain and the cell line used to propagate the virus (Frana et al. 1985). Although cleavage of S does not reveal a hydrophobic sequence at the new amino terminus of S2 like those found at the new amino termini of the cleavage products of the HA and F glycoproteins of orthomyxoviruses and paramyxoviruses, cleavage of coronavirus S is required for infectivity of BCV virions and for MHV-A59-induced cell fusion (Storz et al. 1981; Sturman et al. 1985). Expression of recombinant BCV S2 alone is sufficient to cause receptor-independent fusion of insect cells (Yoo et al. 1991). Interestingly, S glycoproteins of some coronaviruses such as HCV-229E and feline infectious peritonitis virus (FIPV) lack the protease target sequences, and cleavage of their S proteins is not required for infectivity or membrane fusion (de Groot et al. 1989; Raabe et al. 1990). The mechanism by which S glycoproteins induce membrane fusion is not known.

Analysis of amino acid sequences and monoclonal antibody reactivities reveals considerable heterogeneity among the S glycoproteins of different strains, isolates, and mutants of coronaviruses. For IBV and MHV, several "hot spots" for recombination have been identified where insertions or deletions of more than 100 amino acids can result in hypervariable regions (Cavanagh et al. 1988; Parker et al. 1989; Banner et al. 1990; Gallagher et al. 1990). Some MHV-A59 isolates from persistently infected cultures have mutations in the protease target site that prevent cleavage (Gombold et al. 1993). These mutants cause reduced cytopathic effects and may show significant delay in the rate of virus-induced cell fusion (Gallagher et al. 1991). Deletions, insertions, and point mutations in S have been correlated with escape from neutralization by monoclonal antibodies, altered tissue tropism, and attenuated virulence (Gallagher et al. 1990). Monoclonal antibodies mapped to different domains of S neutralize the virus and/or prevent cell fusion (Daniel et al. 1993). Thus, the S glycoprotein interacts with cellular receptors and induces membrane fusion.

The genetic variability of the S glycoproteins of MHV strains is a critically important determinant of the biological properties of the viruses. A large insertion in the S1 protein appears to be the major determinant of the different diseases induced by two closely related porcine coronaviruses, TGEV and PRCV (Laude et al. 1990; Rasschaert et al. 1990). TGEV is predominantly an enteric virus that causes diarrhea in young piglets, and spontaneously emerging PRCV strains cause epidemics of acute respiratory disease that affect pigs of all ages. There is strong sequence identity between TGEV and PRCV in all viral genes, except that isolates of PRCV from different outbreaks have large deletions in S1 (Laude et al. 1993).

The S glycoprotein of coronaviruses can undergo conformational changes that affect viral infectivity. Urea treatment of IBV virions released S1 from virions and reduced viral infectivity. The released S1 bound to membranes of chicken cells, suggesting that the receptor-recognition domain is located within the S1 peptide (Cavanagh and Davis 1986; Cavanagh et al. 1986). Similarly, when purified MHV-A59 virions were treated with trypsin to cleave S to S1 and S2, and then incubated at 37°C (pH 8.0), infectivity was markedly reduced (Sturman et al. 1990). Under these conditions, S1 was released from virions, the remainder of the spikes on the virions aggregated, virions clumped together, and epitopes on S recognized by some monoclonal antibodies were eliminated or masked (Weismiller et al. 1990). Many coronaviruses, including MHV, FIPV, and TGEV, cause cell-cell fusion at neutral or mildly alkaline pH. These viruses, like paramyxoviruses and HIV, which also fuse at neutral or alkaline pH, probably enter cells by fusion at the plasma membrane. Variants of MHV-4 have an acidic pH optimum for fusion, exhibit attenuated neurovirulence, and appear to penetrate in endosomes instead of at the plasma membrane (Gallagher et al. 1990, 1991).

These observations suggest the following model for conformational changes in the S glycoprotein during coronavirus attachment and penetration. The virion binds to its receptor glycoprotein on the plasma membrane at a specific, conformationally determined, but as yet unidentified, site on the S1 glycoprotein. Binding of S to the receptor is followed by a conformational change in S similar to that induced by treatment of virions with urea or pH 8 and 37°C, partially or completely dissociating the S1 from the S2 domain. In the S glycoproteins of some coronaviruses, this change may be facilitated by prior protease cleavage of S to yield S1 and S2. Interaction between a newly exposed hydrophobic region of S2 and the cell membrane would result in fusion of the viral envelope with the cell membrane and penetration of the virus. Several monoclonal antibodies that inhibit fusion have been mapped to the coiled-coil region of S2, suggesting that this site may be associated with membrane fusion (de Groot et al. 1987; Daniel et al. 1993).

Hemagglutinin-Esterase

The gene that encodes the hemagglutinin-esterase (HE) glycoprotein is found only in coronaviruses related to MHV and is absent from viruses in the IBV or HCV-229E/TGEV serogroups (Rottier 1990; Spaan et al. 1990). Coronavirus HE shows strong nucleic acid sequence homology with the HE glycoprotein of influenza C virus (Luytjes et al. 1988; Vlasak et al. 1988b). Coronavirus and influenza C HE glycoproteins both bind to 9-O-acetylated neuraminic acid residues on cell membrane molecules and have esterase activity that can cleave the ester bond of 9-O-acetylated neuraminic acid, destroying the receptor moiety recognized by HE (Vlasak et al. 1988a; Herrler et al. 1991; Schultze et al. 1991b). Thus, like the neuraminidase of influenza A, HE glycoproteins of influenza C and coronaviruses have been called receptor-destroying enzymes. There is no evidence that coronavirus HE is able to induce membrane fusion. Therefore, penetration of a virion bound to a membrane via HE probably depends on the membrane-fusion activity of S.

Among coronavirus strains that encode HE, there is considerable diversity in the extent to which the glycoprotein is expressed and incorporated into virions. BCV expresses large amounts of HE, which can be seen as a fringe of short spikes on the virions (King et al. 1985). Some strains of MHV, including MHV-DVIM and some MHV-JHM isolates, incorporate considerable amounts of HE in the virions, whereas other strains, including MHV-A59, do not express transcripts that encode the HE glycoprotein, so no HE is made or incorporated into the virions (Sugiyama et al. 1986; Yokomori et al. 1989). MHV strains can be infectious in vitro and virulent in vivo either with or without HE. However, the level of expression of HE may affect the pathogenesis of the virus. Inoculation of a MHV-JHM strain that produced little HE into rat brain resulted in selection of a variant that expressed increased amounts of HE mRNA (Taguchi et al. 1985, 1987). It appears likely that virulence and tissue tropism of MHV and related coronaviruses may depend on a complex interplay between the availability of HE glycoprotein on the virion and the diverse receptor-binding and penetration characteristics of the S glycoproteins of different virus strains. Possibly some variant S glycoproteins if expressed on virions without HE would not bind to receptor or penetrate efficiently enough to permit transmissible infection. In that case, expression of HE could provide an accessory way for the virion to bind to the cell and confer a significant selective advantage upon the virus.

RECEPTORS FOR MHV AND RELATED CORONAVIRUSES

CEA-related Receptors for MHV

Characterization of the receptor glycoprotein for MHV was facilitated by the genetic differences in susceptibility to MHV exhibited by different inbred strains of mice. Bang and Warwick (1960) showed that host susceptibility to MHV disease correlates with the ability of the virus to grow in cells derived from different strains of mice. To explore the mechanism of host resistance to MHV, adult BALB/c mice, which are highly susceptible to MHV, were compared with adult SJL/J mice, which are more resistant to MHV than other inbred strains (Stohlman and Frelinger 1978; Knobler et al. 1981; Barthold and Smith 1987, 1992). Inoculation of MHV-JHM intranasally into adult BALB/c and SJL/J mice, the presumed natural route of infection, results in replication of the virus at the site of inoculation in the epithelial cells of the nasal turbinates of both strains (Barthold and Smith 1987). In BALB/c mice, virus quickly spreads to other tissues, including liver, spleen, intestine, and brain, but in SJL/J mice, little virus disseminates beyond the site of inoculation, and many inoculated animals fail to seroconvert. Cell cultures derived from SJL/J mice, such as peritoneal exudate cells or primary glial cultures, are highly resistant to infection with MHV (Collins et al. 1983; Knobler et al. 1984, 1985). The difference in susceptibility of BALB/c and SJL/J mice to infection with MHV-A59 and MHV-4 (a variant of MHV-JHM) was mapped to a single gene, *hv2*, near the proximal end of mouse chromosome 7 (Smith et al. 1984; Knobler et al. 1985).

The binding of MHV to membranes from one of its principal target tissues in vivo was investigated using a solid phase immunoassay. Virus bound to purified brush border membranes (BBM) from the small intestines of adult mice was detected by antiviral antibody (Boyle et al. 1987). MHV-A59 binds in a concentration-dependent manner to BBM from BALB/c mice. In contrast, no binding of virus to BBM from SJL/J mice is detectable. This suggests that the difference in susceptibility of the mouse strains to MHV might reflect differences in the ability of their membrane proteins to serve as a virus receptor. Either the SJL/J mouse lacks a receptor, or its receptor binds virus with such low affinity that binding is not detectable in this immunoassay. To characterize the receptor further, the BBM proteins from different mouse strains were separated by SDS-PAGE and blotted with MHV-A59 virus in a virus overlay protein blot assay (VOPBA; Fig. 2). In liver membranes or intestinal BBM from BALB/c or C3H mice, a broad protein band of 110 kD or 120 kD binds virus, whereas in SJL/J mice no virus-binding protein is detectable (Boyle et al. 1987).

Antireceptor Antibodies

Polyclonal antibody against the candidate MHV receptor was prepared by immunizing SJL/J mice with BALB/c BBM. In immunoblots of BALB/c BBM and liver membrane proteins, this antiserum detects a single band of the same molecular weights as the VOPBA, whereas SJL/J proteins fail to react with the antiserum. An antireceptor monoclonal antibody, MAb-CC1, detects the same 110–120-kD glycoproteins in immunoblots, as well as an additional protein of about 58 kD (Williams et al. 1990). Both the polyclonal antireceptor antibody and MAb-CC1 block virus binding to L2 cells and prevent MHV-A59 infection of several MHV-susceptible murine cell lines, including L2, 17 Cl 1, DBT, and Sac⁻. When infant mice are treated with MAb-CC1 prior to and after intranasal challenge with MHV-A59, the yield of virus from the nose, liver, and brain is markedly diminished compared to those in

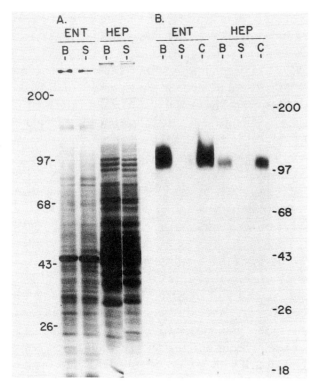

Figure 2 Binding of MHV-A59 to receptor glycoproteins from liver and intestine of susceptible mice. (*A*) Coomassie blue stains of intestinal brush border
membranes and liver membranes from MHV-susceptible BALB/c and
MHV-resistant SJL/J small intestine, and liver. (*B*) Membranes of BALB/c (B),
SJL/J (S), and semi-resistant C3H (C) mice in a virus overlay protein blot assay
(VOPBA). MHV-A59 virus binds to receptor glycoproteins in BALB/c and C3H
intestine and liver but does not bind to homologous glycoproteins in SJL/J tissues. (Reprinted, with permission, from Boyle et al. 1987.)

mice treated with an irrelevant monoclonal antibody, indicating substantial in vivo protection by the antireceptor monoclonal antibody (Fig. 3)
(Smith et al. 1991).

MAb-CC1 was used to purify sufficient receptor glycoprotein from
Swiss-Webster mouse liver for amino-terminal amino acid sequencing.
Antibody (anti-NTR) directed against a synthetic peptide corresponding
to the first 15 amino acids of the receptor protein reacts in immunoblots
with glycoproteins of 100–120 kD and 55–58 kD from liver and BBM
membranes of SJL/J mice as well as those from BALB/c mice (Williams
et al. 1990). This experiment indicates that the MHV-resistant SJL/J

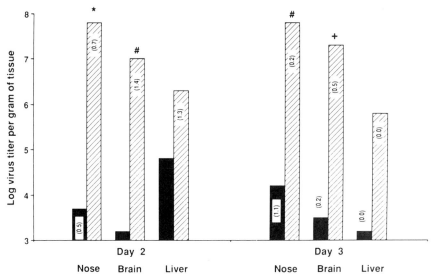

Figure 3 MHV-A59 virus titers in tissues of infant mice treated with blocking anti-receptor MAb-CC1. Newborn animals were treated with MAb-CC1 or buffer intranasally and intraperitoneally daily, beginning at day 1, and then challenged oronasally with MHV-A59 at day 2. Virus in the nose, liver, and brain was titered in suckling CD-1 mice. (Reprinted, with permission, from Smith et al. 1991.)

mice express glycoproteins homologous to the putative MHV receptor glycoprotein of BALB/c mice, suggests that the SJL/J proteins are less functional as virus receptors than the BALB/c proteins, and identifies a difference in apparent molecular weight of about 3–5 kD between the BALB/c and SJL/J proteins.

Further microsequencing of the first 25 amino acids of the affinity-purified MHV receptor showed a 60–72% identity with human members of the carcinoembryonic antigen (CEA) family of glycoproteins and 100% identity with the first 25 amino acids of two murine CEA family members called mmCGM1 and mmCGM2 (Williams et al. 1991). Antibodies directed against human CEA cross-react with immuno-affinity-purified MHV receptor from mouse liver. The CEA family includes a large group of genes that have been placed in the immunoglobulin superfamily because of the tertiary structure of the encoded proteins (Williams and Barclay 1988). Binding of radiolabeled MAb-CC1 to membranes from various tissues of BALB/c mice indicates that the greatest amount of receptor protein is expressed in the small intestine, colon, and liver (Williams et al. 1991). Two CEA-related glycoproteins, human biliary glycoprotein (BGP) and rat ecto-ATPase, are known to be expressed in the same sites (Lin 1989; Hammarstrom et al. 1993). Taken together, the data suggested that the MHV receptor might be a murine member of the CEA family of glycoproteins, possibly a protein homologous to BGP.

Cloning and Expression of MHVR

To isolate the cDNA encoding the putative MHV receptor, a cDNA probe specific for murine BGP was obtained by RNA-polymerase chain reaction (RNA-PCR) amplification of RNA from BALB/c colon with degenerate oligonucleotide primers corresponding to the amino-terminal amino acid sequence of the receptor protein and an oligonucleotide primer derived from a partial cDNA clone that encodes a murine CEA-related protein, mmCGM1, from outbred CD-1 mice (Beauchemin et al. 1989a; Dveksler et al. 1991). Screening of a cDNA library of BALB/c liver yielded a cDNA clone called MHVR1 that encodes the MHVR receptor glycoprotein (Dveksler et al. 1991). On the basis of the charac-teristics of other immunoglobulin superfamily members, the structure of the receptor glycoprotein predicted by its nucleotide sequence includes four immunoglobulin-like (Ig) domains, a transmembrane domain, and a short cytoplasmic domain (Fig. 4). The amino-terminal Ig domain resem-bles a variable Ig domain, and the other three Ig domains resemble con-stant regions (Hammarstrom et al. 1993). The predicted molecular weight of the protein encoded by MHVR1, assuming that most or all of the 16 N-linked glycosylation sites are glycosylated, is approximately 110 kD, which corresponds well with the size of the MHVR glycoprotein detected by MAb-CC1 in BHK cells transfected with MHVR1 (Dveksler et al. 1991).

The MHVR1 clone was transiently expressed in hamster (BHK) and human (RD) cell lines that are resistant to infection with MHV-A59 virions (Dveksler et al. 1991). Expression of MHVR makes the MHVR-transfected hamster and human cells susceptible to infection with MHV-A59, as shown by the development of viral antigens in the cytoplasm (Fig. 5). Anti-MHVR MAb-CC1 protects the transfected cells from infection with MHV-A59 (Fig. 5), confirming that MHVR is the functional receptor in these cells. BHK cell lines stably expressing MHVR are susceptible to infection with many strains of MHV including MHV-A59, -JHM, and -3 (Dveksler et al. 1991; G.S. Dveksler and K.V. Holmes, unpubl.). MAb-CC1 protects the transfected cells from infection with these virus strains (Table 2). Thus, all MHV strains tested share a common receptor, MHVR.

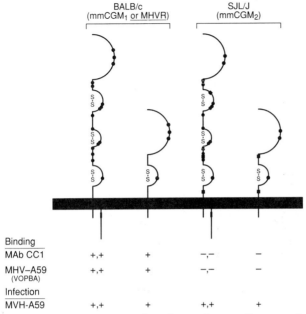

BALB/c
(mmCGM₁ or MHVR)

SJL/J
(mmCGM₂)

Binding				
MAb CC1	+,+	+	−,−	−
MHV–A59 (VOPBA)	+,+	+	−,−	−
Infection				
MVH-A59	+,+	+	+,+	+

Figure 4 Virus receptor functions of naturally occurring isoforms of murine biliary glycoproteins (BGP) from susceptible and resistant mouse strains. MHV-susceptible BALB/c mice express several variants of MHVR (mmCGM1) derived by alternative splicing. On the left is the 110-kD glycoprotein MHVR(4d), which has 4 immunoglobulin-like (Ig) domains, a transmembrane domain, and a short cytoplasmic domain. MHVR(4d)$_L$ is the same, but has a longer cytoplasmic domain. BALB/c mice also express a 58-kD glycoprotein MHVR(2d) that lacks the second and third Ig domains. SJL/J mice express homologous proteins with 29-amino-acid substitutions in the amino-terminal domain, and single amino acid substitutions in the other domains, shown by filled squares. Potential N-linked glycosylation sites are shown by filled circles. Domain 1 of MHVR has one more glycosylation site than domain 1 of mmCGM2. Solid-phase immunoassays demonstrated which glycoproteins bind to antireceptor MAb-CC1 or to MHV-A59 virions and which served as functional receptors for MHV-A59 when expressed in hamster cells.

Unglycosylated MHVR made by in vitro translation or from a recombinant vaccinia virus in the presence of tunicamycin does not bind virus or MAb-CC1 (Pensiero et al. 1992). However, when translation is done in the presence of microsomal membranes, or in cells treated with monensin, the receptor glycoprotein can bind virus and MAb-CC1. These studies show that the viral S glycoprotein and MAb-CC1 bind to a determinant(s) of the MHVR protein that depends on posttranslational processing and/or conformation.

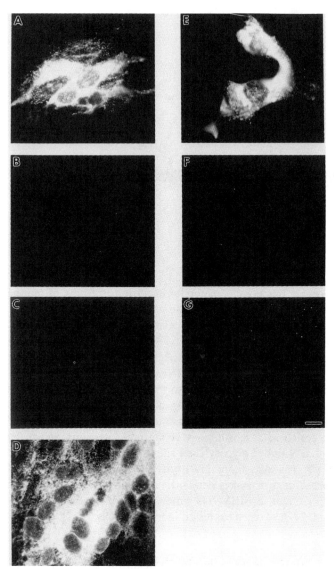

Figure 5 MHV-A59 virus antigen cytoplasm of hamster and human cells transfected with cDNA encoding MHVR glycoprotein. Hamster cells (BHK; *A–D*) and human cells (RD; *E–G*) were transfected with cDNA encoding MHVR receptor glycoprotein (*A, C, D, E,* and *G*), or with plasmid alone (*B* and *F*). Cells in *C* and *G* were pretreated with antireceptor MAb-CC1. All cells were challenged with MHV-A59. Virus antigens were detected by immunofluorescence with anti-MHV antibody. (Reprinted, with permission, from Dveksler et al. 1991.)

Table 2 Functional assays for MHV receptors

Assays for receptor activity	MHV-A59	MHV-JHM	MHV-3
Binds to BALB/c BBM[a]	+	+	+
Binds to SJL/J BBM	–	–	–
Binds to rat BBM	–	–	–
Binds to MHVR(4d) in virus blot	+	+	+
Binds to mmCGM2(4d) in virus blot	–	–	–
Hamster cells transfected with MHVR can be infected by virions	+	+	+
Hamster cells transfected with mmCGM2 can be infected by virions	+	+	+
Hamster cells can be infected by virions	–	–	–
Hamster cells can be infected by co- cultivation with virus-infected mouse cells	–	+	n.d.

n.d. indicates not determined.
[a]BBM indicates purified apical brush border membranes from small intestine of adult mice.

Gene Organization, Transcription, and Polymorphism of Rodent BGPs

The CEA glycoproteins are encoded by a large family of related genes that yield numerous transcripts with complex patterns of alternative splicing (Hammarstrom et al. 1993). Recent studies of the organization of human and rodent CEA-related genes indicate that there are more than 22 different CEA-related genes located in a cluster of about 1.2 Mb on human chromosome 19 in the 19q13.1-19q13.3 region. Related glycoproteins of the mouse are located in a syntenic region of chromosome 7 (Robbins et al. 1991), and the *hv2* gene for MHV resistance maps to this region (Smith et al. 1984; Knobler et al. 1985). Rodent homologs of the seven-Ig-domain CEA glycoprotein or the related five-domain glycoprotein called normal cross-reacting antigens (NCA) have not been identified (Hammarstrom et al. 1993). Humans have a single BGP gene that has multiple transcripts generated by complex patterns of splicing (Barnett et al. 1989). Cloned cDNAs from BALB/c and other mice share the same coding region as MHVR1, but differ in the lengths and sequences of their 5' and 3' untranslated regions (Dveksler et al. 1991; Turbide et al. 1991; McCuaig et al. 1992), suggesting alternative splicing of untranslated regions. In addition, numerous splice variants encode many different BGP isoforms (Fig. 4). For example, cDNAs that encode the 58-kD isoform of MHVR have been cloned from CD-1, BALB/c, and C57BL/6 mice (Dveksler et al. 1991; Yokomori et al. 1991; McCuaig et al. 1992). The coding sequences of these transcripts are identical to MHVR1, but have a 564-nucleotide deletion that results from alternative splicing which joins domains 1 and 4, eliminating domains 2 and 3. The nomenclature for the human and murine BGPs has been changed several times and continues to evolve as additional genes and splice variants are identified (Table 3). For clarity in this discussion of the virus receptor functions of the BGPs, we refer to the four-Ig-domain MHVR splice variant as MHVR(4d) and the two-domain splice variant as MHVR(2d). In addition to this alternative splicing within the extracellular domain, alternative splicing of BGP transcripts generates intracytoplasmic domains of different lengths, which we indicate by subscripts to denote long versus short. A cDNA clone MHVR(4d)$_L$ from CD-1 mouse colon encodes a protein identical to MHVR, except that it has 62 extra amino acids in its cytoplasmic domain (McCuaig et al. 1992). Variants of rat BGPs that differ in the lengths of their cytoplasmic domains have also been cloned (Lin and Guidotti 1989; Lin et al. 1991; Culic et al. 1992). Unlike the glycoproteins with shorter cytoplasmic domains, isoforms with longer cytoplasmic domains have consensus binding sites for ATP and are possible targets for the insulin receptor tyrosine kinase (Margolis et al. 1990; Najjar et al. 1993). In human BGP, short splice differences preceding the transmembrane region and secreted forms have also been detected. Multiple splice variants of a single BGP gene can be coexpressed in a single cell, and the ratios of different splice variants vary in different tissues and at different developmental stages. The complexity of splice variants suggests that the protein products play delicately balanced or regulated roles in essential cellular functions (Hammarstrom et al. 1993).

Two identical cDNA clones that encode a murine BGP variant called mmCGM2(4d) were isolated from SJL/J and CD-1 mice (Dveksler et al. 1993b). In comparison with MHVR, mmCGM2(4d) has 29 amino acid

Table 3 Nomenclature of biliary glycoproteins

Source	Alternative names	Reference
Human	BGPa through BGPi	Barnett et al. (1989)
Rat	Ecto-ATPase	Lin and Guidotti (1989)
	cell CAM-105	Odin et al. (1986)
	C-CAM	Obrink (1991)
Mouse	mmCGM1 and 2	Beauchemin et al. (1989,a,b)
	MHVR	Dveksler et al. (1991)
	BgpA through BgpH	McCuaig et al. (1993)
	Bgp1[a], 1[b], 2	Nedellec et al. (1994)

N-DOMAIN

```
MHVR     EVTIEAVPPQVAEDNNVLLLVHNLPLALGAFAWYKGNTTAIDKEI
                                              ::::::
mmCGM2   EVTIEAVPPQVAEDNNVLLLVHNLPLALGAFAWYKGNPVSTNAEI
```

```
ARFVPNSNMNFTGQAYSGREIIYSNGSLLFQMITMKDMGVTTLDMTDENYRRTQATVRFHVH
::  :::  :::  :  :       ::        :  ::  :   :  : ::     :   :   :
VHFVTGTNKTTTGPAHSGRETVYSNGSLLIQRVTVKDTGVYTIEMTDENFRRTEATVQFHVH
```

Figure 6 Sequences of the amino-terminal domains of the allelic MHVR and mmCGM2 glycoproteins. Amino acid substitutions (29) are indicated by colons. Potential N-linked glycosylation sites are underlined. The amino-terminal domains of CEA-related glycoproteins exhibit the greatest variability in amino acid sequence.

substitutions in the 108 amino acids of domain 1 (Fig. 6) and 5 single amino acid differences scattered through domains 2–4. Like MHVR, mmCGM2(4d) has an isoform generated by alternative splicing that eliminates the middle two Ig domains (mmCGM2[2d]) as well as isoforms with cytoplasmic domains of different lengths (Fig. 4). To determine whether these transcripts were derived by differential splicing or from different genes, RNase protection assays were done with riboprobes that hybridized specifically to either of the amino-terminal domains. These data, together with RNA-PCR with domain-specific oligonucleotides and identification of restriction fragment length polymorphisms, showed that MHVR and mmCGM2 are alleles of a single gene, and that inbred mouse strains express either one or the other (Table 4). The SJL/J mouse is the only inbred line known to encode the mmCGM2 allele. Outbred CD-1 mice express both MHVR and mmCGM2. There is considerable diversity between the amino-terminal domains of MHVR, mmCGM2 (Fig. 6), and homologous BGP proteins of rats and humans. BGP cDNAs encoding amino-terminal domains that vary considerably in sequence have also been cloned from rats (Lin and Guidotti 1989; Lin et al. 1991; Culic et al. 1992), and it appears likely

Table 4 Expression of Bgp1 alleles in inbred and outbred mice

BGP gene expression[a]	BALB/c	SJL/J	C3H	CD1
MHVR (Bgp1[a])	+	–	+	+
mmCGM2 (Bgp1[b])	–	+	–	+

[a]The transcripts of BGP were detected by RNA-PCR from small intestine or colon and by RNase protection assays using oligonucleotides specific for the amino-terminal domain of either MHVR or mmCGM2.

that these represent allelic variation. No allelic variants of BGP in humans have yet been identified.

The most extensive variations in amino acid sequence between different BGP proteins are in the amino-terminal domain, which corresponds to an Ig-variable-like domain (Kodelja et al. 1989; Thompson et al. 1989; Hammarstrom et al. 1993). This variability in the ligand-binding domains of BGPs encoded by different alleles or genes is probably important for their diverse cellular functions.

The genomic organization of BGPs and other CEA-related genes is reviewed by Hammarstrom et al. (1993). In mice, an additional Bgp gene, Bgp2, was found to be an MHV receptor (Nedellec et al. 1994), and a cDNA clone encoding a different amino-terminal domain sequence, mmCGM3, was identified in outbred and inbred mice and in a murine cell line (N. Beauchemin; W. Zimmermann; J.-H. Lu, all pers. comm.). At least two additional amino-terminal domains have been cloned from cosmid clones from inbred mice (N. Beauchemin; M.M.C. Lai, both pers. comm.).

Recently, numerous important and diverse cellular functions for human and rodent CEA-related glycoproteins have been discovered (Table 5) (Benchimol et al. 1989; Lin and Guidotti 1989; Lin et al. 1991; Obrink 1991; Sauter et al. 1991; Turbide et al. 1991; McCuaig et al. 1992; Dveksler et al. 1993b). Particularly interesting are the findings that BGPs can act as cell adhesion molecules, and NCA serves as a receptor for type 1 fimbriae of *Escherichia coli* (Sauter et al. 1991; Hammarstrom et al. 1993). Other cell adhesion glycoproteins in the immunoglobulin superfamily also serve as virus receptors (White and Littman 1989). For example, HIV-1 binds to CD4, poliovirus binds to an Ig-related protein called

Table 5 Functions of rodent biliary glycoproteins

Extracellular hydrolysis of ATP, (ecto-ATPase)	Lin and Guidotti (1989)
Homotypic cellular adhesion	Svalander et al. (1987); Tingstrom et al. (1990); Turbide et al. (1991); McCuaig et al. (1992)
MHV receptor	Dveksler et al. (1991); Yokomori and Lai (1992a,b)
Binds calmodulin	Kostka (1989); Blikstad et al. (1992)
Substrate of the insulin receptor tyrosine kinase	Najjar et al. (1993)
Transporter of bile acids	Sippel et al. (1993)

PVR, and the major group of rhinoviruses binds to ICAM-1 (Jameson et al. 1988; Racaniello 1990). The homophilic and heterophilic interactions of human CEA-related glycoproteins appear to depend on determinants in the amino-terminal domains (Oikawa et al. 1991). The expression of the BGP glycoprotein isoforms in various tissues is differently regulated during embryogenesis and cell transformation (Huang et al. 1990). The mechanisms that regulate expression of CEA-related glycoproteins are not yet well understood.

MHV Receptor Activities of BGP Isoforms in Mice

The various splice variants or alleles of MHVR described above were cloned and transfected into BHK cells or COS cells (Dveksler et al. 1991, 1993b; Yokomori and Lai 1992a,b). The transfected cells were tested for their ability to bind MAb-CC1, polyclonal anti-MHVR antibody, or different strains of MHV, and for susceptibility to infection by these viruses (Fig. 4). BHK cells and COS cells are resistant to infection with MHV-A59 or MHV-JHM virions. When transiently or stably transfected into BHK or COS cells, the two-domain splice variant of MHVR, MHVR(2d), serves as a functional receptor for MHV-A59 and MHV-JHM. This is surprising because in VOPBAs, the MHVR(2d) protein binds MHV-A59 poorly compared to MHR(4d), although in immunoblots, MAb-CC1 binds to both isoforms equally well (Williams et al. 1990). MHVR isoforms with a long cytoplasmic domain also served as a functional receptor for MHV-A59 (Fig. 4) (Dveksler et al. 1993b). Thus, each of the MHVR isoforms tested from the MHV-susceptible strains such as BALB/c, and from semi-resistant strains, including C3H, can function as a receptor for MHV.

The glycoproteins homologous to MHVR that are expressed in MHV-A59-resistant SJL/J mice are encoded by the mmCGM2 allele of murine BGP. To determine if mmCGM2 isoforms can serve as MHV receptors, peritoneal exudate cells and cell lines derived from SJL/J mice were challenged with virus. In low-passage SJL/J embryo fibroblasts, MHV-3, but not MHV-A59 or MHV-JHM, replicates in a small percentage of cells, suggesting that different strains of MHV have different host ranges. Viruses with wider host ranges may use different receptors in different mouse strains, or they may use homologous receptors with higher efficiency than that of virus strains that cannot grow in those cells. Surprisingly, when mmCGM2(2d), mmCGM2(4d), and mmCGM2(4d)$_L$, the isoforms from SJL/J mice, were expressed transiently or in stable lines derived from transfected hamster cells, they served as functional receptors for MHV-A59, MHV-JHM, and MHV-3 (Fig. 4). MAb-CC1, which does not bind to mmCGM2 proteins, failed to protect the mmCGM2-transfected cells from infection with MHV-A59 (Table 2). Overexpression of cloned mmCGM2(2d) in the cell lines derived from SJL/J mice, which already express a limited amount of the mmCGM2 isoforms as shown by RNA-PCR, also rendered them susceptible to infection with MHV-A59 and MHV-JHM (Dveksler et al. 1993b). Possibly the mmCGM2 isoforms are less efficient receptors for MHV-A59 than the MHVR isoforms, and only at higher levels of expression can a relatively inefficient receptor lead to virus infection.

Recently, an additional murine Bgp gene, Bgp2, was cloned and expressed in BHK cells and shown to be an alternative receptor for MHV (Nedellec et al. 1994). Bgp2 is expressed in both BALB/c and SJL/J mice. Although CMT-93 cells express both MHVR and BGP2, anti-MHVR specific Mab-CC1 completely blocks virus infection of CMT-93 cells. Thus, MHVR may be the preferred receptor when coexpressed with Bgp2.

Functional Domains of MHVR

To identify the domain of MHVR that binds MHV S glycoprotein and to determine which parts of MHVR are essential for virus receptor function, a series of deletions of MHVR1 was expressed in BHK cells and the truncated proteins were tested for binding of MHV-A59, MAb-CC1, and polyclonal anti-MHVR and for functional MHV-A59 receptor activity (Fig. 7) (Dveksler et al. 1993a). Anchored MHVR proteins lacking part or all of domain 1 were recognized on the cell surface by polyclonal anti-MHVR but failed to bind virus or MAb-CC1 and did not serve as receptors for MHV-A59. Anchored MHVR proteins from which any other single Ig domain was deleted did bind MHV-A59 virus and MAb-CC1 and did serve as receptors for MHV-A59. Thus, both the S glycoprotein of MHV and MAb-CC1 bind to the amino-terminal domain of MHVR. Similarly, the amino-terminal domains of other Ig superfamily glycoproteins play key roles in binding to a variety of ligands. For example, both HIV and human rhinoviruses bind to the amino-terminal domains of their receptors, CD4 and I-CAM1, respectively. The natural ligands of CD4 and I-CAM1, and the homophilic adhesion of CEA-related proteins, also bind to their amino-terminal domains (Oikawa et al. 1991). Deletions and point mutations within the first domain of MHVR are being used to identify the amino acids required for binding to MHV S glycoprotein and MAb-CC1. Elimination of all three potential N-linked glycosylation sites in the amino-terminal domain of MHVR does not abrogate its virus receptor function (G.S. Dveksler, in prep.).

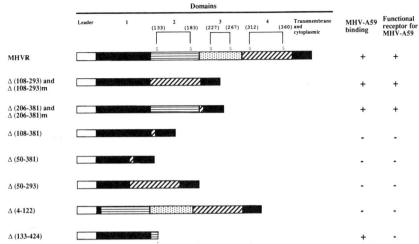

Figure 7 Functions of deletion mutants of MHVR. The domains of MHVR are shown in marked boxes. Numbers in parentheses indicate the positions of cysteine residues. Deletion mutants are designated by Δ followed by the numbers of amino acids missing from MHVR. Point mutations, indicated by m, are at positions 85 and 94 in Δ (108-293) and amino acids 6 and 30 in Δ (206-381). The ability of the proteins to bind MHV-A59 virions and to serve as functional receptors when expressed in hamster cells is shown at right. (Adapted, with permission, from Dveksler et al. 1993a.)

To identify other parts of the MHVR(4d) glycoprotein that may also be required for virus receptor activity, additional deletions and chimeric proteins were tested (Dveksler et al. 1993a). Anchored constructs containing domains 1 and 4 or domains 1 and 2 were able to serve as MHV receptors. In contrast, an anchored construct of domain 1 alone was not a functional receptor, even when expressed on the plasma membrane at very high levels using a vaccinia vector. This protein was recognized by the protective MAb-CC1 but failed to bind virus in a VOPBA. This experiment suggested that all or part of another Ig domain, in addition to the amino-terminal domain, is needed for full receptor function.

To determine the requirements for specificity of the additional domains needed for receptor activity, a chimeric protein containing the amino-terminal domain of MHVR and the second, third, transmembrane, and cytoplasmic domains of the mouse homolog of the poliovirus receptor (mph) was expressed in BHK cells (G.S. Dveksler, in prep.). The MHVR-mph chimera had MHV-A59 receptor activity, and cells expressing it formed syncytia after MHV-A59 infection. Thus, when the virus-binding site on the amino-terminal domain is present, many different Ig-like constant regions can provide the accessory function needed to make the molecule a functional receptor.

Rat BGPs as Receptors for MHV Strains

To explore the role of virus receptors in determining the species specificity or host range of MHV, cDNA clones encoding two rat BGP glycoproteins that differ in the first domain and in the length of their cytoplasmic tails were expressed in COS cell lines and tested for MHV-A59 receptor activity (S. Gagneten, in prep.). Neither of the rat glycoproteins can serve as a functional receptor for MHV-A59. This supports the hypothesis that the specificity of the interactions between the viral S glycoprotein and the BGP-related receptor glycoprotein plays an important role in restricting MHV-A59 infection to murine cells.

Subsequently, other strains of MHV were tested for utilization of rat BGPs as receptors, including MHV-JHM, which is neurotropic, and MHV-3, which is hepatotropic. Both MHV-JHM and MHV-3 can cause acute encephalitis and demyelination following inoculation into the brains of suckling rats, although adult rats are fully resistant to infection with all strains of MHV. Interestingly, MHV-JHM and MHV-3 can use both of the two different rat BGP glycoproteins as receptors (S. Gagneten, in prep.). These observations suggest that the wider host range of MHV-3 in vitro and in vivo might be due to the ability of its S glycoprotein to utilize a greater variety of BGP variants as receptors. Adaptation of coronaviruses to foreign species or to growth in cultured cells may be dependent on selection for viruses whose S glycoproteins can use as receptors the BGP glycoprotein isoforms that are expressed on those cells.

Receptors for Coronaviruses Related to MHV

Rat Coronavirus

There are two rat coronaviruses, Parker's rat coronavirus (RCV-P) and sialodacryadenitis virus (RCV-SDAV), which are closely related to MHV by serology and nucleotide sequence homology (Jacoby 1986). In rats, these RCV strains infect the respiratory epithelium, salivary and lachrymal glands, but, unlike MHV, they do not infect the liver, intestine, or brain. Since MHV-3 can utilize rat BGPs as receptors, it is reasonable to investigate whether rat coronaviruses also use rat BGPs as receptors. RCV-P and RCV-SDAV were used to challenge BHK or COS cells transfected with cDNA clones expressing rat BGP_L or rat BGP_S (Culic et al. 1992; S. Gagneten, in prep.). These rat BGP proteins do not serve as receptors for the rat coronaviruses. The receptor for the RCV strains has not yet been identified.

Human Coronavirus HCV-OC43

HCV-OC43 expresses both HE and S glycoproteins, and binding to cell membranes may be mediated by either of them (Zhang et al. 1992; Künkel and Herrler 1993; Mounir and Talbot 1993). The HE and the S glycoproteins of HCV-OC43 bind to 9-*O*-acetylated neuraminic acid, and binding is reduced by treatment of the cells with neuraminidase (Schultze and Herrler 1992; Künkel and Herrler 1993).

Human coronavirus HCV-OC43 is serologically related to MHV and shares considerable nucleic acid sequence homology with MHV (Künkel and Herrler 1993). In nontransfected, control mouse cells, there is a low incidence of infection with HCV-OC43. This is not an unexpected finding, since the virus was passaged repeatedly in mouse brain during its isolation. In murine cells, HCV-OC43 does not appear to utilize MHVR as its receptor, since HCV-OC43 infection of mouse fibroblasts is not blocked by MAb-CC1. No increase in susceptibility to HCV-OC43 infection was noted in mouse cells transfected with cDNAs encoding human BGPs (R.K. Williams, in prep.). Antibodies directed against the human BGP glycoproteins did not protect mouse cells from infection. Thus, the available evidence suggests that HCV-OC43 does not utilize human or mouse BGP glycoproteins as its receptor. Infection of human rhabdomyosarcoma (RD) cells with HCV-OC43 was reported to be blocked with a monoclonal antibody (W6/32) directed against the 45-kD heavy chain of human HLA class I antigen (Collins 1993). Further work is needed to determine whether cloned MHC class I glycoproteins confer susceptibility to HCV-OC43 upon expression in nonhuman cells.

Bovine Coronavirus and Hemagglutinating
Encephalomyelitis Virus

BCV and HEV, members of the MHV serogroup of coronaviruses, cause enteric infection of cattle and respiratory and neurological disease in swine. Both BCV and HEV express HE glycoproteins that bind to N-acetyl 9-*O*-acetylated neuraminic acid and have hemagglutination and esterase activities (Schultze et al. 1990a,b,c; Schultze and Herrler 1992). In addition, the S glycoprotein of BCV binds to 9-*O*-acetylated neuraminic acid (Schultze et al. 1991a). The ability of these viruses to bind to the carbohydrate moieties on cell membranes is important for virus infectivity. Infectivity of BCV is greatly reduced, but not eliminated, by treatment of cells with acetyl esterase or neuraminidase to remove the carbohydrate recognized by the virus (Schultze and Herrler 1992; Herrler et al. 1991). Esterase inhibitors block hemagglutination and virus infectivity (Vlasak et al. 1988b). The roles of the S and HE glycoproteins in initiation of BCV infection are not yet fully understood. Although it is clear that binding to carbohydrate moieties facilitates infection, it is not yet known whether the S glycoprotein recognizes a specific receptor protein in addition to the 9-*O*-acetylated neuraminic acid. This might represent a second step in the attachment and penetration of BCV.

BCV binds to erythrocytes and to intestinal BBM and cultured cells of many different species (Compton 1988). BCV can infect the intestine of infant mice (Barthold et al. 1990). The wide host range of this virus may be due at least in part to its ability to bind to 9-*O*-acetylneuraminic acid, a moiety that is expressed on cells of many species.

Model for Interactions of MHV Strains with BGP Receptors

Figure 8 shows a model of how the different BGP glycoproteins and their levels of expression may affect their MHV receptor activities. We postulate that most anchored cell lines express at least a low level of BGP as well as whatever cellular accessory proteins interact with BGP for cellular functions such as aiding in adhesion to the substrate. New information about the structures of the viral S glycoproteins and the murine BGP proteins will refine and improve the model. Identification of the receptors for HCV-OC43, RCV, BCV, and HEV will determine whether this model is also applicable to these related coronaviruses.

Specificity and Affinity of Interaction of S with BGP Receptor

The biological diversity of MHV strains depends in large part on differences in the amino acid sequences and, possibly, the conformation and

Figure 8 Model of MHV-receptor interactions. The key shows spike glycoproteins of murine coronavirus strains MHV-A59 or MHV-JHM, and MHV-3, and CEA-related glycoproteins (CGMs) of BALB/c mice (MHVR), SJL/J mice (CGM2), rats (rat BGP), and hamsters (BHK). Cells that naturally express low levels of CGMs (*left*) are susceptible to virus infection if there is effective binding between the virus spikes and receptors. BALB cells are infected by virions of all 3 virus strains, but SJL cells are susceptible only to MHV-3. Rat and hamster cells are resistant to infection. Expression of recombinant MHVR or mmCGM2 at higher levels makes hamster cells susceptible to infection with all 3 virus strains, but rat BGP serves as a receptor only for MHV-3 (*right*, top three figures). Thus, virus strains differ in their ability to use different CGMs as receptors. Lower right panel shows that BHK cells, which are resistant to infection with MHV virions, can be infected by cocultivation with mouse cells infected with MHV-JHM. The hamster BGP may be a relatively poor receptor but may function if there is a large excess of virus spike glycoprotein.

stability of the S glycoproteins of different virus strains. These varied S glycoproteins interact with the rodent BGP receptors in the amino-terminal S1 domain, which is the most variable part of the receptor glycoprotein. A receptor-binding region was localized to the first 330 amino acids of the S1 glycoprotein of MHV (Kubo et al. 1994). Although in Table 2 and Figures 4 and 8 receptor activity is shown as either present or absent, certain BGP splice variants may function more efficiently as receptors than others with the same amino-terminal domain.

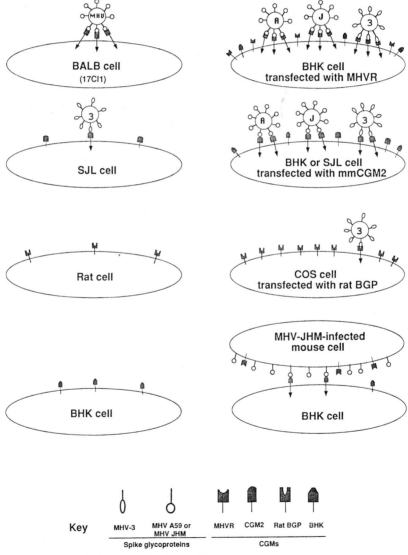

Figure 8 (See facing page for legend.)

Both within the animal and in cell culture, there may be strong selection upon viruses in favor of mutant S glycoproteins that provide optimal interaction with the locally available BGP receptor(s). The high mutation frequency of coronaviruses, together with selection of mutants by variant receptors, may account in part for the wide diversity of MHV S glycoproteins and, accordingly, of virus strains with different biological properties.

The binding specificity of the viral glycoprotein for a BGP isoform is a critical factor in receptor function. This may vary considerably with different virus strains. The S glycoproteins of MHV-A59, MHV-JHM, and MHV-3 can all utilize MHVR(4d) and MHVR(2d) as receptors on mouse tissue culture cells such as the 17 Cl 1 line of spontaneously transformed BALB/c-3T3 cells. Only MHV-3 can infect a small fraction of low-passage SJL/J embryo cells that express mmCGM2 isoforms (C. Cardellichio, in prep.). The model (Fig. 8) predicts that the S glycoprotein of MHV-A59 "fits" the virus binding determinant on the amino-terminal domain of the MHVR receptor very well, but does not fit the mmCGM2 or rat BGP glycoproteins well enough to bind virions and lead to infection. MHV-3 may have a wider host range because it can bind to BGPs of the SJL/J mouse and the rat, even though this binding may be weak and may lead to a low level of infection. The BGP of a species unrelated to mice, such as humans or hamsters, does not fit the S glycoproteins of any MHV strains well enough to lead to infection. In this model, "fitting" represents both hypothetical conformational determinants that would limit access of S to the binding sites on MHVR and the strength of the affinity between the S glycoprotein and receptor. When it becomes available, information about the binding affinities of viral S glycoproteins and BGP isoforms will distinguish between these two important factors.

The surface density of the receptor glycoprotein appears to be another important determinant of cellular susceptibility to MHV infection. In fibroblast cell lines, the level of BGP expression is much lower than that seen in tissues such as intestine, liver, or kidney (Williams et al. 1991). The level of protein expressed in cell lines transfected with BGP cDNA is intermediate between that of normal cell lines and high-expression tissues. Although SJL/J macrophages and embryo fibroblasts are highly resistant to infection with MHV-A59, if additional mmCGM2 is expressed from transfected cDNA, the fibroblasts become susceptible (Dveksler et al. 1993b). This shows that the surface density of the receptor is an important determinant of susceptibility. The importance of receptor density is more readily demonstrable with a relatively poor receptor, such as mmCGM2 that fails to bind virus in VOPBAs, than with a stronger receptor such as MHVR that shows strong binding in VOPBAs.

The surface density of the viral S glycoprotein also affects cellular susceptibility to virus. Table 2 shows that although BHK cells cannot be infected by MHV-A59, MHV-JHM, or MHV-3 virions, they can be infected by cocultivation with MHV-JHM-infected mouse cells (Gallagher et al. 1992). The model suggests that the BHK homolog of BGP binds so poorly to the S glycoprotein of MHV-JHM that virus attachment is only transient, and the virions elute before they can recruit enough BGPs to permit membrane fusion. In contrast to the relatively small number of S glycoproteins on a virion, an infected murine cell presents to the BGP glycoproteins of the BHK cell a large surface covered with adsorbed virions and S glycoprotein in the plasma membrane. Even if membrane fusion is a very unlikely event, in such a local excess of even a weakly binding S protein, fusion may occasionally result. When antibody to the BHK homolog of MHVR becomes available, or when the recombinant BHK homolog can be expressed at high levels, this hypothesis can be tested.

Changes in S Protein

The fusion glycoproteins of influenza virus and other enveloped viruses undergo a conformational change associated with membrane fusion, subsequent to receptor binding (White 1990). Since coronavirus S glycoproteins undergo a conformational change and/or loss of the S1 peptide after urea or pH 8, 37°C, it is possible that attachment to the receptor also triggers this conformational change. The loss of the S1 protein causes virions to become sticky and hydrophobic, as seen with other membrane fusion glycoproteins after activation by altered pH. Different MHV strains may vary in their susceptibility to the conformational change in S glycoproteins, which could affect the specific infectivity of the virus and its efficiency of penetration. For other virus groups such as reovirus and rhinovirus, the rates of disassembly of virions and penetration are closely correlated and vary between strains. Intermediate rates provide optimal survival of infectivity in the environment, coupled with efficient uptake once receptor binding has occurred. More stable viruses uncoat inefficiently, and so have a lower particle-to-pfu ratio, whereas more labile viruses may irreversibly lose the ability to bind to receptors and penetrate into the cell. To explore this hypothesis, analysis of the interactions of S glycoproteins from different MHV strains with various receptor glycoproteins is now feasible.

Viral S glycoproteins that have delayed or reduced membrane fusion activity are commonly associated with persistent infection. Such mutants have a selective advantage because they are much less likely to cause membrane damage leading to cell death than wild-type virus. The variable expression and efficiency of MHV receptors could aid in selection of such attenuated mutants in several ways. In an infected culture or tissue, cells that survive may be those that express the least amount of receptor, or those that express a receptor(s) which provides a relatively inefficient portal of virus entry. When virus infects these cells, synthesis of new viral glycoprotein and virions would be less likely to interact efficiently with receptors in the Golgi or on the plasma membrane and, therefore, less likely to cause fusion and more likely to favor persistent infection. Transfected cell lines that express different murine BGP isoforms are now available for direct studies of selection of virus variants to explore the hypothesis that attenuated mutants may be selected by inefficient receptors.

When virus is inoculated in high multiplicity or in the form of virus-infected cells, some cells that only express inefficient receptors may become infected. Virus infection could spread locally, albeit perhaps inefficiently, and in vivo development of an immune response could arrest replication before disease occurs. This may be what happens when MHV infects rats, whose BGPs are suboptimal receptors. Rarely during such an infection, a mutant S glycoprotein may arise that is better adapted to the receptors expressed by the new host. Such a mutant might then spread within the animal, possibly causing disease, and might have acquired the ability to spread to other members of the same species.

Subsequent Host-dependent Steps in Virus Penetration

Following receptor binding, additional steps are required for penetration and uncoating of virus. For some virus/cell combinations, these events may be the rate-limiting factor in infection. It is important to distinguish between secondary events that involve components of the receptor and subsequent ones that deal with virus replication, such as host-dependent transcription or replication factors. As yet unidentified postbinding host factors play a critical role in the restriction of MHV-JHM replication observed in many murine cell types (Yokomori et al. 1993). Evidence that these host-dependent restriction events are associated with receptors is based on the replication phenotypes of two recombinants that differ in the S glycoprotein. Further study of the early events in replication of these and other MHV strains may identify additional host factors that aid in virus penetration. Examples of receptor-associated secondary steps might include lateral clustering or homophilic aggregation of receptors in the membrane under a bound virion to facilitate penetration, heterophilic interaction of receptor with other proteins in the membrane, or conformational changes of the receptor associated with membrane fusion.

Little is known about whether the BGP proteins undergo conformational changes in association with their virus-receptor or cellular functions. Other immunoglobulin-like proteins do show conformational changes upon binding to ligands, which may induce secondary interactions at other sites on the protein. Since BGP is postulated to be a transporter for taurocholate and bile acids (Sippel et al. 1993), like other transporters, it may have several alternative conformations associated with the membrane. Aggregation of BGP proteins with homologous or heterologous proteins in the membrane could affect their affinity or availability for binding of S glycoprotein.

Significance of Interactions of HE to 9-O-Acetylated Neuraminic Acid

For coronaviruses that have S glycoproteins which utilize BGP receptors relatively inefficiently, either because of weak binding or inefficient secondary steps associated with penetration, expression of the HE glycoprotein could provide a considerable biological advantage. As postulated for the initial binding of the HSV glycoprotein to heparan sulfate (Shieh et al. 1992), binding of coronavirus HE to 9-*O*-acetylated neuraminic acid may hold the virus on the membrane, which then facilitates the interaction of S with its receptor. For viruses with relatively weak S-receptor interactions, HE could be essential, whereas for viruses with more efficient S-receptor interactions, HE could be nonessential. Thus, whether HE confers a selective advantage on a coronavirus would depend on which host receptors are available in the cells or tissues and how efficiently the viral S glycoprotein can utilize those receptors. This might explain why BCV replication is strongly inhibited by removal of neuraminic acid residues from cells (Vlasak et al. 1988b) and why HE-expressing variants of the Wurzburg strain of MHV-JHM appear to have a selective advantage over non-HE-expressing virus during replication in the rat brain, although both types of viruses can replicate in cell culture (Taguchi et al. 1985).

The esterase activity of HE may also be a determinant of coronavirus spread. If cells express the hemagglutinin without any esterase activity, then released virions might remain bound to carbohydrate moieties in the plasma membrane of the cell that produced them, rather than spreading to other cells. When esterase is expressed in an infected cell, the target *N*-acetyl neuraminic acid residues may be removed from cellular macromolecules as they transit the Golgi apparatus. Because cell-surface molecules stripped of this receptor-binding moiety would be less available, HE-bearing virions could spread to adjacent cells.

Biological Significance of Diversity in Virus/Receptor Interactions

The extensive variability in the sequences of S glycoproteins of different MHV strains affects their ability to utilize the various rodent BGP isoforms as receptors. The capacity of using HE as an accessory attachment protein to facilitate weak S/BGP interactions may extend the host range of HE-expressing viruses. Each preparation of MHV contains variants in the S glycoprotein that may affect receptor binding and utilization, as well as variants in the level of HE expressed. Replication of certain variants may be facilitated under conditions in which only a relatively inefficient receptor is available, whereas replication in a particular cell type or cell line tends to select virus populations optimized for interaction with the available receptor(s). Adaptation of enterotropic MHV strains to cell culture has been difficult to achieve. This may reflect differences between receptors utilized in the gut and those available in murine cell lines. Analysis of the amino acid sequences, structure, and receptor-binding specificities of S glycoproteins may suggest improved ways to isolate fastidious MHV virus strains from clinical specimens.

Because the expression of various BGP isoforms can be separately regulated in age-dependent and tissue-dependent fashion, the variability among MHV S glycoproteins could affect the tissue tropism, age, and mouse strain susceptibility to infection with different virus strains. It has long been recognized that the route of virus inoculation can affect the pathogenesis of disease. The tissue-dependent expression of BGP isoforms could present virus inoculated at different sites with BGPs that vary in their efficiency as virus receptors. The initial local replication of virus at different sites of entry could select variant viruses with different potentials for dissemination. As data on the expression of BGP isoforms in different tissues become available, and as the receptor functions of these different BGP glycoproteins are quantitated, the significance of these factors in the route of inoculation can be directly tested.

The above discussion about the variability of interactions of MHV with receptors indicates the importance of careful definition not only of the origins of the virus strains used for experiments, but also of the passage history of the virus. Apparently conflicting observations published by different laboratories working on MHV viruses derived from a common source may be resolved by careful analysis of the passage history and receptor specificities of the virus strains.

AMINOPEPTIDASE N RECEPTORS FOR CORONAVIRUSES
TGEV AND HCV-229E

HCV-229E is the prototype of a group of mammalian coronaviruses that is serologically distinct from the MHV/HCV-OC43 group. In humans, HCV-229E and HCV-OC43 infect the epithelial cells of the human respiratory tract and cause about 20% of colds (McIntosh 1990). Because human coronaviruses are very difficult to isolate in tissue culture, primary human fetal tracheal organ cultures were used to obtain coronaviruses from clinical specimens. Other coronaviruses in the HCV-229E serogroup cause enteric or respiratory diseases of cats (FIPV and FECV), dogs (CCV), pigs (TGEV and PRCV), and several other species (Moestl 1990). These viruses generally cause disease only in a single natural host species.

In solid-phase immunoassays, virions of CCV, FIPV, HCV-229E, and TGEV bind to the purified intestinal BBM of their natural host species, and not to BBM from rodents (Compton 1988). This absence of receptor activity on rodent membranes apparently explains why mice and rats are resistant to infection with this group of coronaviruses.

Surprisingly, in contrast to their failure to bind to rodent membranes, HCV-229E, TGEV, CCV, and FIPV all bind well to BBM from humans, pigs, dogs, and cats (Compton 1988). This suggests that a common virus-binding moiety is expressed on the membranes of each of these species. Since these coronaviruses do not encode HE glycoproteins, virus binding is probably mediated by the S glycoprotein. Although the viruses bind to receptor moieties common to pigs, humans, dogs, and cats, they generally do not infect cells of the foreign species as well as cells of their natural host species. Transfection of infectious viral genomic RNA into cells of a foreign species results in virus replication (R. Levis, in prep.). Virus inoculation does not establish a transmissible infection in these other species. Therefore, it is likely that the replication of these viruses in cells of these other species is blocked or inefficient at one or more of the steps that follow virus binding but precede RNA replication.

Several research groups are investigating the nature of the common coronavirus-binding moiety on the cells of humans, pigs, dogs, and cats. To determine whether HCV-229E recognized any human CEA-related glycoproteins as receptors, rodent cells or COS cells transfected with cDNAs encoding human CEA-related glycoproteins were challenged with HCV-229E. Expression of cloned human CEA-related glycoproteins on membranes of these cells does not make them susceptible to infection with HCV-229E (Yeager et al. 1992). In addition, antibodies to human CEA-related glycoproteins fail to protect human cell lines from infection with HCV-229E. Therefore, CEA-related glycoproteins were not promising candidates for HCV-229E receptors.

The strategy that led to the identification of the first MHV receptor was used to identify receptors for HCV-229E and TGEV. As shown in Table 1 and described in detail below, both HCV-229E and TGEV utilize aminopeptidase N (APN) as their cellular receptor (Delmas et al. 1992; Yeager et al. 1992). APN, also known as CD13, is expressed on membranes of granulocytes, on intestinal brush border, and at synaptic junctions (Look et al. 1989). APN is a metalloprotease that cleaves the amino-terminal amino acid from small peptides and plays an important role in the digestion of peptides in the gut, at synapses, and on myeloid cells (Look et al. 1989). Human APN (hAPN) is a 150-kD glycoprotein. Its cDNA has been cloned, sequenced, and expressed in nonhuman cells (Look et al. 1986). A short amino-terminal cytoplasmic domain is followed by a transmembrane domain and a large extracellular domain consisting of a stalk and a globular region that contains the catalytic site of the enzyme. At the active site of APN is a consensus amino acid sequence that is the binding site for a zinc ion (Ashmun et al. 1992). Enzyme activity is inhibited by chelation of the zinc ion, by small competitive inhibitors that bind to the catalytic site, or by several of the many monoclonal antibodies directed against APN/CD13. APN is the first protease recognized as a virus receptor.

TGEV Receptor

Monoclonal antibodies derived from mice immunized with membranes of porcine cells were screened for the ability to protect the ST line of porcine cells from infection with TGEV (Delmas et al. 1992). Several anti-cell monoclonal antibodies that block TGEV infection precipitate a 150-kD membrane glycoprotein from porcine cells. This purified protein binds the virus. Amino-terminal amino acid sequencing identified the protein as APN. When recombinant pig APN (pAPN) is expressed in cells that are normally resistant to infection, the cells become susceptible to infection and produce infectious virus (Delmas et al. 1992). Thus, for TGEV, as well as for MHV, expression of a functional virus receptor can make resistant cells susceptible to virus infection, and the species-specificity of virus infection is determined, at least in part, at the level of virus receptor specificity. A short amino acid sequence on pAPN was found to be required for TGEV receptor function by using recombinant chimeric pAPN and hAPN glycoproteins (Delmas et al. 1994).

HCV-229E Receptor

Solid-phase binding assays show that HCV-229E binds to membranes from human BBM, human respiratory epithelium, and several human cell lines, including the WI38 and HL60 cell lines (Yeager 1992). Monoclonal antibodies directed against human BBM or membranes from human cell lines were tested for the ability to block infection of WI38 cells with HCV-229E. MAb-RBS blocks infection of WI38 cells (Fig. 9) and other human cell lines and immunoprecipitates a 150-kD glycoprotein from human intestinal brush border membranes (Yeager et al. 1992). Solid-phase immunoassays and fluorescence-activated cell sorting (FACS) show that MAb-RBS specifically recognizes the hAPN glycoprotein on mouse cells transfected with a cDNA clone encoding hAPN derived from granulocytes. Furthermore, expression of hAPN makes mouse cells susceptible to infection with HCV-229E (Fig. 9). These experiments show that, as for MHV and TGEV, one host factor that determines susceptibility to HCV-229E infection is the availability of a functional virus receptor on the cell membrane.

The binding sites on hAPN for MAb-RBS and the S glycoprotein of HCV-229E were investigated using MAb-RBS to block binding to hAPN-transfected mouse cells and to inhibit the enzyme activity of hAPN (Yeager et al. 1992). The virus and antibody compete for binding sites on hAPN, suggesting that they recognize the same site or contiguous sites on hAPN. MAb-RBS inhibits the activity of hAPN, which suggests that the monoclonal antibody, and consequently the virus glycoprotein, may bind at or near the active site of the enzyme. To test this hypothesis, HCV-229E was inoculated onto mouse cells transfected with a mutant hAPN which has a 39-amino-acid deletion that includes the catalytic site of the enzyme (Ashmun et al. 1992). Although the mutant glycoprotein is expressed on the plasma membrane as demonstrated by FACS, the cells are not susceptible to infection (Fig. 9). Therefore, either the virus binds near the active site of the enzyme, or deletion of the 39-amino-acid segment from hAPN causes a conformational change that obscures the virus-binding site (Yeager et al. 1992). In the presence of actinonin and bestatin, small inhibitors of hAPN activity, HCV-229E binding and receptor activity are unimpaired (Yeager et al. 1992). Numerous monoclonal antibodies directed against hAPN/CD13 were tested for inhibition of APN activity, binding to the deletion mutant of hAPN, or blocking of HCV-229E infection of mouse cells transformed with hAPN. Some monoclonal antibodies that bind to the mutant lacking the active site of the enzyme block HCV-229E infection of hAPN-transfected mouse cells. These experiments and the observation that the site on pAPN required for TGEV receptor activity is distinct

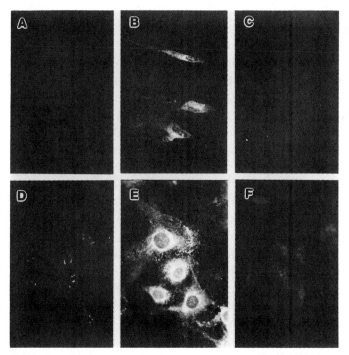

Figure 9 HCV-229E infection of human cells and hAPN-transfected mouse cells. HCV-229E inoculation of the WI38 line of human diploid lung fibroblasts induced the production of viral antigens in the cytoplasm (*B*). Treatment with anti-hAPN MAb-RBS prevented virus infection of WI38 cells (*C*). Mouse cells are resistant to HCV-229E infection (*D*) unless transfected with cDNA encoding hAPN (*E*). Deletion of a segment of 39 amino acids that includes the zinc-binding site and the catalytic site yields a mutant hAPN protein that cannot serve as a receptor for HCV-229E (*F*). (Reprinted, with permission, from Yeager et al. 1992.)

from the enzymatic site (Delmas et al. 1994) suggest that the viral glycoprotein does not bind precisely at the catalytic site of APN and show that the protease activity of APN is not required for its virus receptor activity.

RECEPTORS IN CORONAVIRUS EVOLUTION, DIAGNOSIS, AND PREVENTION

The MHV and HCV-229E serogroups of coronaviruses have evolved to utilize different types of cell membrane glycoproteins as receptors. The virus-binding determinants of the BGP and APN receptors are being mapped in several laboratories. However, at present there is no indication of homology between the virus-binding sites on these two very different membrane proteins. It appears likely that the two serogroups diverged when an ancestral coronavirus developed a mutated S glycoprotein that fortuitously allowed it to bind to an unrelated receptor glycoprotein. Selection would favor the emergence of better adapted viruses that could bind and utilize the new receptor more effectively. Analysis of chimeras of the S glycoproteins of MHV and HCV-229E may indicate the site(s) at which receptors bind. If a single site on S is involved in binding to both types of receptors, then the mutant that gained a new binding specificity may have simultaneously lost the original one. If APN and BGP recognize different sites on the large S1 glycoproteins, then possibly viruses with dual receptor specificities could represent a transitional form between serogroups.

The availability of cell lines that express cloned receptors at high surface density may facilitate the isolation of coronaviruses from infected humans and animals. This is of particular importance in the human coronaviruses, for which only a handful of isolates can be propagated in the laboratory, and for enterotropic MHV strains that cause epizootic disease in mouse colonies but cannot be propagated in culture. Virus isolation using cells that overexpress a receptor may, however, select for mutants in the clinical specimen that do not represent the majority of viruses in the infected tissues. Availability of cloned receptor glycoproteins may make it possible to capture coronaviruses from clinical specimens even if host-dependent blocks subsequent to virus binding prevent their replication in cell culture. Thus, it may be possible to use receptor glycoproteins to trap coronaviruses or glycoproteins for diagnosis of infected tissues.

Prevention of infection is perhaps the greatest potential benefit of understanding virus/receptor interactions. The antireceptor antibody MAb-CC1 inhibits virus replication in vivo and has no deleterious effects on the host cells. Possibly smaller, nonimmunogenic peptides that mimic the binding specificity of MAb-CC1 could be synthesized and used to block virus binding. Peptides that block binding of HCV-229E to hAPN might be used as nose drops in combination with peptides that block the site on ICAM-1 that binds the major group of human rhinoviruses. Such receptor blockade therapy might prevent the spread of rhinovirus and coronavirus colds in families that have one infected person and might even shorten the duration of colds after symptoms have begun. Alternative approaches to receptor blockade for coronaviruses include soluble receptors as competitive inhibitors of virus binding to tissues or some inhibitors of APN activity.

For coronaviruses of veterinary importance, understanding receptor interactions may have implications for epidemiology. For the HCV-229E-related viruses, due to the cross-binding of viruses to APN proteins of some other species, infection across species boundaries may occur more commonly than previously believed. Mutation of S glycoproteins could allow a virus to utilize an APN receptor of a different species, and infection might spread within that species.

An exciting outcome of coronavirus receptor research would be the creation of genetically engineered animals that lack the virus-binding site on the coronavirus receptor. This would be a very desirable goal for coronaviruses such as MHV where enzootic infections interfere with research that requires mice, or such as TGEV where infection causes serious economic losses. Transgenic BALB/c mice that express mmCGM2, the SJL/J allele of murine BGP, in place of MHVR, the BALB/c allele, would have much higher levels of resistance to MHV infection than the highly susceptible BALB/c mice. Because the functions of the BGP glycoproteins during development and in tissues are still being elucidated, it is not yet possible to predict the consequences to the biology of the mouse of the expression of mmCGM2 in place of MHVR. If cell-cell communication in the immune response and other cellular interactions were altered in the transgenic mice, they might not be suitable for research on these topics. It is not clear whether knock-out mice lacking BGP expression completely would survive embryonic development. Further understanding of the gene organization and control of murine CEA-related glycoproteins will facilitate work on the development of MHV-resistant transgenic mouse strains.

ACKNOWLEDGMENTS

The authors are grateful to Robin Levis, Mark de Souza, Sara Gagneten, and Franziska Grieder for review of the manuscript and to Susan Compton, Richard K. Williams, David Wessner, Nicole Beauchemin, Jin-Hua Lu, Charles Scanga, and Christine Cardellichio for helpful discussions. Some of the research discussed was supported by U.S. Public Health Service grants AI-25231 and AI-26075. The opinions expressed herein are those of the authors and do not reflect those of the Uniformed Services University of the Health Sciences or the Department of Defense.

REFERENCES

Abraham, S., T.E. Kienzle, W. Lapps, and D.A. Brian. 1990. Deduced sequence of the bovine coronavirus spike protein and identification of the internal proteolytic cleavage site. *Virology* **176:** 296.

Ashmun, R.A., L.H. Shapiro, and A.T. Look. 1992. Deletion of the zinc-binding motif of CD13/aminopeptidase N molecules results in loss of epitopes that mediate binding of inhibitory antibodies *Blood* **79:** 3344

Bang, F.B. and A. Warwick. 1960. Mouse macrophages as host cells for the mouse hepatitis virus and the genetic basis of their susceptibility. *Proc. Natl. Acad. Sci.* **46:** 1065.

Banner, L.R., J.G. Keck, and M.M. Lai. 1990. A clustering of RNA recombination sites adjacent to a hypervariable region of the peplomer gene of murine coronavirus. *Virology* **175:** 548.

Barnett, T.R., A. Kretschmer, D.A. Austen, S.J. Goebel, J.T. Hart, J.J. Elting, and M.E. Kamarck. 1989. Carcinoembryonic antigens: Alternative splicing accounts for the multiple mRNAs that code for novel members of the carcinoembryonic antigen family. *J. Cell Biol.* **108:** 267.

Barthold, S.W. and A.L. Smith. 1987. Response of genetically susceptible and resistant mice to intranasal inoculation with mouse hepatitis virus JHM. *Virus Res.* **7:** 225.

———. 1992. Viremic dissemination of mouse hepatitis virus-JHM following intranasal inoculation of mice. *Arch. Virol.* **122:** 35.

Barthold, S.W., M.S. de Souza, and A.L. Smith. 1990. Susceptibility of laboratory mice to intranasal and contact infection with coronaviruses of other species. *Lab. Anim. Sci.* **40:** 481.

Beauchemin, N., C. Turbide, D. Afar, J. Bell, M. Raymond, C.P. Stanners, and A. Fuks. 1989a. A mouse analogue of the human carcinoembryonic antigen. *Cancer Res.* **49:** 2017.

Beauchemin, N., C. Turbide, J.Q. Huang, S. Benchimol, S. Jothy, K. Shirota, A. Fuks, and C.P. Stanners. 1989b. Studies on the function of carcinoembryonic antigen. In *The carcinoembryonic antigen gene family* (ed. A. Yachi and J.E. Shively), p. 49. Elsevier Science, New York.

Benchimol, S., A. Fuks, S. Jothy, N. Beauchemin, K. Shirota, and C.P. Stanners. 1989. Carcinoembryonic antigen, a human tumor marker, functions as an intercellular adhesion molecule. *Cell* **57:** 327.

Blikstad, I., T. Wikström, M. Aurivillius, and B. Obrink. 1992. C-CAM (cell-CAM 105) is a calmodulin binding protein. *FEBS Lett.* **302:** 26.

Boyle, J.F., D.G. Weismiller, and K.V. Holmes. 1987. Genetic resistance to mouse hepatitis virus correlates with absence of virus-binding activity on target tissues. *J. Virol.* **61:** 185.

Cavanagh, D. and P.J. Davis. 1986. Coronavirus IBV: Removal of spike glycopolypeptide S1 by urea abolishes infectivity and haemagglutination but not attachment to cells. *J. Gen. Virol.* **67:** 1443.

Cavanagh, D., P.J. Davis, and A.P. Mockett. 1988. Amino acids within hypervariable region 1 of avian coronavirus IBV (Massachusetts serotype) spike glycoprotein are associated with neutralization epitopes. *Virus Res.* **11:** 141.

Cavanagh, D., P.J. Davis, J.H. Darbyshire, and R.W. Peters. 1986. Coronavirus IBV: Virus retaining spike glycopolypeptide S2 but not S1 is unable to induce virus-neutralizing or haemagglutination-inhibiting antibody, or induce chicken tracheal protection. *J. Gen. Virol.* **67:** 1435.

Collins, A.R. 1993. HLA class I antigen serves as a receptor for human coronavirus OC43. *Immunol. Invest.* **22:** 95.

Collins, A.R., L.A. Tunison, and R.L. Knobler. 1983. Mouse hepatitis virus type 4 infection of primary glial cultures from genetically susceptible and resistant mice. *Infect. Immun.* **40:** 1192.

Compton, S.R. 1988. *Coronavirus attachment and replication.* The Uniformed Services University of the Health Sciences, Bethesda, Maryland.

Culic, O., Q.H. Huang, D. Flanagan, D. Hixson, and S.H. Lin. 1992. Molecular cloning and expression of a new rat liver cell-CAM105 isoform. Differential phosphorylation of isoforms. *Biochem. J.* **285:** 47.

Daniel, C., R. Anderson, M.J. Buchmeier, J.O. Fleming, W.J. Spaan, H. Wege, and P.J. Talbot. 1993. Identification of an immunodominant linear neutralization domain on the S2 portion of the murine coronavirus spike glycoprotein and evidence that it forms part of complex tridimensional structure. *J. Virol.* **67:** 1185.

de Groot, R.J., W. Luytjes, M.C. Horzinek, B.A.M. van der Zeijst, W.J. Spaan, and J.A. Lenstra. 1987. Evidence for a coiled-coil structure in the spike proteins of coronaviruses. *J. Mol. Biol.* **196:** 963.

de Groot, R.J., R.W. Van Leen, M.J. Dalderup, H. Vennema, M.C. Horzinek, and W.J. Spaan. 1989. Stably expressed FIPV peplomer protein induces cell fusion and elicits neutralizing antibodies in mice. *Virology* **171:** 493.

Delmas, B. and H. Laude. 1990. Assembly of coronavirus spike protein into trimers and its role in epitope expression. *J. Virol.* **64:** 5367.

Delmas, B., J. Gelfi, E. Kut, H. Sjöström, O. Noren, and H. Laude. 1994. Determinants essential for the transmissible gastroenteritis virus-receptor interaction reside within a domain of aminopeptidase N that is distinct from the enzymatic site. *J. Virol.* **68:** 5216.

Delmas, B., J. Gelfi, R. L'Haridon, L.K. Vogel, H. Sjöström, O. Norén, and H. Laude. 1992. Aminopeptidase N is a major receptor for the entero-pathogenic coronavirus TGEV. *Nature* **357:** 417.

Dveksler, G.S., M.N. Pensiero, C.B. Cardellichio, R.K. Williams, G.S. Jiang, K.V. Holmes, and C.W. Dieffenbach. 1991. Cloning of the mouse hepatitis virus (MHV) receptor: Expression in human and hamster cell lines confers susceptibility to MHV. *J. Virol.* **65:** 6881.

Dveksler, G.S., M.N. Pensiero, C.W. Dieffenbach, C.B. Cardellichio, A.A. Basile, P.E. Elia, and K.V. Holmes. 1993a. Mouse hepatitis virus strain A59 and blocking antireceptor monoclonal antibody bind to the N-terminal domain of cellular receptor. *Proc. Natl. Acad. Sci.* **90:** 1716.

Dveksler, G.S., C.W. Dieffenbach, C.B. Cardellichio, K. McCuaig, M.N. Pensiero, G.S. Jiang, N. Beauchemin, and K.V. Holmes. 1993b. Several members of the mouse carcinoembryonic antigen-related glycoprotein family are functional receptors for the coronavirus mouse hepatitis virus-A59. *J. Virol.* **67:** 1.

Frana, M.F., J.N. Behnke, L.S. Sturman, and K.V. Holmes. 1985. Proteolytic cleavage of the E2 glycoprotein of murine coronavirus: Host-dependent differences in proteolytic cleavage and cell fusion. *J. Virol.* **56:** 912.

Gallagher, T.M., M.J. Buchmeier, and S. Perlman. 1992. Cell receptor-independent infection by a neurotropic murine coronavirus. *Virology* **191:** 517.

Gallagher, T.M., C. Escarmis, and M.J. Buchmeier. 1991. Alteration of the pH dependence of coronavirus-induced cell fusion: Effect of mutations in the spike glycoprotein. *J. Virol.* **65:** 1916.

Gallagher, T.M., S.E. Parker, and M.J. Buchmeier. 1990. Neutralization-resistant variants of a neurotropic coronavirus are generated by deletions within the amino-terminal half of the spike glycoprotein. *J. Virol.* **64:** 731.

Gombold, J.L., S.T. Hingley, and S.R. Weiss. 1993. Fusion-defective mutants of mouse hepatitis virus A59 contain a mutation in the spike protein cleavage signal. *J. Virol.* **67:** 4504.

Hammarstrom, S., W.N. Khan, S. Teglund, M.-L. Hammarstrom, T. Ramos, V. Baranov,

M.M.-W. Yeung, and L. Frangsmyr. 1993. The carcinoembryonic antigen family. In *Structure of antigens* (ed. M.H.V. Van Regenmortel), p. 341. CRC Press, Boca Raton, Florida.

Herrler, G., S. Szepanski, and B. Schultze. 1991. 9-O-acetylated sialic acid, a receptor determinant for influenza C virus and coronaviruses. *Behring Inst. Mitt.* **68:** 177.

Hogue, B.G., B. King, and D.A. Brian. 1984. Antigenic relationships among proteins of bovine coronavirus, human respiratory coronavirus OC43, and mouse hepatitis coronavirus A59. *J. Virol.* **51:** 384.

Holmes, K.V. 1989. Replication of coronaviruses. In *Virology* (ed. B.N. Fields), vol. 2, p. 841. Raven Press, New York.

Huang, J.Q., C. Turbide, E. Daniels, S. Jothy, and N. Beauchemin. 1990. Spatiotemporal expression of murine carcinoembryonic antigen (CEA) gene family members during mouse embryogenesis. *Development* **110:** 573.

Jacoby, R.O. 1986. Rat coronavirus. In *Viral, and mycoplasmal infections of rodents* (ed. P.N. Bhatt, et al.), p. 625. Academic Press, New York.

Jameson, B.A., P.E. Rao, L.I. Kong, B.H. Hahn, G.M. Shaw, L.E. Hood, and S.B. Kent. 1988. Location and chemical synthesis of a binding site for HIV-1 on the CD4 protein, *Science* **240:** 1335.

King, B., B.J. Potts, and D.A. Brian. 1985. Bovine coronavirus hemagglutinin protein. *Virus. Res.* **2:** 53.

Knobler, R.L., M.V. Haspel, and M.B. Oldstone. 1981. Mouse hepatitis virus type 4 (JHM strain) induced fatal central nervous system disease. I. Genetic control and murine neuron as the susceptible site of disease. *J. Exp. Med.* **153:** 832.

Knobler, R.L., D.S. Linthicum, and M. Cohn. 1985. Host genetic regulation of acute MHV-4 viral encephalomyelitis and acute experimental autoimmune encephalomyelitis in (BALB/cKe x SJL/J) recombinant-inbred mice. *J. Neuroimmunol.* **8:** 15.

Knobler, R.L., L.A. Tunison, and M.B. Oldstone. 1984. Host genetic control of mouse hepatitis virus type 4 (JHM strain) replication. I. Restriction of virus amplification and spread in macrophages from resistant mice. *J. Gen. Virol.* **65:** 1543.

Kodelja, V., K. Lucas, S. Barnert, S. von Kleist, J.A. Thompson, and W. Zimmermann. 1989. Identification of a carcinoembryonic antigen gene family in the rat. Analysis of the N-terminal domains reveals immunoglobulin-like, hypervariable regions. *J. Biol. Chem.* **264:** 6906.

Kostka, G. 1989. Characterization and partial purification of a high-molecular-mass, calmodulin-binding, tyrosyl-phosphorylated protein from lymphocyte plasma membranes. *Exp. Cell Res.* **181:** 85.

Kubo, H., Y.K. Yamada, and F. Taguchi. 1994. Localization of neutralizing epitopes and the receptor binding site within the amino-terminal 330 amino acids of the murine coronavirus spike protein. *J. Virol.* **68:** 5403.

Künkel, F. and G. Herrler. 1993. Bovine coronavirus hemagglutinin protein. *Virus Res.* **2:** 53.

Lai, M.M. 1990. Coronavirus: Organization, replication and expression of genome. *Annu. Rev. Microbiol.* **44:** 303.

Laude, H., K. Van Reeth, and M. Pensaert. 1993. Porcine respiratory coronavirus: Molecular features and virus-host interactions. *Vet. Res.* **24:** 125.

Laude, H., D. Rasschaert, B. Delmas, M. Godet, J. Gelfi, and B. Charley. 1990. Molecular biology of transmissible gastroenteritis virus. *Vet. Microbiol.* **23:** 147.

Lin, S.H. 1989. Localization of the ecto-ATPase (ecto-nucleotidase) in the rat hepatocyte plasma membrane. Implications for the functions of the ecto-ATPase. *J. Biol. Chem.* **264:** 14403.

Lin, S.H. and G. Guidotti. 1989. Cloning and expression of a cDNA coding for a rat liver plasma membrane ecto-ATPase. The primary structure of the ecto-ATPase is similar to that of the human biliary glycoprotein I. *J. Biol. Chem.* **264:** 14408.

Lin, S.H., O. Culic, D. Flanagan, and D.C. Hixson. 1991. Immunochemical characterization of two isoforms of rat liver ecto-ATPase that show an immunological and structural identity with a glycoprotein cell-adhesion molecule with M_r 105,000. *Biochem. J.* **278:** 155.

Look, A.T., R.A. Ashmun, L.H. Shapiro, and S.C. Peiper. 1989. Human myeloid plasma membrane glycoprotein CD13 (gp150) is identical to aminopeptidase N. *J. Clin. Invest.* **83:** 1299.

Look, A.T., S.C. Peiper, M.B. Rebentisch, R.A. Ashmun, M.F. Roussel, R.S. Lemons, M.M. Le Beau, C.M. Rubin, and C.J. Sherr. 1986. Molecular cloning, expression, and chromosomal localization of the gene encoding a human myeloid membrane antigen (gp150). *J. Clin. Invest.* **78:** 914.

Luytjes, W., P.J. Bredenbeek, A.F. Noten, M.C. Horzinek, and W.J. Spaan. 1988. Sequence of mouse hepatitis virus A59 mRNA 2: Indications for RNA recombination between coronaviruses and influenza C virus. *Virology* **166:** 415.

Luytjes, W., L.S. Sturman, P.J. Bredenbeek, J. Charite, B.A.M. van der Zeijst, M.C. Horzinek, and W.J. Spaan. 1987, Primary structure of the glycoprotein E2 of coronavirus MHV-A59 and identification of the trypsin cleavage site. *Virology* **161:** 479.

Margolis, R.N., M.J. Schell, S.I. Taylor, and A.L. Hubbard. 1990. Hepatocyte plasma membrane ECTO-ATPase (pp120/HA4) is a substrate for tyrosine kinase activity of the insulin receptor. *Biochem. Biophys. Res. Commun.* **166:** 562.

McCuaig, K., C. Turbide, and N. Beauchemin. 1992. mmCGM1a: A mouse carcinoembryonic antigen gene family member, generated by alternative splicing, functions as an adhesion molecule. *Cell Growth Differ.* **3:** 165.

McCuaig, K., M. Rosenberg, P. Nedellec, C. Turbide, and N. Beauchemin. 1993. Expression of the Bgp gene and characterization of mouse colon biliary glycoprotein isoforms. *Gene* **127:** 173.

McIntosh, K. 1990. Coronaviruses. In *Virology* (ed. B.N. Fields), vol. 2, p.857. Raven Press, New York.

Moestl, K. 1990. Coronaviridae, pathogenetic and clinical aspects: An update. *Comp. Immun. Microbiol. Infect. Dis.* **13:** 169.

Mounir, S. and P.J. Talbot. 1993. Molecular characterization of the S protein gene of human coronavirus OC43. *J. Gen. Virol.* **74:** 1981.

Najjar, S.M., D. Accili, N. Philippe, J. Jernberg, R. Margolis, and S.I. Taylor. 1993. pp120/ecto-ATPase, an endogenous substrate of the insulin receptor tyrosine kinase, is expressed as two variably spliced isoforms. *J. Biol. Chem.* **268:** 1201.

Nedellec, P., G.S. Dveksler, E. Daniels, C. Turbide, B. Chow, A.A. Basile, and K.V. Holmes. 1994. Bgp2, a new member of the carcinoembryonic antigen-related gene family, encodes an alternative receptor for mouse hepatitis virus. *J. Virol.* **68:** 4525.

Obrink, B. 1991. C-CAM (cell-CAM 105)—A member of the growing immunoglobulin superfamily of cell adhesion proteins. *Bioessays* **13:** 227.

Odin, P., A. Tingstrom, and B. Obrink. 1986. Chemical characterization of cell-CAM 105, a cell-adhesion molecule isolated from rat liver membranes. *Biochem. J.* **236:** 559.

Oikawa, S., C. Inuzuka, M. Kuroki, F. Arakawa, Y. Matsuoka, G. Kosaki, and H. Nakazato. 1991. A specific heterotypic cell adhesion activity between members of carcinoembryonic antigen family, W272 and NCA, is mediated by N-domains. *J. Biol. Chem.* **266:** 7995.

Parker, S.E., T.M. Gallagher, and M.J. Buchmeier. 1989. Sequence analysis reveals extensive polymorphism and evidence of deletions within the E2 glycoprotein gene of several strains of murine hepatitis virus. *Virology* **173**: 664.

Pensiero, M.N., G.S. Dveksler, C.B. Cardellichio, G.S. Jiang, P.E. Elia, C.W. Dieffenbach, and K.V. Holmes. 1992. Binding of the coronavirus mouse hepatitis virus A59 to its receptor expressed from a recombinant vaccinia virus depends on posttranslational processing of the receptor glycoprotein. *J. Virol.* **66**: 4028.

Raabe, T., B. Schelle-Prinz, and S.G. Siddell. 1990. Nucleotide sequence of the gene encoding the spike glycoprotein of human coronavirus HCV 229E. *J. Gen. Virol.* **71**: 1065.

Racaniello, V.R. 1990. Cell receptors for picornaviruses. *Curr. Top. Microbiol. Immunol.* **161**: 1.

Rasschaert, D. and H. Laude. 1987. The predicted primary structure of the peplomer protein E2 of the porcine coronavirus transmissible gastroenteritis virus. *J. Gen. Virol.* **68**: 1883.

Rasschaert, D., M. Duarte, and H. Laude. 1990. Porcine respiratory coronavirus differs from transmissible gastroenteritis virus by a few genomic deletions. *J. Gen. Virol.* **71**: 2599.

Robbins, J., P.F. Robbins, C.A. Kozak, and R. Callahan. 1991. The mouse biliary glycoprotein gene (Bgp): Partial nucleotide sequence, expression, and chromosomal assignment. *Genomics* **10**: 583.

Rottier, P.J. 1990. Background paper. Coronavirus M and HE: Two peculiar glycoproteins. *Adv. Exp. Med. Biol.* **276**: 91.

Sauter, S.L., S.M. Rutherfurd, C. Wagener, J.E. Shively, and S.A. Hefta. 1991. Binding of nonspecific cross-reacting antigen, a granulocyte membrane, to *Escherichia coli* expressing type 1 fimbriae. *Infect. Immun.* **59**: 2485.

Schmidt, I., M. Skinner, and S. Siddell. 1987. Nucleotide sequence of the gene encoding the surface projection glycoprotein of coronavirus MHV-JHM. *J. Gen. Virol.* **68**: 47.

Schultze, B. and G. Herrler. 1992. Bovine coronavirus uses N-acetyl-9-0-acetylneuraminic acid as a receptor determinant to initiate the infection of cultured cells. *J. Gen. Virol.* **73**: 901.

Schultze, B., H.J. Gross, R. Brossmer, and G. Herrler. 1991a. The S protein of bovine coronavirus is a hemagglutinin recognizing 9-O-acetylated sialic acid as a receptor determinant. *J. Virol.* **65**: 6232.

Schultze, B., K. Wahn, H.D. Klenk, and G. Herrler. 1991b. Isolated HE-protein from hemagglutinating encephalomyelitis virus and bovine coronavirus has receptor-destroying and receptor-binding activity. *Virology* **180**: 221.

Schultze, B., H.J. Gross, R. Brossmer, H.D. Klenk, and G. Herrler. 1990a. Hemagglutinating encephalomyelitis virus attaches to N-acetyl-9-O-acetylneuraminic acid-containing receptors on erythrocytes: Comparison with bovine coronavirus and influenza C virus. *Virus Res.* **16**: 185.

Schultze, B., H.J. Gross, H.D. Klenk, R. Brossmer, and G. Herrler. 1990b. Differential reactivity of bovine coronavirus (BCV) and influenza C virus with N-acetyl-9-O-acetylneuraminic acid (Neu5, 9Ac2)-containing receptors. *Adv. Exp. Med. Biol.* **276**: 115.

Schultze, B., G. Hess, R. Rott, H.D. Klenk, and G. Herrler. 1990c. Isolation and characterization of the acetylesterase of hemagglutinating encephalomyelitis virus (HEV). *Adv. Exp. Med. Biol.* **276**: 109.

Shieh, M.T., D. WuDunn, R.I. Montgomery, J.D. Esko, and P.G. Spear. 1992. Cell surface receptors for herpes simplex virus are heparan sulfate proteoglycans. *J. Cell Biol.* **116**: 1273.

Sippel, C.J., F.J. Suchy, M. Ananthanarayanan, and D.H. Perlmutter. 1993. The rat liver ecto-ATPase is also a canalicular bile acid transport protein. *J. Biol. Chem.* **268:** 2083.

Smith, A.L., C.B. Cardellichio, D.F. Winograd, M.S. deSouza, S.W. Barthold, and K.V. Holmes. 1991. Monoclonal antibody to the receptor for murine coronavirus MHV-A59 inhibits virus replication in vivo. *J. Infect. Dis.* **163:** 879.

Smith, M.S., R.E. Click, and P.G. Plagemann. 1984. Control of mouse hepatitis virus replication in macrophages by a recessive gene on chromosome 7. *J. Immunol.* **133:** 428.

Spaan, W., D. Cavanagh, and M.C. Horzinek. 1988. Coronaviruses: Structure and genome expression. *J. Gen. Virol.* **69:** 2939.

————. 1990. Coronaviruses. In *Immunochemistry of viruses.* II. *The basis for serodiagnosis and vaccines* (ed. M.H.V. van Regenmortel and A.R. Neurath), p. 359. Elsevier, Amsterdam.

Stohlman, S.A. and J.A. Frelinger. 1978. Resistance to fatal central nervous system disease by mouse hepatitis virus strain JHM. I. Genetic analysis. *Immunogenetics* **6:** 277.

Storz, J., R. Rott, and G. Kaluza. 1981. Enhancement of plaque formation and cell fusion of an enteropathogenic coronavirus by trypsin treatment. *Infect. Immun.* **31:** 1214.

Sturman, L.S. and K.V. Holmes. 1983. The molecular biology of coronaviruses. *Adv. Virus Res.* **28:** 35.

Sturman, L.S., C.S. Ricard, and K.V. Holmes. 1985. Proteolytic cleavage of the E2 glycoprotein of murine coronavirus: Activation of cell-fusing activity of virions by trypsin and separation of two different 90K cleavage fragments. *J. Virol.* **56:** 904.

————. 1990. Conformational change of the coronavirus peplomer glycoprotein at pH 8.0 and 37°C correlates with virus aggregation and virus-induced cell fusion. *J. Virol.* **64:** 3042.

Sugiyama, K., R. Ishikawa, and N. Fukuhara. 1986. Structural polypeptides of the murine coronavirus DVIM. *Arch. Virol.* **89:** 245.

Svalander, P.C., P. Odin, B.O. Nilsson, and B. Obrink. 1987. Trophectoderm surface expression of the cell adhesion molecule cell-CAM 105 on rat blastocysts. *Development* **100:** 653.

Taguchi, F., S.G. Siddell, H. Wege, and V. ter Meulen. 1985. Characterization of a variant virus selected in rat brains after infection by coronavirus mouse hepatitis virus JHM. *J. Virol.* **54:** 429.

Taguchi, F., S. Siddell, H. Wege, P. Massa, and V. ter Meulen. 1987. Characterization of JHMV variants isolated from rat brain and cultured neural cells after wild type JHMV infection. *Adv. Exp. Med. Biol.* **218:** 343.

Thompson, J.A., E.M. Mauch, F.S. Chen, Y. Hinoda, H. Schrewe, B. Berling, S. Barnert, S. von Kleist, J.E. Shively, and W. Zimmermann. 1989. Analysis of the size of the carcinoembryonic antigen (CEA) gene family: Isolation and sequencing of N-terminal domain exons. *Biochem. Biophys. Res. Commun.* **158:** 996.

Tingstrom, A., I. Blikstad, M. Aurivillius, and B. Obrink. 1990. C-CAM (cell-CAM 105) is an adhesive cell surface glycoprotein with homophilic binding properties. *J. Cell Sci.* **96:** 17.

Turbide, C., M. Rojas, C.P. Stanners, and N. Beauchemin. 1991. A mouse carcinoembryonic antigen gene family member is a calcium-dependent cell adhesion molecule. *J. Biol. Chem.* **266:** 309.

Vlasak, R., W. Luytjes, W. Spaan, and P. Palese. 1988a. Human and bovine coronaviruses recognize sialic acid-containing receptors similar to those of influenza C viruses. *Proc. Natl. Acad. Sci.* **85:** 4526.

Vlasak, R., W. Luytjes, J. Leider, W. Spaan, and P. Palese. 1988b. The E3 protein of bovine coronavirus is a receptor-destroying enzyme with acetylesterase activity. *J. Virol.* **62:** 4686.

Wege, H., S. Siddell, and V. ter Meulen. 1982. The biology and pathogenesis of coronaviruses. *Curr. Top. Microbiol. Immunol.* **99:** 165.

Weismiller, D.G., L.S. Sturman, M.J. Buchmeier, J.O. Fleming, and K.V. Holmes. 1990. Monoclonal antibodies to the peplomer glycoprotein of coronavirus mouse hepatitis virus identify two subunits and detect a conformational change in the subunit released under mild alkaline conditions. *J. Virol.* **64:** 3051.

White, J.M. 1990. Viral and cellular membrane fusion proteins. *Annu. Rev. Physiol.* **52:** 675.

White, J.M. and D.R. Littman. 1989. Viral receptors of the immunoglobulin superfamily. *Cell* **56:** 725.

Williams, A.F. and A.N. Barclay. 1988. The immunoglobulin superfamily-domains for cell surface recognition. *Annu. Rev. Immunol.* **6:** 381.

Williams, R.K., G.S. Jiang, and K.V. Holmes. 1991. Receptor for mouse hepatitis virus is a member of the carcinoembryonic antigen family of glycoproteins. *Proc. Natl. Acad. Sci.* **88:** 5533.

Williams, R.K., G.-S. Jiang, S.W. Snyder, M.F. Frana, and K.V. Holmes. 1990. Purification of the 110-kilodalton glycoprotein receptor for mouse hepatitis virus (MHV)-A59 from mouse liver and identification of a nonfunctional, homologous protein in MHV-resistant SJL/J mice. *J. Virol.* **64:** 3817.

Yeager, C. 1992. "Identification of APN as a cellular receptor for human coronavirus HCV-229E." Ph.D. thesis. Uniformed Services University, Bethesda, Maryland.

Yeager, C.L., R.A. Ashmun, R.K. Williams, C.B. Cardellichio, L.H. Shapiro, A.T. Look, and K.V. Holmes. 1992. Human aminopeptidase N is a receptor for human coronavirus 229E. *Nature* **357:** 420.

Yokomori, K. and M.M. Lai. 1992a. The receptor for mouse hepatitis virus in the resistant mouse strain SJL is functional: Implications for the requirement of a second factor for viral infection. *J. Virol.* **66:** 6931.

———. 1992b. Mouse hepatitis virus utilizes two carcinoembryonic antigens as alternative receptors. *J. Virol.* **66:** 6194.

Yokomori, K., L.R. Banner, and M.M. Lai. 1991. Heterogeneity of gene expression of the hemagglutinin-esterase (HE) protein of murine coronaviruses. *Virology* **183:** 647.

Yokomori, K., M. Asanaka, S.A. Stohlman, and M.M. Lai. 1993. A spike protein-dependent cellular factor other than the viral receptor is required for mouse hepatitis virus entry. *Virology* **196:** 45.

Yokomori, K., N. La Monica, S. Makino, C.K. Shieh, and M.M. Lai. 1989. Biosynthesis, structure, and biological activities of envelope protein gp65 of murine coronavirus. *Virology* **173:** 683.

Yoo, D.W., M.D. Parker, and L.A. Babiuk. 1991. The S2 subunit of the spike glycoprotein of bovine coronavirus mediates membrane fusion in insect cells. *Virology* **180:** 395.

Zhang, X.M., K.G. Kousoulas, and J. Storz. 1992. The hemagglutinin/esterase gene of human coronavirus strain OC43: Phylogenetic relationships to bovine and murine coronaviruses and influenza C virus. *Virology* **186:** 318.

22

Distribution of the Poliovirus Receptor in Human Tissue

Marion Freistadt
Louisiana State University Medical Center
Department of Microbiology, Immunology, and Parasitology
New Orleans, Louisiana 70112-1293

INTRODUCTION
General

The purpose of this chapter is to discuss the distribution of the poliovirus receptor (PVR) in human tissues with regard to its role in poliovirus (PV) pathogenesis; that is, in causing poliomyelitis. After the historical background of this problem is discussed, the identification of the PVR gene is summarized. A description of the present state of knowledge concerning the PVR protein(s) follows. A discussion of the current unresolved scientific issues closes the chapter. The PVR gene and its gene product(s) have turned out to be surprisingly complex; experimental results have often raised more questions than they answer. In the interest of precision, I use the abbreviation "PVR" when discussing issues relevant to the cloned reagent and the full phrase "PV receptor" when referring to the biological activity.

Viruses can bring about tissue destruction, and therefore disease, in various ways: cytolysis, immune damage, toxic products, and cell transformation (Dulbecco and Ginsberg 1988). It is thought that PV kills neurons by direct cellular killing (Bodian 1959). Therefore, pathogenesis by virulent strains of PV is the direct effect of a characteristic, restricted range of cytopathic viral replication. The well-accepted premise of current molecular studies of viruses is that there are both virus-encoded and host-encoded determinants of virulence and, thus, disease. For both virus-encoded and host-encoded determinants of virulence, these specific molecules can contribute to viral life cycles in two distinct ways: by mediating viral host range or by mediating tissue tropism. The term "host-range determinant" refers to a characteristic that affects the range of species that a virus can infect, whereas "tissue tropism determinant" indicates a characteristic that imparts tissue- or cell-type-specific replication within a susceptible species. Each step in a viral life cycle, from

Cellular Receptors for Animal Viruses
© 1994 Cold Spring Harbor Laboratory Press 0-87969-429-7/94 $5 + .00

entry to maturation, is influenced by different host molecules, and each of these molecules may affect each aspect of virulence: host range or tissue tropism.

Virus-encoded Determinants of Poliovirus Virulence

Although the topic of this paper is the role of a cell-surface molecule in mediating PV pathogenesis, a brief historical description of the study of virus-encoded determinants of PV pathogenesis precedes the main discussion. In early work on poliomyelitis victims and in experimental non-human primate studies, autopsy studies showed that PV replication is primarily restricted to the afflicted tissues: specific parts of the central nervous system (CNS)—motor cortex, cerebellum, brain stem, and spinal cord (Bodian 1959). The other areas in which PV was detected (gut, associated lymph) were, in general, consistent with the epidemiological evidence for the oral/fecal route of transmission. Experimental infections in primates confirmed the interpretation that PV replicates exclusively in tissue types that are relevant to the disease. Thus, there are tissue tropism determinants, contributed by both the virus and the host cell, that permit replication in susceptible tissues such as gut and CNS and preclude replication in other tissues such as liver and kidney.

It is the inability of the attenuated, Sabin vaccine strains to replicate in the CNS, while replicating in the gut, that is the basis of the protective immunity (Nomoto and Wimmer 1987; Racaniello 1988; Wimmer et al. 1993 and references therein). Thus, vaccine strains of PV differ from virulent strains in their range of tissue-specific replication; i.e., they lack tissue tropism determinants for neurovirulence. Although it was clear when the vaccine strains were developed that the differences between virulent and attenuated strains are complex (Sabin 1955), it was not until the application of molecular methods and the development of mouse model systems for PV that the mechanistic studies of these issues became feasible (Kitamura et al. 1981; Racaniello and Baltimore 1981). Work from many laboratories, involving the construction of recombinant molecular chimeras between virulent and attenuated strains and their subsequent testing in primates, has identified the virus-encoded molecular determinants of neurovirulence (Almond 1987; Nomoto and Wimmer 1987; Racaniello 1988 and references therein). Additionally, molecular recombinant PVs can be analyzed in two mouse model systems: one that uses intracerebral injection of PV(2) (La Monica et al. 1987; Ren et al. 1991) and another that utilizes transgenic mice expressing the human PVR (Ren et al. 1990; Koike et al. 1991b). Presumably, these determinants are similar or identical to the tissue-tropism determinants in a normal virulent PV infection. It is striking that for all three PV serotypes, strongly attenuating mutations are found in regions encoding viral capsid proteins. This suggests that the initial interactions between PV and host cell molecules are crucial in the determination of tissue-specific replication.

A clear example of a virus-encoded determinant of host range was also recently identified. The three serotypes of PV(1, 2, and 3) infect primates. PV(2), but not PV(1) and PV(3), can additionally infect mice, causing a paralysis similar to the human disease, poliomyelitis, although only via intracerebral injection. Thus, PV(2) has (minimally) one additional host-range determinant permitting replication in mice. (Mouse-adapted strains do not lose their ability to replicate in primate cells, suggesting that a single virus can recognize more than one receptor.) Through the use of molecular recombinant viruses, the virus-encoded determinant permitting PV(2) to replicate in mouse brains has been identified as residing in an eight-amino-acid segment in the BC loop of viral capsid protein VP1. This short segment can be molecularly transferred into PV(1), allowing the virus to infect mice (Martin et al. 1988; Murray et al. 1988). Since the cell-surface receptor is the primary trait restricting PV replication in murine cells (see below), this finding suggests that this eight-amino-acid segment interacts with the murine receptor.

Host-encoded Determinants of Poliovirus Virulence

In contrast, the study of host determinants of these processes has been more difficult. Both early work and recent molecular studies have amply demonstrated that host-encoded cell-surface receptors can have roles in mediating viral pathogenesis for many different viruses (Maddon et al. 1986; Moore et al. 1987). Experimental evidence for a "PV receptor substance" with which PV interacts appeared in the literature in 1959 (Holland and McLaren 1959; McLaren et al. 1959). The initial studies utilized a simple assay in which minces or homogenates from susceptible or nonsusceptible cultured cells were tested for their ability to bind PV. "Virus binding" or PV receptor activity was simply defined by assessing the ability of homogenates to reduce the titer of PV samples. PV receptor activity was found in homogenates from susceptible cells but not from nonsusceptible cells. Although the biochemical nature of the PV receptor remained unknown for many years, this striking demonstration of a biochemical entity mediating a biological phenomenon was a landmark event.

This work was then extended to the study of animal tissues (Holland 1961). Homogenates of susceptible and nonsusceptible tissues from primates (Holland 1961), as well as tissue homogenates from non-susceptible species (Kunin and Jordan 1961), were compared for their ability to inactivate PV. A reasonable correlation of PV tropism with PV receptor activity confirmed the idea that the PV receptor would be exclusively limited to susceptible cells in both tissue- and species-specific manners.

Not all studies supported the tissue-specific aspect of the dogma, however; one study found PV-absorbing activity in minces from heart, muscle, gut, brain, lung, liver, testis, and spleen of a rhesus monkey (Kunin and Jordan 1961). The differences between the studies may have been due to different experimental procedures; in particular, the purity of fractions being tested differed quite widely.

By testing for conditions that destroyed the PV-inactivation activity, the PV receptor was deduced to be proteinaceous (heat-labile [Kunin and Jordan 1961], papain- and trypsin-sensitive [Holland 1962; Holland and McLaren 1961]). It was further determined to be an integral membrane protein due to its lack of release by EDTA and solubilization by nonionic detergents (Crowell and Landau 1983). A more recent study (yet prior to the identification of PVR) showed an inhibition of PV binding to HeLa cell membranes by the sialic-acid-specific wheat germ lectin, suggesting that PV receptor activity is a glycoprotein (Tomassini et al. 1989). Other recent studies have confirmed (Kaplan et al. 1990) and characterized the glycosylation of PVR (Bernhardt et al. 1994). Further attempts to purify the "PV-inactivating activity" were unsuccessful; the activity was lost during experimental manipulation.

Another important event in the history of the identification of PVR, and its role in pathogenesis, came from viral RNA transfection studies of nonsusceptible cultured cells. In these experiments, it was found that nonsusceptible cells, such as mouse cells, can support a single round of viral replication following transfection of viral RNA (Holland et al. 1959a,b). This suggested that, at least for these cells, the resistance to PV was due solely to a block at the cell surface—a block that a putative PV receptor would overcome. Similar results were obtained for vertebrate cell culture lines from many species, suggesting that the PV receptor was the sole host-range block between vertebrate species.

The situation for tissue tropism is not as clear because, with only a few exceptions (Kaplan et al. 1989), the majority of cultured primate cell lines are susceptible to PV, regardless of tissue of origin. This observation was interpreted to mean that when primate cells are cultured, the expression of the PV receptor becomes unregulated.

The PV-binding studies, when considered with other experimental observations, led to the hypothesis that a cell-surface molecule that is specific for PV exists and, furthermore, is the primary mediator of both host-range and tissue-tropic restrictions to PV replication. Further attempts to purify the activity, solely on the basis of PV binding, have not been successful. Although a cloned reagent is now available (see below), the reason for the loss of activity has not been adequately explained. Several interpretations are possible. PV receptor activity may require a lipid bilayer, an additional protein cofactor, multimerization, or membrane fluidity to inactivate PV.

IDENTIFICATION OF THE PVR GENE

Further biochemical identification of the PV receptor required three innovations: the development of a monoclonal antibody (MAb) that specifically blocks PV replication by blocking PV entry, the development of a transfection assay for PV receptor function, and the recovery of susceptible cells using a rosetting assay with a blocking MAb. The work of several different laboratory groups, working independently as well as collaboratively, culminated in the identification of the PVR gene and its gene product.

Using intact HeLa cells as antigen, three groups (Minor et al. 1984; Nobis et al. 1985; Koike et al. 1990) screened mouse MAbs for their ability to protect HeLa cells from PV infection. The MAbs are not against PV antigens. This important development implicitly revealed (since it protected intact cells) that a single specific epitope or molecule (likely a receptor) that PV recognizes is on the cell surface of HeLa cells. This was the first step toward the identification of PVR. Although several independent hybridomas that produce PV-blocking MAbs have been reported in the literature, they likely corresponded to the same or very close epitopes. This is in contrast to anti-CD4 antibodies, whose binding sites cluster into several distinct regions on the CD4 molecule, each pertaining to different aspects of HIV uptake (Ryu et al. 1990; Wang et al. 1990). It is possible that in the future, other categories of blocking anti-PVR antibodies will be identified. Although the development of this antibody was an important breakthrough, disappointingly, none of the antibodies led directly to an understanding of the biochemical nature of the receptor. The antibodies were not useful biochemically; at the time, attempts to utilize them for immunoprecipitation, Western blotting, or immunoaffinity purification were not successful. More recently, anti-PVR blocking MAbs have been successfully utilized in biochemical studies (Koike et al. 1990; Bernhardt et al. 1994).

The second requirement for identification of the receptor was the development of a transfection assay. In these assays, human DNA is transfected into cells, in this case mouse L cells, that are initially resistant to PV. After the transfected DNA is permitted to be transcribed and protein is produced, the cells are challenged with PV. The supernatant is subsequently assayed for PV production in a standard plaque assay. If progeny virions are detected in the supernatant, a gene encoding a PV receptor was taken up by the resistant cells. Using this assay, it was demonstrated that a specific, single gene encoding a PV receptor is present in the human genome (Mendelsohn et al. 1986). If more than one gene product had been required for an active receptor, as is the case for some receptors, such as the IL-2 receptor, a simple transfection experiment likely would not have been successful.

The recovery of the gene itself was complicated by the fact that PV is a lytic virus, destroying the cells it infects. To overcome this difficulty, a third innovation was required: the use of one of the blocking MAbs (D171) in a rosetting assay to identify stably transfected cells expressing the receptor, in the absence of infection. In the rosetting assay, cell-surface expression of an antigen, in this case PVR, is visualized by the formation of characteristic clusters, or rosettes, of anti-mouse immunoglobulin antibody-conjugated red blood cells after prior incubation with D171. Rosetted colonies were singly recovered from culture plates and expanded; then a subculture was challenged with PV. A further complication was the identification of the human gene from the mouse background. This required the use of human Alu-containing probes to identify the human sequences. The combination of these two powerful applications, the blocking MAbs and the transfection followed by a rosetting assay, have resulted in the identification of the PVR gene (Mendelsohn et al. 1989).

The PVR gene is a novel member of the immunoglobulin superfamily (Williams and Barclay 1988), encoding three Ig-type ectodomains in the arrangement V-C-C, from the amino-terminal, membrane-distal end. There are nine sites for potential N-linked glycosylation. Two cDNAs, termed H20A and H20B, result from alternative splicing of primary transcripts from this single-copy gene, and both are active in the PV receptor function. Each has identical extracellular and transmembrane domains. The two cDNAs differ only at their 3′ ends, in the regions encoding the extreme carboxyl terminus of the cytoplasmic domains and 3′-untranslated regions. In the cytoplasmic tails, there are 15 amino acid residues in common, after which the sequence diverges, resulting in a 25-residue tail for H20B and a 50-residue tail for H20A. The molecular masses of the deduced polypeptide chains (in the absence of glycosylation) are approximately 43 kD and 45 kD, respectively. Two additional, alternatively spliced mRNAs from the gene, termed β and γ, result in secreted forms of PVR (Koike et al. 1990). Using cosmid clones of the PVR gene, transgenic mice expressing the human PVR have been generated (Ren et al. 1990; Koike et al. 1991b). The finding that these mice are susceptible to PV(1), which normally does not infect mice, and that they get a disease resembling human poliomyelitis is overwhelming evidence that PVR mediates PV infection in vivo and that the absence of PVR is the host-encoded, host-range determinant for PV replication in mice.

Two other related molecules should be mentioned. A mouse homolog to the human PVR, termed MPH, has been identified (Morrison and Racaniello 1992). Although some negative controls were not carried out in this work, it seems clear that MPH is not the receptor for PV(2). In separate work, another MAb, AF3, that blocks PV replication was developed (Shepley et al. 1988). AF3 recognizes a molecule that is distinct from PVR by several criteria. Recently, AF3 has been shown to be specific for CD44 (Shepley and Racaniello 1994); this finding and its possible role in poliomyelitis are discussed elsewhere (Shepley, this volume).

USE OF CLONED REAGENT TO STUDY DISTRIBUTION
OF mRNA

Surprisingly, although PVR is clearly the physiologically relevant receptor in mediating poliomyelitis, studies of its distribution in human tissues have not revealed the mechanism of PV tissue tropism. The availability of the cloned reagent for PVR permitted the immediate testing of some long-held hypotheses concerning the receptor for PV. One of the most important issues to be addressed was the role of the receptor in mediating the tissue tropism of PV. Ostensibly, if the cell-surface receptor is the primary determinant of viral tissue tropism, one would expect to find a precisely parallel distribution between receptor and viral replication. However, when studied by Northern blot analysis, PVR mRNA of the correct size is found in many human tissues. This was originally demonstrated for only one nonsusceptible tissue, kidney (Mendelsohn et al. 1989); however, later work revealed a widespread distribution in human tissues, including brain, leukocytes, liver, and placenta (Koike et al. 1990).

When the detection of alternatively spliced forms of PVR, encoding secreted forms, was reported, it was speculated that the explanation for expression of PVR in inappropriate tissues may be the secreted forms (which would not be active as viral receptors). The sizes of all four mRNAs, as determined by Northern blot analysis, are quite similar.

However, using mRNA-specific polymerase chain reaction (PCR) primers, the tissue distribution of the secreted forms was shown to be identical to that of the cell-surface forms (Koike et al. 1990). Similarly, using RNA from the transgenic mice expressing the human gene, PVR, two groups (Ren et al. 1990; Koike et al. 1991b) have shown that PVR mRNA is present in many tissues. Although this finding may be an artifact of the mouse system, it is pertinent to note that these independently derived transgenic mice, which both use the natural PVR promoter, demonstrated qualitatively similar phenomena. Thus, data from experiments with both human and PVR-expressing transgenic mouse tissue appeared to support the notion that PVR expression exceeds PV tissue tropism and, therefore, PVR is not the primary host-encoded tissue tropism determinant.

A more detailed study by in situ hybridization with nucleic acid probes of PVR with transgenic mouse tissues raised even more questions (Ren and Racaniello 1992a). This work revealed a much more limited expression of PVR (CNS, thymus, lung, kidney, and adrenal), and within these tissues, PVR expression is restricted to specific cell types. For example, in the kidney, PVR is expressed in the epithelial layer of Bowman capsule, but not in the renal cortex. Within the CNS, PVR is expressed ubiquitously and exclusively in neurons. Since Northern blot analysis generally cannot distinguish cell-type heterogeneity with tissues, it is not surprising to find that a more precise methodology, in situ hybridization, reveals a more limited expression of a molecule; however, it is more difficult to resolve the striking absence of PVR from many tissues (in this recent work) with the apparently ubiquitous expression previously described. Furthermore, the in situ hybridization experiments were carried out using PVR sequences that would react with all four mRNAs. As detailed below, there are several possible ways to reconcile these contradictory data. However, it is important to realize that there is not a complete description of PVR mRNA expression in human tissues. In situ hybridization of human tissues with mRNA-specific nucleic acid probes will be required before a simple description of PVR mRNA expression is complete.

The current knowledge of PVR mRNA expression is fragmentary and contradictory. To the extent that it is understood, it leaves open the question of the role of the host cell receptor in mediating PV tissue tropism. However, the available data support the finding that there are "ectopic" sites of expression of PVR mRNA (Mendelsohn et al. 1989), although likely not as many as was thought. This suggests, contrary to the original hypothesis (Holland 1961), that the receptor is not the primary host-encoded mediator of the tissue-specific replication of PV.

IDENTIFICATION AND DISTRIBUTION OF PVR PROTEIN

Western Blot Analysis in Human Tissues

The complexity of PVR mRNA expression has raised many questions about its gene products. To identify the PVR gene product, polyclonal antisera were raised in several laboratories (Freistadt et al. 1990; Zibert et al. 1991). These groups used several bacterial fusion proteins as antigens and produced several useful antisera. Western blot analysis was carried out to determine, first, whether the protein expression paralleled the mRNA expression and, second, whether tissue-specific differences that could explain the tissue tropism of PV would be visible.

Using one of these antisera, PVR protein was detected in many tissues including kidney, liver, intestine, cerebellum, and motor cortex by Western blot analysis (Freistadt et al. 1990). Thus, to a first approximation, PVR protein appears to be ubiquitously expressed in human tissues. The molecular mass of the protein detected by these methods is approximately 69 kD. The specificity of the antisera was demonstrated in competition experiments in which the reactivity was competed away by an independently expressed form of PVR, but not by an unrelated competitor.

This analysis is complicated by several findings. In these experiments, more than one reactive species was detected. Generally, a doublet or triplet of protein from 55 kD to 69 kD was detected. Since PVR is a glycoprotein (Kaplan et al. 1990; Zibert et al. 1991), the simplest interpretation of this size heterogeneity is that the various forms are glycosylation intermediates. More recent work using HeLa cells (Bernhardt et al. 1994) has revealed an 80-kD, glycosylated species which is likely to be the fully processed form. Furthermore, although PVR-reactive material was found ubiquitously, a substantial amount of variation was apparent. This variability took several forms: size, abundance, immunoreactivity, and subunit arrangement. In some tissues (CNS), the smaller forms (55 kD) predominated, whereas the larger forms (69 kD) predominated in other tissues, such as kidney. The lowest amounts of PVR protein were found in CNS samples (20 μg of total protein was required for detection in Western analysis), and much more was found in kidney (1 μg yielded a strong signal).

A tissue-specific difference in immunoreactivity was noted when the forms of the protein were studied in Western analysis using polyclonal antisera generated against different parts of the molecule. Using the antiserum anti-1i, which was generated against domains 1, 2, and 3, the forms of the protein in the kidney were more reactive than CNS forms. However, using the antiserum anti-4a, which was generated against domain 1, the species in the CNS were more reactive than forms in the kidney and other nonneuronal tissues. This suggests that in the form of PVR in the motor cortex, domain 1 is more able to react with the anti-domain-1 antiserum than is the form in the kidney. Since the antisera were generated against bacterial proteins, they should react exclusively with peptide epitopes. Taken together, these findings suggest that, in the motor cortex, domain 1 of PVR is under-glycosylated relative to its form in other tissues. The accumulated data from mutagenesis experiments (Freistadt and Racaniello 1991; Koike et al. 1991a; Selinka et al. 1991, 1992; Morrison and Racaniello 1992) show that the amino-terminal 163 amino acids, when fused to the transmembrane and cytoplasmic domains, are sufficient to confer susceptibility to PV. It may be that the residues in domain 1 that are crucial for PV receptor function in humans are covered by glycosylation in nonsusceptible tissues. However, PV was able to bind (using the classic assay described above; Holland and McLaren 1959) to all tissues when tested in the PVR-expressing transgenic mouse model (Ren et al. 1990).

A final type of heterogeneity was detected by comparing the electrophoretic migration of the proteins in the presence or absence of reducing agents. The 55-kD form in the kidney had much slower mobility (migrating as ~150 kD) in the absence of reducing agent, whereas the 69-kD form in the motor cortex had unchanged or slightly increased mobility under similar conditions (Freistadt et al. 1990). This suggests that in the kidney, the PVR exists as a multimer, either bound to itself or to another molecule, whereas the form in the motor cortex is likely to be monomeric. This may be important if a monomeric form of PVR is required for viral uptake.

Considered together, these data suggest that the form of PVR in the motor cortex is the active form and is able to bind and take up PV. However, a number of difficulties remain with the current understanding of PVR protein expression. None of the putative active forms was detected in samples of ileum or intestine, where PV replicates. This may be a problem of abundance. Furthermore, none of these antisera are isoform-specific; that is, they do not distinguish between the gene products formed from the four mRNAs. They recognize common residues and thus cannot distinguish between cell-surface and secreted forms of PVR protein.

Similar to the understanding of PVR mRNA, the knowledge of PVR protein expression thus remains fragmentary. A clear understanding of the role of PVR in mediating PV tissue tropism awaits a precise description using isoform-specific immunocytochemical analyses with human tissues. Preliminary immunocytochemical experiments revealed D171-reactive protein in the human olfactory bulb, a brain tissue not susceptible to PV (D. Stoltz and M. Freistadt, unpubl.). If cell-surface PVR is still detected in cells that do not support PV replication, its competency to bind and take up PV will need to be assessed.

Studies on the Expression of PVR in Human Blood Cells

One cell type that was not considered in the descriptive work of PVR expression is blood cells. Since several reports show that PV replicates in human blood cell lines (Kitamura et al. 1985; Okada et al. 1987; Lopez-Guerrero et al. 1991), various primary blood cell types were screened for their expression of PVR. This was carried out using two-color immunofluorescence with an anti-PVR MAb (D171) and lineage-specific markers followed by flow cytometric analysis (Freistadt et al. 1993). PVR expression was absent from platelets and polymorphonuclear leukocytes. However, PVR cell-surface expression was found on the majority of cells of one blood cell type, the mononuclear phagocyte (CD14$^+$; MP). Furthermore, at least one cell type from peripheral blood mononuclear cells, purified by density centrifugation through Ficoll-hypaque (Boyum 1968), likely MPs, supported PV replication (Freistadt et al. 1993). More recent, dual-labeling studies confirm that CD14$^+$ cells support PV replication (K. Eberle and M. Freistadt, unpubl.).

This finding provides a possible resolution for some of the contradictory data about PVR expression. PVR expression in MPs could explain the apparent ubiquity of PVR mRNA and protein in tissues, when analyzed by Northern and Western blots. Tissue samples from cadavers contain blood cells; thus, the PVR-reactive mRNA and protein could have been contributed by MPs. In addition, this finding is important with regard to many unexplained phenomena in PV pathogenesis. The primary site of PV replication in a normal human infection has not been identified. It was originally defined as "oropharyngeal and intestinal mucosa." More recent work suggests that M cells, a phagocytic cell type in the lumen of intestinal mucosa, perhaps associated with Peyer's patches, can take up PV nonspecifically (Sicinski et al. 1990). These cells may deliver PV via transendothelial transcytosis to the associated lymph tissue. If resident macrophages (CD14$^+$ cells) support PV replication, this may provide a route both for excretion via feces and for subsequent steps in the infection process, such as viremia. In addition, these cells may constitute the elusive sites of extraneuronal replication, responsible for shedding PV after the viremia has been cleared by antibodies (Bodian 1959). Finally, the mechanism(s) by which PV enters the CNS remains to be elucidated (Bodian 1959). Until recently, two models were prevalent: (1) During viremia PV could cross the blood brain barrier or (2) PV could enter other tissues (like muscle), replicate, and then travel up nerves by retrograde transport to the CNS (Ren and Racaniello 1992b). The demonstration of PVR expression in primary circulating MPs and PV replication in human blood cells suggests a third possibility: PV could be carried by MPs into the CNS. These bone-marrow-derived cells have the capacity to diapedese into the CNS and differentiate into microglia, the resident macrophages (Junqueira and Carneiro 1971).

Other Sites of Cell-surface PVR Expression

Some other studies bear mentioning here. The finding of PVR on leukocytes resulted in its being considered by the Fifth International Workshop on Human Leukocyte Differentiation Antigens (M. Freistadt and E. Wimmer, pers. comm.). Although PVR was not given a CD designation, a blind panel analysis revealed other sites of PVR expression. These analyses were carried out using semi-quantitative flow cytometry with D171 in primary human tissues. In these studies, PVR was confirmed on MPs and was also found on PHA-stimulated leukocytes, high CD34+ bone marrow cells, and thymic epithelium. These findings may have important consequences for both normal and pathogenic function of PVR.

In independent experiments, PVR expression in denervated and degenerating human muscle fibers was studied (M.C. Dalakas and M. Leon-Monzon, pers. comm.). In these tissues, which were obtained from human muscle biopsies, PVR expression was detected by means of immunofluorescence microscopy. These findings suggest that PVR is present in human muscle cells and that it may function at the neuromuscular junction. This is consistent with the detection of high polioviral replication in PVR-expressing transgenic mouse skeletal muscle (Ren and Racaniello 1992a). This finding may be important when considering the route of PV entry into the CNS.

CONCLUSION: REMAINING QUESTIONS

Although spectacular progress has recently been achieved in our understanding of the mechanism by which PV initiates the infection process, further work remains to be carried out before a full understanding of PV pathogenesis is attained. Some of the work is descriptive, whereas other experimentation will be directed toward acquiring insight into the mechanisms by which PVR mediates paralytic poliomyelitis. Ultimately, an understanding of the normal endogenous function of PVR is sought.

Precise Tissue Distribution of PVR Protein

Much purely descriptive work remains to be carried out in order to obtain an accurate and precise understanding of PVR expression in human tissues. For the questions concerning mRNA distribution, in situ hybridization using isoform-specific probes with human tissues is required. It is still not known whether PVR protein correlates with mRNA levels. Some experiments suggest that translation regulation of this mRNA occurs in cell-free translational systems (A. Zibert and E. Wimmer, unpubl.); however, it is not clear whether this finding is physiologically relevant. To precisely determine the tissue localization of PVR protein, immunocytochemical analyses with isoform-specific reagents should be carried out with human tissues. In addition to sorting out questions such as whether PVR protein expression has cell-type limitation within specific tissues, such studies should reveal whether PVR has differential subcellular localization (cell surface, secreted, or vesicular). Immunoelectron microscopic analysis may be required. Furthermore, a determination of the nature of PVR glycosylation and whether it differs between tissues is required. An initial characterization of PVR glycosylation revealed that PVR protein bears sialylated complex-type oligosaccharides (Bernhardt et al. 1994).

Significance of Ectopic Expression

At this stage in our understanding, it appears likely that once a descriptive study is complete, ectopic (relative to PV replication) sites of PVR expression will be confirmed. At that point, it will be important to establish the significance of this expression. First, it will be necessary to confirm that these proteins are competent to bind PV. Using recombinant expressed forms of PVR, it was recently shown that solubilized PVR is capable of inducing a conformational alteration (135S particle formation) that inactivates PV (Kaplan et al. 1990). It may be possible to develop an in situ PV-binding assay, based on the ability of cells in tissues to induce 135S particles. However, it may become necessary to clone cDNA from the specific sites and test them for PVR function in transfection studies, since the PVR cDNAs studied so far have been derived from tissue-culture cells. There may be minor differences in PVR mRNAs in tissues that can account for differences in susceptibility to PV.

Blocks to PV replication may be at the level of entry or later steps. If PVR is active (i.e., if it binds and inactivates PV), entry may be blocked subsequent to binding PV—either in uptake or uncoating. An isoform of CD44, the molecular identified by the PV-blocking MAb, AF3, may function to overcome this block (Shepley, this volume), since AF3 reactivity correlates well with PV replication. However, a functional assay for this activity may be difficult to develop. It may be possible to develop a transfection assay using PVR-expressing, but PV-resistant, cells, similar to the assay used to identify PVR. Several findings suggest that there may be more than one tissue-specific block, subsequent to entry, to PV replication. Although the three serotypes of PV have attenuating mutations in the capsid region, other attenuating mutations are scattered throughout the PV genome (Almond 1987; La Monica et al. 1987; Nomoto and Wimmer 1987; Ren et al. 1991). For example, it is likely that the sequence surrounding and including the major attenuating mutation in the 5′ untranslated region (nucleotide 472 in PV[3]) interacts with important host factors for translation: These host factors may vary between tissues (Svitkin et al. 1988). In the case of PVR-expressing transgenic mice, PV tissue tropism is clearly mediated by different mechanisms. The absence of PVR (when analyzed by in situ hybridization) from many nonneuronal tissues, such as liver, certainly restricts PV replication during viremia. However, within the CNS of transgenic mice, PVR expression is restricted to the correct cell type (neurons but not glia) but is not correctly restricted among neurons; i.e., it is present in all neurons, not exclusively in susceptible cells (motor neurons). Thus, within the CNS, there must be additional postreceptor blocks. One experimental system shows promise as a way to identify differences between PVR-expressing susceptible and nonsusceptible cells. PV-binding and PVR-expressing, but PV-resistant, cells from dispersed kidney tissue of PVR-expressing transgenic mice become susceptible to PV infection within 24 hours of culturing (Ren and Racaniello 1992a). This may provide an opportunity to delineate the nature of the block in those cells. Another intriguing possibility is that there are cases where PV replicates but does not kill cells. In the PVR-expressing transgenic mice, PV replication in the absence of cell lysis was detected in the anterior horn of the spinal cord (Ren and Racaniello 1992a).

Once this work is completed, it will be interesting to compare this information to the situation of other viral receptors. There probably is no universal rule regarding the role of cell-surface receptors in mediating viral tissue tropism; in fact, there is a striking diversity in the extent of correlation between viral receptor expression and viral replication. At one extreme is influenza virus, which uses the ubiquitous sialic acid as its receptor, but whose full viral life cycle requires a protease found in a very limited number of cell types. At the other extreme is Epstein-Barr virus (EBV); the expression of its receptor, CR2, correlates well with EBV infection in B lymphocytes (Moore et al. 1987).

PVR is unique among viral receptors in that it was initially identified as a viral receptor and, to date, 5 years after its identification as a novel molecule, the normal function remains unidentified. It is hoped that further studies concerning the distribution and other properties of PVR will shed light on its endogenous function.

REFERENCES

Almond, J.W. 1987. The attenuation of poliovirus neurovirulence. *Ann. Rev. Microbiol.* **41:** 153.

Berhardt, G., J.A. Bibb, J. Bradley, and E. Wimmer. 1994. Molecular characterization of the cellular receptor for poliovirus. *Virology* **199:** 105.

Bodian, D. 1959. Poliomyelitis: pathogenesis and histopathology. In *Viral and rickettsial infections of man* (ed. F.L. Horsfall and I. Tamm), p. 479. Lippincott, Philadelphia.

Boyum, A. 1968. Separation of leukocytes from blood and bone marrow. *Scand. J. Clin. Lab. Invest.* (suppl. 97) **21:** 77.

Crowell, R.L. and B.J. Landau. 1983. Receptors in the initiation of picornavirus infections. In *Comprehensive virology* (ed. H. Fraenkel-Conrat and R.R. Wagner), vol. 18, p. 1. Plenum Press, New York.

Dulbecco, R. and H.S. Ginsberg. 1988. *Virology.* Lippincott, Philadelphia.

Freistadt, M.S. and V.R. Racaniello. 1991. Mutational analysis of the cellular receptor for poliovirus. *J. Virol.* **65:** 3873.

Freistadt, M.S., H.B. Fleit, and E. Wimmer. 1993. Poliovirus receptor on human blood cells: A possible extraneural site of poliovirus replication. *Virology* **195:** 798.

Freistadt, M.S., G. Kaplan, and V.R. Racaniello. 1990. Heterogeneous expression of poliovirus receptor-related proteins in human cells and tissues. *Mol. Cell. Biol.* **10:** 5700.

Holland, J.J. 1961. Receptor affinities as major determinants of enterovirus tissue tropisms in humans. *Virology* **15:** 312.

――――. 1962. Irreversible eclipse of poliovirus by HeLa cells. *Virology* **16:** 163.

Holland, J.J. and L.C. McLaren. 1959. The mammalian cell-virus relationship. II. Adsorption, reception, and eclipse by HeLa cells. *J. Exp. Med.* **109:** 487.

――――. 1961. The location and nature of enterovirus receptors in susceptible cells. *J. Exp. Med.* **114:** 161.

Holland, J.J., L.C. McLaren, and J.T. Syverton. 1959a. The mammalian cell virus relationship III. Production of infectious poliovirus by nonprimate cells exposed to poliovirus ribonucleic acid. *Proc. Soc. Exp. Biol. Med.* **100:** 843.

――――. 1959b. The mammalian cell virus relationship. IV. Infection of naturally insusceptible cells with enterovirus ribonucleic acid. *J. Exp. Med.* **110:** 65.

Junqueira, L.C. and J. Carneiro. 1971. *Basic histology.* LANGE Medical Publications, Los Altos, California.

Kaplan, G., M.S. Freistadt, and V.R. Racaniello. 1990. Neutralization of poliovirus by cell receptors expressed in insect cells. *J. Virol.* **64:** 4697.

Kaplan, G., A. Levy, and V.R. Racaniello. 1989. Isolation and characterization of HeLa cell lines blocked at different steps in the poliovirus life cycle. *J. Virol.* **63:** 43.

Kitamura, N., B.L. Semler, P.G. Rothberg, G.R. Larsen, C.J. Adler, A.J. Dorner, E.A. Emini, R. Hanecak, J. Lee, S. van der Werf, C.W. Anderson, and E. Wimmer. 1981. Primary structure, gene organization and polypeptide expression of poliovirus RNA. *Nature* **291:** 547.

Kitamura, Y., M. Masuda, and H. Yoshikura. 1985. Effect of myelocytic maturation of HL60 cells on replication of influenza and polioviruses. *Virology* 141: 299.

Koike, S., I. Ise, and A. Nomoto. 1991a. Functional domains of the poliovirus receptor. *Proc. Natl. Acad. Sci.* 88: 4104.

Koike, S., C. Taya, T. Kurata, S. Abe, I. Ise, H. Yonekawa, and A. Nomoto. 1991b. Transgenic mice susceptible to poliovirus. *Proc. Natl. Acad. Sci.* 88: 951.

Koike, S., H. Horie, I. Ise, A. Okitsu, M. Yoshida, N. Iizuka, K. Takeuchi, T. Takegami, and A. Nomoto. 1990. The poliovirus receptor protein is produced both as membrane-bound and secreted forms. *EMBO J.* 9: 3217.

Kunin, C.M. and W.S. Jordan. 1961. In vitro adsorption of poliovirus by noncultured tissues. Effect of species, age and malignancy. *Am. J. Hyg.* 73: 245.

La Monica, N., J.W. Almond, and V.R. Racaniello. 1987. A mouse model for poliovirus neurovirulence identifies mutations that attenuate the virus of humans. *J. Virol.* 61: 2917.

Lopez-Guerrero, J.A., C. Cabanas, C. Bernabeu, M. Fresno, and M.A. Alonso. 1991. Effects of poliovirus replication on undifferentiated and differentiated monocytic U937 cells: Comparative studies with human macrophages. *Intervirology* 32: 137.

Maddon, P.J., A.G. Dalgleish, J.S. McDougal, P.R. Clapham, R.A. Weiss, and R. Axel. 1986. The T4 gene encodes the AIDS virus receptor and is expressed in the immune system and the brain. *Cell* 47: 333.

Martin, A., C. Wychowski, T. Couderc, R. Crainic, J. Hogle, and M. Girard. 1988. Engineering a poliovirus type 2 antigenic site on a type 1 capsid results in a chimeric virus which is neurovirulent for mice. *EMBO J.* 7: 2839.

McLaren, L.C., J.J. Holland, and J.T. Syverton. 1959. The mammalian cell-virus relationship I. Attachment of poliovirus to cultivated cells of primate and non-primate origin. *J. Exp. Med.* 109: 475.

Mendelsohn, C.L., E. Wimmer, and V.R. Racaniello. 1989. Cellular receptor for poliovirus: Molecular cloning, nucleotide sequence, and expression of a new member of the immunoglobulin superfamily. *Cell* 56: 855.

Mendelsohn, C., B. Johnson, K.A. Lionetti, P. Nobis, E. Wimmer, and V.R. Racaniello. 1986. Transformation of a human poliovirus receptor gene into mouse cells. *Proc. Natl. Acad. Sci.* 83: 7845.

Minor, P.D., P.A. Pipkin, D. Hockley, G.C. Schild, and J.W. Almond. 1984. Monoclonal antibodies which block cellular receptors of poliovirus. *Virus Res.* 1: 203.

Moore, M.D., N.R. Cooper, B.F. Tack, and G.R. Nemerow. 1987. Molecular cloning of the cDNA encoding the Epstein-Barr virus/C3d receptor (complement receptor type 2 of human B lymphocytes. *Proc. Natl. Acad. Sci.* 84: 9194.

Morrison, M.E. and V.R. Racaniello. 1992. Molecular cloning and expression of a murine homolog of the human poliovirus receptor gene. *J. Virol.* 66: 2807.

Murray, M.G., J. Bradley, X.-F. Yang, E. Wimmer, E.G. Moss, and V.R. Racaniello. 1988. Poliovirus host range is determined by a short amino acid sequence in neutralization antigenic site I. *Science* 241: 213.

Nobis, P., R. Zibirre, G. Meyer, J. Kühne, G. Warnecke, and G. Koch. 1985. Production of a monoclonal antibody against an epitope on HeLa cells that is the functional poliovirus binding site. *J. Gen. Virol.* 66: 2563.

Nomoto, A. and E. Wimmer. 1987. Genetic studies of the antigenicity and the attenuation phenotype of poliovirus. *Symp. Soc. Gen. Microbiol.* 35: 107.

Okada, Y., G. Toda, H. Oka, A. Nomoto, and H. Yoshikura. 1987. Poliovirus infection of established human blood cell lines: Relationship between the differentiation stage and susceptibility or cell killing. *Virology* 156: 238.

Racaniello, V.R. 1988. Poliovirus neurovirulence. *Adv. Virus Res.* **34:** 217.

Racaniello, V.R. and D. Baltimore. 1981. Molecular cloning of poliovirus and determination of the complete nucleotide sequence of the viral genome. *Proc. Natl. Acad. Sci.* **78:** 4887.

Ren, R. and V.R. Racaniello. 1992a. Human poliovirus receptor gene expression and poliovirus tissue tropism in transgenic mice. *J. Virol.* **66:** 296.

————. 1992b. Poliovirus spreads from muscle to the central nervous system by neural pathways. *J. Infect. Dis.* **166:** 747.

Ren, R.B., F. Costantini, E.J. Gorgacz, J.J. Lee, and V.R. Racaniello. 1990. Transgenic mice expressing a human poliovirus receptor: A new model for poliomyelitis. *Cell* **63:** 353.

Ren, R.B., E.G. Moss, and V.R. Racaniello. 1991. Identification of two determinants that attenuate vaccine-related type 2 poliovirus. *J. Virol.* **65:** 1377.

Ryu, S.-E., P.D. Kwong, A. Truneh, T.G. Porter, J. Arthos, M. Rosenberg, X. Dia, N. Xuong, R. Axel, R.W. Sweet, and W.A. Hendrickson. 1990. Crystal structure of an HIV-binding recombinant fragment of human CD4. *Nature* **348:** 419.

Sabin, A.B. 1955. Characteristics and genetic potentialities of experimentally produced and naturally occurring variants of poliomyelitis virus. *Ann. N.Y. Acad. Sci.* **61:** 924.

Selinka, H.C., A. Zibert, and E. Wimmer. 1991. Poliovirus can enter and infect mammalian cells by way of an intercellular adhesion molecule 1 pathway. *Proc. Natl. Acad. Sci.* **88:** 3598.

————. 1992. A chimeric poliovirus/CD4-receptor confers susceptibility to poliovirus on mouse cells. *J. Virol.* **66:** 2523.

Shepley, M.P. and V. Racaniello. 1994. A monoclonal antibody that blocks poliovirus attachment recognizes the lymphocyte homing receptor CD44. *J. Virol.* **68:** 1301.

Shepley, M.P., B. Sherry, and H.L. Weiner. 1988. Monoclonal antibody identification of a 100-kDa membrane protein in HeLa cells and human spinal cord involved in poliovirus attachment. *Proc. Natl. Acad. Sci.* **85:** 7743.

Sicinski, P., J. Rowinski, J.B. Warchol, Z. Jarzabek, W. Gut, B. Szczygiel, K. Bielecki, and G. Koch. 1990. Poliovirus type 1 enters the human host through intestinal M cells. *Gastroenterology* **98:** 56.

Svitkin, Y.V., T.V. Pestova, S.V. Maslova, and V.I. Agol. 1988. Point mutations modify the response of poliovirus RNA to a translation initiation factor: A comparison of neurovirulent and attenuated strains. *Virology* **166:** 394.

Tomassini, J.E., T.R. Maxson, and R.J. Colonno. 1989. Biochemical characterization of a glycoprotein required for rhinovirus attachment. *J. Biol. Chem.* **264:** 1656.

Wang, J., Y. Van, T.P.J. Garrett, J. Liu, D.W. Rodgers, R.L. Garlick, G.E. Tarr, Y. Husain, E.L. Reinherz, and S.C. Harrison. 1990. Atomic structure of a fragment of human CD4 containing two immunoglobulin-like domains. *Nature* **348:** 411.

Williams, A.F. and A.N. Barclay. 1988. The immunoglobulin superfamily. Domains for cell surface recognition. *Annu. Rev. Immunol.* **6:** 381.

Wimmer, E., C.U.T. Hellen, and X. Cao. 1993. Genetics of poliovirus. *Annu. Rev. Genet.* **27:** 353.

Zibert, A., H.C. Selinka, S.O. Elroy, B. Moss, and E. Wimmer. 1991. Vaccinia virus-mediated expression and identification of the human poliovirus receptor. *Virology* **182:** 250.

23

Transgenic Mouse for the Study of Poliovirus Pathogenicity

Satoshi Koike,[1] Junken Aoki,[1] and Akio Nomoto[1,2]
[1]Department of Microbiology
The Tokyo Metropolitan Institute of Medical Science
Honkomagome, Bunkyo-ku, Tokyo 113, Japan
[2]Department of Microbiology
Institute of Medical Science
The University of Tokyo, Shirokanedai
Minato-ku, Tokyo 108, Japan

Poliomyelitis is an acute disease of the central nervous system (CNS) caused by poliovirus. Poliovirus is a human enterovirus that belongs to the Picornaviridae family and is classified into three stable serotypes, 1, 2, and 3 (Paul 1971). Humans are the only natural host of poliovirus, although poliovirus can be experimentally transferred to monkeys, in which it also causes a paralytic disease. Other animal species are not susceptible to most poliovirus strains. Because of this characteristic species specificity of poliovirus, monkeys and chimpanzees have been used as animal models for the studies of poliovirus pathogenicity.

In the 1950s, an outline of the pathology of poliomyelitis was established. According to this outline (Bodian 1955; Sabin 1956), poliovirus infection is initiated by ingestion of virus followed by its primary multiplication in the oropharynx and intestine (alimentary phase). Extensive viral multiplication is evident in tissues of the tonsils and Peyer's patches of the ileum (lymphatic phase). From these sites, the virus moves into deep cervical and mesenteric lymph nodes, and then into the blood (viremic phase). Poliovirus invades the CNS through the blood-brain barrier or by the axonal pathway, and paralytic poliomyelitis occurs as a result of the destruction of neurons in the CNS, especially motor neurons in the anterior horn of the spinal cord and neurons of the motor cortex and the brain stem (neurological phase). Although many tissues are exposed to the virus during the viremic phase, sites of poliovirus replication are limited to certain tissues. Thus, poliovirus seems to have distinct tissue tropism, which plays an important role in the development of poliomyelitis. Susceptibility of tissues to poliovirus in vivo must be

Cellular Receptors for Animal Viruses
© 1994 Cold Spring Harbor Laboratory Press 0-87969-429-7/94 $5 + .00

determined by many factors, as described below. Molecular mechanisms of this tissue tropism have not been elucidated.

To control poliomyelitis, attenuated poliovirus strains have been developed and effectively used as oral live vaccines; that is, Sabin 1 (type 1), Sabin 2 (type 2), and Sabin 3 (type 3) (Sabin and Boulger 1973). In the alimentary tract of humans, the attenuated Sabin strains can replicate enough to elicit neutralizing antibodies. The attenuated viruses have poor replicating capacity in the CNS and they seldom or never invade the neurons in the CNS. Because inoculation of virus into the CNS of monkeys has been the only method to evaluate neurovirulence of poliovirus, a large number of monkeys have been used to assess neurovirulence levels of vaccine candidate strains (Sabin and Boulger 1973) and of oral poliovirus vaccine lots (WHO 1990).

Molecular genetic approaches were carried out to elucidate the molecular mechanisms of poliovirus attenuation (Almond 1987; Nomoto and Wimmer 1987; Nomoto and Koike 1992). The analyses, including monkey neurovirulence tests, have revealed that the loci influencing attenuation phenotype are spread over wide areas of the genomes and that strong determinants for attenuation reside in the 5′-proximal portion of the genomes of all three poliovirus serotypes, particularly the nucleotide positions 480, 481, and 472 of poliovirus types 1, 2, and 3, respectively (Evans et al. 1985; Omata et al. 1986; Kohara et al. 1988; Kawamura et al. 1989; Westrop et al. 1989; Macadam et al. 1991). However, many other neurovirulence determinants spread over the genomes remain to be elucidated.

Although the monkey model has been effectively used for evaluating neurovirulence levels of poliovirus as described above, this animal model has inherent disadvantages, including (1) extremely high costs of breeding; (2) high risk of zoonosis because of close evolutionary relatedness between humans and monkeys; (3) species extinction of monkeys; and (4) marked individual difference in experiments. These situations made it difficult to obtain statistically reliable results from monkey neurovirulence tests. It is, therefore, desirable to develop a new animal model for studying poliovirus pathogenesis.

An alternative strategy to study poliovirus pathogenicity is to use mouse-adapted polioviruses. Virus strains such as type 2 Lansing and MEF-1 can replicate in mice and cause a paralytic disease which is clinically and pathologically similar to human poliomyelitis (Jubelt et al. 1980). It was demonstrated that chimera polioviruses carrying a part of the viral capsid protein derived from the Lansing strain can infect mice (La Monica et al. 1986; Martin et al. 1988; Murray et al. 1988). Such polioviruses were tested for their neurovirulence in mice (La Monica et al. 1987; Moss et al. 1989; Martin et al. 1991; Ren et al. 1991). Although the mouse neurovirulence tests on these polioviruses identified the determinants that attenuated the virus in primates, the mouse tests are applicable only to mouse-adapted polioviruses whose infection is mediated by binding to a receptor molecule that is different from a human receptor for poliovirus (PVR). Therefore, it is possible that determinants concerning mouse adaptation of poliovirus are regarded as those of neurovirulence phenotype (La Monica et al. 1986; Martin et al. 1991; Moss and Racaniello 1991).

New technologies have emerged over the past decade that may allow the replacement of the monkey model of poliomyelitis with transgenic animals which express selected human genes. The host-range restriction of poliovirus is considered to be primarily determined by a cell-surface receptor that is common to all three poliovirus serotypes (Crowell and Landau 1983). Thus, transgenic animals expressing the human gene for PVR may be susceptible to poliovirus infection.

PVR AS A DETERMINANT FOR HOST RANGE OF POLIOVIRUS

The genomic and complementary DNAs for a human PVR have been isolated from HeLa S3 cells (Mendelsohn et al. 1989; Koike et at. 1990). The PVR gene is approximately 20 kb in length and is located at band q13.1-13.2 of human chromosome 19 as a single-copy gene. This appears to be identical to the locus of poliovirus sensitivity (*PVS*) (Miller et al. 1974; Siddique et al. 1988). Nucleotide sequence analysis of cDNAs revealed that PVR belongs to a member of the immunoglobulin (Ig) superfamily. There are at least four mRNA isoforms of approximately 3.4 kb (mRNAs for PVRα, PVRβ, PVRγ, and PVRδ) generated by alternative splicing from the primary transcript (Koike et al. 1990). Of these, two membrane-bound forms, PVRα and PVRδ, which correspond to H20A and H20B (Mendelsohn et al. 1989), respectively, are functional receptor molecules. They have an identical amino acid sequence within a putative signal peptide, three Ig-like domains, and a transmembrane domain, but different sequences within a cytoplasmic domain that resulted from an alternative splicing. Molecular masses of PVRα and PVRδ calculated from the deduced amino acid sequences were approximately 45 kD and 43 kD, respectively (Mendelsohn et al. 1989). There are eight putative N-linked glycosylation sites in the extracellular domain. Antibodies against PVR detected them as integral membrane glycoproteins of approximately 80 kD (Zibert et al. 1991; Bernhardt et al. 1994; S. Koike et al., unpubl.). Two other mRNA isoforms, PVRβ and PVRγ, lack a region encoding a transmembrane domain and therefore are soluble forms of PVRs. Indeed, PVRβ was proved not to be a functional PVR (Koike et al. 1990). Further molecular genetic analysis has revealed that the poliovirus-binding site resides in the amino-terminal Ig-like domain (Koike et al. 1991a; Selinka et al. 1991). Experimental evidence indicated that two N-linked carbohydrate chains, if attached to this domain, were dispensable with respect to poliovirus infection (Koike et al. 1992a; Zibert and Wimmer 1992). The physiological function of PVR is not known at present.

Mouse L cells are not permissive for poliovirus infection. However, mouse L-cell transformants carrying the human PVR gene (Koike et al. 1990) or the PVR cDNA (Mendelsohn et al. 1989; Koike et al. 1990) are permissive for the infection of all three serotypes of poliovirus. This observation indicates that mouse L cells have cellular factors supporting poliovirus replication except for PVR.

ESTABLISHMENT OF TRANSGENIC MOUSE STRAINS
AS NEW EXPERIMENTAL ANIMAL MODELS

To date, two research groups (Ren et al. 1990; Koike et al. 1991b) have succeeded in producing poliovirus-sensitive transgenic (Tg) mice by introducing a human PVR gene. Founders were derived by microinjection of the PVR DNA into the genomes of (C57BL6/J x CBA/J) F_2 zygotes (TgPVR1-7, TgPVR1-17, and TgPVR3-8) (Ren et al. 1990), strain ICR (ICR-PVRTg1, ICR-PVRTg5, and ICR-PVRTg21) and C57BL/10 (B10-PVRTg8) (Koike et al. 1991b). Of these, TgPVR1-17 mice (Ren et al. 1991) and ICR-PVRTg1 mice (Koike et al. 1991b; Horie et al. 1994) have so far been extensively investigated for their susceptibility to poliovirus and distribution of PVR.

The Tg mice as an experimental animal model for the study of poliovirus pathogenicity should possess the following characters: (1) the mice show clinical and pathological signs similar to poliomyelitis displayed by humans and monkeys; (2) neurovirulence tests using the mice discriminate viruses with different neurovirulence levels.

The Tg mice are susceptible to all three poliovirus serotypes, and show a flaccid paralysis in limbs and die after inoculation of poliovirus by various routes such as intracerebral, intraspinal, intraperitoneal, intravenous (Ren et al. 1990; Koike et al. 1991b), intramuscular (Ren and Racaniello 1992a,b), and oral routes (Table 1). Latency periods were 3–10 days after inoculation in most paralytic cases (Horie et al. 1994). Susceptibility of the Tg mice to poliovirus is different depending on inoculation routes, virus strains, and mouse lines used (Ren et al. 1990; Koike et al. 1991b). The different susceptibilities of ICR-PVRTg1 mice

Table 1 Amount of poliovirus required to cause paralysis in ICR-PVRTg1 mice

Route of inoculation	Mahoney strain	Sabin 1 strain
Intraspinal	n.t.[a]	>1[b]
Intracerebral	>1~2	>6
Intraperitoneal	>4~5	>7
Intravenous	>4~5	>7
Oral	>6~7	>8

[a]Not tested.
[b]Logarithmic value of pfu.

to poliovirus inoculation by various routes are summarized in Table 1. The mice are very sensitive to poliovirus when viruses are inoculated into the CNS. The mice are less sensitive when virus is inoculated via peripheral routes such as intraperitoneal and intravenous routes. The mice are also sensitive to oral inoculation of poliovirus, although the sensitivity is not as high as in humans and chimpanzees (Table 1) (Bodian 1955, 1956). Similar low rate of "virus take" from the alimentary canal is well known for monkeys.

Regardless of inoculation routes, poliovirus finally invades the neurons in the brain stem and spinal cord. Histological lesions including neuronal degeneration and cellular infiltration are observed mainly in the brain stem and spinal cord of paralyzed mice. Poliovirus antigens or poliovirus genome RNA is always detected in neurons but not in glia cells in these sites of paralyzed mice (Fig. 1A) (Koike et al. 1991b; Ren and Racaniello 1992a; Horie et al. 1994). This indicates that the paralysis of mice is due to direct destruction of neurons in the brain stem and spinal cord. Similar conditions have been found in these tissues of monkeys (Hashimoto et al. 1984; Couderc et al. 1989). The clinical and pathological similarities between Tg mice and monkeys strongly suggest that the mouse model can become a new animal model for the study of poliovirus pathogenicity.

With any route of infection, many more doses of virus were required for the attenuated strain to cause paralysis as compared with the virulent strain (Table 1) (Koike et al. 1991b). Developments of the disease caused by the virulent and attenuated strains are also different from each other. In mice intracerebrally inoculated with the virulent Mahoney strain of the type 1 poliovirus, disease developed very rapidly, and all mice died within 24 hours after the onset of paralysis in all limbs or, in some cases, in the front limbs (Horie et al. 1994). These observations support a strong neurovirulence phenotype of this virus in the Tg mice. On the other hand, most Tg mice inoculated with the attenuated Sabin 1 virus developed paralysis in the hind limbs and then later in the front limbs (Horie et al.

A

B

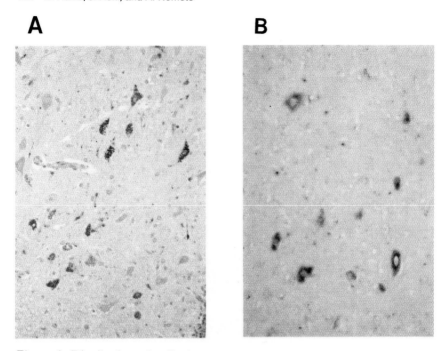

Figure 1 Distribution of poliovirus antigens and PVR mRNA. (*A*) Poliovirus antigens (brown spots) were detected at neurons in the medulla oblongata of a paralyzed ICR-PVRTg1 mouse after inoculation of poliovirus Mahoney strain intracerebrally as described by Koike et al. (1991b). (*B*) PVR mRNA was detected by in situ hybridization. PVR RNA probe labeled with digoxigenin-UTP was hybridized to a section of medulla oblongata of an ICR-PVRTg1 mouse. After hybridization and subsequent washing, a hybridization signal in the section was detected using anti-digoxigenin antibody conjugated with alkaline phosphatase. Color reaction was performed with 5-bromo-4-chloro-3-indolyl phosphate and nitroblue tetrazolium.

1994). In this case, development of the disease was relatively slow, and the mice survived for 1–5 days with signs of paralysis. Some mice survived with signs of paralysis indefinitely. The results supported a less neurovirulent phenotype of the Sabin 1 virus in the Tg mice. Thus, the virulent and attenuated phenotypes of poliovirus strains are obviously preserved in the Tg mice.

In contrast to the high sensitivity of ICR-PVRTg1 mice, TgPVR1-17 mice are less susceptible to poliovirus infection: 5×10^5 pfu of the Mahoney virus is required for paralysis by the intracerebral route. In addition, TgPVR1-17 mice orally inoculated with 1×10^9 pfu of the Mahoney virus do not show paralysis (Ren et al. 1990). ICR-PVRTg21 and ICR-PVRTg5 (Koike et al. 1991b) are less sensitive than ICR-PVRTg1. The reason for this difference in susceptibility is not known.

The differences in genetic background or amount of PVR expressed may influence the sensitivity.

TISSUE TROPISM OF POLIOVIRUS IN TRANSGENIC MICE

Susceptibility of animal tissues to poliovirus must be governed by many factors, such as physical accessibility of virus to cells, virus entry ability into cells, and virus replication ability in the subsequent steps. Furthermore, all these steps of virus replication involve host immunological and physiological conditions. Thus, mechanisms for the development of poliomyelitis are very complicated and therefore difficult to elucidate. One possible approach to solve this problem is to determine the distribution of the PVR in susceptible and nonsusceptible tissues and to compare it with poliovirus dissemination routes.

Distribution of Human PVR in Transgenic Mice and Humans

Adsorption of virus to the cell surface is the essential step to initiate virus infection. Holland (1961) proposed after measuring the binding activity of tissue homogenates to poliovirus that the receptor affinity is a major determinant of the tissue tropism of poliovirus infection. Since then, more elegant techniques to determine the tissue distribution of PVR have been developed and applied to clarify the molecular mechanisms for tissue-specific pathogenesis of poliovirus.

Expression of the PVR gene in Tg mice has so far been examined by several methods, including Northern blot hybridization, in situ hybridization, and Western blotting. However, detection of PVR protein by immunohistochemical analysis has not been carried out. Northern blot analysis with human PVR cDNA as a probe was carried out to analyze human PVR transcripts expressed in various tissues of Tg mice (Fig. 2A) (Ren et al. 1990; Koike et al. 1991b). The cDNA probe detected human PVR mRNAs at a position corresponding to a length of approximately 3.4 kb of poly(A)$^+$ RNA from almost all tissues tested. The brain and spinal cord consistently expressed high levels of PVR mRNA in any lines of Tg mice, whereas liver and small intestine expressed low levels. Thus, expression patterns of human PVR mRNA in different transgenic mouse lines were similar but not identical to each other (Ren et al. 1990; Koike et al. 1991b). Polymerase chain reaction (PCR) analysis established for identification of PVR mRNA isoforms (Koike et al. 1990) revealed that mRNA species for PVRα (functional PVR), PVRβ, and PVRγ exist in RNA of all tissues tested (Koike et al. 1991b; Ren and Racaniello 1992a). This indicates that mRNA for functional PVR,

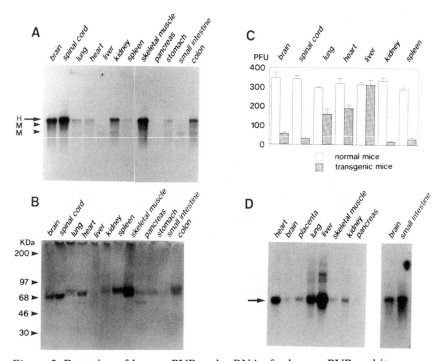

Figure 2 Detection of human PVR and mRNAs for human PVR and its mouse homologs. (*A*) Northern blot analysis of human PVR mRNA and mouse PVR homolog mRNA in ICR-PVRTg1. Poly(A)⁺ RNA was prepared from the tissues of ICR-PVRTg1 mice. Human PVR cDNA probe was used for the hybridized reaction. Filter was washed with 1x SSC containing 0.1% SDS at 65°C. An arrow with H indicates a position of human PVR mRNA, and arrowheads with M indicate positions of mouse PVR homolog mRNAs cross-hybridized to the human PVR cDNA probe. (*B*) Western blot analysis of human PVR in ICR-PVRTg1. Membrane fractions of various tissues of ICR-PVRTg1 were prepared and blotted onto a nitrocellulose filter. Human PVR was detected by an ^{125}I-labeled anti-PVR monoclonal antibody, 5H5. (*C*) Poliovirus-binding activity of tissues of ICR-PVRTg1. One ml of 5% tissue homogenates of ICR-PVRTg1 in phosphate-buffered saline was incubated with 300 pfu of poliovirus Mahoney strain for 1 hr at 37°C. The virus titer of the mixture was determined by plaque assay. (*D*) Northern blot analysis of human PVR mRNA. Multiple tissue Northern blot filter (Clontech) was used for the detection of PVR mRNAs (*left*). Poly(A)⁺ RNAs from the human brain and small intestine (Clontech) were used for the Northern blot hybridization experiment (*right*). Experimental conditions are the same as in *A* except that filters were washed with 0.1x SSC containing 0.1% SDS. The arrow indicates the position of PVR mRNA.

PVRα, is expressed in almost all tissues, including nonsusceptible tissues.

Expression of PVR mRNAs in TgPVR1-17 mice was more precisely determined by in situ hybridization (Ren and Racaniello 1992a). High-level expression of PVR mRNAs was observed in neurons of the central and peripheral nervous systems. In ICR-PVRTg1, we observed that the PVR mRNA is expressed at high levels in the neurons in the brain stem and spinal cord (Fig. 1B). PVR mRNA was not detected in the glia cells. These data clearly indicate that human PVR genes are effectively expressed in the neurons of the Tg mice, the final targets of poliovirus. Besides these tissues, PVR mRNA is expressed in TgPVR1-17 mice at high levels in developing T lymphocytes in the thymus, epithelial cells of Bowman's capsule and tubules in the kidney, alveolar cells in the lung, and endocrine cells in the adrenal cortex (Ren and Racaniello 1992a).

Detection of PVR mRNA by Northern blot hybridization and in situ hybridization, however, does not provide information concerning the alternative splicing of PVR mRNA and posttranslational modification of PVR protein. Accordingly, we employed Western blotting of membrane fractions from various tissues of ICR-PVRTg1 (Fig. 2B). The amounts of PVR detected (Fig. 2B) roughly correlated with those of PVR mRNA (Fig. 2A), indicating that the membrane-bound form of PVR is expressed in these tissues. Interestingly, apparent molecular weights of PVRs in different tissues were not identical. In the brain and spinal cord, an approximately 70-kD band was observed. In many other tissues, however, the bands migrated to positions larger than 70 kD (Fig. 2B). Additional faster-migrating bands were detected in some tissues. PVR was not detected in the liver.

To examine whether this heterogeneity of the PVR molecule affects the poliovirus-binding activity, we determined the binding activity of the tissue homogenates to poliovirus according to the method of Holland (1961). It has been shown that PVR fractions convert native 160S poliovirus particles to "A particle" (135S) by binding, and that A particle is not infectious any more (Frickes and Hogle 1990; Kaplan et al. 1990; Koike et al. 1992b). As shown in Figure 2C, tissue homogenates prepared from brain, spinal cord, heart, lung, kidney, and spleen show binding activity to poliovirus. This suggests that the PVRs of higher molecular weights also have poliovirus-binding activity. However, it is not known whether this heterogeneity affects poliovirus infection in steps other than binding. Poliovirus-binding activity of tissue homogenates from TgPVR1-17 was demonstrated in a similar experiment (Ren et al. 1990).

Distribution of human PVR mRNA in human tissues and in Tg mice
was compared by Northern blot hybridization. Distribution of PVR
mRNA in human tissues is shown in Figure 2D. PVR mRNA expression
was detected in all human tissues tested. Human PVR mRNAs were expressed at high levels in the liver, lung, heart, and small intestine, and at
low levels in the brain. Thus, the expression pattern of PVR mRNA in
humans is greatly different from those in mice (Fig. 2A,D). The regulation mechanisms of the human PVR gene introduced in mice may not be
the same as those in humans. cis-Acting elements on the human PVR
gene may not function properly in mice, or the transgene may not contain
all the cis-acting elements. The expression pattern of the mouse PVR
homolog (Morrison and Racaniello 1992) indicated by arrowheads with
M in Figure 2A is similar to that of PVR mRNA in humans (Fig. 2D).
Differences in the expression patterns in humans and Tg mice may result
in different poliovirus pathogenesis. If this is the case, the results obtained from the experiments with Tg mice may not always reflect the
phenomena in primates. The expression pattern of PVR molecules in various tissues of primates should be elucidated.

Dissemination of Poliovirus in Transgenic Mice

Investigation of the dissemination route after oral administration is of
great interest, because it may mimic the natural infection in humans. We
investigated virus replication in the tissues of ICR-PVRTg1 mice after
administration of 3×10^8 pfu of light-sensitive poliovirus Mahoney strain
via oral routes. In this condition, about 80–90% of Tg mice developed
paralysis. Ten mice were sacrificed every day, and the virus titers of the
tissue homogenates were determined. The results are shown in Table 2.

The virus was recovered in the small intestine one day after administration of the virus. Therefore, the small intestine was considered to be
the primary multiplication site of the virus. Some Tg mice excreted up to
several hundred pfu of poliovirus in the feces (Table 3). This indicated
that poliovirus replicated in the alimentary tract of the mice, although the
multiplication rate was very low compared to a chimpanzee model
(Bodian 1955; Nathanson and Bodian 1961). This may be due to the low
expression level of PVR in the small intestine in ICR-PVRTg1 (Fig.
2A,B). Two days after administration and later, viremia was observed in
many Tg mice. This indicated that the poliovirus was circulating in the
mouse bodies. Levels of viruses recovered from most "nontarget" tissues
were usually very low. In one Tg mouse, extensive multiplication of
virus in the pancreas was exceptionally observed (mouse 25 in Table 2).
A large amount of poliovirus appeared in the lung, brain, and spinal cord

of Tg mice. Extensive multiplication of poliovirus in lung has not been reported in chimpanzees (Bodian 1955, 1956; Sabin 1956). Poliovirus first invaded the brain of the CNS two days after administration. Five days after administration, when the paralysis was observed, a large amount of virus was recovered from the spinal cord. The results suggested that poliovirus invades the brain first and spreads caudally to the spinal cord through the brain stem. Attempts to find the virus replication sites by immunohistochemistry and in situ hybridization in the extraneuronal sites were not successful, probably because the multiplication rate of the virus in these sites was too low to be detected by these methods. Therefore, further investigations are needed to identify the pathway of dissemination.

Ren and Racaniello (1992b) reported virus entry into the CNS by axonal pathway after the inoculation of the virus into the muscle of a limb. Multiplication of the virus in skeletal muscle was observed, although the expression level of PVR was low. Initial paralysis occurred only in the inoculated limb, and paralysis was not observed in mice that had been denervated. A similar result was observed in monkeys inoculated with the neurotropic MV strain intramuscularly (Nathanson and Bodian 1961). Localization of initial paralysis to the inoculation site was also observed in humans in "the Cutter incident" (Nathanson and Langmuir 1963). This incident occurred after injection of imperfectly inactivated vaccine to children. These results indicated that direct axonal pathways from the inoculated muscle to soma of motor neurons were operative in Tg mice, monkeys, and humans. However, involvement of this route after oral infection has not been proved in chimpanzees. Indeed, the virus was not isolated from the muscle of chimpanzees during previremic and viremic periods (Bodian 1955, 1956). In the case of ICR-PVRTg1 (Table 2), only a small amount of the virus was recovered from the skeletal muscle, and the initial invasion sites in the CNS appear to be in the brain. This observation is inexplicable if virus spreads by axonal pathway from the muscle, because the virus should have appeared in the spinal cord earlier than in the brain by this route (Ren and Racaniello 1992b). These data suggest that orally administered poliovirus invades the CNS through the blood-brain barrier.

As shown in Table 2, a large amount of virus was detected in tissues of the CNS and the lung of many ICR-PVRTg1 mice, but relatively smaller amounts of virus in other sites. These observations indicate that poliovirus effectively replicates in tissues of the CNS and the lung but not in other tissues. In some tissues, the degree of poliovirus susceptibility correlates well with the expression level of PVR (Fig. 2B). For example, poliovirus effectively replicated in the CNS where a large

Table 2. Dissemination of poliovirus in ICR-PVRTg1 after oral administration

days after administration	1									2									
Mouse No.	1	2	3	4	5	6	7	8	9	10	11	12	13	14	15	16	17	18	19
brain (-brain stem)								2.3	4.2				1.5	4.4	5.7	6.5	6.5	6.1	6.5
brain stem								1.7				0.4			1.4	3.4	3.5		3.4
spinal cord								2.6		0.3						1.9	1.2	2.9	
lung								3.1	6.6				2.9		4.6	5.7	5.3	6.5	6.4
heart								3.3					1.5				1.2		
spleen								3.7		0.2	2.7	1.7			1.3	0.6	1.1	1.4	1.3
pancreas	N.T.d		N.T.					1.2	5.5			1.0			1.0			3.0	
kidney								3.7					2.3					1.7	1.7
liver								1.7	4.4				2.8					1.1	1.7
stomach								1.1	3.1		0.6	3.6	0.9	0.9	1.4	1.6	0.9	1.8	1.2
small intestine	1.2	2.3	2.5	1.8	1.7	2.5	1.5	1.7	3.7		1.0	2.0			1.1				
colon						0.7	0.5		1.9		0.2	1.0			0.4		1.3	1.5	
skeletal muscle b							1.0		2.5		1.0	1.0					1.7		
plasma a									4.3			3.6			1.3			1.7	2.0

amount of membrane-bound PVR was produced, and hardly replicated in the liver where no detectable amount of PVR was produced. However, poliovirus multiplication rates do not correlate with expression levels of PVR in tissues of the lung, kidney, and skeletal muscle. These observations could also pertain to humans, because the liver, which is not identified as a poliovirus replication site, produces a large amount of PVR mRNAs (Fig. 2D). Furthermore, distribution of PVR mRNAs in Tg mice and humans differs, as mentioned above. Nevertheless, poliovirus causes a similar paralytic disease in humans and Tg mice. These results indicate that susceptibility of tissues to poliovirus is not determined only by tissue distribution of PVR. Tissue tropism of poliovirus may also be determined by the stage of virus invasion into tissues from blood stream

3								4						5									
20	21	22	23	24	25	26	27	28	29	30	31	32	33[c]	34	35	36	37[c]	38[c]	39[c]	40[c]	41[c]	42[c]	43[c]
		6.2	1.5	7.0	7.0	7.2	7.1				4.9	7.0	7.0	2.0		6.4	6.8	6.9	6.9	6.4	6.7	6.7	7.0
		5.4	1.1	4.8	3.0	5.2	5.4				6.4	7.0	7.2			6.8	7.6	7.4	7.4	7.3	6.9	7.5	6.9
		3.6	1.1	2.3	1.7	0.9	1.9			1.0	5.0	3.7	7.3	2.4		6.3	7.5	7.5	7.7	7.6	7.3	7.6	7.5
		4.9	4.5	6.0	6.5	5.8	5.9	4.2	1.1	1.6		5.4	5.5	2.8			1.1	4.0	4.5	4.7	4.7	5.3	5.5
			1.2		2.6							1.2	1.3	2.9				1.6	1.3		2.7	1.1	
				2.1	5.6	2.1	1.3				3.5		3.2	3.2			2.5	3.3	2.7	3.6	2.6	2.4	
				2.1	7.5		1.6				5.9	1.1	1.1	3.0				1.1	4.7	1.0	2.6	4.2	1.1
				1.7	4.0						3.1			2.5					2.0		2.0	2.1	
				1.7	4.5						3.4		3.0	3.1			1.7	3.0		3.1	4.4	3.1	N.T.
	0.6		2.4	1.2	4.0		1.8	1.6			4.9			2.8	0.6			2.4	3.0	1.3	3.4		1.8
1.6			1.7	1.7	4.5		1.7				5.1		1.7	2.9			1.7			4.1	2.5	3.6	
0.4	0.5			1.2	3.8						4.0			2.0	1.3					3.7		2.4	2.2
			2.0	1.7	1.7						1.7	1.7	2.3	1.7	2.6		2.4			3.1	1.7		1.7
			1.7	2.3	4.1	2.4	4.2	1.0				1.7	2.5	1.7	2.2	1.0	2.7	3.4		3.6	4.6		

Results of mice in which poliovirus was not detected were not shown. $\log_{10}$pfu/tissue.
[a] $\log_{10}$pfu/ml.
[b] Skeletal muscle isolated from hindlimbs.
[c] Paralyzed.
[d] Not tested.

and/or by virus replication efficiency after entry into cells. Tissue-specific distribution of every host cell factor supporting poliovirus replication may solve the latter problem.

MOUSE NEUROVIRULENCE TESTS

Since the development of the disease and the dose of viruses required for paralysis are different in individual virus strains, Tg mice could be used for the identification of attenuation determinants and safety tests for oral live vaccine lots. It is a great advantage of the mouse system that planned production, control of genetic background, and control of pathogens can be done. These characteristics of the mouse system can overcome problems associated with the monkey system. Therefore, we believe that Tg

Table 3 Recovery of poliovirus excreted from ICR-PVRTg1 mice

Tg mice No.	Days after administration													
	1	2	3	4	5	6	7	8	9	10	11	12	13	14
1	–	–	–	+	–	d								
2	–	–	–	–	–	–	d							
3	–	–	–	+	–	–	–	–	–	–	–	–	–	–
4	–	++	+	+	–	d								
5	–	++	++	+	+	d								
6	–	+	++	–	–	d								
7	–	++	–	–	–	d								
8	+	+	–	–	–	d								
9	–	+	–	–	–	d								

(–) Virus not detected; (+) 10 to 100 pfu; (++) more than 100 pfu; (d) died.

mice provide a much better animal model for studying poliovirus neurovirulence than monkeys.

Recombinant viruses between the Mahoney and Sabin 1 strains were subjected to neurovirulence tests using the Tg mice, ICR-PVRTg1 (Horie et al. 1994). The genome structures of the recombinant viruses are shown in Figure 3. Mice inoculated with these viruses were observed for death up to 14 days and LD_{50} values were estimated (Fig. 3). LD_{50} values seemed not to change even if the observation period was longer. The LD_{50} values for the Mahoney (PV1(M)pDS306) and Sabin 1 (PV1 (Sab)IC-0) viruses were $10^{2.0}$ and more than $10^{6.3}$ pfu, respectively. Most other recombinant viruses showed intermediate neurovirulence levels.

Allele replacement of the Mahoney genome segment upstream of 1122 by the corresponding Sabin 1 segment was most effective in increasing mouse LD_{50} values ($10^{2.0}$–$10^{4.8}$ pfu), and similar replacements of other genome segments resulted in changes of the values to a lesser extent (virus Nos. 1, 2–5 in Fig. 3). On the other hand, allele replacements of the Sabin 1 genome segments by the corresponding Mahoney segments resulted in decreasing mouse LD_{50} values (virus Nos. 6–10). Of these, replacement of a genome region upstream of 1122 was most effective in changing the mouse LD_{50} value. These data are compatible with those obtained in monkey neurovirulence tests and indicate that the strong neurovirulence determinant(s) resides in the genome region of the 5′-proximal 1122 nucleotides. The relative neurovirulence levels of individual viruses estimated by monkey and Tg mouse systems are similar to each other (Omata et al. 1986; Kohara et al. 1988; Horie et al. 1994). Mouse neurovirulence tests with intracerebral inoculation of poliovirus

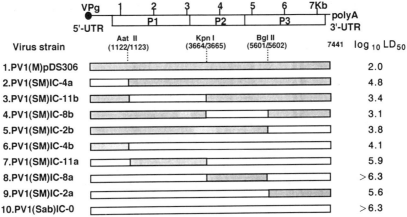

Figure 3 Genome structures of the recombinant type 1 polioviruses. Length of the genome of type 1 poliovirus is shown at the top of the figure in kilobases from the 5' terminus. Restriction enzyme sites used for the in vitro recombination between segments of the Mahoney and Sabin 1 strain genomes are shown. The genome structures of the recombinant viruses are shown as a combination of the Mahoney (PV1(M)pDS306) and the Sabin 1 (PV1(Sab)IC-0) sequences represented by shadowed and open boxes, respectively. The results of the neurovirulence tests using ICR-PVRTg1 mice are shown in LD_{50} logarithmic values at the right margin. (VPg) A genome linked protein; (UTR) untranslated region.

can therefore be used to distinguish most polioviruses with a wide range of neurovirulence levels, from the virulent Mahoney to attenuated Sabin 1 viruses.

ACKNOWLEDGMENTS

We thank Hiromichi Yonekawa for critical reading of the manuscript and for valuable suggestions. We also thank Yuko Kato, Etsuko Suzuki, and Atsuko Fujisawa for help in preparing the manuscript.

REFERENCES

Almond, J.W. 1987. The attenuation of poliovirus neurovirulence. *Annu. Rev. Microbiol.* **41:** 153.

Bernhardt, G., J.A. Bibb, J. Bradley, and E. Wimmer. 1994. Molecular characterization of the cellular receptor for poliovirus. *Virology* **199:** 105.

Bodian, D. 1955. Emerging concept of poliomyelitis infection. *Science* **122:** 105.

———. 1956. Poliovirus in chimpanzee tissues after virus feeding. *Am. J. Hyg.* **64:** 181.

Couderc, T., C. Christodoulou, H. Kopecka, S. Marsden, L.E. Taffs, R. Crainic, and F.

Horaud. 1989. Molecular pathogenesis of neural lesions induced by poliovirus type 1. *J. Gen. Virol.* **70:** 2907.

Crowell, R.L. and B.J. Landau. 1983. Receptors in the initiation of picornavirus infections. *Compr. Virol.* **18:** 1.

Evans, D.M.A., G. Dunn, P.D. Minor, G.C. Schild, A.J. Cann, G. Stanway, J.W. Almond, K. Currey, and J.V. Maizel, Jr. 1985. Increased neurovirulence associated with a single nucleotide change in a noncoding region of the Sabin type 3 poliovaccine genome. *Nature* **314:** 548.

Frickes, C.E. and J.M. Hogle. 1990. Cell-induced conformational change of poliovirus: Externalization of the amino terminus of VP1 is responsible for liposome binding. *J. Virol.* **64:** 1934.

Hashimoto, I., A. Hagiwara, and T. Komatsu. 1984. Ultrastructural studies on the pathogenesis of poliomyelitis in monkeys infected with poliovirus. *Acta Neuropathol.* **64:** 53.

Holland, J.J. 1961. Receptor affinities as major determinants of enterovirus tissue tropisms in humans. *Virology* **15:** 312.

Horie, H., S. Koike, T. Kurata, Y. Sato-Yoshida, I. Ise, Y. Ota, S. Abe, K. Hioki, H. Kato, C. Taya, T. Nomura, S. Hashizume, H. Yonekawa, and A. Nomoto. 1994. Transgenic mice carrying the human poliovirus receptor: New animal model for study of poliovirus neurovirulence. *J. Virol.* **68:** 681.

Jubelt, B., O. Narayan, and R.T. Johnson. 1980. Pathogenesis of human poliovirus infection in mice. I. Clinical and pathological studies. *J. Neuropathol. Exp. Neurol.* **39:** 138.

Kaplan, G.M., M.S. Freistadt, and V.R. Racaniello. 1990. Neutralization of poliovirus by cell receptors expressed in insect cells. *J. Virol.* **64:** 4697.

Kawamura, N., M. Kohara, S. Abe, T. Komatsu, K. Tago, M. Arita, and A. Nomoto. 1989. Determinants in the 5′ noncoding region of poliovirus Sabin 1 RNA that influence the attenuation phenotype. *J. Virol.* **63:** 1302.

Kohara, M., S. Abe, T. Komatsu, K. Tago, M. Arita, and A. Nomoto. 1988. A recombinant virus between the Sabin 1 and Sabin 3 vaccine strains of poliovirus as a possible candidate for a new type 3 poliovirus live vaccine strain. *J. Virol.* **62:** 2828.

Koike, S., I. Ise, and A. Nomoto. 1991a. Functional domains of poliovirus receptor. *Proc. Natl. Acad. Sci.* **88:** 4104.

Koike, S., I. Ise, Y. Sato, H. Yonekawa, O. Gotoh, and A. Nomoto. 1992a. A second gene for the African green monkey poliovirus receptor that has no putative N-glycosylation site in the functional N-terminal immunoglobulin-like domain. *J. Virol.* **66:** 7059.

Koike, S., I. Ise, Y. Sato, K. Mitsui, H. Horie, H. Umeyama, and A. Nomoto. 1992b. Early events of poliovirus infection. *Semin. Virol.* **3:** 109.

Koike, S., C. Taya, T. Kurata, S. Abe, I. Ise, H. Yonekawa, and A. Nomoto. 1991b. Transgenic mice susceptible to poliovirus. *Proc. Natl. Acad. Sci.* **88:** 951.

Koike, S., H. Horie, I. Ise, M. Yoshida, N. Iizuka, K. Takeuchi, T. Takegami, and A. Nomoto. 1990. Poliovirus receptor protein is produced both as membrane-bound and secreted forms. *EMBO J.* **9:** 3217.

La Monica, N., J.W. Almond, and V.R. Racaniello. 1987. A mouse model for poliovirus neurovirulence identifies mutations that attenuate the virus for humans. *J. Virol.* **61:** 2917.

La Monica, N., C. Meriam, and V.R. Racaniello. 1986. Mapping of sequences required for mouse neurovirulence of poliovirus type 2 Lansing. *J. Virol.* **57:** 515.

Macadam, A.J., S.R. Pollard, G. Ferguson, G. Dunn, R. Skuce, J.W. Almond, and P.D. Minor. 1991. The 5′ noncoding region of the type 2 poliovirus vaccine strain contains determinants of attenuation and temperature sensitivity. *Virology* **181:** 451.

Martin, A., C. Wychowski, T. Couderc, R. Crainic, J. Hogle, and M. Girard. 1988. Engineering a poliovirus type 2 antigenic site on a type 1 capsid results in a chimaeric virus which is neurovirulent for mice. *EMBO J.* **7:** 2839.

Martin, A., D. Benichou, T. Couderc, J.M. Hogle, C. Wychowski, S. van der Werf, and M. Girard. 1991. Use of type 1/type 2 chimeric polioviruses to study determinants of poliovirus type 1 neurovirulence in a mouse model. *Virology* **180:** 648.

Mendelsohn, C.L., E. Wimmer, and V.R. Racaniello. 1989. Cellular receptor for poliovirus: Molecular cloning, nucleotide sequence, and expression of a new member of the immunoglobulin superfamily. *Cell* **56:** 855.

Miller, D.A., O.J. Miller, V.G. Dev, S. Hashmi, R. Tantravahi, L. Medrano, and H. Green. 1974. Human chromosome 19 carries a poliovirus receptor gene. *Cell* **1:** 167.

Morrison, M.E., and V.R. Racaniello. 1992. Molecular cloning and expression of a murine homolog of the human poliovirus receptor gene. *J. Virol.* **66:** 2807.

Moss, E.G. and V.R. Racaniello. 1991. Host range determinants located in the interior of the poliovirus capsid. *EMBO J.* **10:** 1067.

Moss, E.G., R.E. O'Neill, and V.R. Racaniello. 1989. Mapping of attenuating sequences of an avirulent poliovirus type 2 strain. *J. Virol.* **63:** 1884.

Murray, M.G., J. Bradley, X.F. Yang, E. Wimmer, E.G. Moss, and V.R. Racaniello. 1988. Poliovirus host range is determined by a short amino acid sequence in neutralization antigenic site 1. *Science* **241:** 213.

Nathanson, N. and D. Bodian. 1961. Experimental poliomyelitis following intramuscular virus infection. 1. The effect of neural block on a neurotropic and a pantropic strain. *Bull. Johns Hopkins Hosp.* **108:** 308.

Nathanson, N. and A.D. Langmuir. 1963. The Cutter incident — Poliomyelitis following formaldehyde-inactivated poliovirus vaccination in the United States during the spring of 1955. III. Comparison of the clinical character of vaccinated and contact cases occurring after use of high rate lots of Cutter vaccine. *Am. J. Hyg.* **78:** 61.

Nomoto, A. and S. Koike. 1992. Molecular mechanisms of poliovirus pathogenesis. In *Molecular neurovirology* (ed. R.P. Roos), p. 251. Humana Press, Totowa, New Jersey.

Nomoto, A. and E. Wimmer. 1987. Genetic studies of the antigenicity and the attenuation phenotype of poliovirus. In *SGM40, molecular basis of virus disease* (ed. W.C. Russell and J.W. Almond), p. 107. Cambridge University Press, England.

Omata, T., M. Kohara, S. Kuge, T. Komatsu, S. Abe, B.L. Semler, A. Kameda, H. Itoh, M. Arita, E. Wimmer, and A. Nomoto. 1986. Genetic analysis of the attenuation phenotype of poliovirus type 1. *J. Virol.* **58:** 348.

Paul, J.R. 1971. *A history of poliomyelitis.* Yale University Press, New Haven, Connecticut.

Ren, R. and V.R. Racaniello. 1992a. Human poliovirus receptor gene expression and poliovirus tissue tropism in transgenic mice. *J. Virol.* **66:** 296.

————. 1992b. Poliovirus spreads from muscle to the central nervous system by neural pathways. *J. Infect Dis.* **166:** 747.

Ren, R., E.G. Moss, and V.R. Racaniello. 1991. Identification of two determinants that attenuate vaccine-related type 2 poliovirus. *J. Virol.* **65:** 1377.

Ren, R., F. Costantini, E.J. Gorgacz, J.J. Lee, and V.R. Racaniello. 1990. Transgenic mice expressing a human poliovirus receptor: A new model for poliomyelitis. *Cell* **63:** 353.

Sabin, A.B. 1956. Pathogenesis of poliomyelitis. Reappraisal in the light of new data. *Science* **123:** 1151.

Sabin, A.B. and L.R. Boulger. 1973. History of Sabin attenuated poliovirus oral live vaccine strains. *J. Biol. Stand.* **1:**115.

Selinka, H.-C., A. Zibert, and E. Wimmer. 1991. Poliovirus can enter and infect mammalian cells by way of an intracellular adhesion molecule 1 pathway. *Proc. Natl. Acad. Sci.* **88:** 3598.

Siddique, T., R. Mckinney, W. Hung, R.J. Bartlett, G. Bruns, T.K. Mohandas, H. Ropers, C. Wiltert, and A.D. Poses. 1988. The poliovirus sensitivity (PVS) gene is on chromosome 19q12-q13.2. *Genomics* **3:** 156.

Westrop, G.D., D.M.A. Evans, G. Dunn, P.D. Minor, D.I. Magrath, F. Taffs, S. Marsden, K.A. Wareham, M. Skinner, G.C. Schild, and J.W. Almond. 1989. Genetic basis of attenuation of the Sabin type 3 oral poliovaccine. *J. Virol.* **63:** 1338.

World Health Organization (WHO). 1990. Requirements for poliomyelitis vaccine. *WHO Tech. Rep. Ser.* **800:** 30.

Zibert, A. and E. Wimmer. 1992. N glycosylation of the virus binding domain 1 is not essential for function of the human poliovirus receptor. *J. Virol.* **66:** 7368.

Zibert, A., H.-C. Selinka, O. Elroy-Stein, B. Moss, and E. Wimmer. 1991. Vaccinia virus-mediated expression and identification of the human poliovirus receptor. *Virology* **182:** 250.

24

Lymphocyte Homing Receptor CD44 and Poliovirus Attachment

Michael P. Shepley
Department of Microbiology
Columbia University College of Physicians and Surgeons
New York, New York 10032

IDENTIFICATION OF CELLULAR PROTEINS INVOLVED
IN POLIOVIRUS ATTACHMENT

Poliovirus, the causative agent of poliomyelitis, is a member of the Picornaviridae, a family of single-stranded RNA viruses that cause a variety of human diseases (Ginsberg 1980). Infection of susceptible cells begins when the viral capsid, which consists of 60 copies of each of four proteins arranged in icosahedral symmetry, binds to a receptor site on the cell surface. Most strains of poliovirus infect only primates and replicate primarily in the intestine, tonsils, deep cerebellar nuclei, brain stem, motor cortex, and anterior spinal gray matter (Bodian 1949). Results of studies utilizing organ minces and homogenates suggest that the tissue tropism and species specificity of poliovirus are determined primarily by the presence or absence of unique virus-binding activity (Holland 1961).

During the 1980s, several monoclonal antibodies, directed against the surface of susceptible cells, were isolated that blocked poliovirus binding and infection (Minor et al. 1984; Nobis et al. 1985; Shepley et al. 1988). Antibodies 280 and D171 specifically blocked poliovirus infection and were subsequently found to be directed against the same protein (Minor et al. 1984; Nobis et al. 1985; V. Racaniello, pers. comm.). A third monoclonal antibody, AF3, which preferentially blocked type 2 poliovirus, detected a 100-kD glycoprotein only in cells and tissues permissive to poliovirus infection (Shepley 1988; Shepley et al. 1988). Antibody D171 was utilized to isolate and clone poliovirus receptor (PVR) cDNA, which encodes a new member of the immunoglobulin superfamily (Mendelsohn et al. 1989). This cDNA confers poliovirus binding and infectivity onto mouse L cells for all three serotypes of virus.

Examination of the expression pattern of the PVR, however, indicates that a more complex relationship exists between PVR expression and virus tropism because PVR mRNA and protein are expressed in a wide range of tissues, including those that poliovirus does not normally infect (Mendelsohn et al. 1989; Freistadt et al. 1990; Koike et al. 1993). Furthermore, inoculation of transgenic mice, expressing human PVR, with poliovirus results in replication mainly in neurons in the brain and spinal cord, and in skeletal muscle cells, despite expression of PVR mRNA in other sites, including developing T lymphocytes of the thymus, Bowman's capsule and tubules in the kidney, alveolar cells of the lung, endocrine cells in the adrenal cortex, and intestine and spleen (Ren and Racaniello 1992). The tissue tropism of poliovirus therefore appeared to be controlled by cellular factors other than PVR, either at the cell surface or in the cytoplasm, that determine the outcome of infection. Consequently, the 100-kD protein identified by antibody AF3 appears to be a candidate for an additional determinant of poliovirus tropism because, unlike PVR expression, the organ- and tissue-type expression of the 100-kD protein correlates with poliovirus tropism (Shepley et al. 1988).

Antibody AF3 was isolated by its ability to block poliovirus infection in HeLa cells, and it was subsequently found to identify a 100-kD glycoprotein only in cells and tissues permissive to poliovirus infection. In an immunohistochemical survey of the human brain stem, antibody AF3 binding precisely correlated with those areas that are damaged by poliomyelitis of the brain stem, including the periaqueductal motor nuclei, suggesting that the 100-kD protein may be involved in the pathogenesis of poliomyelitis and in the cellular function of the PVR site (Bodian 1949; Shepley 1988; Shepley et al. 1988). The 100-kD protein, now known to be CD44, was subsequently shown to be incapable of binding poliovirus (Shepley and Racaniello 1994). Thus, a 100-kD variant of CD44 appears to be involved in poliovirus attachment in vitro and is expressed in a manner that precisely correlates with poliovirus tropism in vivo, yet only the protein encoded by the PVR cDNA cloned by Mendelsohn et al. (1989) binds poliovirus. One possibility is that a second cell-surface protein, such as CD44, may be required, with PVR, for entry of poliovirus into susceptible tissues. This is a particularly strong possibility, since infectious particles can be generated in a number of receptor-deficient cells transfected with poliovirus cDNA or mRNA, demonstrating that the block to replication is not at the level of the cytoplasm (Holland et al. 1959a,b; Racaniello and Baltimore 1981).

THE CD44 FAMILY OF PROTEINS

CD44, a member of the cartilage link family of proteins (Stamenkovic et al. 1989), is a heterogeneously glycosylated, multifunctional family of molecules identified initially with a number of monoclonal antibodies

(Dalchau et al. 1980; Hughes et al. 1981; Carter 1982; Telen et al. 1983 1984; Jalkanen et al. 1986a,b, 1987, 1988; Haynes et al. 1989 1991). The CD44 family of proteins comprises three general size classes: The major species found in hematopoietic (CD44H) and nonhematopoietic cells have molecular masses ranging from 80 kD to 110 kD (Dalchau et al. 1980; Hughes et al. 1983; Isacke et al. 1986; Jalkanen et al. 1988; Omary et al. 1988; Shimizu et al. 1989; Stamenkovic et al. 1989, 1991; Dougherty et al. 1991); a species primarily associated with epithelial cells (CD44E) has molecular masses ranging from 130 kD to 160 kD (Omary et al. 1988; Picker et al. 1989a; Stamenkovic et al. 1989, 1991; Dougherty et al. 1991); and a minor species associated with a variety of cell types is modified by chondroitin sulfate resulting in molecular masses ranging from 180 kD to 215 kD (Jalkanen et al. 1988; Omary et al. 1988; Stamenkovic et al. 1989, 1991). Antibody AF3 reacts with the hematopoietic isoform, CD44H, which is considered to play major roles in lymph node homing for circulating lymphocytes, binding of hyaluronic acid, lymphocyte activation, and homotypic and heterotypic cell adhesion (Jalkanen et al. 1986a,b; Huet et al. 1989; Idzerda et al. 1989; Shimizu et al. 1989; Aruffo et al. 1990; Beltisos et al. 1990; Denning et al. 1990; Koopman et al. 1990). CD44H has a predicted extracellular domain of 248 amino acids, a 21-amino-acid transmembrane domain, and a 72-amino-acid cytoplasmic domain (Stamenkovic et al. 1989). Due to highly variable glycosylation, CD44H has an apparent molecular mass range of 80 kD to 110 kD.

IN VITRO STUDIES OF CD44H AND POLIOVIRUS ATTACHMENT

The 100-kD protein recognized by antibody AF3 was identified as CD44H by partial internal amino acid sequence derived from a 65-kD fragment resulting from cyanogen bromide cleavage of immunoaffinity-purified 100-kD protein (Shepley and Racaniello 1994). CD44H cDNA was cloned, and stable L-cell transformants were generated, which were used to further elucidate the role of CD44H in poliovirus attachment (Shepley and Racaniello 1994). The first two questions to address were (1) whether CD44H cDNA encoded for the AF3 epitope and (2) whether CD44H could act as a receptor for poliovirus. As shown in Table 1, antibody AF3 and the previously described anti-CD44 antibodies P3H9 and A3D8 reacted with mouse L cells transformed with CD44H cDNA but did not react with L cells transformed with PVR cDNA, demonstrating that CD44H cDNA encodes the AF3 epitope. The anti-PVR monoclonal antibody 711C did not react with L cells transformed with CD44H cDNA. Monolayers of L-cell transformants, expressing human

Table 1 Antibody immunoreactivity of transformant cell lines

Cell line	Antibodies			
	AF3	P3H9[a]	A3D8[a]	711C[b]
CD44H-pcDNA1/NEO.33.2[c]	+[d]	+	+	−
CD44H-pcDNA1/NEO.13.1[c]	+	+	+	−
PVR-pcDNA1/NEO.1	−	−	−	+
PVR-pSVL.20B	−	−	−	+
HeLa	+	+	+	+
L	−	−	−	−

[a]Anti-CD44 monoclonal antibodies.
[b]Anti-PVR monoclonal antibody.
[c]Independently derived L cell transformants.
[d]Determined by indirect immunofluorescence.

CD44H, were then inoculated with poliovirus to determine whether the cDNA conferred permissivity to infection with poliovirus onto receptor-deficient murine cells. As shown in Table 2, CD44H-L-cell transformants were not susceptible to poliovirus infection, demonstrating that CD44H did not act as a receptor for poliovirus.

Furthermore, binding of ^{125}I-labeled AF3 to HeLa cells, which express CD44, was inhibited by the anti-CD44 antibodies A3D8 and IM7, demonstrating functional overlap among the epitopes (Fig. 1). Finally, antibodies A3D8 and IM7, which react with epitopes that functionally overlap with that of antibody AF3, also inhibit poliovirus binding to HeLa cells. As shown in Figure 2, antibody A3D8 inhibited radiolabeled poliovirus binding as effectively as antibody AF3, IM7 inhibited virus to a lesser extent, the anti-PVR antibody 711C inhibited poliovirus binding maximally, and two irrelevant antibodies had no effect. Thus, antibodies to CD44 which inhibit ^{125}I-labeled AF3 binding to HeLa cells can also inhibit poliovirus binding to HeLa cells, yet CD44H cannot act as a receptor for the virus (Shepley and Racaniello 1994; M.P. Shepley, unpubl.). From these and other observations, a picture has begun to emerge of the role of CD44H in poliovirus attachment.

A SUBSET OF CD44H MOLECULES APPEARS TO INTERACT WITH PVR

Antibody A3D8 inhibits poliovirus binding as well as antibody AF3, yet A3D8 binds a wider molecular-weight range of CD44 (80–100 kD) compared to AF3 (100 kD). Furthermore, ^{125}I-labeled AF3-binding assays demonstrate that AF3 reacts, with high affinity, to less than 5% of the total CD44H expressed by HeLa cells (Shepley 1988). ^{125}I-labeled AF3-

Table 2 Susceptibility of CD44H transformants to poliovirus infection

Cell line	Time postinoculation			
	day 0	day 1	day 2	CPE day 4
CD44H-pcDNA1/NEO.33.2	<1[a]	<1	<1	–[b]
PVR-pcDNA1/NEO.1	<1	4×10^4	5×10^5	+
PVR-pSVL.20B	<1	4×10^4	5.5×10^6	+
L	<1	<1	<1	–

[a]pfu/ml on HeLa cells.
[b]Cytopathic effect determined by MTT/INT assay (Shepley et al. 1988).

binding assays, on the CD44H-L-cell transformants, demonstrate that
AF3 binds to the same small fraction of CD44H molecules with the same
affinity as was previously determined for HeLa cells (M.P. Shepley, unpubl.). Thus, the same magnitude of inhibition of poliovirus binding is

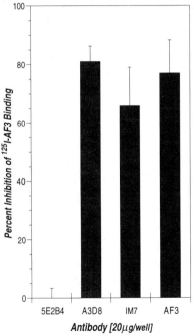

Figure 1 Competition between ^{125}I-labeled AF3 and anti-CD44 monoclonal
antibodies for binding to HeLa cells. All antibodies were preincubated with
HeLa cell monolayers at 400-fold higher concentration as compared to [125]I-
labeled AF3. Antibodies A3D8 and IM7 are anti-CD44 monoclonal antibodies.
5E2B4 is an irrelevant monoclonal antibody. ^{125}I-labeled AF3 was added at 10^5
cpm (~ 50 ng of immunoglobulin) per well. One standard deviation is indicated.

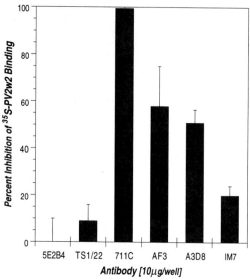

Figure 2   Inhibition of radiolabeled poliovirus type 2w2 binding to HeLa cells by monoclonal antibodies. The ability of antibody AF3 to inhibit virus binding to HeLa cell monolayers was compared with the anti-CD44 antibodies A3D8 and IM7 and the anti-PVR antibody 711C. 5E2B4 and TS1/22 are irrelevant monoclonal antibodies. All antibodies were preincubated with monolayers, after which 1.5×10^4 cpm of ^{35}S-labeled PV2w2 was added in the presence of antibody. One standard deviation is shown.

achieved whether a small, specific population of CD44 (that which reacts with AF3) or a much larger population of CD44 (that which reacts with A3D8) is induced to inhibit poliovirus binding. This suggests that the small population of specifically glycosylated CD44H species, the 100-kD species named $_{AF3}$CD44H, is primarily involved in the CD44H/PVR interaction. This hypothesis is particularly interesting, given the speculation by some investigators that differential glycosylation may alter the function of subpopulations of CD44 (Hardingham and Fosang 1992).

Immunohistochemical data also support the hypothesis that $_{AF3}$CD44H is a functionally distinct species. The anti-CD44 antibody F-10-44-2, which binds the same protein as antibody A3D8 (Telen et al. 1986), reacts with the white matter of human brain (McKenzie et al. 1982). The Hermes series of antibodies, which also bind to the same CD44 protein (Picker et al. 1989b), react with white matter, the periaqueductal gray matter of the brain stem, the anterior horn gray matter of the spinal cord, and much less so with posterior horn gray matter (Vogel et al. 1992). In contrast, antibody AF3 does not react with the white matter of the human brain stem, but it does react with the periaqueductal motor nuclei of the brain stem, as well as other brain stem nuclei which poliovirus infects (Shepley 1988; Shepley et al. 1988). Thus, $_{AF3}$CD44H appears to be a functionally distinct species of CD44H that is expressed in a pattern consistent with poliovirus tropism.

It is interesting that the anti-CD44 antibodies A3D8 and IM7 inhibit ^{125}I-labeled AF3 binding so well, since the antibodies most likely recognize different epitopes. If AF3 binds a different epitope than either antibodies A3D8 or IM7, how do A3D8 and IM7 inhibit ^{125}I-labeled AF3 binding? One possibility is that binding of A3D8 and IM7 may result in conformational changes in a spatially distinct AF3 epitope. Alternatively, the AF3 epitope and the A3D8 and IM7 epitopes may overlap. The AF3 epitope may only be present in the 100-kD species, but the A3D8 and IM7 epitopes may be present in many species of CD44H. When all three epitopes are present simultaneously, as in the 100-kD species, antibodies A3D8 and IM7 are able to inhibit AF3 binding. This hypothesis is particularly interesting, since the AF3 epitope would be situated within a cluster of overlapping epitopes previously identified by antibodies A3D8, IM7, and the Hermes 2 antibodies (Picker et al. 1989b), which can induce CD44-mediated modulation of other cellular events.

MOLECULAR BASIS OF THE CD44H-PVR INTERACTION

How CD44H interacts with PVR remains unknown, but several possibilities are consistent with the data. First, CD44H and PVR may be noncovalently associated. In this case, antibody AF3 or other CD44 antibodies would inhibit poliovirus binding by steric hindrance. It has been suggested that CD44 directly associates with LFA-3 in a noncovalent manner, providing LFA-3, which is anchored to the membrane by a phosphoinositol linkage, indirect anchorage to the cytoskeleton (Shimizu et al. 1989). It is not likely that the activity of AF3 results from nonspecific steric hindrance that would occur by binding of an antibody to an abundant cell-surface protein, because there are only approximately 4,100 $_{AF3}$CD44H molecules per HeLa cell compared to approximately 100,000 PVR molecules (Shepley 1988 and unpubl.). Second, CD44 may be associated with PVR only after it interacts with poliovirus. Antibodies to CD44 would block subsequent processes leading to viral entry. This hypothesis appears unlikely, since AF3 inhibits radiolabeled poliovirus binding to the same degree as inhibition of plaque formation of the virus, indicating that AF3 inhibits virus binding directly (Shepley et al. 1988). Third, CD44 may interact through other cellular elements without direct association with PVR. For example, an anti-CD44 antibody has been described that triggers CD44 on T lymphocytes to promote T-cell adhesion through the LFA-1 pathway (Koopman et al. 1990). Although lymphocyte adhesion is mediated through LFA-1, the anti-CD44 induction of adhesion is dependent on protein kinase C and an intact cytoskeleton. The PVR protein is sufficient to confer poliovirus binding and susceptibility to mouse cells (Mendelsohn et al. 1989). However, if $_{AF3}$CD44H is involved in steps other than virus binding directly, then a murine homolog of $_{AF3}$CD44H may also provide a similar function.

To further study the role of $_{AF3}$CD44H in poliovirus attachment to PVR, a large number of stable L-cell transformants that express both CD44H and PVR were isolated. These cell lines, however, could not be used to study the $_{AF3}$CD44H/PVR interaction, because their growth rate was greatly reduced in proportion to the level of expression of both proteins. High-level dual-expressing cells did not survive subcloning. Intermediate expressers could be cloned but quickly lost most surface expression as their growth rate increased. The use of inducible promoter systems did not overcome the growth inhibition, because low levels of promoter activity occurred in the absence of inducer. Other systems are being sought that may be used to determine the nature of the $_{AF3}$CD44H/PVR interaction.

Examples of the involvement of multiple cell-surface proteins in viral binding and entry have begun to emerge for other viruses (Spear et al. 1992; Callebaut et al. 1993; for review, see 1994). HIV-1 appears to require a second human cell factor in addition to the receptor, CD4, for entry of virus into cells. Although expression of human CD4 in a variety of human cell types results in susceptibility to HIV-1 infection (Maddon et al. 1986), murine cells expressing human CD4 cannot be infected, apparently due to a block subsequent to binding which can, in some cells, be overcome by expression of human CD26 (Callebaut et al. 1993). Adenovirus has been demonstrated to utilize the vitronectin-binding proteins $\alpha_v\beta_3$ and $\alpha_v\beta_5$ for viral entry, yet these proteins do not act as receptors for the virus, since antibodies to these cellular proteins do not block virus binding (Wickham et al. 1993). It is not surprising that multicomponent receptor/entry sites exist for viruses because most, if not all, cell-surface proteins interact with other cellular components. Once cellular proteins have been identified as being involved in viral attachment and/or entry, the next challenge is to elucidate the complexity of the interaction in terms of both viral pathogenesis and cellular function.

The finding that $_{AF3}$CD44H is involved in poliovirus attachment provides insight into the interaction of PVR with other cellular components and will facilitate understanding of the cellular function of PVR and the pathogenesis of poliomyelitis. These results may also lead to an elucidation of the structure/function relationships among the diversely glycosylated group of CD44 molecules and a new opportunity to study the processes underlying CD44-mediated cellular events.

ACKNOWLEDGMENTS

The author thanks Dr. Baruj Benacerraf of the Dana-Farber Cancer Institue (DFCI) for financial support, and Dr. Robert Finberg (DFCI) for space and equipment. The author also thanks Drs. Bernard Fields, Richard Colonno, Hamish Young, David Johnson, Patrick Hogan, and Vincent Racaniello for advice and critical input. M.P.S. was the recipient of a fellowship from the Dana-Farber Cancer Institute and the Jimmy Fund, and an Individual National Research Service Award from the National Institutes of Health. This work was also supported by a grant to Dr. Vincent Racaniello from the American Cancer Society.

REFERENCES

Aruffo, A., I. Stamenkovic, M. Melnick, C.B. Underhill, and B. Seed. 1990. CD44 is the principal cell receptor for hyaluronate. *Cell* **61:** 1303.

Beltisos, P.C., E.K. Hildreth, and J.T. August. 1990. Homotypic cell aggregation induced by anti-CD44(Pgp-1) monoclonal antibodies and related to CD44(Pgp-1) expression. *J. Immunol.* **144:** 1661.

Bodian, D. 1949. Histopathologic basis of clinical findings in poliomyelitis. *Am. J. Med.* **6:** 563.

Callebaut, C., B. Krust, E. Jacotot, and A.G. Hovanessian. 1993. T cell activation antigen, CD26, as a cofactor for entry of HIV in CD4+ cells. *Science* **262:** 2045.

Carter, W.G. 1982. The cooperative role of the transformation-sensitive glycoproteins, GP140 and fibronectin, in cell attachment and spreading. *J. Biol. Chem.* **257:** 3249.

Dalchau, R., J. Kirkley, and J. Fabre. 1980. Monoclonal antibody to a human brain-granulocyte-T lymphocyte antigen probably homologous to the W 3/13 antigen in rat. *Eur. J. Immunol.* **10:** 745.

Denning, S.M., P.T. Le, K.H. Singer, and B.F. Haynes. 1990. Antibodies against the CD44 p80, lymphocyte homing receptor molecule augment human peripheral blood T cell activation. *J. Immunol.* **144:** 7.

Dougherty, G.J., P.M. Lansdorp, D.L. Cooper, and R.K. Humphries. 1991. Molecular cloning of CD44R1 and CD44R2, two novel isoforms of the human CD44 lymphocyte "homing" receptor expressed on hemopoietic cells. *J. Exp. Med.* **174:** 1.

Freistadt, M., G. Kaplan, and V.R. Racaniello. 1990. Heterogeneous expression of poliovirus receptor-related proteins in human cells and tissues. *Mol. Cell. Biol.* **10:** 5700.

Ginsberg, H.S. 1980. Picornaviruses. In *Microbiology* (ed. B.D. Davis et al.), p. 1096. Harper and Row, Hagerstown, Maryland.

Hardingham, T.E. and A.J. Fosang. 1992. Proteoglycans: Many forms and many functions. *FASEB J.* **6:** 861.

Haynes, B.F., H.-X. Liao, and K.L. Patton. 1991. The transmembrane hyaluronate receptor (CD44): Multiple functions, multiple forms. *Cancer Cells* **3:** 347.

Haynes, B.F., M.J. Telen, L.P. Hale, and S.M. Denning. 1989. CD44–A molecule involved in leukocyte adherence and T-cell activation. *Immunol. Today* **10**: 423.

Haywood, A.M. 1994. Virus receptors: Binding, adhesion strengthening, and changes in viral structure. *J. Virol.* **68**: 1.

Holland, J.J. 1961. Receptor affinities as major determinants of enterovirus tissue tropism in humans. *Virology* **15**: 312.

Holland, J.J., L.C. McLaren, and J.T. Syverton. 1959a. Mammalian cell-virus relationship. III. Poliovirus production by non-primate cells exposed to poliovirus ribonucleic acid. *Proc. Soc. Exp. Biol. Med.* **100**: 843.

————. 1959b. Mammalian cell-virus relationship. IV. Infection of naturally insusceptible cells with enterovirus ribonucleic acid. *Proc. Soc. Exp. Biol. Med.* **110**: 65.

Huet, S., H. Groux, B. Caillou, H. Valentin, A.M. Prieur, and A. Bernard. 1989. CD44 contributes to T cell activation. *J. Immunol.* **143**: 798.

Hughes, E.N., A. Colombatti, and J.T. August. 1983. Murine cell surface glycoproteins. *J. Biol. Chem.* **258**: 1014.

Hughes, E.N., G. Mengod, and J.T. August. 1981. Murine cell surface glycoproteins. *J. Biol. Chem.* **256**: 7023.

Idzerda, R.L., W.G. Carter, C. Nottenberg, E.A. Wayner, W.M. Gallatin, and T. St. John. 1989. Isolation and DNA sequence of a cDNA clone encoding a lymphocyte adhesion receptor for high endothelium. *Proc. Natl. Acad. Sci.* **86**: 4659.

Isacke, C.M., C.A. Sauvage, R. Hyman, J. Lesley, R. Schulte, and I.S. Trowbridge. 1986. Identification and characterization of the human Pgp-1 glycoprotein. *Immunogenetics* **23**: 326.

Jalkanen, S.T., R.F. Bargatze, J. de los Toyos, and E.C. Butcher. 1987. Lymphocyte recognition of high endothelium: Antibodies to distinct epitopes of an 85-95-kD glycoprotein antigen differentially inhibit lymphocyte binding to lymph node, mucosal, or synovial endothelial cells. *J. Cell Biol.* **105**: 983.

Jalkanen, S.T., R.F. Bargatze, L.R. Herron, and E.C. Butcher. 1986a. A lymphoid cell surface glycoprotein involved in endothelial cell recognition and lymphocyte homing in man. *Eur. J. Immunol.* **16**: 1195.

Jalkanen, S.T., A.C. Steere, R.I. Fox, and E.C. Butcher. 1986b. A distinct endothelial cell recognition system that controls lymphocyte traffic into inflamed synovium. *Science* **233**: 556.

Jalkanen, S.T., M. Jalkanen, R. Bargetze, M. Tammi, and E.C. Butcher. 1988. Biochemical properties of glycoproteins involved in lymphocyte recognition of high endothelial venules in man. *J. Immunol.* **141**: 1615.

Koike, S., H. Horie, Y. Sato, I. Ise, C. Taya, T. Nomura, I. Yoshioka, H. Yonekawa, and A. Nomoto. 1993. Poliovirus-sensitive transgenic mice as a new animal model. *Dev. Biol. Stand.* **78**: 101.

Koopman, G., Y. van Kooyk, M. de Graaff, C.J. Meyer, C.G. Figdor, and S.T. Pals. 1990. Triggering of the CD44 antigen on T lymphocytes promotes T cell adhesion through the LFA-1 pathway. *J. Immunol.* **145**: 3589.

Maddon, P.J., A.G. Dalgleish, J.S. McDougal, P.R. Clapham, R.A. Weiss, and R. Axel. 1986. The T4 gene encodes for the AIDS virus receptor and is expressed in the immune system and in the brain. *Cell* **47**: 333.

McKenzie, J.L., R. Dalchau, and J.W. Fabre. 1982. Biochemical characterization and localization in brain of a human brain-leukocyte membrane glycoprotein recognized by a monoclonal antibody. *J. Neurochem.* **39**: 1461.

Mendelsohn, C.L., E. Wimmer, and V.R. Racaniello. 1989. Cellular receptor for poliovirus: Molecular cloning, nucleotide sequence, and expression of a new member of the immunoglobulin superfamily. *Cell* **56:** 855.

Minor, P.D., P.A. Pipkin, D. Hockley, G.C. Schild, and J.W. Almond. 1984. Monoclonal antibodies which block cellular receptors for poliovirus. *Virus Res.* **1:** 203.

Nobis, P., R. Zibbire, G. Meyer, J. Kuhne, G. Warnecke, and G. Koch. 1985. Production of a monoclonal antibody against an epitope on HeLa cells that is the functional poliovirus receptor site. *J. Gen. Virol.* **66:** 2563.

Omary, M.B., I.S. Trowbridge, M. Letarte, M.F. Kagnoff, and C.M. Isacke. 1988. Structural heterogeneity of human Pgp-1 and its relationship with p85. *Immunogenetics* **27:** 460.

Picker, L.J., M. Nakache, and E.C. Butcher. 1989a. Monoclonal antibodies to human lymphocyte homing receptors define a novel class of adhesion molecules on diverse cell types. *J. Cell Biol.* **109:** 927.

Picker, L.J., J. de los Toyos, M.J. Telen, B.F. Haynes, and E.C. Butcher. 1989b. Monoclonal antibodies against the CD44 [In(Lu)-related p80], and Pgp-1 antigens in man recognize the Hermes class of lymphocyte homing receptors. *J. Immunol.* **142:** 2046.

Racaniello, V.R. and D. Baltimore. 1981. Clones poliovirus complementary DNA is infectious in mammalian cells. *Science* **214:** 916.

Ren, R. and V.R. Racaniello. 1992. Human poliovirus receptor gene expression and poliovirus tissue tropism in transgenic mice. *J. Virol.* **66:** 296.

Shepley, M.P. 1988. "Monoclonal antibody identification of a 100 kD membrane protein in HeLa cells and human spinal cord involved in poliovirus attachment." Ph.D. thesis, Harvard Medical School, Cambridge, Massachusetts.

Shepley, M.P. and V.R. Racaniello. 1994. A monoclonal antibody that blocks poliovirus attachment recognizes the lymphocyte homing receptor CD44. *J. Virology* **68:** 1301.

Shepley, M., B. Sherry, and H. Weiner. 1988. Monoclonal antibody identification of a 100 kD membrane protein in HeLa cells and human spinal cord involved in poliovirus attachment. *Proc. Natl. Acad. Sci.* **85:** 7743.

Shimizu, Y., G. Van Seventer, R. Siraganian, L. Wahl, and S. Shaw. 1989. Dual role of the CD44 molecule in T cell adhesion and activation. *J. Immunol.* **143:** 2457.

Spear, P.G., M.T. Shieh, B.C. Herold, D. WuDunn, and T.I. Koshy. 1992. Heparin sulfate lycosaminoglycans as primary cell surface receptors for herpes simplex virus. *Adv. Exp. Med. Biol.* **313:** 341.

Stamenkovic, I., M. Amiot, J.M. Pesando, and B. Seed. 1989. A lymphocyte molecule implicated in lymph node homing is a member of the cartilage link protein family. *Cell* **56:** 1057.

Stamenkovic, I., A. Aruffo, M. Amiot, and B. Seed. 1991. The hematopoietic and epithelial forms of CD44 are distinct polypeptides with different adhesion potentials for hyaluronate-bearing cells. *EMBO J.* **10:** 343.

Telen, M.J., G.S. Eisenbarth, and B.F. Haynes. 1983. Human erythrocyte antigens. *J. Clin. Invest.* **71:** 1878.

Telen, M.J., T.J. Palker, and B.F. Haynes. 1984. Human erythrocyte antigens: II. The In(Lu) gene regulates expression of an antigen on a 80-kilodalton protein of human erythrocytes. *Blood* **64:** 599.

Telen, M.J., H. Shehata, and B.F. Haynes. 1986. Human medullary thymocyte p80 antigen and In(Lu)-related antigen reside on the same protein. *Hum. Immunol.* **17:** 311.

Vogel, H., E.C. Butcher, and L.J. Picker. 1992. H-CAM expression in the human nervous system: Evidence for a role in diverse glial interactions. *J. Neurocytol.* **21:** 363.

Wickham, T.J., P. Mathias, D.A. Cheresh, and G.R. Nemerow. 1993. Integrins $\alpha_v\beta_3$ and $\alpha_v\beta_5$ promote adenovirus internalization but not virus attachment. *Cell* **73:** 309.

25

Antibody-dependent Enhancement of Infection: A Mechanism for Indirect Virus Entry into Cells

Scott B. Halstead
Rockefeller Foundation
New York, New York 10018

A review of receptor-mediated virus entry into vertebrate cells provides a provocative opportunity to consider the growing literature on an important mechanism of indirect entry of viruses into cells and a newly described phenomenon, antibody-dependent enhancement (ADE) of viral infection. To supplement this relatively brief treatment, the interested reader may wish to consult three recent reviews. The review by Halstead (1982) considers enhanced disease and/or infection in immune hosts and in vitro systems. Not all examples are mediated unequivocally by antibody. Porterfield (1986) provides a crisp summary of in vitro mechanisms in ADE, and Burke (1992) focuses his review on the burgeoning literature on in vitro ADE by the human immunodeficiency virus type 1 (HIV-1) and related retroviruses. The AIDS epidemic has brought a new urgency to studying direct and indirect mechanisms of viral infections—all the more urgent because antibodies, the most effective weapon available to prevent viral diseases, are peculiarly ineffective in containing HIV infection.

The consummate biologic importance of antibody-enhanced (or other ligand-enhanced) cellular infection by viruses or other intracellular organisms resides in the contributions of this mechanism to enhanced clinical disease in human beings or other vertebrates and to the survival and evolution of intracellular microorganisms. Since the earlier general reviews, in vitro ADE has been described in a number of new viral groups (hantaviruses [hemorrhagic fever with renal syndrome], Yao et al. 1992; nonproductive influenza A infection, Tamura et al. 1991; productive infection, Ochiai et al. 1988, 1990, 1992; nonproductive infection for the lentivirus, caprine arthritis-encephalitis virus, Jolly et al. 1989; respiratory syncytial virus infection of monocyte/macrophage cell lines, Gimenez et al. 1989; Krilov et al. 1987; infection by the BK papovavirus, Traavik et al. 1988; feline infectious peritonitis virus [FIPV], Olsen et al. 1992; and HIV-1 and related viruses, for review, see Burke 1992). Dendritic cells are beginning to emerge as a distinct class of FcR-bearing cells which may play a role in viral pathogenesis and ADE. In this review, these cells are not considered apart from cells of mononuclear phagocyte lineage.

In vitro antibody-enhanced infections or underneutralization of viruses, probably due to ADE, have been described in the literature since the 1930s (Halstead 1982). The first explicit descriptions of the phenomenon were by Hawkes (1964) and Hawkes and Lafferty (1967). These authors conjectured that enhanced plaque formation of Murray Valley encephalitis (MVE) virus by avian anti-MVE on chick embryo "fibroblasts" (CEF) was due to the stabilization of viral infectivity by antibody. It remained for Kliks and Halstead (1980, 1983) to demonstrate that CEF monolayers were "contaminated" with 2% functional mononuclear phagocytes. At a relatively low multiplicity of infection (moi), MVE virions by themselves did not infect mononuclear phagocytes. The other chick fibroblastic cells were permissive to MVE infection at rates that were comparable to several other widely used cell culture assay systems. The addition of MVE antibody at low dilutions efficiently directed viruses to mononuclear phagocytes. Antibody-mediated infections in this small population accounted for the 20–30% increase in infected cells observed under these conditions.

The explanation of the Hawkes-Lafferty phenomenon had been made possible by studies on the immune enhancement of dengue virus infection in peripheral blood mononuclear phagocytes (Halstead et al. 1973; Halstead and O'Rourke 1977a). These studies had defined the phenomena of immune-enhanced viral infection of cells as possessing several attributes (Table 1): (1) Cells are infected in the presence of antibody or cells are infected which are derived from an immune host. In vivo, this may translate to an enhanced susceptibility to infection which is de-coupled from the number of infectious particles in an infectious inoculum. (2) Cells may be infected more quickly. This can be illustrated most clearly at low incubation temperatures. In vivo, the incubation period from infection to onset of disease may be shortened. (3) There are increased numbers of productively infected cells. This phenomenon may be derivative of attributes 1 and/or 2. In vivo, this translates into increased viremia and/or increased severity of disease. (4) Cell tropism may be altered. This is a largely hypothetical attribute of enhanced infection. The in vivo correlate might be an altered disease course, e.g., atypical measles or neurologic AIDS.

In vitro and in vivo studies demonstrate that indirect virus-cell entry

Table 1 Attributes of immune-enhanced viral infections compared with non-immune controls

In vitro	In vivo correlates
Increased infectivity	increased susceptibility to infection
Increased rate of infection	shortened incubation period to disease
Increased numbers of	increased viremia
productively infected cells	increased severity of disease
Altered cell tropism	"new" disease

is controlled by many factors, some interconnected. These are listed in Table 2. Each is discussed briefly.

LIGAND

Infection enhancement may result when bivalent ligands bind to receptors on viruses and on cells. Ligand binding increases the forces that bring viruses in close approximation to other usually normal cell-virus receptors. For the most part, in well-studied systems, virus entry into cells follows the normal route by mechanisms described by Marsh and Helenius (1989).

Table 2 Factors controlling indirect entry of viruses into animal cells

Ligand	Cells	Virus
Antibody	FcR-bearing	infective agent eliciting infection
Ig class	FcR-type virus R	moi
Ig subclass	age	temperature
Fc receptor-	activation	nonenhanceable viruses
vertebrate class		
idiotype	tissue source	intratypic variants
specificity com-		
plement		
nonneutralizing	primary cell	autologous immune enhancement
concentration		
enhancing (Enh)		
titer		sensitizing infection or immunization
Enh peak titer	cell line	intra-genus viruses
Enh power	C′ R-bearinq	intra-group viruses
Complement	virus R	chemically altered viruses
Non-antibody		killed viruses
		subunit antigens

Bivalent ligands described to date include immunoglobulin G (IgG), immunoglobulin M (IgM) plus complement, IgG plus complement, complement alone, an unidentified factor in unheated plasma and, with simian immunodeficiency virus (SIV), soluble CD4.

Antibody

The best-studied, possibly the most powerful and ubiquitous ligand which enhances the infection of animal viruses is antibody. In both natural and experimental settings, there is a corresponding requirement for an appropriate receptor on the cell surface; e.g., Fc receptors for IgG immunoglobulins and complement receptors when IgM serves as an intermediate ligand.

Immunoglobulin Class

Most published studies on ADE have used antiviral IgG as a source of enhancing antibody. It is known that a number of cell types also carry FcR for IgA, IgE, and IgM. Whether any of these latter immunoglobulin types contribute significantly to ADE is unknown at the present time. In early studies in rhesus monkeys, whole sera obtained 14 days after dengue 2 infection contained neutralizing antibodies (PRNT) when assayed in continuous rhesus monkey kidney cells, but when assayed on rhesus peripheral blood mononuclear cells (PBMC), weak ADE was noted at dilutions between 1:160 and 1:2560 (Halstead 1982). When IgM and IgG were assayed separately, the IgG fraction exhibited *only* ADE to a serum-equivalent dilution of 1:10,240 whereas decomplemented IgM only neutralized virus. However, when fresh complement was added, the IgM fraction neutralized dengue 2 to a serum equivalent dilution of 1:40, but enhanced infection in rhesus PBMC to a serum-equivalent dilution of 1:800. ADE, due to IgG, was unaffected by complement. When whole serum was assayed in PBMC in the presence of complement, virus was neutralized at low dilution (1:10 and 1:40), and weak ADE was noted at higher dilutions (1:160–1:2560). These studies show that early IgM is very efficient at neutralizing dengue virus, but at high dilutions *in the presence of complement,* IgM can mediate ADE. Cardosa et al. (1983) have studied this phenomenon and shown that the IgM/virus/complement complex attaches to C3 receptors and initiates virus entry into cells via this ligand/receptor interaction.

Whereas low concentrations of IgM antibodies can mediate ADE in an autologous system, it is well to remember that in vivo, at least in the dengue system, infection enhancement by IgM could be expected to occur only *very* early in the immune response and then only transiently. In whole serum, anti-dengue IgM effectively ablated the pro-ADE effect of IgG (Halstead and O'Rourke 1977b; Halstead 1982). The reason early anti-dengue IgG enhanced, but failed to neutralize, dengue 2 has not been further investigated. It seems likely that this reflects the rather poor avidity and conformational "fit" of early IgG idiotypes to critical virion epitopes.

In a non-FcR-bearing cell system studied extensively by Robinson, Montefiori, and colleagues (Robinson et al. 1988), C3R is required and IgG antibody/complement/virus complexes mediate infection. This system uses MT-2 cells (continuous human lymphoblast cell line) which are permissive to HIV and SIV. IgG-complement-mediated ADE might represent a significant infection mechanism and pathway in vivo if cells bearing both C3R and CD4+ contribute significantly to HIV infection and disease.

Ig Subclass

In humans, IgG1 and IgG3 are principally responsible for ADE, whereas in mice, IgG2a is principally responsible. This reflects receptors on the mononuclear phagocyte cell system used: Human PBMC have IgG1 and IgG3 receptors. There is a large family of Fc receptors that have parallel functions but are only loosely related structurally. These are discussed below. Mouse macrophages have at least three types of FcR: FcRI which binds to IgG2a; FcRII which binds to IgG2b, and FcRIII which binds to IgG3 (Porterfield 1986).

Phylogenetic Class of Fc Terminus

Hawkes (1964) and Hawkes and Lafferty (1967) observed that avian antisera enhanced viral plaque formation on CEF and chorioallantoic membranes (CAM). However, enhancement was not observed when the same reagents were assayed on pig kidney cell cultures or in suckling mice. Mouse and rabbit antisera failed to enhance viral plaque or pock formation on CEF and CAM. This latter phenomenon is explained by the structural similarities between Fc termini and FcR receptors at the level of phylogenetic class (Kliks and Halstead 1983). Fc/FcR interactions do not occur regularly when antibody source and cells providing the FcR differ between avians and mammals. Curiously, guinea pig anti-MVE enhanced MVE plaque formation on CEF (Kliks and Halstead 1983).

Idiotype Specificity

Controversy continues to surround the idiotype specificity that mediates ADE and the corresponding epitopes on viral surfaces. A fundamental fact established repeatedly, both with polyclonal and monoclonal antibodies, is that antibodies directed at epitopes which neutralize viruses efficiently, can, in general, produce ADE when tested at concentrations below the neutralization threshold (Halstead 1982; Porterfield 1986; Burke 1992; Matsuda et al. 1989). The importance of antibody concentration is discussed below.

It is well established that ADE occurs when antibodies, even at relatively high concentrations, are directed against virion epitopes which are not thought to mediate attachment to and entry through the plasma membrane. The classic example is infections with dengue 1, 3, or 4 viruses, which raise antibodies against dengue subgroup or flavivirus group epitopes that can enhance dengue 2 infection in vitro and are thought to enhance infection and disease in vivo (Halstead 1982). In fact, the most powerful risk factor ever identified for the occurrence of dengue hemorrhagic fever/dengue shock syndrome (DHF/DSS) in humans was the circulation of antibodies raised by heterotypic dengue viral infections that exhibited dengue 2 ADE when undiluted serum was tested in human PBMC in vitro (Kliks et al. 1989). In contrast, even small amounts of cross-reactive dengue 2 neutralizing antibody raised during primary infections due to dengue 1, 3, or 4 viruses down-regulated secondary dengue 2 infections to produce inapparent disease. In vitro, a wide range of heterotypic polyclonal and monoclonal antibodies have been shown to produce ADE in the flavivirus, togavirus, and influenza virus families (Halstead 1982; Porterfield 1986; Ochiai et al. 1990, 1992).

Antibodies that fail to neutralize at low dilutions underlie ADE. Several putative examples of diseases in which nonneutralizing antibodies might contribute to ADE have been described in human beings. Measles, respiratory syncytial virus (RSV), and parainfluenza 3 virus (PIV3) infections in individuals who had previously received one or more doses of a formalin-killed vaccine resulted in severe disease (Halstead 1982; Porterfield 1986; Burke 1992). In the paramyxoviruses, formalin was shown to destroy selectively the fusion (F) protein (Norrby 1975; Mertz et al. 1980). Antibodies raised in vaccinated subjects failed to neutralize homologous live virus (Norrby et al. 1975; Murphy et al. 1986). This has been attributed to the absence of anti-F. Subsequent exposure to live measles virus, live-attenuated measles vaccine, or live RSV or PIV3 resulted in severe systemic disease or local Arthus-like lesions. There is some evidence that enhanced virus infection is the basis of vaccine-related severe RSV disease (Chin et al. 1969); ADE has been demonstrated in human pulmonary macrophages and a human monocytoid cell line (Gimenez et al. 1989; Krilov et al. 1989). For measles and parainfluenza 3, ADE has not been demonstrated in vitro or in vivo. Enhanced growth of influenza A virus has been demonstrated in the lungs of mice vaccinated with inactivated heterotypic influenza A vaccines and challenged intranasally with live virus (Webster and Askonas 1980). Following immunization with killed virus preparations or subunit vaccines, diseases due to Aleutian disease of mink, FIPV, equine infectious anemia (EIA), and caprine infectious arthropathy have all been enhanced in an appropriate host using criteria described in Table 1.

Implied in each of the above examples of immunologically enhanced disease is that nonneutralizing antibodies have been raised. Idiotype specificity is well established in the dengue, paramyxovirus and FIPV (Corapi et al. 1992), and EIA (Issel et al. 1992) models, but is less clearly established in other systems. Despite some uncertainty concerning idiotype specificity, the most reliable risk factor for ADE in vivo is the circulation of nonneutralizing, virion-directed antibodies. As discussed below, nonneutralization is more a function of concentration of antibody molecules than the epitopes toward which they are directed.

Concentration

A large number of studies have shown that homotypic neutralizing antibodies, polyclonal or monoclonal, produce ADE at dilutions above the neutralization end point. Dengue neutralizing antibodies passively transferred to human infants by mothers with multiple previous dengue infections can produce severe disease in such infants when primary infections occur in the first few months of life (Kliks et al. 1988). Apparently competent neutralizing antibodies to FIPV, when transferred in colostrum from dame to kitten, enhance the infectability and the resultant disease when kittens are subsequently exposed to wild-type virus (Weiss and Scott 1981). Passive transfer of antibody by other routes has produced the same result (Pederson and Boyle 1980; Weiss and Scott 1981). In the FIPV model, it appears that enhanced disease occurs at antibody dilutions which, in vitro, competently neutralize virus (Olsen et al. 1992). In the dengue model, enhanced disease occurred in 13 infants developing DHF/DSS during primary dengue 2 infections when passively acquired dengue 2 neutralizing antibodies, raised by mothers from several earlier dengue infections, had been catabolized to dilutions of 1:5 or lower (measured in non-Fc-bearing cells). This was also the time when peak enhancement titers had been achieved (Kliks et al. 1988). DHF/DSS occurred when infants experienced a dengue 2 infection during a critical time window of only a few weeks. This "window" was the period when infants circulated maternal antibodies at enhancing dilutions. Earlier in life, higher concentrations of these same antibodies neutralized virus. There is no report in the literature of mothers who were monotypically immune to dengue 2 whose infants developed DHF/DSS when subsequently infected with this virus.

It appears that maternal antibody to measles does not sensitize infants to "atypical measles," although severe and fatal measles *does* occur in infants who acquire measles infections shortly after the protective efficacy of maternal antibody wanes. There is reasonable evidence that maternal antibody is responsible for the bronchiolitis that occurs when infants acquire RSV infections within the first 6 months of life (Halstead 1982).

Enhancing Titer

As illustrated in Figure 1, measurements of viral infections in PBMC cultures have three parameters. The highest dilution of antibody that produces significant and reproducibly enhanced infections is called the "enhancing titer." With respect to in vivo phenomena, it is important to point out that many sera, when tested at low dilutions, neutralize; infection enhancement is only demonstrable at higher dilutions. Many authors interpret the highest dilution at which ADE can be demonstrated as a measure of biologic potency. It is not. In vivo, antibodies that neutralize in undiluted serum will neutralize regardless of the enhancing titer of this same serum when diluted. It is a general rule that sera which competently neutralize to relatively high titer will demonstrate extremely high enhancing titers.

Peak Enhancement Titer

The dilution of sera at which fold enhancement is greatest is labeled peak enhancement titer (Fig. 1). Those infants who developed severe disease during primary dengue 2 infections acquired their infections at a time when it was estimated that peak infection enhancement would occur.

Enhancing Power

The fold increase in the number of cells infected or the amount of virus produced at peak enhancement in antibody-supplemented assays as compared with controls is expressed as "power." As illustrated in Figure 1, over many dilutions at the low range, enhancing and neutralizing

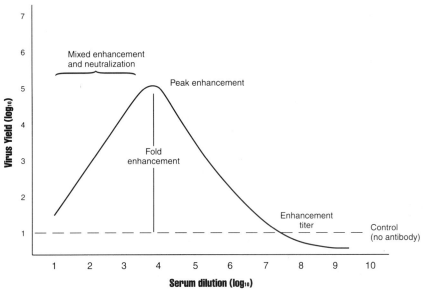

Figure 1 Diagram defining the various parameters of antibody-dependent infection enhancement. The reagents used are virus, antibody, and cultured mononuclear phagocytes. At low dilution of serum, little or no virus growth is observed; at a higher dilution, enhanced viral growth occurs (peak enhancement). At still higher dilution, the enhancement effect is gradually lost (enhancement titer).

antibodies are mixed. Under these conditions, infection enhancement is suboptimal. At some dilution of antibody, optimal viral infections occur; at still higher dilutions, the concentration of infectious antibody/virus complexes is not great enough to saturate the system. Power must also reflect the abundance of virus receptors on FcR-bearing cells, the efficiency of entry of virus, the viability of virus after reaching the cytosol, and competence to complete all steps to achieve assembly and final release of virions.

Enhanced internalization of virus does not always lead to enhanced infection. Visna virus immune complexes, when exposed to sheep peritoneal macrophages, cells which appear to lack any visna virus receptor, result in enhanced uptake of virus, but its destruction in the phagolysome (Jolly et al. 1989).

Complement

HIV and SIV can enter cells in a two-step process that involves first the formation of IgG/virus complexes which activate complement to C3R with subsequent entry of virus via the CD4$^+$ receptor. Robinson et al. (1987) found an infection-enhancing factor in seropositive sera that increased HIV replication in cells of a transformed lymphoblastoid line, MT-2. Two activities were needed to mediate HIV-1 enhancement: antibodies and complement (Robinson et al. 1988). The required complement component was heat-labile and cobra-venom-labile, present in C1q-deficient serum, but not present in C3-deficient or factor-B-deficient serum. Thus, complement-dependent ADE is mediated by the alternative pathway.

Sera from virtually all HIV-1-infected humans taken at any stage of HIV disease have this type of enhancing activity (Robinson et al. 1989a,b). Antibodies in sera from infected nonhuman primates, HIV-1-infected chimpanzees, and SIV-infected rhesus macaques also enhanced viral infection (Robinson et al. 1989b; Montifiori et al. 1990). SIV immunoglobulin/complement/virus complexes have been detected when sera are raised in monkeys immunized with various SIV vaccine preparations (Montifiori et al. 1990). Animals inoculated with detergent-inactivated whole virus, formalin-inactivated whole virus, or glycoprotein-enriched subunit vaccines all raised enhancing antibodies that mediate infection via C3R. Human monoclonal HIV antibodies have been tested in an attempt to differentiate "enhancing" from "neutralizing" epitopes (Bugge et al. 1990). Epstein-Barr virus infection of B lymphocytes mediates HIV-1 infection enhancement via induced type 2 complement receptor (Tremblay et al. 1990).

Non-antibody Enhanced Infection

Complement

Montefiori et al. (1989) have reported that in the absence of antibody components of the human alternative complement pathway, C3 and factor B can restore infectivity to HIV-1 virions grown in MT-2 cells in the presence of N-linked glycosylation blockers. Fresh, nonimmune serum from normal chimpanzees can also increase HIV-1 infection via the alternative complement pathway, as can fresh normal human serum (Robinson et al. 1987, 1989b).

Other

Allen et al. (1990) have reported a paradoxical effect of soluble CD4 in enhancing rather than blocking SIV in MOLT-4 clone 8 T-lymphoblastoid cells. In the same system, soluble CD4 totally blocked infection by HIV-1/IIIB. Pretreatment of cells with anti-CD4 monoclonal antibodies did not block receptor-enhanced SIV infection, suggesting that a second cell receptor was involved. The soluble CD4 may bind the virion glycoprotein with entry mediated via a secondary binding protein such as the fusogenic region of the SIV transmembrane protein.

Halstead (1982) has discussed a group of unexplained infection-enhancement phenomena, each involving cell systems which were thought not to possess Fc receptors. Included were: (1) increased infectivity for *Escherichia coli* protoplasts of antibody-treated bacteria; (2) enhanced plaque formation of a pike fry rhabdovirus when assayed on fathead minnow monolayers, which resulted when fish antibodies were stored at $-20°C$ for more than a year and was ablated by the addition of anti-rabbit serum or complement; and (3) low-level plaque enhancement of flaviviruses at high dilutions of antisera in non-FcR-bearing cells, stable pig kidney, or rhesus monkey kidney cells. The tentative explanation of this phenomenon is a slight antiviral effect observed at low dilutions of control serum but not at high dilutions of experimental sera.

CELLS

FcR-bearing

With the few exceptions noted, the sine qua non of antibody-dependent and non-complement-dependent enhancement of viral infection is the existence of *permissive* FcR-bearing cells. FcR can be naturally distributed or can be induced following infection by one of several members of the herpesvirus family (Bell et al. 1990; McKeating et al. 1990). A large family of distinct classes of Fc receptors exist. They have been partially defined by monoclonal antibodies. Each receptor is differentially represented on cells in various tissues. Gamma interferon can increase type 1 Fc receptor density (Kontny et al. 1988). Among the reasonably characterized immunoglobulin Fc receptors, there are three for IgG (FcRI, FcRII, FcRIII), at least one for IgM, one for IgE, and one for IgA (Unkeless et al. 1988). In humans, Fc receptors have been detected on T, B, and NK lymphocytes, polymorphonuclear leukocytes, mononuclear phagocytes, and dendritic cells, including Langerhans cells. Monocytes bear two Fc receptors. Fc receptors are also found at high density on epithelial cells of the intestinal tract (Kobayashi et al. 1989). FcRI numbers are augmented by gamma interferon, and such augmentation can be shown to increase dengue viral ADE (Kontny et al. 1988).

Mouse macrophages have at least three types of FcR; FcRI, FcRII, and FcRIII, which bind to IgG_2a, to IgG_2b and complexes of IgG_1, and to IgG_3 complexes, respectively (Unkeless et al. 1988). In humans, IgG_1 and IgG_3 appear to mediate ADE, whereas in mice, IgG_2a and IgG_1 are important (Porterfield 1986; Burke 1992).

Fc receptors can be induced in non-Fc receptor-bearing cells and convert such cells to being permissive to antibody-dependent enhancement (Bell et al. 1990; McKeating et al. 1990).

Cytophilia

Although noncomplexed monomeric IgG_1 and IgG_3 occupy FcR furtively, this weak and brief interaction merely reflects the concentration of immunoglobulins in the extracellular medium. Attempts to "stick" monomeric enhancing antibody on human or monkey PBMC prior to the addition of virus have failed (Halstead and O'Rourke 1977b). When antibody was incubated for 1 hour at 37°C and PBMC were washed in a different IgG-containing medium, no ADE occurred unless antibody was added back to the reaction mixture. In contrast, despite extensive washing to remove original serum or loosely bound IgG, PBMC from dengue-immune rhesus monkeys or human beings are permissive to dengue infection in vitro (Halstead et al. 1973). Using silica, these cells have been identified as monocytes (Halstead 1982). Enhanced infection was reduced or ablated by treatment with trypsin or anti-IgG prior to addition of dengue virus. Hohdatsu et al. (1991) have demonstrated that macrophages obtained from cats immune to FIPV carry cytophilic antibody and are more permissive to FIPV infection than macrophages from non-immune cats. These results appear to be explained by the existence of a cytophilic antibody which is firmly attached to monocytes in vivo. How and under what circumstances this antibody becomes bound to PBMC remains a mystery.

The incubation of human anti-yellow-fever serum with U937 continuous human monocytoid cells resulted in irreversible cytophilic attachment of antibody which could not be eluted off at 37°C (Schlesinger and Brandriss 1981). This may be related to the finding of Anderson and Abraham (1980) that monomeric IgG myeloma immunoglobulins showed a higher affinity for U937 Fc receptors than did aggregated immunoglobulin of the same subclass. Thus, in U937, but not PBMC, monomeric immunoglobulin may become cell-associated in vitro.

Age

In the dengue system, ADE is optimal when human or rhesus PBMC are held in culture for 24 hours at 37°C before adding virus and antibody

(Halstead and O'Rourke 1977b). In cells infected at 48–96 hours, a sharp decline in viral replication was observed. Similar results were obtained in PBMC which were plated onto glass or plastic surfaces. Under both conditions, but especially the latter, monocytes differentiate into macrophages. Splenic, thymic, and lymph node macrophages from rhesus monkeys showed a similar reduction in permissiveness when held in culture for 2–4 days prior to infection (Halstead et al. 1977). Bone marrow mononuclear phagocytes showed no such maturational phenomenon, being equally permissive on days 0 and 4 after removal from their rhesus monkey host. This may reflect the fact that the progeny of stem cells in vitro are relatively immature cells.

Activation

The effects of macrophage activation on viral replication have been examined in a number of studies, the majority of which report that activated macrophages are more restrictive (Mogenson 1979; Morahan et al. 1985). There are some contrary reports. Van der Groen et al. (1976) found Semliki forest virus replicated better in protease-peptone-elicited macrophages than in resident macrophages, and Hotta and colleagues reported increased yields of dengue viruses in macrophages activated by extracts of bacterial and parasitic cell walls and peptidoglycans (Hotta and Hotta 1982; Wiharta et al. 1985). Cardosa et al. (1986) showed that IgG-West Nile virus complexes grew better in BCG-infected mouse peritoneal macrophages than in resident or thioglycolate-elicited macrophages. In contrast, in the IgM/complement/West Nile virus system, virus grew better in thioglycolate-elicited macrophages than in the others (Cardosa et al. 1986). Ochiai et al. (1992) observed better ADE of influenza A NWS strain in resident than in thioglycolate-induced mouse peritoneal macrophages. With HIV-1 viruses, Shadduck et al. (1991) failed to demonstrate FcR-mediated ADE when they added virus and antibody to PBMC 1–6 days after isolation from blood or to human macrophages 2–4 days after removal from the peritoneal cavity. Weakly plastic-adherent PBMC were removed by a 1-hour incubation of cells on plastic surfaces. Homsy et al. (1990), on the other hand, incubated PBMC on plastic surfaces for 3 days, trypsinized and washed off weakly adherent cells, and then incubated adherent cells for an additional 7–8 days prior to HIV infection.

Both RSV and PIV3 grew well in PBMC cultures incubated for 7 days, as compared with cells infected after only 1 day in culture (Krilov et al. 1987). For PIV3, reduced growth was correlated with the ability of infected young peripheral blood monocytes to produce interferon compared to older cells, but the opposite effect was seen with RSV.

The effect of macrophage activation has even been demonstrated in vivo when two susceptible rhesus monkeys were inoculated with *Cornybacterium parvum* and an additional two animals were inoculated with pertussis vaccine intravenously. Three days later, the four animals were infected with dengue 2 (S.B. Halstead, unpubl.). Viremias were measured daily and compared with sham-inoculated controls. Viremia levels were significantly higher in animals given substances known to stimulate and activate the mononuclear phagocyte system.

Clearly, age or differentiation of cells in vitro plus activation (a separate process) of monocytes/macrophages have a profound effect on ADE, although not in predictable or yet understandable ways.

Tissue Source

For many of the animal diseases for which ADE may be operative in vivo, the sites of replication of virus in the intact animal are known to be one or more varieties of tissue macrophages (Halstead 1982; Stott et al. 1984; McGuire et al. 1986; Porterfield 1986; Burke 1992). In vitro systems rarely employ these biologically relevant cells. Usually, monocytes are obtained from peripheral blood. Several workers have used macrophages obtained by lavage of the peritoneal cavity. Most such techniques activate these cells. Whether such activation affects virus growth and ability to demonstrate ADE has been carefully studied in some, but not all, systems (see above).

Differential infection permissiveness and susceptibility to ADE of HIV strains have been described between PBMC and tissue macrophages (Burke 1992). This is a frontier area in present-day research on ADE. Particularly interesting is the possibility that antibody directs virus to a different subpopulation of cells than infection in the absence of antibody.

Primary Cells Versus Cell Line

Reference has been made above to differences in FcR on primary versus monocytoid cell lines. Differences in C' receptors have also been described previously (Burke 1992). Finally, primary cells and cell lines may differ in the distribution and density of viral receptors. The number of human and other mammalian mononuclear phagocyte cell lines is too large to be reviewed here. Suffice it to say, great care must be taken in extrapolating results from surrogate models to predict or interpret in vivo phenomena.

Virus Receptor

The majority of studies on ADE in HIV and SIV infections, plus several elegant studies in the dengue model (Gollins and Porterfield 1985), have demonstrated that in ADE the entry of the virus into the cytosol is critically dependent on the normal virus receptor and the process of endocytosis.

For both HIV-1 and dengue, bispecific Fab antibodies together with some method of blocking normal cell viral receptors have shown that virus/IgG complexes do not trigger infection via a phagocytic event (Takeda and Ennis 1990; Connor et al. 1991). In other words, antibody attracts virus to the cell surface, following which virus attaches to normal cell receptors. The most easily characterized system involves HIV-1 and its receptor molecule CD4. A bivalent antibody to a human FcR and to HIV-1 gp120 links virus to FcR. If anti-CD4 or soluble CD4 is added to block the CD4 receptor, no increase in cellular infection occurs. Although this experiment may not trigger FcR endocytosis, essentially the same result is obtained by attempting ADE in the presence of sCD4 or anti-CD4 (Zeira et al. 1990). A study of ADE with influenza A by Ochiai et al. (1992) suggests that influenza infection is via hemagglutinin (HA) receptors and depends on protease cleavage of the HA spike protein.

Convincing experiments demonstrating the mode of entry of virus into cells have not been published for most viruses that participate in ADE. Most authors assume infection is via Fc-mediated endocytosis; yet several different kinds of outcomes of the attachment to cells of virus/IgG complexes to FcR are evident. In visna-maidi, a lentivirus that produces a chronic disease in sheep and goats, immune complexes formed between anti-visna IgG and visna virus bind quickly to sheep macrophage FcR; apparently the entire complex is subsequently internalized. Antibody had the effect of enhancing uncoating but delaying subsequent replication in macrophages. F(ab)$_2$ fragments similarly delayed viral replication, but not to the same extent as intact IgG (Jolly et al. 1989). Contrary to the author's interpretation that immune complexes were destroyed in phagolysosomes, the fact that visna/F(ab)$_2$ complexes were infectious suggests that entry of virus from immune complexes into cells can occur via normal cell receptors.

C′R-bearing Cells: Virus Receptor

Few experiments similar to the one described above have been done with IgM-C′ or IgG-C′-mediated infections of PBMC by dengue or HIV-1 viruses. There is suggestive evidence that ADE does not occur when viral receptors are blocked by ligand or antibody (Kimura et al. 1986; Clapham et al. 1989).

VIRUS

Infective Agent: Sensitizing Versus Eliciting Viruses

In systems requiring two infections or an immunization process to sensitize to ADE, the virus whose cell entry is enhanced is referred to as the eliciting virus or infection, and the initial infection or immunization is referred to as the sensitizing virus or infection or the sensitizing immunization.

Eliciting Virus Multiplicity of Infection

The moi has been studied carefully in the dengue system (Halstead and O'Rourke 1977b). Serial tenfold dilutions of virus were tested in human and monkey PBMC. When moi ranged between 0.001 and 0.1, infection of cells occurred regularly in the presence of antibody with three- to tenfold lower infection in the absence of antibody. When the moi was raised to between 1 and 100, the differential effect of adding antibody was often lost. Day of peak infection is related directly to moi. In the dengue system, moi in the range 0.01–0.05 resulted in peak extracellular virus yields between days 2 and 4 after infection.

Temperature

Hawkes and Lafferty (1967) found that infection enhancement could be optimized when reactants were held at 4°C for 30–90 minutes. At 37°C, enhancement was optimal if reactants were incubated on PBMC for less than 6 minutes. Longer periods of incubation pushed the reaction in the direction of neutralization. To measure ADE with HIV, incubation of antibody and HIV with or without C' on FcR-bearing or CR-bearing cells is commonly done at 4°C (Robinson et al. 1988; Homsy et al. 1990). Strangely, systematic comparison of results at other temperatures and various time periods appears not to have been done.

Non-enhanceable Viruses

Burke et al. (1988) have published data suggesting that in human beings, prior dengue infection does not enhance the severity of a secondary dengue 1 infection. It is important to note that there is no in vitro correlate of this observation. Dengue 1 infections can be enhanced in vitro by dengue antibodies when assayed in a macrophage-like cell line (Morens and Halstead 1990).

In the confusing and controversial HIV literature, the role of viral strains in FcR-mediated or C'R-mediated infection enhancement has not been resolved. Shadduck et al. (1991) may have failed to demonstrate FcR-mediated ADE due to one or more of the following factors: the strains of HIV-1 used, their prior passage history, or the method of preparing virus seeds.

Intratypic Variants

Genetic, but not antigenic, studies have shown that DHF/DSS epidemics have resulted when the eliciting infection is due to a Southeast Asian topotype (Rico-Hesse 1990). Preliminary data from Kliks (1990) suggest that in the presence of polyclonal enhancing antibody, Southeast Asian dengue 2 topotypes grow in primary human PBMC better than Caribbean dengue 2 strains under the same antibody and cell-culture conditions. Morens and Halstead (1987) have reported preliminary evidence that under ADE conditions, the replicative ability of dengue 2 strains in PBMC varies directly with the severity of infection in the hosts from whom virus strains were recovered. The test system employed dengue 4 monoclonal antibodies.

Probably the most important in vivo risk factor for DHF/DSS that has been identified is the absence of cross-reactive (heterotypic) neutralizing antibodies in individuals with a single previous dengue infection who were subsequently infected with dengue 2. As Kliks et al. (1989) have shown, of 40 Thai school children studied during what probably were predominantly secondary dengue 2 infections, 32 had *no* clinical illness. The majority of these well children had low-level dengue 2 neutralizing antibodies raised from their initial dengue infection, whereas the 8 children who developed clinical illness with secondary dengue infections circulated only dengue 2 enhancing antibodies measured at no serum dilution. These were measured by testing undiluted serum for enhancing or neutralizing antibodies in human PBMC.

The implications of this study are profound. Assuming that differences in immune responses measured do not derive from human genetic heterogeneity, this study suggests that shared epitopes between sensitizing and eliciting dengue serotypes, perhaps in the cell-receptor/fusion domain, result in *benign* (in fact, inapparent) sequential infections. Virus pairs that lack these shared epitopes, which constitute a minority of circulating viruses, result in secondary dengue infections that are antibody-enhanced and clinically severe.

Autologous Immune Enhancement

The lentiviruses as a group tend to infect macrophages, have high rates of mutation in their envelope protein genes, and (by mechanisms not yet well understood) elicit antibodies which are inefficient at neutralizing virus (Wigzell 1988). Aleutian disease of mink virus, a coronavirus, and lactate dehydrogenase virus, a togavirus, share these properties. The degree to which continuing infection and subsequent disease course are dependent on antibody-mediated infection of FcR-bearing cells is not clear. The mechanisms by which nonneutralizing antibodies are produced and the biological relevance of ADE to in vivo infections are research questions of paramount importance, particularly in the face of the continuing HIV pandemic.

Sensitizing Infections or Immunization (Passive/Active)

Intra-genus Viruses

So far as is known, DHF/DSS is not regularly caused by sequential flavivirus infection outside the dengue subgroup. Yellow fever, Japanese encephalitis, and West Nile viruses circulate in dengue-endemic areas but are not epidemiologically associated with DHF/DSS. There has been one report of a DHF-like illness in a dengue-infected individual previously given Japanese encephalitis vaccine (Okuno et al. 1989). Adult males who were yellow fever-immune when given the S1 live-attenuated dengue 2 virus had enhanced vaccine infectivity (higher seroconversion rates) but were not more symptomatic than nonimmune dengue vaccine recipients (Bancroft et al. 1984).

Intra-group Viruses

In the dengue system, sequential infections with DEN 1-2, DEN 3-2, DEN 4-2 produced DHF/DSS, but the attack rate decreased in descending order (Sangkawibha et al. 1984). The large Cuban and Venezuelan DHF/DSS epidemics were due to dengue 1-2 infection sequences. Secondary dengue 3 and secondary dengue 4 infections result in DHF/DSS, but the role that sensitizing dengue types or strains play in the outcome of secondary dengue 3 and 4 infections is not known.

Considerable evidence attests that ADE in FcR-bearing cells is the underlying mechanism which converts dengue fever syndrome to DHF/DSS. Dengue is the prototype of the heterotypic infection model of ADE. Some authors have suggested that sequential infection with antigenically drifted influenza A strains may result in disease enhancement. Compelling epidemiological and clinical data are missing (Ochiai et al. 1990, 1992; Tamura et al. 1991). As discussed in earlier reviews (Halstead 1982; Porterfield 1986; Burke 1992), putative candidates for in vivo immunologically enhanced infections fall into two additional groups: vaccine-enhanced disease (see below) and autologous immune enhancement (see above).

Chemically Altered Viruses: Killed and Subunit Vaccines (Vaccine-enhanced Diseases)

Candidates include the paramyxoviruses, measles, RSV, PIV3, FIPV (Vennema et al. 1990), caprine arthritis-encephalitis (McGuire et al. 1986), Aleutian disease of mink (Porter et al. 1972), EIA (Issel et al. 1992), blue tongue virus in cattle (Stott et al. 1984), and influenza A (Webster and Askonas 1980). As discussed earlier (Halstead 1982), early deaths in postexposure rabies-immunized humans and animals appears to be due to accelerated destructive immune response and is, therefore, an efferent rather than an afferent immune-enhancement phenomenon. Except for measles and PIV3, studies show that mononuclear phagocytes are important sites of viral growth in vivo, and ADE in monocytes/macrophages has been demonstrated in vitro.   Two kinds of antigens stimulate ADE in vivo: chemically modified killed virions and virion subunit vaccines. The prototype for chemical alteration is formalin treatment of the paramyxoviruses, which selectively destroys the fusion protein (Norrby 1975; Mertz et al. 1980). Such vaccines raise antibodies (Murphy et al. 1986) that do not neutralize infections in vitro or in vivo and might lead to enhanced infections of FcR-bearing cells, although this mechanism has not been demonstrated in relevant models. The precise damage done by formalin to other viruses is less clear; interestingly, in these less defined models, ADE in monocytes/macrophages in vivo is well established.

Subunit vaccines, whether given as peptides or as genes inserted into live-virus vectors, can sensitize to ADE in vivo as in FIPV (Vennema et al. 1990) or EIA (Issel et al. 1992). In most cases, except for FIPV, antibodies raised to subunit antigens have weak or no neutralizing activity in in vitro test systems.

CONCLUSION

From a wealth of experimental evidence, it seems likely that pathogenicity is established when vertebrate viruses successfully enter, survive, and replicate in cells of mononuclear phagocyte and dendrocyte lineage. These FcR-bearing cells with phagocytic and/or antigen-presenting functions appear to serve as sentinels to microbial invasion, whether at parenteral or body-surface routes of infection. Ultimately, viral diseases are differentiated by replication in secondary target organs and tissues. It is not surprising, therefore, that a wide spectrum of viruses successfully replicate in mononuclear phagocytes, primary cells, or cell lines. It is also not surprising that viruses and other intracellular pathogens have exploited accessory molecules designed to attach to microorganisms as well as to the surfaces of mononuclear phagocytes and dendrocytes. What *is* surprising is the relative dearth of research by microbiologists on the mechanisms of entry, survival, and replication of microorganisms in these frontier cells in the context of the accessory molecules, particularly, in vivo. Although in vitro phenomena clearly provide the easiest access to dissect out "two-step" virus-cell entry mechanisms, the relevance of much of the recent literature is questionable. Most authors reason from in vitro data to in vivo infection and disease. In fact, much of in vitro research may be on epiphenomena. To avoid irrelevance, the scientific community will be well advised to seek and be guided by in vivo/in vitro correlates.

REFERENCES

Allen, J.S., J. Strauss, and D.W. Buck. 1990. Enhancement of SIV infection with soluble receptor molecules. *Science* **247:** 1084.

Anderson, C.L. and G.N. Abraham. 1980. Characterization of the Fc receptor for IgG on a human macrophage cell line, U937. *J. Immunol.* **125:** 2735.

Bancroft, W., R.M. Scott, K. Eckels, C. Hoke, T. Simms, K.D.T. Jesuani, P. Summers, D. Dubois, D. Tsuolos, and P. Russell. 1984. Dengue virus type 2 vaccine reactogenicity and immunogenicity in soldiers. *J. Infect. Dis.* **149:** 1005.

Bell, S., M. Cramage, L. Borysiewicz, and T. Minson. 1990. Induction of immunoglobulin G Fc receptors by recombinant vaccinia viruses expressing glycoproteins E and I of herpes simplex virus type 1. *J. Virol.* **64:** 2181.

Bugge, T.H., B.O. Lindhardt, L.L. Hansen, P. Kusk, E. Hulgaard, K. Holmback, P.J. Klasse, J. Zeuthen, and K. Ulrich. 1990. Analysis of a highly immunodominant epitope in the human immunodeficiency virus type 1 transmembrane glycoprotein gp41, defined by a human monoclonal antibody. *J. Virol.* **64:** 4123.

Burke, D.S. 1992. Human HIV vaccine trials: Does antibody-dependent enhancement pose a genuine risk? *Perspect. Biol. Med.* **35:** 511.

Burke, D.S., A. Nisalak, D.E. Johnson, and R.M. Scott. 1988. A prospective study of dengue infections in Bangkok. *Am. J. Trop. Med. Hyg.* **38:** 172.

Cardosa, M.J., J.S. Porterfield, and S. Gordon. 1983. Complement receptor mediates enhanced flavivirus replication in macrophages. *J. Exp. Med.* **185**: 258.

Cardosa, M.J., S. Gordon, S. Hirsch, T.A. Springer, and J.S. Porterfield. 1986. Interaction of West Nile virus with primary murine macrophages: Role of cell activation and receptors for antibody and complement. *J. Virol.* **57**: 952.

Chin, J., R.L. Magoffin, L.A. Shearer, J.H. Schieble, and E.H. Lennette. 1969. Field evaluation of a respiratory syncytial virus vaccine and a trivalent parainfluenza virus vaccine in a pediatric population. *Am. J. Epidemiol.* **89**: 449.

Clapham, P.R., J.N. Weber, D. Whitby, K. McIntosh, A.G. Dalgleish, P.J. Maddon, K.C. Deen, R.W. Sweet, and R.A. Weiss. 1989. Soluble CD4 blocks infectivity of diverse strains HIV and SIV for T cells and monocytes but not for brain and muscle cells. *Nature* **337**: 368.

Connor, R.I., N.B. Dinces, A.L. Howell, J.L. Romet-Lemonne, J.L. Pasquali, and M.W. Fanger. 1991. Fc receptors for IgG (Fc Rs) on human monocytes and macrophages are not infectivity receptors for human immunodeficiency virus type 1 (HIV-1): Studies using bi-specific myeloid cell surface molecules including Fc R. *Proc. Natl. Acad. Sci.* **88**: 9593.

Corapi, W.V., C.W. Olsen, and F.W. Scott. 1992. Monoclonal antibody analysis of neutralization and antibody-dependent enhancement of feline infectious peritonitis virus. *J. Virol.* **66**: 6695.

Giminez, H.B., H.M. Keir, and P. Cash. 1989. In vitro enhancement of respiratory syncytial virus infection of U937 cell by human serum. *J. Gen. Virol.* **70**: 89.

Gollins, S.W. and J.S. Porterfield. 1985. Flavivirus infection enhancement in macrophages: An electron microscopic study of viral cellular entry. *J. Gen. Virol.* **66**: 1969.

Halstead, S.B. 1982. Immune enhancement of viral infection. *Prog. Allergy* **31**: 301.

Halstead, S.B. and E.J. O'Rourke. 1977a. Antibody-enhanced dengue virus infection in primate leukocytes. *Nature* **265**: 739.

―――. 1977b. Dengue viruses and mononuclear phagocytes. I. Infection enhancement by nonneutralizing antibody. *J. Exp. Med.* **146**: 201.

Halstead, S.B., J.S. Chow, and N.J. Marchette. 1973. Immunological enhancement of dengue virus replication. *Nat. New Biol.* **243**: 24.

Halstead, S.B., E.J. O'Rourke, and A.C. Allison. 1977. Dengue viruses and mononuclear phagocytes. II. Identity of blood and tissue leukocytes supporting in vitro infection. *J. Exp. Med.* **146**: 218.

Hawkes, R.A. 1964. Enhancement of the infectivity of arboviruses by specific antisera products in infected fowls. *Aust. J. Exp. Biol. Med. Sci.* **42**: 465.

Hawkes, R.A. and K.J. Lafferty. 1967. The enhancement of virus infectivity by antibody. *Virology* **33**: 250.

Hohdatsu, T., M. Nakamura, Y. Ishizuka, H. Yamada, and H. Koyama. 1991. A study on the mechanism of antibody-dependent enhancement of feline infectious peritonitis virus infection in feline macrophages by monoclonal antibodies. *Arch. Virol.* **120**: 207.

Homsy, J., M. Meyer, and J.A. Levy. 1990. Serum enhancement of human immunodeficiency virus (HIV) infection correlates with disease in HIV-infected individuals. *J. Virol.* **64**: 1437.

Hotta, H. and S. Hotta. 1982. Dengue virus multiplication in cultures of mouse peritoneal macrophages: Effects of macrophage activators. *Microbiol. Immunol.* **26**: 665.

Issel, C.J., D.W. Horohor, D.F. Lea, M.V. Adams, Jr., S.D. Hagins, J.M. McManus, A.C. Allison, and R.C. Montelaro. 1992. Efficacy of inactivated whole virus and subunit vaccines in preventing infection and disease caused by equine infectious anemia virus. *J. Virol.* **66**: 3398.

Jolly, P.E., D.L. Huso, D. Shefer, and O. Narayan. 1989. Modulation of lentivirus replication by antibodies: Fc portion of immunoglobulin molecule is essential for enhancement of binding, internalization and neutralization of visna virus in macrophages. *J. Virol.* **63:** 1811.

Kimura, T., S.W. Gollins, and J.S. Porterfield. 1986. The effect of pH on the early interactions of West Nile with P338D1 cells. *J. Gen. Virol.* **69:** 1247.

Kliks, S. 1990. Antibody-enhanced infection of monocytes as the pathogenic mechanism for severe dengue illness. *AIDS Res. Hum. Retroviruses* **6:** 993.

Kliks, S.C. and S.B. Halstead. 1980. An explanation for enhanced virus plaque formation in chick embryo cells. *Nature* **285:** 504.

———. 1983. Role of antibodies and host cells in plaque enhancement of Murray Valley encephalitis virus. *J. Virol.* **46:** 394.

Kliks, S.C., S. Nimmannitya, A. Nisalak, and D.S. Burke. 1988. Evidence that maternal dengue antibodies are important in the development of dengue hemorrhagic fever in infants. *Am. J. Trop. Med. Hyg.* **38:** 411.

Kliks, S.C., A. Nisalak, W.E. Brandt, L. Wahl, and D.S. Burke. 1989. Antibody-dependent enhancement of dengue virus growth in human monocytes as a risk factor for dengue hemorrhagic fever. *Am. J. Trop. Med. Hyg.* **40:** 444.

Kobayashi, K., M.J. Blaser, and W.R. Brown. 1989. Identification of a unique IgG Fc binding site in human intestinal epithelium. *J. Immunol.* **143:** 2567.

Kontny, U., I. Kurane, and F.A. Ennis. 1988. Gamma interferon augments Fc receptor-mediated dengue virus infection of human monocytic cells. *J. Virol.* **62:** 3928.

Krilov, L.R., R.M. Hendry, E. Godfrey, and K. McIntosh. 1987. Respiratory virus infection of peripheral blood monocytes: Correlation with ageing of cells and interferon production *in vitro. J. Gen. Virol.* **68:** 1749.

Krilov, L.R., L.J. Anderson, L. Marcoux, V.R. Bonagura, and J.F. Wedgwood. 1989. Antibody-mediated enhancement of respiratory syncytial virus infection in two monocyte/macrophage cell lines. *J. Infect. Dis.* **162:** 777.

Marsh, M. and A. Helenius. 1989. Virus entry into animal cells. *Adv. Virus Res.* **36:** 107.

Matsuda, S., M. Gidlund, F. Chiodi, A. Cafaro, A. Nygren, B. Morein, K. Nilsson, E.M. Fenyo, and H. Wigzell. 1989. Enhancement of human immunodeficiency virus (HIV) replication in human monocytes by low titres of anti-HIV antibodies in vitro. *Scand. J. Immunol.* **30:** 425.

McGuire, T.C., D.S. Adams, G.C. Johnson, P. Klevjer-Anderson, P.D. Barbee, and J.R. Gorham. 1986. Acute arthritis in caprine arthritis-encephalitis virus challenge exposure of vaccinated or persistently infected goats. *Am. J. Vet. Res.* **47:** 537.

McKeating, J.A., P.D. Griffiths, and R.A. Weiss. 1990. HIV susceptibility conferred to human fibroblasts by cytomegalovirus-induced Fc receptor. *Nature* **343:** 659.

Mertz, D.C., A. Scheid, and P.W. Choppin. 1980. Importance of antibodies to the fusion proteins of paramyxoviruses to the prevention of the spread of infection. *J. Exp. Med.* **151:** 275.

Mogensen, S.C. 1979. Role of macrophages in natural resistance to virus infections. *Microbiol. Rev.* **43:** 1.

Montefiori, D.C., W.E. Robinson, Jr., and W.M. Mitchell. 1989. Antibody-independent, complement-mediated enhancement of HIV-1 infection by mannosidase I and II inhibitors. *Antiviral Res.* **11:** 137.

Montefiori, D.C., M. Murphey-Corb, R.C. Desrosiers, and M.D. Daniel. 1990. Complement-mediated, infection-enhancing antibodies in plasma from vaccinated macaques before and after inoculation with live simian immuno-deficiency virus. *J. Virol.* **64:** 5223.

Morahan, P.S., J.R. Connor, and K.R. Leary. 1985. Viruses and the versatile macrophage. *Br. Med. Bull.* **41:** 15.

Morens, D.M. and S.B. Halstead. 1987. Disease severity–related antigenic differences in dengue 2 strains detected by dengue 4 monoclonal antibodies. *J. Med. Virol.* **22:** 169.

———. 1990. Measurement of antibody-dependent infection enhancement of four dengue virus serotypes by monoclonal and polyclonal antibodies. *J. Gen. Virol.* **71:** 2909.

Murphy, B.R., G.A. Prince, E.E. Walsh, H.W. Kim, R.H. Parrott, V.G. Hemming, W.J. Rodriguez, and R.M. Chanock. 1986. Dissociation between serum neutralizing and glycoprotein antibody responses of infants and children who received inactivated respiratory syncytial virus vaccine. *J. Clin. Microbiol.* **24:** 197.

Norrby, E. 1975. Occurrence of antibodies against envelope components after immunization with formalin inactivated and live measles vaccine. *J. Biol. Stand.* **3:** 375.

Norrby, E., G. Enders-Ruckle, and V. ter Meulen. 1975. Differences in the appearance of antibodies to structural components of measles virus after immunization with inactivated and live virus. *J. Infect. Dis.* **132:** 262.

Ochiai, H., M. Kurokawa, K. Hayashi, and S. Niwayama. 1988. Antibody-mediated growth of influenza A NWS virus in macrophage-like cell line, P388D1. *J. Virol.* **62:** 20.

Ochiai, H., M. Kurokawa, V. Kuroki, and S. Niwayama. 1990. Infection enhancement of influenza A H1 subtype viruses in macrophage-like P388D1 cells by cross-reactive antibodies. *J. Med. Virol.* **30:** 258.

Ochiai, H., M. Kurokawa, S. Matsui, T. Yamamoto, Y. Kuroki, C. Kishimoto, and K. Shiraki. 1992. Infection enhancement of influenza A NWS virus in primary murine macrophages by anti-hemagglutinin monoclonal antibody. *J. Med. Virol.* **36:** 217.

Okuno, Y., T. Harada, M. Ogawa, Y. Okamoto, and K. Maeda. 1989. A case of dengue hemorrhagic fever in a Japanese child. *Microbiol. Immunol.* **33:** 649.

Olsen, C.W., W.V. Corapi, C.K. Ngichabe, J.D. Baines, and F.W. Scott. 1992. Monoclonal antibodies to the spike protein of feline infectious peritonitis virus mediate antibody-dependent enhancement of infection of feline microphages. *J. Virol.* **66:** 956.

Pedersen, N.C. and J.F. Boyle. 1990. Immunologic phenomena in the effusive form of feline infectious peritonitis. *Am. J. Vet. Res.* **41:** 868.

Porter, D.D., A.E. Larsen, and H.G. Porter. 1972. The pathogenesis of Aleutian disease of mink. II. Enhancement of tissue lesions following administration of killed virus vaccine or passive antibody. *J. Immunol.* **109:** 1.

Porterfield, J.S. 1986. Antibody-dependent enhancement of viral infectivity. *Adv. Virus Res.* **31:** 335.

Rico-Hesse, R. 1990. Molecular evolution and distribution of dengue viruses type 1 and 2 in nature. *Virology.* **174:** 479.

Robinson, W.E., Jr., D.C. Montefiori, and W.M. Mitchell. 1987. A human immunodeficiency virus type 1 (HIV-1) infection-enhancing factor in sero-positive sera. *Biochem. Biophys. Res. Commun.* **149:** 693.

———. 1988. Antibody-dependent enhancement of human immunodeficiency virus type 1 infection. *Lancet* **1:** 790.

Robinson, W.E., Jr., D.C. Montefiori, D.H. Gillespie, and W.M. Mitchell. 1989a. Complement-mediated, antibody-dependent enhancement of HIV-1 infection *in vitro* is characterized by increased protein and RNA synthesis and infectious virus release. *J. Acquired Immune Defic. Syndr.* **2:** 33.

Robinson, W.E., Jr., D.C. Montefiori, W.M. Mitchell, A.M. Prince, H.J. Alter, G.R. Dreesman, and J.W. Eichberg. 1989b. Antibody-dependent enhancement of human immunodeficiency virus type 1 (HIV-1) infection *in vitro* by serum from HIV-1-infected and passively immunized chimpanzees. *Proc. Natl. Acad. Sci.* **86:** 4710.

Sangkawibha, N., S. Rojanasuphot, S. Ahandrik, S. Viriyapongse, S. Jatanasen, V. Salitul, B. Phanthumachinda, and S.B. Halstead. 1984. Risk factors in dengue shock syndrome: A prospective-epidemiologic study in Rayong, Thailand. I. The 1980 outbreak. *Am. J. Immunol.* **120:** 653.

Schlesinger, J.J. and M.W. Brandriss. 1981. Growth of 17D yellow fever virus in a macrophage-like cell line, U937: Role of Fc and viral receptors in antibody-mediated infection. *J. Immunol.* **127:** 659.

Shadduck, P.P.. J.B. Weinberg, A.F. Haney, J.A. Bartlett, A.J. Langlois, D.P. Bolognesi, and T.J. Matthews. 1991. Lack of enhancing effect of human anti-human immunodeficiency virus type 1 (HIV-1) antibody on HIV-1 infection of human blood monocytes and peritoneal macrophages. *J. Virol.* **65:** 4309.

Stott, J.L., G.A. Anderson, M.M. Jochim, T.L. Barber, and B.I. Osburn. 1984. Clinical expression of blue tongue disease in cattle. *Proc. Annu. Meet. U.S. Anim. Health Assoc.* **86:** 126.

Takeda, A. and F.A. Ennis. 1990. FcR-mediated enhancement of HIV-1 infection by antibody. *AIDS Res. Hum. Retroviruses* **6:** 999.

Tamura, M., R.G. Webster, and F.A. Ennis. 1991. Antibodies to HA and NA augment uptake of influenza A viruses into cells via Fc receptor entry. *Virology* **182:** 211.

Traavik, T., L. Uhlin-Hansen, T. Flaegstad, and H.E. Christie. 1988. Antibody-mediated enhancement of 3K virus infection in human monocytes and a human macrophage-like cell line. *J. Med. Virol.* **24:** 283.

Tremblay, M., S. Meloche, R.P. Sekaly, and M.A. Wainberg. 1990. Complement receptor 2 mediates enhancement of HIV-1 infection in Epstein-Barr virus-carrying B cells. *J. Exp. Med.* **171:** 1791.

Unkeless, J.C., E. Scigliano, and V.H. Freedman. 1988. Structure and function of human and murine receptors of IgG. *Annu. Rev. Immunol.* **6:** 251.

Van der Groen, G., P.A.R. Van den Berghe, and S.R. Pattyn. 1976. Interaction of mouse peritoneal macrophages with different arboviruses in vitro. *J. Gen. Virol.* **34:** 353.

Vennema, H., J. Raoul, R.J. de Groot, D.A. Harbour, M. Dalderup, T. Gruffydd-Jones, M.C. Horzinek, and W.J. Spaan. 1990. Early death after feline infectious peritonitis virus challenge due to recombinant vaccinia virus immunization. *J. Virol.* **64:** 1407.

Webster, R.G. and B.A. Askonas. 1980. Cross-protection and cross-reactive cytotoxic T cells induced by influenza virus vaccines in mice. *Eur. J. Immunol.* **10:** 396.

Weiss, R.C. and F.W. Scott. 1981. Antibody-mediated enhancement of disease in feline infectious peritonitis: Comparisons with dengue hemorrhagic fever. *Comp. Immunol. Microbiol. Infect. Dis.* **4:** 175.

Wigzell, H. 1988. Immunopathogenesis of HIV infection. *J. Acquired Immune Defic. Syndr.* **1:** 559.

Wiharta, A.S., H. Hotta, S. Hotta, T. Matsumura, M. Tsuji, and Sujidi. 1985. Increased multiplication of dengue virus in mouse peritoneal macrophage cultures by treatment with extracts of Ascaris-Parascaris parasites. *Microbiol. Immunol.* **29:** 337.

Yao, J.S., H. Kariwa, I. Takashima, K. Yoshimatsu, J. Arikawa, and N. Hashimoto. 1992. Antibody-dependent enhancement of hantavirus infection in macrophage cell lines. *Arch Virol.* **122:** 107.

Zeira, M., A.. Rendal, and J.E. Groopman. 1990. Inhibition of serum-enhanced HIV-1 infection of U937 monocytoid cells by recombinant soluble CD4 and anti-CD4 monoclonal antibody. *AIDS Res. Hum. Retroviruses* **6:** 629.

Index

9-*O*-Acetylated neuraminic acid
    binding of gHE and gS of BCV and HEV, 423–424, 429–430
    binding of gHE and gS of HCV-OC43, 423
Acetylcholine receptor (α-1), 4, 228
Acetyl esterase. *See* Bovine coronavirus
ADE. *See* Antibody-dependent enhancement of infection
Adenovirus
    multiple cell-surface proteins in viral binding, 488
    pH dependence, 222
    renewed interest in cloning T2 and T5 receptor genes, 82
    shared receptor with coxsackievirus B3, 2, 82
    virus/receptor relationships, 7–8, 229
    vitronectin as entry accessory factor, 8
African green monkey kidney cells (Vero C1008). *See* Epithelial cells
African swine fever virus, 229
AIDS. *See* CD4 receptor; Human immunodeficiency viruses;Receptor-mediated virus entry
Aleutian disease of mink virus, 411, 499
Alphaviruses
    anti-Id antibodies as antireceptor antibodies, 144–147
    early studies of receptors, 143–144
    laminin receptor as chicken receptor, 153–156
    laminin receptor as mammalian receptor, 147–153
    role of E1 and E2 in altering receptor-binding domain, 157–159
    search for mosquito cell receptors, 155–157
    structure, 142–143
ALSV. *See* Avian leukosis and sarcoma viruses

Amantadine, 9–10, 305–308, 311–317
ε-Amino-η-caproic acid, 264
Aminopeptidase N receptor, 1
    in coronavirus diagnosis and prevention, 434–435
    HCV-229E, 431–434
    TGEV, 431–434
    virus/receptor relationships, 5, 229
Antibody 280, 481. *See also* Polioviruses; Poliovirus receptors
Antibody AF3, 481–488. *See also* CD44, lymphocyle homing receptor; Polioviruses; Poliovirus receptors
Antibody D171, 481. *See also* Polioviruses; Poliovirus receptors
Antibody-dependent enhancement (ADE) of infection, 493–512
    antibody and normal cell receptor relationships, 507
    antibody-enhancing titer, 500
    antibody-Fc receptor, vertebrate class, 497
    antibody-idiotype specificity, 498–499
    antibody-Ig class, 496–497
    antibody-Ig subclass, 497
    antibody-nonneutralizing concentration, 499–500
    autologous immune enhancement, 510
    complement, 501–502
    cytophilic antibodies: effect on ADE, 504
    intratypic variants, 509–510
    macrophage activation: effect on ADE, 505
    non-antibody complement, 502
    non-antibody, other than complement, 502
    non-enhanceable viruses, 508–509
    permissive FcR-bearing cells, 503–512
    sensitizing infections or immunization, 510–511
    tissue macrophage: importance of source, 506
    vaccine-enhanced disease, 511

"A" particle, 81, 86, 116–117, 471. *See also*
  Poliovirus receptors; Transgenic mice
  studies
APN. *See* Aminopeptidase N receptor
Aprotinin, 264
Arenaviridae, 247
Astroglial cell lines, U87 and U373, 22, 24
Aujeszky's disease, 365
Avian leukosis and sarcoma viruses. *See also*
  Leukosis virus
  blockage of ALSV-A infection, 67–68
  comparing and contrasting of ALSV-A and
    CD4, 69–70
  expression of ALSV-A susceptibility factor,
    63–65
  model system for retrovirus infection, 62–63
  receptor locus for ALSV-A: *tva*, 69

B-cell lymphomas, 375
BCV. *See* Bovine coronavirus
BFA. *See* Brefeldin A
bFGF. *See* Fibroblast growth factor
BGP. *See* Biliary glycoprotein
Biliary glycoprotein (BGP)
  human receptors, 411–412
  receptor interactions with MHV strains, 424–
    425
  murine variant receptors, 416–417
  rodent receptors, 415–419
  splice variant receptors, 415–416
  tissue-dependent expression of isoforms, 430
Blue tongue virus, 511
BLV. *See* Bovine leukosis virus
Bovine coronavirus
  cleavage, 247
  receptor-independent fusion, 405
  receptors, 423–424
  role of acetyl esterase in infectivity reduction,
    423
  role of gHE in interaction of gS with its
    receptor, 429
  virus/receptor relationships, 5, 229
Bovine leukosis virus, 16, 69–70
Brefeldin A, 333–335
Bunyaviruses, basolateral release, 330
Burkitt's lymphoma, 373

CaMKII kinase, 109
Canine coronavirus (CCV), 431
Canine distemper virus, 182
Canyon hypothesis, 110
Caprine arthritis-encephalitis virus, 493, 499,
  511
Carboxypeptidase N, 257
Carcinoembryonic antigen, 4, 229, 411–415
Cardioviruses, 84
Cartilage link family, 482

Cationic amino acid transporter, mouse, 1, 50–
  55
C'C" ridge, 38–39, 42–43
CD4 receptor. *See also* Receptor-mediated
  virus entry; Retroviruses, type C;
  Retrovirus receptors
  comparison with ALSV-A, 69–70
  conformational changes, 20
  contacts with class II MHC proteins, 42–43
  cytoplasmic contact, 44
  in endocytosis, 217
  in HIV entry, 19–21, 36–39
  homology with V domain of hPVR, 115
  inducement of gp120 shedding, 39
  interactions with $p56^{lck}$, 218
  likely second role, 33, 89
  possible strategies to inhibit HIV infection,
    40
  recombinant soluble CD4 (sCD4)
    enhancement of infection, 24
    role in entry, 21
    use in therapy, 25
  structure, 33–36
  V domain fusion to domains 3–4 of CD4,
    111
CD13. *See* Aminopeptidase N receptor
CD14+. *See* Poliovirus receptors
CD26, 22, 181
CD34+, 456
CD44, lymphocyte homing receptor
  CD44H and $_{AF3}$CD44H
    molecular basis of interaction with PVR,
      487–488
  in PV attachment and infection, 483–487
  in poliovirus infection, 8, 451, 457
  virus/receptor relationships, 77, 481–482
CD46. *See* Measles virus; Membrane cofactor
  protein
CD55. *See* Decay accelerating factor
CD4-D1D2, 33–36
CD4-D3D4, 33–36
CEA. *See* Carcinoembryonic antigen
CEA-related glycoproteins
  BGP regulation during embryogenesis and
    cell transformation, 419
  BGPs as cell adhesion molecules, 418
  cellular functions, 418
  NCA as a receptor, 418
Chimera polioviruses
  ability to infect mice, 464
  virus-encoded PV virulence, 446
Chymotrypsin, 263–264
Class II MHC molecules, 42. *See also* CD4
  receptor
Clathrin. *See* Endocytosis
Coated vesicles
  in bulk membrane turnover, 216
  in fluid-phase endocytosis, 216
  formation, 216–219
  in receptor-mediated endocytosis, 216

Coronaviridae, 246–247
Coronaviruses. *See also* Bovine coronavirus;
    Mouse hepatitis virus
  basolateral release, 330
  disease diagnosis and prevention, 434–436
  MHV receptor, 408–422
  MHV-related receptors, 422–424
    bovine coronavirus, 423–424
    hemagglutinin encephalomyelitis virus,
        423–424
    human coronavirus HCV-OC43, 423
    rat coronavirus, 422
    sialodacryadenitis virus, 422
    virus/receptor interactions, 403–436
      role of HE glycoprotein, 403–408
      role of S glycoprotein, 403–408
Coxsackieviruses
  B3-RD variant, 87
  CBV5 relationship to SVDV, 8
  shared receptors, 82
  virus/receptor relationships, 4, 8, 76–77, 229
Cryoelectron microscopy, 342
Cutter incident, 473
Cytomegaloviruses
  human (HCVM)
    associated diseases, 370
    cellular receptors, 370–372
    cleavage, 249, 262
    latent infection, 365–366
    viral/receptor relationships, 5, 228
  mouse (MCVM) virus/receptor relationships,
        4, 228

Decay accelerating factor (CD55), 1–2
Dengue virus
  cause of hemorrhagic fever, 9
  receptor-mediated virus entry, 494, 496–500,
      504–510

Eastern equine encephalitis virus. *See also* Al-
    phaviruses
  ability to cause encephalitis in man, 142
  isolation from hematophagous arthropods and
      from mosquitoes, 141
EBV. *See* Epstein-Barr virus
Echo viruses
  localization of gene receptors on human
      chromosome 19, 79
  relationships to receptors, 4–5, 77
  type 1, 2, 86, 229
  type 7 (6, 11, 12, 20, 21), 2
  type 8, 86
EEE. *See* Eastern equine encephalitis virus
EGF. *See* Epidermal growth factor receptor
Elastase, 263
EMCV. *See* Encephalomyocarditis virus

Encephalitis, 366. *See also* Alphaviruses
Encephalitis, measles inclusion body. *See*
    Measles virus; Membrane cofactor
    protein, CD46
Encephalomyocarditis virus, 5, 7, 77, 86, 229
Endocytic pathway, 218, 231
Endocytic signals, 217–219
Endocytosis. *See also* Receptor-mediated virus
    entry
  constitutive, 215–217
  phagocytic, 215–217
  receptor-mediated, 81, 216
  and viral entry, 221–235, 245
Endoproteinases, 16, 257–263
Endosomes
  early, 219
  late, 219
  in membrane fusion in influenza viruses, 62,
      281
  pH factor, 219–221
  in virus entry, 281
Enteric viruses. *See* Coronaviruses; Coxsack-
    ieviruses; Polioviruses; Reoviruses
Enteroviruses
  enterovirus (EV) 70, 8
  acid-pH-resistance factor, 81
Epidermal growth factor (EGF) receptor, 4,
    229
Epithelial cells
  apical and basolateral (polarized) domains,
      323–336
    Caco-2, 324, 328, 331, 333
    Vero C1008, 324, 328, 331–333
    virus entry, 326–328
    virus release from infected cells, 328–335
  growth on porous supports, 324–326
Epstein-Barr virus
  binding, 373–376
  cellular receptors, 374–377
    complement receptors, 374
    short consensus repeats (SCRs), 374
  entry, 377–379
    endocytosis, 377
    pH independence, 230
    viral envelope fusion, 379
  latent infection, 365–366
  role in diseases, 373
Equine infectious anemia, 499, 511

Factor X, 258
Familial hypercholesteremia (FH)
  incubation of HRV-2 with FH fibroblasts,
      131
  infection with HRV-2, 133
  receptor-associated protein (RAP), 135
Fc receptor, 86, 228
Feline infectious bronchitis virus (FIBV), 404
Feline infectious peritonitis virus, 406

Feline infectious peritonitis virus (*continued*)
  antibody-dependent enhancement (ADE),
    494, 499, 504, 511
  binding, 431
  cleavage of glycoproteins, 247, 406
Feline leukemia virus type B, 18
FeLV-B. *See* Feline leukemia virus type B
Fibroblast growth factor, 367
FIPV. *See* Feline infectious peritonitis virus
Flaviviridae, 246
FM. *See* Fort Morgan virus
FMDV. *See* Foot and mouth disease virus
Foot and mouth disease virus
  sensitivity to neuraminidase, 84
  structure, 196
  unique feature, 78
  virus/receptor relationships, 4, 77, 229
Fort Morgan virus, 141. *See also* Alphaviruses
Fowl plague virus
  A/Udorn/72, 313, 316–317
  cleavage, 260, 262–265
  endocytic fusion, 232
  Rostock, 313, 316–317
  Weybridge, 313, 317
FPV. *See* Fowl plague virus
Furin, 260–265
  accumulation in *trans* Golgi network (TGN),
    261–262
  glycoprotein activation, 262
Fusion peptide, 191
Fusion pore
  formation and opening, 292–295
  M2 TM domain, 311–312, 315–316
Fusion (F) proteins in cleavage, 241, 250,
  262–263, 266

Galactosyl ceramide
  alternative receptor site to CD4, 7, 16, 24
  virus/receptor relationships, 5, 228
GALV. *See* Gibbon-ape leukemia virus
Gibbon-ape leukemia virus. *See* Avian
    leukosis and sarcoma viruses;
    Retrovirus receptors, human;
    Retroviruses, type C
Glycoprotein B, 249, 262, 368
Glycoprotein C, 326–327, 366–368
Glycoprotein 120/gp41 oligomer
  C′ C″ ridge role in gp120/CD4 interaction,
    38–40
  conformational changes, 20–21, 42
  free gp120, 36–39
  gp160, precursor, 39
  in HIV entry, 19–21, 36–39
  of sCD4 in uncoupling, 21, 25
Glycoprotein HE of coronaviruses
  accessory attachment protein, 430
  binding to 9-*O*-acetylated neuraminic acid,
    429–430

  role of esterase activity in viral spread, 429–
    430
  tissue tropism, 408
Glycoproteins. *See also specific glycoproteins*
  in coronavirus/receptor interactions, 403–407
  in EBV infection, 374–381
  in HMCV infection, 370–374
  in poliovirus, 79
Glycoprotein S of coronaviruses
  binding specificity, 426
  conformational changes, 406, 427–428
  interaction with BGP receptor, 424–427
  membrane fusion, 406, 427–428
  mutants, 406
  role of surface density in MHV infection,
    426–427
  spike, 404
  tissue tropism, 406
Glycoprotein 120 shedding, 39–41. *See also*
    CD4 receptor
Glycosaminoglycans, 8
G protein, 330

HA. *See* Hemagglutinin
HA-mediated membrane fusion, 281–296
HCAT-1. *See* Human cationic amino acid
    transporter 1
HCV-229E. *See* Human coronavirus 229E
HCV-OC43. *See* Human coronavirus OC43
Hemagglutinating encephalomyelitis virus
    receptors, 423–424
Hemagglutinin (HA). *See also* Influenza
    viruses
  biosynthesis, 305–306
  conformational changes, 282–292, 307–308,
    314–316
  fusion, 306
Hemagglutinin membrane. *See* Influenza
    viruses, hemagglutinin protein
Hemagglutinin neuraminidase (HN), 243
Hemorrhagic fever, 9, 493
Heparan sulfate proteoglycan
  binding of HSV infection cells, 8, 367
  virus/receptor relationship, 228
Heparin-specific proteoglycan
  in HCMV infection, 370–371
  in HSV infection, 368–370
Hepatitis, autoimmune chronic active. *See*
    Measles virus; Membrane cofactor
    protein, CD46
Hermes 2 antibodies, 487. *See also* CD44,
    lymphocyte homing receptor;
    Polioviruses; Poliovirus receptors
Herpes simplex viruses
  basolateral release, 330
  early events in entry, 366–370
    cellular receptors, 367–368
    pH-independent direct fusion, 368

hSV-1
  bFGF not receptor, 367
  latent infection, 365–366
  virus entry in polarized epithelial cells, 236–237
Herpesviridae, 249
Herpesviruses. *See also* Cytomegaloviruses; Epstein-Barr virus; Herpes simplex viruses; Varicella-zoster virus
  bovine, type 1 (BHV-1), 369
  early events in infection, 365–381
  human, type 7 (HHV-7), relationship to receptor, 4, 18
HEV. *See* Hemagglutinating encephalomyelitis virus
HIV. *See* Human immunodeficiency viruses
Hodgkin's disease, 373
HRV. *See* Rhinoviruses, human
HSPG. *See* Heparin-specific proteoglycan
HSV. *See* Herpes simplex viruses
HTLV-1. *See* Human T-cell leukemia virus type 1
Human cationic amino acid transporter 1, 52
Human chromosome 19, 79, 415, 465. *See also* Echoviruses; Polioviruses; Rhinoviruses, human
Human coronavirus 229E
  aminopeptidase N (APN) receptors, 431–434
  membrane fusion, 404–406
Human coronavirus OC43, 404, 423
Human immunodeficiency viruses. *See also* Antibody-dependent enhancement (ADE) of infection; CD4 receptor; Retrovirus receptors, human
  alternative receptors, 7, 22–24
  assembly of particles in polarized epithelial cells, 329
  entry, 19–21
    constitutive endocytic activity, 230
    endocytosis, 233–234
    pH independence, 224
    role of envelope glycoprotein, 39–42
  HIV-1
    binding, 181, 488
    cleavage/fusion, 248, 262–265
    conformational changes, 15–16
    interaction with CD4⁻, 180
  HIV-2
    alternative receptor, 24
    cleavage/fusion, 248
    pH independence, 224
    secondary receptors, 21–23
Human parainfluenza virus III, 262–263
Human T-cell leukemia virus type 1, 17, 55–56
Hybrid receptors with HPVR
  antigenic hybrid viruses and receptor binding, 115–116
  MPH fusion, 113
  mutational analysis and model of the V

domain, 113–115
  homolog scanning between hPVR and MPH, 114
  N-glycosylation sites, 115
  V domain fusion with ICAM and CD4, 111
Hygromycin B. *See* Avian leukosis and sarcoma viruses

IBV. *See* Infectious bronchitis virus
ICAM-1 (intercellular adhesion molecule 1)
  antigenic hybrid viruses and receptor binding, 115–116
  HRV virion can bind 60 molecules, 84
  interaction with rhinoviruses, 195–210
  structure, 199–202
  V domain fusion to domains 3–5, 111
  Ig-like domains, 33
Immunoglobulin G (IgG). *See* Antibody-dependent enhancement (ADE) of infection
Infectious bovine rhinotracheitis, 365
Infectious bronchitis virus, 247, 404–406
Infectious mononucleosis, 370, 373
Infectious subvirion particle. *See* Reoviruses, characterization of ISVPs
Influenza, 493. *See also* Influenza viruses
Influenza viruses. *See also* Endocytosis
  apical budding, 328–329
  avian strains, 254–256
  bacterial coinfection, 256–257
  entry, 62
  hemagglutinin (HA) protein
    cleavage, 306
    comparison to retrovirus env proteins, 61
    in infection, 243, 252–256
    in membrane fusion, 188–192, 281–296
    parallels to "A" particles in picornaviruses, 81
    parallels to HIV, 41
    proteases, 257–260
    receptor binding site, 7, 187–188
  influenza A
    inhibitory effect of drug amantadine, 9
    protease activation of infectivity, 258, 507
    role of M2 ion channel protein, 303–318
  influenza C, HEF, 245
  polarized cell growth, 325
ISVP. *See* Infectious subvirion particle

JA-1, transformed mouse L-cell line, 105

100 kD protein. *See* CD44; Polioviruses; Poliovirus receptors

Kex2 protease, 260, 263
Knockout mice, 89

Lassa virus cleavage site, 247
LCM. *See* Lymphocytic choriomeningitis
virus
LDLR. *See* Low-density lipoprotein receptor
Leukemia viruses
bovine, 5, 228
feline, type B (FeLV-B), 18, 51, 228, 230
gibbon ape (GALV), 4, 16, 18, 50–51, 230
human T-cell, type 1 (HTLV-1), 17, 228
radiation, 228
Leukosis virus. *See also* Avian leukosis and
sarcoma viruses
avian, subgroup A (ALV-A), 4, 16
bovine (BLV), 16
LFA-1 integrin receptor, 201, 488. *See also*
CD44, lymphocyte homing receptor;
Polioviruses; Poliovirus receptors
LFA-3 integrin receptor, 487. *See also* CD44,
lymphocyte homing receptor;
Polioviruses; Poliovirus receptors
Ligand blots. *See* Rhinoviruses, human
Lovo cells, 263
Low-density lipoprotein receptor. *See also*
Avian leukosis and sarcoma viruses;
Rhinoviruses, human
correlation of overexpression with increased
HRV binding, 133
infection of LDLR-deficient human
fibroblasts with HRV-2, 133
internalization and delivery, 136
pH factor, 219–221
techniques for identification of HRV binding
protein, 131
Lymphocytic choriomeningitis virus, cleavage
site, 247

α_2-Macroglobulin receptor/LDLR-related
protein (α_2MR/LRP), 1. *See also*
Rhinoviruses, human
Madin-Darby canine kidney cells
polarized budding, 323–328
virus release, 328
Mannose-6-phosphate, role in HSV infection,
8
Marek's disease, 365
MCAT-1. *See* Cationic amino acid transporter,
mouse
MDCK. *See* Madin-Darby canine kidney cells
Measles. *See* Measles virus; Membrane cofactor protein, CD46
Measles virus
agglutination of monkey erythrocytes, 168
antibody-dependent enhancement of infec-

tion, 498–500, 511
identification of receptor, 169–172, 181
infection of primates, 166–167
Membrane cofactor protein, CD46
determination of measles virus host
specificity, 169–182
CD46 function, 174–176
CD46 structure, 173–174
hemagglutinin gp required for viral attachment, 166
Mengovirus, 78, 196
MHCI antigen role in HCMV infection, 371
MHV. *See* Mouse hepatitis virus
β_2-Microglobulin (β2m) role in HCMV infection, 371
MLV. *See* Murine leukemia viruses
Moesin
possible measles virus receptor, 181
virus/receptor relationship, 5
Mouse hepatitis virus
antireceptor antibodies, 409–412
cleavage of E2, 247
host resistance, 408–409
virus binding in intestine membranes, 409
virus binding in liver membranes, 409
interactions with BGP receptors, 424–425
receptors, 408–422
BGP receptor activities, 419–420, 422,
424–427
CEA-related, 408–412
cloning and expression of MHVR, 412–414
functional domains of MHVR, 420–421
related coronavirus receptors, 422–424
virus/receptor relationships, 4, 229, 403–408,
424–425
M protein, 330, 335, 455
M1 protein, 307–310
M2 protein, 303–318, 356
effects of antibodies, 304–305
ion channel activity blocked by amantadine,
305–308
pH regulation of ion channel activity, 312–
313, 316–318
structure, 303–304
MuLV. *See* Murine leukemia viruses
Murine coronavirus, 408–412. *See also* Mouse
hepatitis virus
Murine leukemia viruses. *See also*
Retroviruses, type C
amphotropic (MLV-A), 16, 25, 49–51, 53
ecotropic (MLV-E), 16, 49–55, 230
xenotropic, 49–50
Murray Valley encephalitis virus, 495
MVE. *See* Murray Valley encephalitis virus

Nasopharyngeal carcinoma, 373
NDV. *See* Newcastle disease virus
Neuraminidase, 423

Newcastle disease virus, 242, 250, 252, 258, 262–263

Orthomyxoviridae, 243–246
  function of hemagglutinin, 243–246
  fusion, 245

Paget's bone disease. *See* Measles virus; Membrane cofactor protein, CD46
Panencephalitis, subacute sclerosing. *See* Measles virus; Membrane cofactor protein, CD46
Panning, 105
Parainfluenza 3 virus, 498–499, 505, 511
Paramyxoviridae, 241–243, 250
  fusion (F) protein, 241
  Sendai virus, 241
  tropism, 258
Peptidyl chloromethylketones, 264–265
Pestivirus des petits ruminants, 182
Peyer's patches, 390–392, 455, 463
pH factor
  in coronavirus infection, 407
  in EBV infection, 377
  effects on endosomes, 219–221
  effects of M2 protein, 310–311
  in fusion, 245, 247, 258, 260, 281–296
  in HCMV infection, 372
  in influenza virus conformational changes, 41, 62
  interactions with early and late endosomes, 219–220
  pH-dependent viruses, 215, 221–223, 227, 246, 368
  pH-independent viruses, 223–224
  regulation of the M2 protein ion channel activity, 312–313, 316–317
Phocine distemper virus, 182
Pichinde virus cleavage site, 247
Picornaviruses
  anti-idiotypic antibodies, 78
  early events in infection, 80–82
    acid pH factor, 81
    virus eclipse, 80, 90
    virus uncoating, 81, 90
  pathogenesis of infection, 87–90
    current status, 89–90
    importance of second receptor function, 88
    transgenic mice studies of PV infection, 88
  receptors, 75–90
    creation of chimeric receptor molecules, 85
    interest in carbohydrate composition, 85
    purification, characterization and gene cloning, 84–87
    specificity of virus attachment, 82–84, 89–90

viral chemotherapy, 83
virion attachment sites (VAS), 75–79
  development of antiviral compounds, 79
  host range viral mutants, 79–87
PIV3. *See* Parainfluenza 3 virus
Plasmin, 258, 264
p56[lck] T-lymphocyte-specific protein tyrosine kinase, 44. *See also* CD4 receptor
Polarity of virus budding, 251
Polioencephalitis, a mouse-adapted PV strain, 119
Poliomyelitis. *See* Picornaviruses; Polioviruses; Poliovirus receptors; Transgenic mice studies
Polioviruses. *See also* CD44, lymphocyte homing receptor; Picornaviruses; Poliovirus receptors
  apical domain release, 331–335
  characterization of PV1(M) mutants, 118–119
  entry in polarized epithelial cells, 327–328, 330
  formation of PV A particles in uncoating, 116–117
  host-encoded virulence
    studies of PV-inactivation activity, 448–449
  virus-encoded virulence
    host range determinant, 119–120, 446–447, 465–466
    identification via recombinant molecular chimeras, 446
  tissue tropism, 445–449, 453–455, 458, 463, 474–475, 482
Poliovirus receptors, 101–122. *See also* Polioviruses; Transgenic mice studies
  antigenic hybrid viruses and receptor binding, 115–116
  determinant for host range of poliovirus, 465–466
  domains of hPVR in virus binding and uptake, 111–113
  gene is member of immunoglobulin superfamily, 105, 450–465
    cDNAs H20A and H20B active in receptor function, 450
    mRNA isoforms, 105, 454, 465, 469–472
    N-linked glycosylation sites, 107–108, 465–466
    role of MPH and AF3 molecules, 451
  genetics, 104–107
  history of receptor identification, 446–450
  identification and distribution of PVR protein, 105–106, 453–455
    expression in human blood cells, 455–456
    expression in human muscle cells, 456
    polyclonal antisera studies, 453–455
  interactions with the poliovirion, 110–111
  likely hPVR binding site, 104, 110–111
  monkey PVR (mPVR), 105

Poliovirus receptors (*continued*)
  multiple cell-surface proteins in viral binding, 481–489
  murine PVR homolog (MPH), 106
  neutralizing antigenic sites (N-Ags), 102
  pre-hPVR signal peptide, 109
  properties of PVR-related proteins, 107–109
  serotype polymorphism of receptor-binding site, 117–118
  soluble receptor-resistant (srr) PV mutants, 117
  virus modifying function, 6
Poliovirus sensitivity, 465–466. *See also*
    Polioviruses; Poliovirus receptors
Porcine respiratory coronavirus, 404, 406
PRCV. *See* Porcine respiratory coronavirus
Proteases
  bacterial, 257
  secretory
    aerosin, 258
    factor X, 258
    kallikrein, 258
    plasmin, 258
    thrombin, 258
    tryptase Clara, 258
    urokinase, 258
  subtilisin-like endoproteases
    furin, 260
    Kex2, 260
Proteolytic cleavage, 241–266
PRV. *See* Pseudorabies virus
Pseudorabies virus, 369
Punta Toro virus basolateral release, 330
PVR. *See* Poliovirus receptors
PVR cDNA, 481. *See also* Polioviruses;
    Poliovirus receptors
PVR mRNA, 481. *See also* Polioviruses;
    Poliovirus receptors
PVS. *See* Poliovirus sensitivity

Receptor-mediated virus entry, 493–512
Reoviridae, 5, 249–250
Reoviruses
  characterization of cores, 349–351
    initiation of transcription, 351
    transition from ISVP to core, 349–351
  characterization of ISVPs, 348–349
    interaction with lipid bilayers, 349, 355
    metastasis to ISVP*, 344, 349, 357, 361
  characterization of virions, 344–348
  early steps in infection, 341–361
  endocytic uptake, 353–355
    cleavage by proteases within lysosomes, 354
    proteolysis, 353–355
  host immune response infection, 397–400
    role of cytotoxic T lymphocytes (CTL), 397–398
    role of monoclonal antibodies, 398–399
    role of T cells, 398
  infected epithelial cells, 335
  pathogenesis, 389–400
    entry into the host, 390–393
    spread throughout the host, 393–396
    tropism determined by S1 gene, 396–397
  penetration of vacuolar membrane, 355–358
  persistent versus lytic infections, 358–360
  receptor attachment, 352–353
  type 1
    apical binding to M cells, 390
    hematogenous spread, 393–395
  type 3
    apical binding to M cells, 391
    neuron spread, 393–396
Respiratory syncytial virus, 494, 498–500, 505, 511
Retroviral vectors for gene delivery, 25
Retroviridae, 248–249, 329
Retroviruses, type C
  determination of host range, 49–50
  identification of receptors, 50
  possible role of transporters in fusion, 53–54
  receptor function in infected cells, 55
  role of transporters in envelope binding, 52
  some related proteins may serve as receptors, 51
  virus-induced leukemia in mice, 49
Retrovirus receptors, human, 15–26
  attachment, 15
  binding sites, 15
  cellular receptors for type C, 49–56
  conformational changes following binding, 15, 20, 40
  diversity, 16–21
  entry, 15
  Env glycoproteins, 61
    surface (SU) proteins, 61
    transmembrane (TM) proteins, 61
  feline endogenous C-type, 26
  interference groups, table, 19
Rhinoviruses, human
  antigenic hybrid viruses and receptor binding, 115–116
  conformational changes in virion, 202–210
  gene receptors on human chromosome 19, 79
  HRV-14
    canyons that bind, 78–79, 110, 196–199
    comparison of HRV-14/ICAM-1 interaction with PV/hPVR interaction, 116
    receptor-mediated uncoating, 203
    shared receptor with coxsackieviruses of group A, 82
  HRV-16, 204, 208
  HRV-87, 84
  HRV-89, 199
  HRV-2 binding experiments, 130–138
  major receptor group
    interaction with receptor ICAM-1, 2, 195–210

virus/receptor relationships, 77, 229
minor receptor group
  attachment to cells via the LDLR, 2, 131
  entry into cell, 129–138
  protein identification techniques, 130
Rift Valley fever virus basolateral release, 330
Rinderpest virus, 182
Rosetting, 105, 449–450
Ross River (RR) polyarthritis human
    epidemic, 158
Ross River virus, 157–158. *See also* Alphaviruses
Rotaviruses
  porcine, group A, 5
  posttranslational proteolytic cleavage, 249–250
Rous sarcoma virus, 54
RR. *See* Ross River virus
RSV. *See* Respiratory syncytial virus

Sabin vaccine, 446, 464
Semliki Forest virus. *See also* Alphaviruses;
    Endocytosis
  binding constant, 143
  major histocompatibility complex (MHC)
      antigens as receptors, 143, 227
  receptor-mediated virus entry, 180, 505
  studies with cleavage-deficient PEZ, 246
Sendai virus
  apical budding, 328, 336
  identification of first paramyxovirus receptor,
      167
  pH independence, 223
  proteolytic activation, 241, 251, 258, 263
SF. *See* Semliki Forest virus
Sialic acid
  first paramyxovirus receptor identified, 167
  presence of residues on membrane
      glycoproteins, 327
  receptor for influenza virus, 187–188, 292
  receptor for reoviruses, 352
Simian immunodeficiency virus
  entry, 19–21
  entry in polarized epithelial cells, 326
  receptor-mediated entry, 496, 501–502, 507
Simian virus 5 cleavage site variants, 242
Simian virus 40 apical domain release, 331–333
SIN. *See* Sindbis virus
Sindbis virus. *See also* Alphaviruses
  AR339, nonvirulent strain, 143
  AR86, neurovirulent strain, 143
  binding to BHK cells, 147–153
  can cause polyarthritis in man, 142
  cleavage site, 262
  decreased pH threshold for fusion, 233
SIV. *See* Simian immunodeficiency virus
SJL/J receptor
  encoding of mm CGM2 allele, 417

murine BGP variant, 416–417
Spike proteins
  activation cleavage by host proteases, 241–266
  in coronavirus infection, 404–408
Subtilisin-like endoproteases, 260–263, 306
SV5. *See* Simian virus 5
SV40. *See* Simian virus 40

Tacaribe virus cleavage site, 247
T-cell receptor relation to CD4, 24, 33
TGEV. *See* Transmissible gastroenteritis virus
Theiler murine encephalitis virus, 77, 79, 229
Togaviridae
  fusion, 246
  Semliki Forest virus, 143, 246
Transgenic mice studies
  comparison of hPVR in Tg mice with PVR in
      humans, 469, 472
  comparison with PV monkey studies, 475–476
  infection of mice by hPVR genomic clones,
      76, 105, 120
    demonstration of PV infection symptoms,
        466–469
    susceptibility to all three PV serotypes, 466
  measles virus infection, 182
  neurovirulence tests, 475–477
  poliovirus infection pathogenesis, 88–89
  poliovirus virulence
    monkey neurovirulence studies, 464
    tissue tropism, 451–454, 458
  PV dissemination routes in Tg mice, 472–473
    axonal pathway, 473
    blood-brain barrier, 473
    Cutter incident, 473
  virus-encoded PV virulence, 446
Transmembrane (TM) envelope protein, 15
Transmissible gastroenteritis virus
  aminopeptidase N (APN) receptors, 431–434
  binding, 431
  cleavage of glycoproteins, 247
  role of S1 glycoprotein, 404, 406
Tropism
  organ, 251
  paramyxovirus, 258
  poliovirus, 76, 445–449, 453, 455, 458, 463,
      474–475, 482
  reovirus, 396–397
  tissue, 326, 406, 408
Tunicamycin, 52, 55, 85
tv-a, 69. *See also* Avian leukosis and sarcoma
    viruses

Vaccinia virus
  evidence of constitutive endocytic activity,
      230

Vaccinia virus (*continued*)
  expression of HIV-1 *gag* (core) polyprotein, 329
  expression of human furin, 262
Varicella-zoster virus, 230, 249
VCAM-1
  counterreceptor to integrin VLA-4, 201
  virus/receptor relationships, 4, 77, 86
VEE. *See* Venezuelan equine encephalitis virus
Venezuelan equine encephalitis virus, 155–157. *See also* Alphaviruses
Vesicular stomatitis virus
  basolateral budding, 328–330
  entry in polarized epithelial cells, 325–326
  pH dependence, 222
Viral receptors. *See also* Retrovirus receptors, human; *see specific viruses and receptors*

antibody-dependent entry, 9
diversity, 1–3
entry accessory factor, 8
listing, 4
secondary receptors, 8, 21–23
Viremia, 49, 101. *See also* Polioviruses
Visna virus receptor-mediated virus entry, 501, 507
VLA-2, 4, 77, 86
VLA-4, 201
VSV. *See* Vesicular stomatitis virus
VZV. *See* Varicella-zoster virus

West Nile virus, 230, 510

Yellow fever, 510

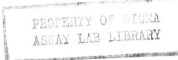